**SYMPOSIUM INTERNATIONAL
SUR LE MESURAGE, LES PROPRIÉTÉS
ET L'UTILISATION DU GAZ NATUREL**

*INTERNATIONAL SYMPOSIUM
ON MEASUREMENTS PROPERTIES
AND UTILISATION OF NATURAL GAS*

Publisher's Note
To expedite publication of this preprint volume, the text has been reproduced directly from a reduction of the original copy submitted by the authors. The publisher, in reproducing the papers as received from the authors, disclaims any and all responsibilities for the contents of individual papers.

Note de l'éditeur
Les textes ont été reproduits directement par réduction des documents originaux remis par les auteurs. En reproduisant les documents remis par les auteurs, l'éditeur dégage sa responsabilité en ce qui concerne le contenu des mémoires individuels.

SYMPOSIUM INTERNATIONAL SUR LE MESURAGE, LES PROPRIÉTÉS ET L'UTILISATION DU GAZ NATUREL

INTERNATIONAL SYMPOSIUM ON MEASUREMENTS PROPERTIES AND UTILISATION OF NATURAL GAS

Montréal, Québec (Canada)
November 25th, 26th and 27th 1987

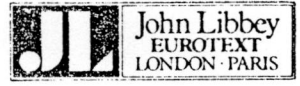

British Library Cataloguing in Publication Data

Symposium International sur le Mesurage, les Propriétés et l'Utilisation du Gaz Naturel
    1. Natural Gas. Production and Use
    I. Title
665.7
ISBN 0-86-196-1890-0

Editions John Libbey Eurotext
6, rue Blanche, 92120 Montrouge, France (1) 47 35 85 52
John Libbey & Company Ltd
80/84 Bondway, London SW8 1SF, England (01) 582 5266

© 3ᵉ trimestre 1988, Paris

Comité organisateur
Organization committee

Pierre L. Gauthier
Directeur, Développement et assistance technologique
Director, Development and Assistance in technology
Gaz Métropolitain, inc.

Kébir Ratnani
Conseiller senior, Développement et assistance technologique
Senior Adviser, Development and Assistance in technology
Gaz Métropolitain, inc.

Roland Francœur
Conseiller principal,
Développement et assistance technologique
Senior Adviser,
Development and Assistance in technology
Gaz Métropolitain, inc.

Jean-Guy Chouinard
Conseiller senior, Développement et assistance technologique
Senior Adviser, Development and Assistance in technology
Gaz Métropolitain, inc.

Tapan K. Bose
Directeur du groupe de recherche sur les dielectriques
Director of the dielectric group
Université du Québec à Trois-Rivières

Remerciements
Aknowledgments

Nous désirons remercier tout particulièrement Mesdames Guylaine Lehoux et Ginette Despatie de Gaz Métropolitain et Mesdames Claire Bournival et Aline Simoneau de l'Université du Québec à Trois-Rivières pour leur précieuse aide dans l'organisation de ce symposium.

We would like to express our sincere thanks to Mrs. Guylaine Lehoux, Mrs. Ginette Despatie of Gaz Métropolitain and Mrs. Claire Bournival and Mrs. Aline Simoneau of Université du Québec à Trois-Rivières for their valuable help in organizing this symposium.

SYMPOSIUM INTERNATIONAL SUR LE MESURAGE, LES PROPRIÉTÉS ET L'UTILISATION DU GAZ NATUREL

Préface

Le Symposium international sur le mesurage, les propriétés et l'utilisation du gaz naturel, organisé par Gaz Métropolitain, inc. et l'Université du Québec à Trois-Rivières, a eu lieu les 25, 26 et 27 novembre 1987 au Palais des Congrès de Montréal (Québec), au Canada.

Le gaz naturel capte l'intérêt non seulement du monde de la recherche et du développement dans le domaine industriel, mais aussi des milieux académiques. En fait, plusieurs problèmes demeurent sans réponse. Entre autres, il est nécessaire de déterminer de façon précise les propriétés thermodynamiques du gaz naturel pour le mesurage du débit, la calorimétrie et la détermination du facteur de compression du gaz. A cet effet, de nouvelles techniques expérimentales ont été mises au point pour atteindre un mesurage de précision, de qualité supérieure. Avec l'augmentation de la consommation du gaz naturel, toute amélioration en termes de précision correspond nécessairement à un accroissement des revenus pour l'industrie du gaz, qui peut se chiffrer en millions de dollars.

L'amélioration des connaissances permet de bien cerner l'importance des hydrates du gaz pour la conception et l'exploitation des installations de production et des gazoducs souterrains et sous-marins. La mise au point de méthodes empêchant la formation d'hydrates s'avère également essentielle. De plus, il faut intensifier la recherche sur l'utilisation des compteurs à turbine pour le gaz. Avec la hausse du coût de la matière première, le développement de meilleures méthodes d'étalonnage est important pour un mesurage précis du débit.

L'industrie du gaz se doit également d'améliorer son efficacité énergétique tout en préservant la qualité de l'environnement. Pour résoudre certains problèmes, il faut intensifier la recherche sur l'efficacité du processus de combustion. On ouvre tous les jours de nouvelles avenues pour promouvoir la consommation du gaz naturel dans le secteur industriel. Par exemple, la génération d'ondes infrarouges à partir du gaz naturel offre énormément d'attraits pour le séchage industriel.

Ce sont là, en partie, quelques-uns des sujets qui ont été traités durant le Symposium par les chefs de file de chacun des domaines de recherche. En tout, plus de vingt-trois conférenciers de renom y représentaient sept pays différents. Nous croyons que les lecteurs sauront trouver matière à réflexion sur les derniers développements de la recherche en technologie gazière effectuée par ces représentants de l'industrie et de l'enseignement.

Nous avons reçu l'aide inestimable de plusieurs collègues pour l'organisation du Symposium et la publication de ces actes. Nous désirons remercier particulièrement Messieurs Kébir Ratnani, Jean-Guy Chouinard, Roland Francoeur et Mesdames Johanne Morissette et Monique Taïeb.

Pierre L. Gauthier, Gaz Métropolitain
Tapan K. Bose, Université du Québec à Trois-Rivières

Mars 1988

INTERNATIONAL SYMPOSIUM ON MEASUREMENTS, PROPERTIES AND UTILIZATION OF NATURAL GAS.

Preface

The International Symposium on Measurements, Properties and Utilization of Natural Gas was organized on behalf of Gaz Métropolitain Inc. and Université du Québec à Trois-Rivières and held on November 25th, 26th and 27th, 1987 at the Montreal Convention Center, Québec, Canada.

Natural gas is attracting a wide interest not only in industrial research and development units but also from academic circles. From a fundamental point of view there are vast array of problems which still have to be solved. Accurate measurement of the thermodynamic properties of natural gas is necessary for gas flow measurement, gas calorimetry and compressibility factor determination. New experimental techniques are being developed for precision measurements which are orders of magnitude better than what the industry was used to. With the increased use of natural gas any improvement in precision would mean millions of dollars to gas industry.

Better understanding is necessary to appreciate the importance of gas hydrates in the design and operation of production facilities and of underground and sub-sea pipelines. Methods have to be developed for inhibiting hydrate formation. More research needs to be done for the use of turbine meter in gas industry. With the increase in cost of the raw material, better calibration methods needs to be developed for accurate flow measurement.

The gas industry needs to develop energy efficiency and pollution control. To address some of these problems more research needs to be done in the efficiency of the combustion process. New avenues are being developed everyday for the increased use of natural gas in the industry. The generation of infrared from natural gas has great potential in the field of industrial drying.

Many of the above subjects are represented in the contributions to this symposium. Articles in this proceedings are to the most part written by the leaders in their respective fields of research. We believe the readers will get some insight on the state of art of gas research carried out both in the industrial and academic sectors.

In the organization of this symposium and eventually in editing the proceedings we received invaluable help from many colleagues.

We would particularly like to thank Mr. Kebir Ratnani, Mr. Jean-Guy Chouinard, Mr. Roland Francoeur, Mrs. Monique Taieb and Mrs. Johanne Morissette.

Montreal and Trois-Rivières
March 1988

Pierre Gauthier
Tapan K. Bose

Table des matières
Table of contents

Préface VII
Preface IX

UTILISATION DU GAZ NATUREL
NATURAL GAS UTILIZATION

Haute température
High temperature

Allocution d'ouverture
Opening address
Pierre L. GAUTHIER 5

Utilisations performantes du gaz naturel dans les procédés hautes températures; exemples en métallurgie
Efficient uses of natural gas for the high temperatures processes; examples in the metallurgical industry
P. BANCOURT 9

Energy considerations of the glass industry
C.W. HIBSCHER 55

Thermal enhanced reciprocating engine cogeneration systems
F.E. BECKER, F.A. DI BELLA, J.C. BALSAVICH 79

Chauffage des bains industriels
Industrial water heating

Getting into hot water efficiently
J.A. DAVIES 89

Le chauffage par le gaz naturel en Industrie
The heating by natural gas in industry
F. LAURENT 97

Wet catalytic oxidation process for industrial effluent treatment
Y. HARADA 145

Moyenne température et qualité de l'air
Medium temperature and indoor air quality

A new high emittance infrared heater
T.M. SMITH MARSDEN 181

Les applications du procédé gaz contact au traitement des déchets industriels
Gaz contact process in the treatment of industrial waste
L. GAURIER 197

Systèmes de combustion industriels
Industrial combustion systems

New technologies to increase combustion efficiency and reduce NOx emission
N. BRAIS 233

New technologies in thermal processing
J. WHITE 263

Regenerative burner systems; case histories on industrial furnaces
R.T. CHAPMAN 289

Pulse firing — Utilization in industry
T. MARTIN 297

MESURAGE DU GAZ NATUREL
NATURAL GAS MEASUREMENTS

Mesure du débit
Flowrate measurements

Allocution d'ouverture
Opening address
T.K. BOSE 315

An overview of the field of gas flowrate measurements
R. MILLER 323

Gas flow measurements: Calibrations and traceabilities
G.E. MATTINGLY 331

Use of turbine meters for high accuracy gas flowrate measurements
R.A. FURNESS 351

New directions in gas flow meter research at the gas research institute
C.H. GRIFFIS 389

Importance of accurate thermodynamic correlations for gas flow measurement
K.R. HALL, K.N. MARSH, J.C. HOLSTE 405

Accurate measurements of fluid densities
J.C. HOLSTE, K.R. HALL, K.N. MARSH 417

Turbine meter based dispenser for natural gas motor vehicles
E.J. FARKAS 449

Propriétés du gaz naturel
Natural gas properties

Importance of hydrates to the gas industry
D.B. Robinson 483

L'odorisation dans l'industrie gazière aujourd'hui
J.P. Coquand 513

Accurate measurements and prediction of compressibility factors in the gas industry
M. Jaeschke 525

SÉANCES D'AFFICHAGE
POSTER SESSIONS

Microwave ground thawing device
G.E. Coburn, W. Rahman 559

Simulation des installations de combustion submergée
M. Fournier, C. Guy, P.J. Carreau, J.R. Paris 571

GNV : système d'injection à commande électronique
M. Perrault, M. Gou, G. Allard, C. Guernier 583

Performance of orifice meters in field conditions
W. Studzinski, J. Szabo, J. Eastwood, R. Rans, D. Bell 591

L'utilisation du gaz naturel dans les procédés d'incinération
Using natural gas in the incineration process
X. D'Hubert 615

Thermal performance studies of gas heating systems
M. Zaheer-Uddin, P. Fazio, P. Roozmon 623

The influence of type of heating systems on thermal comfort
P. Fazio, F. Haghighat, M. Auger 625

Indoor emissions from combustion appliances : Development of a predictive model
F. Haghighat, P. Fazio, J. Payer 627

Mesure précise du facteur de supercompressibilité du gaz naturel par une méthode optique
J.M. St-Arnaud, T.K. Bose, M.J. Achtermann 631

Modelisation de l'odorisation d'une conduite
J. Goyette, J. Sochanski 651

Adsorption du méthane à haute pression sur les charbons actifs
R. Chahine, T.K. Bose 669

A simplified virial equation applied to natural gas mixtures
D.R. McGregor, J.C. Holste, K.R. Hall 695

PVT Measurements of carbon dioxide — methane mixtures
C.A. Hwang, J.C. Holste, K.R. Hall, K.N. Marsh 707

GERG sample measurements
H. Brugge, C.A. Hwang, J.C. Holste, K.R. Hall, K.N. Marsh .. 719

Liquid enthalpies of the C_8 — Hydrocarbons ethylbenzene and isoctane
D. Möller, J.C. Holste, K.R. Hall, B.E. Gammon, K.N. Marsh .. 731

UTILISATION DU GAZ NATUREL
NATURAL GAS UTILIZATION

Haute température
High temperature

TRANSTECH INTERNATIONAL 87

Allocution d'ouverture

Monsieur Pierre L. Gauthier
Directeur du Groupe DATECH, Gaz Métropolitain

Distingués invités,

Mesdames,

Messieurs,

Il m'est très agréable de vous souhaiter la plus cordiale bienvenue à cette Foire internationale de l'innovation et des technologies nouvelles: Transtech 87.

Cet événement majeur m'apparaît très important en raison même de son objet d'abord. Depuis maintenant une décennie, la question de l'énergie est passée au premier plan des préoccupations des sociétés, suivie de très près par la technologie.

La question de l'énergie en sous-tend d'aussi importantes, comme la rationalisation des coûts, l'amélioration des efficacités, l'augmentation de la productivité, tout cela en vue d'une meilleure position concurrentielle sur les marchés nationaux et internationaux. C'est dans ce contexte qu'entrent en jeu les technologies nouvelles, d'autant plus nouvelles qu'elles font de plus en plus appel à une source d'énergie encore trop méconnue: le gaz naturel.

Des événements comme celui auquel nous avons l'honneur d'être associé, constituent des occasions uniques, tant pour les promoteurs que pour les participants, d'être confrontés aux immenses possibilités qu'offrent les nouvelles technologies gazières, que ce soit dans le domaine de la distribution ou dans celui de l'utilisation proprement dite. Transtech se veut en effet le carrefour, non seulement québécois, canadien ou même nord-américain, mais international, de l'innovation et des technologies nouvelles.

Ce Symposium est également important par la diversité et la qualité des participants. Réunissant des spécialistes de l'énergie, qui proviennent tant des industries consommatrices que des industries productrices d'énergies et des universitaires, Transtech 87 permettra de fructueux échanges. Les exposés qui se succéderont au cours des trois prochains jours seront donnés par quelques-uns des experts les plus prestigieux à l'heure actuelle dans le domaine gazier et ce, à travers le monde. Vous constaterez que les applications industrielles dont il sera plus particulièrement question aux sessions A, répondent toutes aux préoccupations suivantes:

- recherche des économies d'énergie;
- satisfaction de la clientèle par l'amélioration des équipements existants ou l'introduction de nouveaux équipements;
- recherche de nouveaux emplois du gaz naturel pour remplacer d'autres énergies moins économiques du point de vue du client.

Pour Gaz Métropolitain, de tels événements sont indispensables et devront se renouveler. Les technologies quelles qu'elles soient, et gazières en particulier, requièrent généralement de nombreux efforts si l'on veut en accroître la notoriété.

Je tiens également à remercier tous ceux et celles qui n'ont pas "ménagé leur énergie" cette fois, en déployant tous les efforts requis pour organiser et mener à bien cet événement. Je salue en particulier Monsieur Tapan Bose, de l'Université du Québec à Trois-Rivières, qui a su si bien nous seconder tout au long de l'organisaniôt de ce Symposium, et à qui je vais bientôt laisser la parole. Je remercie également le Ministère de l'Energie et des Ressources du Québec, Trans Québec & Maritimes, SOQUIP et Western Gas Marketing de leur appui financier à Transtech 87.

Sans plus tarder, je déclare ouvert le Symposium international sur le mesurage, les propriétés et l'utilisation du gaz naturel et souhaite qu'il soit un grand succès!

TRANSTECH INTERNATIONAL 87

Opening Address

Mr. Pierre L. Gauthier
Director of the DATECH Group, Gaz Métropolitain

Distinguished guests,

Ladies and Gentlemen,

It is with great pleasure that I welcome you all here today to the International Market for Innovation and New Technologies: Transtech 87.

Given the main topic, I feel that this major event is of great importance. For the last decade, energy has become the leading subject of concern to our society, followed very closely by technology.

The subject of energy includes other underlying and equally important issues such as cost rationalization, improved efficiency and increased productivity in order to ensure a greater competitive position on domestic and international markets. It is in this context that new technologies come into play, and the newer they are, the more they require an energy source that is still not fully appreciated: natural gas.

Events such as this, which we are proud to be associated with, provide a unique opportunity for promoters and participants alike to learn about the vast possibilities offered by new gas technologies, whether for distribution or for use. Transtech, in fact, is not just a Québec, Canadian or even North American forum, it is an international forum for innovation and new technologies.

This symposium is also important because of the diversity and quality of the participants. Transtech 87 will afford energy specialists from consuming and from producing industries as well as university representatives an opportunity to exchange ideas. Over the next three days, some of the leading gas experts in the world today will be making their presentations. As you can see, the industrial applications that will be discussed more specifically during the A sessions will all address the following concerns:

- energy savings;

- client satisfaction through improvements to existing equipment or through the introduction of new equipment;

- new uses for natural gas to replace other less economical energy sources from the client's viewpoint.

For Gaz Métropolitain, events like these are essential and many more are needed. A great deal of effort is generally required to create technologies of all kinds, particularly gas technologies, if they are to become better known.

I would like to take this opportunity to thank all those who spared no effort, or dare I say "energy", to organize this event and make it a success. My very sincere thanks to Mr. Tapan Bose of the Université du Québec à Trois-Rivières, who will be our next speaker, for his excellent support in organizing this Symposium. I would also like to thank the Ministry of Energy and Resources of Québec, Trans-Québec & Maritimes, SOQUIP and Western Gas Marketing for their financial assistance to Transtech 87.

I now declare open the International Symposium on Measurements, Properties and Utilization of Natural Gas and wish it every success!

CONGRES DE MONTREAL

TRANSTEC 87

=ooOoo=

UTILISATIONS PERFORMANTES DU GAZ NATUREL
DANS LES PROCEDES HAUTES TEMPERATURES
EXEMPLES EN METALLURGIE

—=—=—=—

par M. Pascal BANCOURT

Chef du Service Techniques et Applications Industrielles

Centre d'Essais et de Recherches sur les Utilisations du Gaz

GAZ DE FRANCE

—=—=—=—

Cet exposé présente d'abord les équipements de chauffe apparus le plus récemment en FRANCE :

- brûleur-jet,

- brûleur à double récupérateur,

- tubes radiants autorécupérateurs,

ainsi que leurs applications dans les différents secteurs de la métallurgie : forge, fonderie des métaux non ferreux, traitement thermique.

Chaque équipement est traité avec un ou deux exemples industriels précisant les économies d'énergie réalisées par rapport à des équipements plus traditionnels.

Dans une seconde partie, l'exposé présente l'Unité de Fusion Rapide, nouveau four de fusion des métaux non ferreux mis au point par le Centre de Recherches du GAZ DE FRANCE.

—=—=—=—

1 - INTRODUCTION

Qu'il s'agisse de la fusion des métaux, de leur réchauffage avant déformation, de leur traitement thermique, la métallurgie est un des domaines priviligiés des hautes températures.

Il serait trop long et peut-être fastidieux de passer en revue toutes les applications possibles du gaz dans ce secteur de l'industrie. Elles sont, en effet, nombreuses dans les enceintes thermiques depuis la température de fusion de l'acier (brûleur oxy-gaz dans les fours à arc) jusqu'à celle du zinc (fours de galvanisation), sans compter des applications particulières comme :

- le travail à la flamme (oxycoupage par exemple),

- l'utilisation du méthane comme matière première, pour la génération d'atmosphère dans les fours de traitement thermique.

La suite de cet exposé présente plus particulièrement des produits nouveaux, faisant l'objet d'un développement industriel significatif en FRANCE, grâce à la coopération instaurée entre le GAZ DE FRANCE, distributeur d'énergie et les constructeurs d'équipements thermiques.

Ces produits ont pour but d'améliorer les installations utilisant le gaz naturel sur deux points essentiels :

- l'économie d'énergie,

- la productivité.

Ils utilisent les avantages du gaz naturel par rapport à d'autres énergies :

- puissance,

- propreté,

- facilité du réglage,

qui permettent de concevoir des installations ou des équipements à la fois performants et fiables.

Ce texte se limitera à trois produits qui ont trouvé des applications dans les différents secteurs de la métallurgie que sont la fonderie, la forge et le traitement thermique.

.../...

2 - BRULEUR-JET ET APPLICATIONS

Les brûleurs à grande vitesse de sortie des produits de la combustion (> 100 m/s) ou brûleurs-jet trouvent naturellement leur place dans les fours de traitement thermique à des températures modérées (entre 500 et 1 000°C), la vitesse des gaz brûlés est en effet appréciable pour favoriser :

- les échanges convectifs, prépondérants à ce niveau de température,

- le brassage de l'atmosphère et donc d'homogénéité de température requise en traitement thermique.

2.1 DESCRIPTION DU BRULEUR MGV

Il existe plusieurs types de brûleurs jets, maintenant largement développés dans l'industrie. Le brûleur Métallique à Grande Vitesse (MGV) présente toutefois la caractéristique essentielle d'une conception entièrement métallique alors que, généralement, la chambre de combustion est construite en matériaux réfractaires céramiques. Cette disposition permet de mieux supporter les chocs thermiques résultant des arrêts et remises en marche fréquents.

Ce matériel est disponible pour des puissances de 25 à 400 kW PCI avec une pression d'alimentation en air et en gaz de 50 mbar environ.

Le principe de ce brûleur est présenté par la coupe de la figure n° 1.

Le gaz est injecté en deux points : en B radialement pour réaliser un prémélange partiel, puis axialement en C.

L'air de combustion admis à l'arrière du brûleur est introduit pour une faible partie en B afin de réaliser le prémélange partiel air-gaz. L'autre partie remonte jusqu'au nez du brûleur où des trous tangentiels A assurent sa mise en rotation.

Cette disposition protège les enveloppes métalliques constituant le brûleur.

.../...

La combustion s'amorce dans la chambre C ; il y a donc préchauffage de l'air de combustion permettant d'élever la température de la flamme et d'obtenir ainsi, à la puissance nominale des vitesses de produits de combustion supérieures à 150 m/s avec une poussée spécifique élevée.

Le brûleur est équipé d'une électrode d'allumage et d'une cellule UV de détection de flamme.

Pour les puissances inférieures ou égales à 75 kW, ce brûleur a été développé en version autorécupérateur.

Dans ce cas, les produits de combustion délivrés dans l'enceinte thermique sont aspirés autour de l'enveloppe extérieure et préchauffent ainsi l'air de combustion.

Ce dernier principe a été développé pour une enceinte thermique particulière, le tube radiant, utilisé pour chauffer les fours de traitement thermique sous atmosphère contrôlée, comme le montre la figure n° 2.

2.2 UTILISATION DU BRULEUR MGV EN CHAUFFAGE DIRECT

Exemple d'un four de recuit

2.21 DESCRIPTION

Le premier exemple d'application brûleur-jet MGV est un four de recuit d'homogénéisation et de stabilisation. Construit dans un atelier de traitement thermique à façon, le cahier des charges devait répondre aux exigences suivantes :

- une grande souplesse d'exploitation,
- un volume de laboratoire important,
- une montée rapide en température,
- être économe en énergie.

Le four, présenté en coupe à la figure n° 3 a été construit avec les caractéristiques suivantes :

- un volume utile de 82 m³ (8 m x 3,2 m x 3,2 m),

.../...

- deux soles mobiles, dont l'une est dans le four et l'autre en attente, pouvant supporter des charges allant jusqu'à 50 tonnes : chaque sole, en réfractaire lourd, pèse 30 tonnes,

- un équipement thermique de 16 brûleurs MGV de 140 kW de puissance unitaire, soit 2 240 kW de puissance totale installée,

- une isolation par blocs réfractaires fibreux de 300 mm de côté.

Les deux portes du four coulissent latéralement, puis sont plaquées sur les parois à l'aide d'excentriques mus par des vérins pneumatiques.

Les brûleurs sont placés sur un des grands côtés du four, face à une série de carneaux situés dans la sole. Cette disposition, en limitant l'effet de sole froide rencontré sur de nombreuses installations, favorise les transferts thermiques par conduction et accélère l'homogénéisation de la température des pièces à traiter.

L'équipement de chauffe est réparti en trois zones de régulation de température :

Zone 1	4 brûleurs	560 kW
Zone 2	8 brûleurs	1 120 kW
Zone 3	4 brûleurs	560 kW

Il existe une possibilité de fonctionner en demi-puissance, c'est-à-dire avec 2, 4 et 2 brûleurs.

Les produits de combustion sont évacués par quatre ouvertures placées en voûte du four. Une gaine collecte les fumées vers la cheminée. Afin de maintenir le four en légère surpression, la cheminée est équipée d'un clapet automatique commandé par un capteur de pression placé dans l'enceinte du four. L'ensemble est équipé d'une régulation de température avec la possibilité de programmer la vitesse désirée de montée en température ainsi que la durée et la température des paliers de maintien.

2.22 RESULTATS THERMIQUES

Des bilans thermiques du four ont été réalisés durant trois traitements de normalisation. Deux cycles de chauffage, à une température de 780°C, ont été effectués sur des charges de 10,125 tonnes et 6,4 tonnes de fontes grises. Le troisième cycle réalisé à 930°C concerne une charge de 8,4 tonnes d'acier allié.

On résume les résultats enregistrés dans le tableau suivant :

TRAITEMENTS	1	2	3
Température (°C)	780	780	930
Charges (tonnes)	10.125	6.4	8.4
Durée montée (heures, mn)	7 h 45	7 h 20	10 h 17
maintien (heures, mn)	3 h 00	3 h 00	0 h 52
Consommation (kWh PCI)	15 296	13 171	14 687

Lors des essais, le rendement moyen de combustion était de 55 %, alors que la régulation de pression du four n'était pas opérationnelle. La limitation des entrées d'air parasite qu'elle procure, améliore ce rendement de 5 % environ, à cette température.

Les pertes par les parois, en fibreux, sont inférieures à 5 % de la consommation totale alors que les pertes par la sole en réfractaire lourd représentent en moyenne 40 %. Il est donc intéressant de citer et comparer les consommations spécifiques par tonne de produit brut (sole plus pièces) et par tonne de produit net (pièces seules). A l'examen du tableau ci-dessous, on constate que les différences de consommation entre charge brute et nette correspondent à la quantité de chaleur emmagasinée dans la sole.

Cette valeur est très importante, mais la résistance mécanique doit être calculée en fonction des charges supportées, le plus souvent inégalement réparties. En conséquence, la sole ne peut être réalisée qu'en réfractaire lourd de haute densité.

.../...

TRAITEMENTS	1	2	3
Consommation spécifique sur brut (kWh/PCI/t)	305	283	303
Consommation spécifique sur net (kWh/PCI/t)	1 510	2 058	1 748

. RESULTATS D'EXPLOITATION

Ce four a remplacé deux fours anciens de volume à peu près moitié, construits en réfractaires traditionnels et équipés de brûleurs classiques au fioul.

Avec le nouveau four décrit, l'accélération possible des cycles de traitement, rendue possible par l'association des brûleurs-jet et de réfractaire fibreux a permis à l'industriel d'augmenter sa production mensuelle de 180 à 300 t/mois, tandis que sa facture énergétique baissait de 35 % environ.

Parallèlement, les grandes vitesses des gaz brûlés conduisent à des mouvements de convection qui améliorent l'homogénéité de la température du four (± 10°C) et donc de la charge : il en résulte une meilleure qualité du produit.

Enfin, l'automatisation poussée permet un meilleur emploi du personnel posté, conduisant aussi à réduire les coûts d'exploitation.

2.3 APPLICATION DU BRULEUR MGV AU TUBE RADIANT AUTORECUPERATEUR

Exemple d'un four de carbonitruration

Dans un atelier intégré de l'industrie automobile, le tube radiant présenté à la figure n° 2, équipe 5 fours à passage, à peu près identiques, destinés à traiter des pièces de pignonnerie, brutes de forge, avant rectification, assemblage et montage (boîtes de vitesse). Il s'agit de fours à passage sous atmosphère contrôlée, de carbonitruration ou de cémentation.

L'exemple choisi est relatif à un four de carbonitruration.

.../...

2.31 - Description du four et des équipements

Il s'agit d'un four poussant à 2 files de chacune 17 plateaux. Le volume du laboratoire est de 8 m^3 pour des dimensions externes de 11,3 m de long, 2,2 m de large et 2 m de haut.

La production peut atteindre 1,45 t/h avec un enfournement de plateaux de 50 kg supportant 70 kg de pièces. La température maximale est de 890°C.

L'atmosphère est du type azote-méthanol.

Ce four est équipé d'un bac de trempe à huile incorporé.

Il fonctionne 5 jours par semaine, en 3 postes de 8 h, avec maintien de température sous atmosphère en fin de semaine.

L'équipement de chauffe est constitué de 27 tubes radiants autorécupérateurs MGV 35, de 35 kW de puissance unitaire.

Ils sont répartis en 5 zones de régulation de température de la façon suivante :

Zone 1   11 tubes (dont 3 sous la charge)
(entrée des charges)

Zone 2   9 tubes (dont 3 sous la charge)

Zone 3   3 tubes

Zone 4   2 tubes

Zone 5   2 tubes
(sortie des pièces)

La régulation est du type TOUT ou RIEN.

.../...

2.32 - Résultats

Le rendement de combustion moyen est de 70 %(PCI).

A la capacité nominale du four (1,12 t/h), la consommation spécifique est de 479 kWh/(PCI)/t. Elle n'est plus que de 370 kWh(PCI)/t pour une production horaire de 1,45 t.

Auparavant, l'industriel disposait de fours de géométrie et de caractéristiques de production identiques, mais équipé de tubes radiants "classiques" en   . Leur rendement de combustion n'excédait pas 50 %(PCI) dans cette gamme de température de la carbonitruration.

La figure n° 4 présente l'évolution de la consommation spécifique en fonction de la production des fours selon leur équipement de chauffe.

A production égale, les tubes radiants autorécupérateurs permettent des économies d'énergie de l'ordre de 50 %.

3 - BRULEUR A DOUBLE RECUPERATION "BDR" ET APPLICATIONS

Ce brûleur fait partie des brûleurs à récupération destinés à procurer d'importantes économies d'énergie pour le chauffage des fours à charge à haute températue.

Son principe, présenté à la figure n° 5, est de récupérer le maximum d'énergie sur les produits de combustion pour préchauffer l'air comburant. Le transfert de chaleur s'effectue à travers deux échangeurs d'une conception volontairement simple pour obtenir un produit d'un coût raisonnable.

3.1 CONCEPTION ET FONCTIONNEMENT DU BRULEUR BDR

Le premier échangeur, accolé à l'enceinte du four, est du type "en doigt de gant". Il est constitué d'un caisson isolé avec des réfractaires fibreux dans lequel circulent les produits de combustion issus du four.

.../...

L'air comburant y est admis froid et circule dans l'échangeur en acier réfractaire.

On notera que la partie supérieure de l'échangeur au contact des produits de combustion les plus chauds, est refroidie par la circulation de l'air.

Le deuxième échangeur, disposé en série avec le précédent, se compose d'un double espace annulaire, dans lequel l'air de combustion, avant son admission au brûleur, circule à contre-courant des produits de combustion évacués à l'arrière du brûleur.

Le mélangeur est un simple cône perforé. Il est doté d'une électrode d'allumage. La détection de flamme est effectuée par une cellule UV.

La combustion est intensive. La qualité du mélange air-gaz, due à une admission de l'air en rotation, permet un fonctionnement correct à 20 % de la puissance nominale.

Dans la cheminée, se trouve un système d'injection d'air (éducteur) permettant de créer une dépression. En réglant son débit, on parvient ainsi à maintenir l'enceinte thermique en légère surpression, évitant ainsi des entrées d'air parasite, source de pertes considérables.

La disposition générale du brûleur BDR offre :

- une grande surface d'échanges thermiques permettant les performances indiquées dans les deux applications suivantes,

- l'absence de parties métalliques à trop haute température, assurant ainsi la fiabilité de l'ensemble,

- la possibilité de choisir, en fonction de la conception du four, le point de prélèvement des fumées entrant dans le premier échangeur. Cette possibilité favorise les échanges convectifs et l'homogénéité de la température du four par rapport aux brûleurs à récupération où les produits de combustion sont repris directement au nez du brûleur (brûleurs autorécupérateurs).

Ce brûleur a été construit dans une gamme de puissance allant de 70 à 900 kW. Il existe également certaines versions sans deuxième échangeur, lorsque celui-ci ne se justifie plus économiquement.

.../...

3.2 APPLICATION DU BRULEUR BDR A UN FOUR DE FORGE

Le brûleur BDR a été créé et essayé à la fin de l'année 1984. En août 1985, sa première application industrielle a concerné un petit four de réchauffage d'acier avant forgeage.

3.21 - Description du four

Il s'agit d'un four dormant, d'un volume intérieur de 2,8 m^3, représenté en coupe à la figure n° 6.

La sole est en béton réfractaire, les parois latérales et la voûte, en briques réfractaires. Des modules de fibreux sont collés en voûte. La porte "guillotine" est garnie de fibreux.

Le four est équipé d'un seul brûleur de 500 kW de puissance nominale. Il est placé sur une face latérale, le premier échangeur, d'une longueur de 1,7 m, étant horizontal au niveau de la sole et le brûleur avec le deuxième échangeur étant installé au-dessus de celui-ci.

La régulation est du type TOUT ou PEU avec les valeurs suivantes :

- TOUT : 515 kW ; facteur d'air n = 1,08

- PEU :   85 kW ; facteur d'air n = 1,15

Un contact d'ouverture de la porte du four commande le passage du brûleur en régime PEU. Ce régime est maintenu tant que la porte n'est pas refermée.

3.22 - Résultats

On présente ci-dessous le bilan thermique de ce four pendant une opération de réchauffage d'une charge de 2,37 t d'acier ordinaire à 1 225°C :

ACTIF   - combustion du gaz   1 309 kWh(PCI)
               - oxydation de la charge   58 kWh

.../...

PASSIF
- chaleur utile 548 kWh
- pertes aux fumées 403 kWh
- pertes diverses 416 kWh
  (parois, ouvertures,
  air parasite)

Ce bilan thermique conduit donc à :

- un rendement de combustion de 71 %(PCI),

- un rendement de chauffage de 40 %,

- une consommation spécifique de 552 kWh(PCI)/t.

3.23 - Développement du brûleur BDR en forge

A la suite de ces résultats, trois autres fours de forge ont été équipés en 1986 de brûleurs de ce type. L'un d'entre eux, un four à sole tournante de 4 t/h a été modernisé au moyen de 5 brûleurs BDR de 500 kW de puissance unitaire. Ses performances sont comparables à celles qui viennent d'être décrites.

3.3 APPLICATION DU BRULEUR BDR AUX FOURS A CREUSET

Parallèlement au développement en forge, ce brûleur a trouvé aussi une application en fonderie pour le chauffage des fours à creuset à gaz, dont les rendements de chauffage sont traditionnellement assez bas.

3.31 - Description du four

L'adaptation du brûleur BDR a été menée sur un four à creuset de fusion d'alliage d'aluminium de 200 kg de capacité. Un brûleur BDR de 150 kW a été installé comme il est indiqué à la figure n° 7.

Il s'agit d'un four briqueté utilisé par l'industriel 8 heures par jour pour fondre essentiellement un alliage AS9U3 (88 % Al, 9 % Si, 3 % Cu), puis à le porter à la température de 730°C, convenant pour la coulée.

.../...

La charge est placée dans un creuset : le chauffage est donc indirect. Par ailleurs, les fusions se succèdent pendant la durée du travail, la première étant réalisée le matin "four froid", après l'arrêt de la nuit, alors que les suivantes sont effectuées "four chaud".

3.32 - Résultats

Les résultats suivants proviennent de relevés pratiqués chez l'industriel avec une charge composée pour moitié environ de lingots de 5 kg, et pour l'autre moitié de jets, masselottes et retours provenant des postes de moulage.

La charge exacte et la durée de la fusion sont reportées dans la colonne "conditions d'essais". On sait en effet que ces conditions peuvent considérablement influencer les résultats thermiques.

DEPART FOUR FROID		DEPART FOUR CHAUD	
CONDITIONS DE L'ESSAI	CONSOMMATION SPECIFIQUE kWh(PCI/t	CONDITIONS DE L'ESSAI	CONSOMMATION SPECIFIQUE kWh(PCI)/t
190 kg 142 mn	1 186	184 kg 84 mn	745
190 kg 143 mn	1 291	181 kg 78 mn	783

Ces résultats correspondent à :

- un rendement de combustion de 72 %(PCI) en fin de fusion, lorsque les fumées entrent dans le brûleur à la température maximale (1 025°C), l'excès d'air étant de 10 %,

- un rendement de chauffage de 41 %(PCI).

Habituellement, dans des conditions d'utilisation similaires, la consommation spécifique des fours à creuset est égale ou supérieure à 1 000 kWh(PCI)/t.

3.33 - Développement du brûleur BDR en four à creuset

Le développement de ce brûleur en fonderie a commencé en même temps qu'en forge.

Un atelier de 8 fours de ce type a été installé en 1986.

Ces fours sont utilisés pour effectuer principalement du maintien en température de métal liquide près des machines à mouler sous pression, tout en effectuant une fusion le matin à la prise du travail et en fondant quelques lingots en cours de journée (utilisation en fusion-maintien).

Le développement de ce type de four se poursuit vers la fusion des alliages cuivreux, mais aussi pour du simple maintien en température d'alliages légers, sans fusion. Dans ces deux cas, la puissance du brûleur BDR doit être adaptée aux besoins thermiques. Au total, c'est une douzaine de fours de ce type qui ont été installés en 1986 en FRANCE.

4 - UNITE DE FUSION RAPIDE ET DE MAINTIEN

En fonderie de métaux non ferreux, dès lors que des productions importantes et suivies d'un même alliage sont nécessaires, le four à creuset décrit ci-dessus, ne convient plus. Le métal est alors fondu par chauffage direct dans un four à bassin dont la capacité s'échelonne entre 700 kg et plusieurs dizaines de tonnes. Par l'intermédiaire de poches de transfert, il peut ensuite être réparti vers les différents postes de moulage de l'atelier, où il est stocké dans un four de maintien, en général à creuset, parfois à bassin de faible capacité.

De longue date, thermiciens et constructeurs se sont préoccupés d'améliorer le rendement thermique de ces fours à bassin. Celui-ci est en effet assez faible pour les alliages légers, en raison de la faible émissivité de l'aluminium liquide, limitant son pouvoir d'absorption du rayonnement.

.../...

Les méthodes retenues pour récupérer la chaleur perdue dans les fumées étaient :

- préchauffage de la charge : on contraint en général les fumées à circuler à contre-courant de la charge dans une trémie de chargement ; la solution peut être encore améliorée par l'utilisation de brûleurs-jet, favorisant les échanges convectifs,

- préchauffage de l'air de combustion, au moyen d'échangeurs adaptés.

L'une ou l'autre de ces méthodes conduit à un rendement de chauffage compris entre 40 et 50 %.

Les conditions françaises de la concurrence entre les énergies et plus particulièrement celle de l'électricité, dont les rendements atteignent 60 à 70 % en four à induction, ont conduit le GAZ DE FRANCE à combiner les deux méthodes décrites ci-dessus pour proposer un nouveau type de four à bassin, l'Unité de Fusion Rapide et de maintien (U.F.R.).

4.1 DESCRIPTION DE L'UFR

Il s'agit d'un four à deux cellules juxtaposées, une de fusion et l'autre de maintien, associées à un récupérateur de chaleur sur les produits de combustion.

La figure n° 8 présente une vue en perspective de ce four avec les principales cotes. La figure n° 9 présente les coupes du four de fusion et du récupérateur ainsi que du four de maintien avec ses deux augets de puisage.

La présence d'augets de puisage faisait partie du cahier des charges de la première réalisation effectuée dans un petit atelier et destinée à alimenter en métal liquide 6 postes de moulage en coquille disposés autour du four. Ces augets sont couverts durant les périodes de maintien.

La cellule de fusion, en forme de tunnel, est chauffée par un brûleur d'une puissance nominale de 750 kW (actuellement réglé à 320 kW) et placé à l'une des extrémités.

.../...

La sole inclinée est pourvue, en partie basse, du côté du brûleur, d'un chenal permettant au métal fondu de s'écouler par gravité. Il passe ainsi dans le bassin de maintien.

La cellule de maintien a une longueur totale sensiblement égale à celle de la cellule de fusion. Elle comporte deux brûleurs radiants dits à "flamme plate" de 65 kW chacun, disposés en voûte.

Après retrait du couvercle, le four est chargé par le haut, la chambre de fusion étant totalement remplie de lingots, de jets, de masselottes ou de retours. Dès l'allumage du brûleur de fusion, la partie du métal la plus proche est fondue tandis que les produits de combustion vont préchauffer le reste de la charge. Ces gaz de combustion sont ensuite prélevés en partie haute à l'extrémité de la cellule pour être dirigés, en-dessous, vers le récupérateur.

Ce récupérateur en "doigt de gant" préchauffe l'air de combustion du brûleur de fusion. Les gaz de combustion sont rejetés à une température inférieure tandis que la température des produits de combustion est augmentée, améliorant ainsi le rendement.

Les produits de combustion issus des brûleurs de la cellule de maintien circulent à contre-courant du métal fondu par le chenal la reliant à la cellule de fusion. Ils contribuent au préchauffage de la charge avant d'être ensuite utilisés dans le récupérateur. En période de maintien particulièrement longue, la quantité de chaleur peut être suffisante pour amorcer la fusion de la charge sans mise en route du brûleur de fusion.

Le brûleur de fusion est allumé suivant une procédure automatique déclenchée sur demande manuelle des utilisateurs. L'arrêt est déterminé par un régulateur comparant la température de consigne à celle mesurée par un thermocouple placé dans le conduit de fumées à l'entrée du récupérateur. Le brûleur n'est rallumé pour la fusion suivante que sur commande de l'utilisateur.

Les deux brûleurs de maintien sont également mis en service suivant une procédure automatique.

Leur fonctionnement est piloté en permanence par un régulateur TOUT ou RIEN qui compare la température de consigne à celle mesurée par une canne pyrométrique immergée dans le bain.

.../...

4.2 RESULTATS

On peut charger dans la cellule de fusion 600 kg environ de lingots et 350 kg environ de masselottes, jets et retours des postes de moulage.

Le tableau suivant donne quelques exemples de la consommation spécifique et du rendement de ce four, exprimés relativement au Pouvoir Calorifique Inférieur (PCI) du gaz naturel. Ces exemples sont relatifs à des alliages de type aluminium-silicum contenant jusqu'à 10 % de silicium.

Les consommations indiquées incluent celles des brûleurs de la cellule de maintien.

PUISSANCE	TEMPERATURE DE METAL	TEMPS DE FUSION	CONSOMMATION SPECIFIQUE	RENDEMENT COMBUSTION	RENDEMENT CHAUFFAGE
416 kW	763 °C	45 min	670 kWh/t	73 %	50 %
388 kW	758 °C	45 min	571 kWh/t	72 %	58 %
334 kW	752 °C	53 min	678 kWh/t	73 %	52 %
296 kW	724 °C	61 min	538 kWh/t	76 %	64 %

On peut remarquer que les rendements de chauffage sont comparables à ceux obtenus en fusion par induction.

Cette unité est en exploitation depuis maintenant deux années. Elle est utilisée quotidiennement de la façon suivante :

- 8 heures de production (augets découverts),

- 16 heures de maintien (augets couverts) pendant lesquels la consommation horaire est de 23 kWh(PCI).

Dans ces conditions, pour un tonnage journalier fondu de 5 t, relativement faible par rapport aux possibilités (12 t/jour en tenant compte des durées de chargement et de décrassage), la consommation spécifique moyenne en exploitation est de 720 kWh(PCI)/t.

.../...

Par ailleurs, la perte au feu, différence entre la masse de métal enfourné et la masse de métal coulé est de 1,7 % en moyenne, mesurée sur 6 semaines d'exploitation.

4.3 DEVELOPPEMENT

D'autres fonderies françaises ont choisi de s'équiper de ce type de four, économe en énergie et présentant une bonne qualité de métal coulé. C'est ainsi que seront mises prochainement en service, cinq unités de fusion d'alliages d'aluminium et une unité de fusion de zamak.

Pour ce dernier alliage, des essais ont montré que la consommation spécifique était de 134 kWh(PCI)/t pour du métal porté à 409°C, avec une perte au feu de 1,2 % et un taux de cendre de 0,41 %.

La plus importante des unités prochainement mises en service aura un débit de fusion d'alliage d'aluminium de 3,2 t/h pour une capacité de maintien de 29 t.

Cette capacité de maintien, disproportionnée avec le débit de fusion est fixée par l'utilisateur afin de lui permettre de recevoir directement d'usines d'affinage du métal liquide acheminé par route.

Dans le cas de cette unité basculante, trois brûleurs d'une puissance unitaire maximale de 900 kW seront installés côte à côte à l'une des extrémités de la cellule de fusion.

Ils seront alimentés en air préchauffé par l'intermédiaire de trois échangeurs en doigt de gant logés sous la sole.

5 - CONCLUSION

Economiser l'énergie, augmenter la production des installations, accroître la qualité des produits, sont des préoccupations permanentes et universelles des industriels de la métallurgie, où la plupart des procédés s'effectuent à haute température.

.../...

Cet état d'esprit est particulièrement présent en FRANCE où la grande majorité des combustibles est importée et en particulier le gaz naturel.

Cette situation a conduit les industriels français de l'équipement thermique à présenter à leurs clients les matériels ou procédés gaz performants que ceux-ci attendent. Fournisseurs d'équipements ou utilisateurs de gaz naturel, leur démarche est encouragée par le GAZ DE FRANCE, Société distributrice du gaz naturel, qui souhaite que cette énergie soit utilisée de façon optimale.

Les trois équipements présentés dans cette communication, brûleur-jet métallique, brûleur à double récupération et unité de fusion rapide, ne sont que des exemples parmi les matériels en développement les plus récemment apparus en France.

Les résultats des différentes applications de ces équipements en fonderie, réchauffage avant forgeage ou traitement thermique des métaux, sont les meilleurs garants du maintien de la compétitivité du gaz naturel dans la métallurgie française.

=ooOoo=

Voir figures de ce chapitre à la suite du texte en version anglaise

MONTREAL CONGRESS

TRANSTEC 87

=ooOoo

EFFICIENT USES OF NATURAL GAS
FOR THE HIGH TEMPERATURES PROCESSES
EXAMPLES IN THE METALLURGICAL INDUSTRY

—=—=—=—

by Mr Pascal BANCOURT

Head of the Industrial Utilizations Section

Gas Utilizations Research Station

Research and Development Division

GAZ DE FRANCE

—=—=—=—

S U M M A R Y

—=—=—=—

First, this paper presents the heating devices which have recently appeared in France :

- the jet burner,

- the double recuperative burner,

- the self-recuperative radiant tube,

as well as their utilizations in different sectors of the metallurgical industry : forge, non-ferrous alloys melting, heat treatment.

Each piece of equipement is explained in detail and some examples make clear the energy savings obtained in comparison with more conventional devices.

In the second part of the lecture, the quick-melting and holding unit for non-ferrous alloys designed by the GAZ DE FRANCE Research Center, is presented.

1 - INTRODUCTION

Whether metals are being melted or heated before deformation or treatment, metallurgy is a field in which high temperatures are all-important.

It would take too long and perhaps be tedious to discuss all the possible applications of gas in this industrial sector. Gas has many such applications in various types of furnaces, from the melting temperature of steel (gas-oxygen burners in electric arc furnaces) to the temperature of zinc (galvanizing furnaces), without considering special applications such as:

- flame-work (e.g. oxygas cutting),

- the use of methane as a raw material for generating the right atmosphere in heat-treatment furnaces.

This paper will mainly present new products developed for FRENCH industry through the cooperation between GAZ DE FRANCE, the energy distributor, and manufacturers of heating systems.

These products are designed to improve two important aspects of installations using natural gas; their purpose is to:

- save energy,

- increase productivity.

Gas is used to make these products:

- more powerful,

- cleaner,

- easier to control

than those using other types of energy, which makes it possible to design efficient and reliable installations or systems.

This text will be limited to three products, applied in the following sectors of metallurgy: Foundry, forge and heat treatment.

2 - THE JET BURNER AND ITS APPLICATIONS

High-velocity metal burners (velocity of combustion products > 100 m/s), or jet burners, are of course used in heat-treatment furnaces requiring moderate temperatures (between 500 and 1000°C). If the burned gases move at a high speed:

* Convective heat transfer essential at these temperatures, are increased,

* The atmosphere is stirred, improving the homogeneity of the temperature needed for heat treatment.

2.1 DESCRIPTION OF THE "MGV" BURNER

Several types of jet burners have been developed by the industry. The "MGV" burner (brûleur Métallique à Grande Vitesse) or high-velocity metal burner is basically different from other burners in that it is made entirely of metal, whereas combustion chambers are generally made of refractory ceramics. This design improves resistance to thermal shocks resulting from frequent stops and starts.

This type of burner is manufactured for ratings ranging from 25 to 400 kW ncv, with an air and gas pressure of about 50 mbar.

The section in figure No. 1 shows the principle of this burner.

The gas is injected at two points: Radially at B (to obtain a partial premixture) then axially at C.

A small part of the combustion air entering at the back of the burner goes through B to obtain a partial air-gas premixture. The other part goes to the burner nozzle, where the tangential holes A rotate it.

This arrangement protects the metal structure of the burner.

Combustion takes place in chamber C; in other words, the combustion air is preheated to raise the temperature of the flame and obtain - at the burner rating - a combustion products velocity exceeding 150 m/s with a high specific thrust.

The burner is equipped with an ignition electrode and an ultraviolet flame safety device.

For ratings lower than or equal to 75 kW, a self-recuperative version of this burner has been developed. Combustion products entering the heat chamber are circulated around the casing to preheat the combustion air.

This principle was developed for a specific heating unit, the radiant tube, used to heat heat-treatment furnaces in a controlled atmosphere, as shown in figure No. 2.

2.2 USE OF THE "MGV" BURNER FOR DIRECT HEATING

Example of an annealing furnace

2.21 DESCRIPTION

The first example of the application of the "MGV" jet burner is an annealing furnace, used to homogenize and stabilize cast iron. The furnace was built in a heat-treatment shop and the specifications had to meet the following requirements:

- it must be suitable for very flexible operation,

- it must have a large-volume working chamber,

- it must be able to withstand quickly rising temperatures,

- it must save energy.

The furnace (a section is shown in figure 3) has the following characteristics:

- a useful volume of 82 m3 (8 m x 3.2 m x 3.2 m),

- two mobile hearths (one in the furnace and one stand-by) able to support loads of up to 50 tons: Each hearth, equipped with a heavy refractory lining, weighs 30 tons,

- a heating system consisting of 16 "MGV" burners, each with a rating of 140 kW, i.e. a total output of 2,240 kW,

- an insulation consisting of fibrous refractory blocks with 300 mm sides.

The two oven doors slide open laterally and are flattened against the walls by means of pneumatic cams.

The burners are mounted one one of the long sides of the furnace, opposite a series of flues in the hearth. This arrangement, which limits the effect of the cold hearth (present in so many installations), improves conductive heat transfer and quickly homogenizes the temperature of the parts to be treated.

The heating system is arranged in three temperature-regulation zones:

```
Zone 1     4 burners      560 kW
Zone 2     8 burners    1,120 kW
Zone 3     4 burners      560 kW
```

It is possible to operate at half-rating i.e. with 2, 4 and 2 burners.

The combustion produts are discharged through four openings in the roof of the furnace. There, the flue gases are collected in a flue and channeled to the chimney stack. To keep a slight excess pressure in the furnace, the stack has been equipped with an automatic valve controlled by a pressure sensor mounted in the furnace. The system is equipped with a temperature regulator. It is possible to program the speed at which the temperature should rise, the time during which the temperature should be held, and the temperature of the holding phase.

2.22 FURNACE THERMAL CHARACTERISTICS

The heat balance of the furnace were recorded during three normalizing treatments. Twice, loads of 10.125 tons and 6.4 tons of gray cast iron were heated to a temperature of 780°C. The third time, a load of 8.4 tons of alloyed steel was heated to 930°C.

The results are summarized on the following table:

TREATMENT	1	2	3
Operating temperature (°C)	780	780	930
Loads (tons)	10.125	6.4	8.4
Temperature rise (hours, minutes)	7:45	7:20	10:17
Holding time (hours, minutes)	3:00	3:00	0:52
Heat consumption (kWh ncv)	15,296	13,171	14,687

During tests, the average combustion efficiency was 55%, while the furnace pressure regulator of the furnace was not yet installed. Because this regulator reduces spurious air ingress, its use at the above temperatures improves the efficiency by about 5%.

Less than 5% of the total consumption is lost through the fiber walls, whereas on the average 40% is lost through the heavy-refractory hearth. It is, therefore, of interest to compare the specific consumption per gross ton of product (hearth + parts) with the specific consumption per net ton of product (parts only). Looking at the table below, one can see that the consumption differences between gross and net load are the equivalent of the quantity of heat stored in the hearth.

This is a large value indeed, but the hearth's mechanical resistance must be calculated considering the loads supported, often unequally distributed. Consequently, the hearth can only be made of dense, heavy refractory materials.

TREATMENT	1	2	3
gross specific heat consumption (kWh/t ncv)	305	283	303
net specific heat consumption (kWh/t ncv)	1,510	2,058	1,748

* OPERATING RESULTS

This furnace replaces two older-design furnaces of about half its volume, made of traditional refractory bricks and equipped with traditional fuel-oil burners.

The acceleration of the treatment (made possible by the combination of jet burners and a fibrous refractory lining) in the new furnace described here, has enabled the manufacturer to increase his production from 180 to 300 t/month and to lower his fuel bills by about 35%.

Moreover, the high velocity of the combustion products improves convection, increasing the homogeneity of the furnace temperature ($\pm$ 10°C) and therefore of the load temperature, all of which results in a better product.

Finally, a high degree of automation makes more efficient use of human resources, thereby reducing operating expenses.

2.3 APPLICATION OF THE "MGV" BURNER TO THE SELF-RECUPERATIVE RADIANT TUBE

Example of a carbonitriding furnace

In an integrated workshop of the automobile industry, the radiant tube shown in figure No. 2 is fitted in five almost identical through-type furnaces for treating gear parts straight from the forge before grinding, assembly and mounting (gear boxes). The furnaces are of the controlled atmosphere, carbonitriding or case-hardening type.

For our example we have chosen a carbonitriding furnace.

2.31 - Description of the furnace and its fittings

The furnace is of the continuous type, equipped with 2 lines of 17 trays each. The volume of the working chamber is 8 m3 and its overall dimensions are: Length 11.3 m, width 2.2 m and height 2 m.

Production can reach 1.45 t/h, processing a load of trays weighing 50 kg carrying parts weighing 70 kg. Its maximum temperature is 890°C.

The atmosphere is of the nitrogen-methanol type.

This furnace is equipped with a built-in oil-hardening tank.

It is used 5 days per week in three daily 8-hour shifts. The temperature of the atmosphere is maintained during the weekend.

The heating system consists of 27 "MGV-35" self-recuperative radiant tubes, each with a rating of 35 kW.

They are spread as follows over 5 temperature regulation zones:

Zone 1 (entrance)   11 tubes (3 beneath the load)

Zone 2   9 tubes (3 beneath the load)

Zone 3   3 tubes

Zone 4   2 tubes

Zone 5 (exit)   2 tubes

An ON-OFF controller is used.

2.32 - Results

The average combustion efficiency is 70% (ncv).

At the rated capacity of the furnace (1.12 t/h), the specific consumption is 479 kWh/(ncv)/t. For an hourly production of 1.45 t it is only 370 kWh/(ncv)/t.

Previously, the manufacturer used furnaces of the same shape and production characteristics but equipped with "traditional" radiant tubes made. Their combustion efficiency was never higher than 50% (ncv) at the carbonitriding temperatures used.

Figure No. 4 shows changes of specific heat consumption with furnace production, depending on their heating system.

For the same production, self-recuperative radiant tubes save about 50% energy.

3 - THE "BDR" DOUBLE RECUPERATION BURNER AND ITS APPLICATIONS

This "BDR" burner (Brûleur Double Récupération) is one of the range of recuperative burners used to save large quantities of energy when heating high-temperature charge furnaces.

Its principle, shown in figure No. 5, is to recover as much energy as possible from the flue gases and use it to preheat the combustion air. Heat is transferred by means of two heat exchangers whose design has intentionally been kept simple to keep them reasonably cheap.

3.1 DESIGN AND OPERATION OF THE BDR BURNER

The first heat exchanger, mounted on the furnace, is of the single-ended type. It consists of an insulated housing lined with fibrous refractory materials in which the furnace combustion products circulate.

The combustion air enters cold and circulates in the exchanger, which is made of refractory steel.

The upper part of the exchanger, in contact with the hottest combustion products, is cooled by means of air circulation.

The second heat exchanger, mounted behind the first one, consists of a double annular space in which the combustion air (before entering the burner) circulates in counter-flow with the combustion products discharged from the back of the burner.

The mixer is a simple perforated cone. It is equipped with an ignition electrode. An ultraviolet cell is used as a flame safety device.

Combustion is intense. Due to the fact that the air rotates when entering, air and gas are mixed so well that the furnace can operate properly at 20% of the rating.

The stack contains an air injection system (eductor) used to create a partial vacuum. By adjusting its flow rate, the user can slightly increase the furnace pressure, thus preventing spurious air ingress and eliminating this source of considerable energy losses.

The following characteristics are part of the general design of the "BDR" burner:

- a large heat-transfer surface to produce the output required for the two applications below,

- no metal parts at too high a temperature, thus ensuring the reliability of the BDR,

- the possibility of selecting the point at which the flue gases enter in the first exchanger, depending on the design of the furnace. This solution improves convective heat transfers and the temperature homogeneity as compared with recuperative burners whose combustion products are directly recirculated from the burner nozzle (self-recuperative burners).

This burner is manufactured in a rating range from 70 to 900 kW. Several versions are available without a second burner (when a second burner is not economically justified).

3.2 APPLICATION OF THE "BDR" BURNER TO A FORGE FURNACE

The "BDR" burner was developed and tested at the end of 1984. In August 1985, it was used for the first time industrially, in a small furnace to heat steel before forging.

3.21 - Description of the furnace

The furnace is a batch type furnace with an inner volume of 2.8 m3 (shown by the section in figure No. 6).

The hearth is made of refractory concrete, the sidewalls and the roof are made of refractory bricks. Fiber modules are stuck to the roof. The "guillotine" door is lined with fibers.

The furnace is equipped with a single burner of 500 kW (burner rating). It is mounted on one of the sides. The first exchanger, 1.7 m long, is mounted horizontally at hearth level. The burner and the second exchanger are mounted above it.

A threee position control is used, set at the following values:

- FULL : 515 kW: air factor n = 1.08

- PARTIAL: 85 kW: air factor n = 1.15

By pushing the switch to open the furnace door, the user sets the burner at PARTIAL. This setting is maintained as long as the door remains open.

3.22 - Results

Below we show the results of this furnace when heating a charge of 2.37 t of normal steel to 1,225°C:

INPUT	- gas combustion	1,309 kWh (ncv)
	- load oxidation	58 kWh
OUTPUT	- useful heat	548 kWh
	- flue gas losses	403 kWh
	- various losses (walls, opening of the door, ingress air)	416 kWh

Therefore:

- A combustion efficiency of 71% (ncv)

- a heating efficiency of 40%,

- a specific heat consumption of 552 kWh (ncv)/t.

3.23 - Development of the "BDR" forge burner

In 1986, following these results, four other forge furnaces were equipped with such burners. One of them, a rotating furnace producing 4 t/h, was modernized using 5 "BDR" burners of 500 kW each. Its performance is comparable to the above example.

3.3 APPLICATION OF THE "BDR" BURNER TO THE CRUCIBLE FURNACE

At the time it was adapted to forges, this burner was also used for heating gas-fired crucible furnaces, whose heating efficiency is traditionally low.

3.31 - Description of the furnace

The "BDR" burner was adapted to a crucible furnace for melting aluminium alloys with a capacity of 200 kg. An "BDR" burner of 150 kW was installed (as shown in figure No. 7).

The furnace is brick lined and used 8 hours per day to melt an AS9U3 alloy (88% Al, 9% Si, 3% Cu), and raise it to a temperature of 730°C (i.e. the temperature used for casting).

The load is put in the crucible: Consequently it is heated indirectly. Moreover, the loads are melted one after another during the working day, so that the first load of the day is melted "with a cold furnace" (after the night's idle time), whereas the following loads are melted "with a hot furnace".

3.32 - Results

The following results were recorded at the forge with a load consisting of about 50% 5 kg ingots, and of about 50% runner heads, feeder heads and scrap from moulding stations.

The exact size of the charge and the melting time are noted in the "test conditions" column. As we know, these conditions can greatly affect thermal results.

WHEN STARTING WITH A COLD FURNACE		WHEN STARTING WITH A HOT FURNACE	
TEST CONDITIONS	SPECIFIC HEAT CONSUMPTION kWh(ncv/t)	TEST CONDITIONS	SPECIFIC HEAT CONSUMPTION kWh(ncv)/t
190 kg 142 min	1,186	184 kg 84 min	745
190 kg 143 min	1,291	181 kg 78 min	783

Therefore, these results give:

- a combustion efficiency of 72% (ncv) when the melting is finished, when combustion products enter the burner at the maximum temperature (1,025°C) and with 10 % excess air,

- a heating efficiency of 41% (ncv).

Under similar operating conditions, the specific heat consumption of crucible furnaces is normally equal to or greater than 1,000 kWh (ncv)/t.

3.33 - Development of the "BDR" burner for crucible furnaces

This burner was developed simultaneously for foundries and for forges.

In 1986 a workshop was set up with 8 furnaces of this type.

These furnaces are mainly used to maintain the temperature of liquid metal close to pressure moulding machines, while executing a melting operation in the morning at shift start and melting some ingots during the day (i.e. it is used to melt and maintain load temperatures).

The development of this type of furnace continues. It has been adapted to melting copper alloys, but is also used to maintain the temperature of light alloys (without melting them). In both cases the power of the "BDR" burner must be adapted to the required heat. Twelve such furnaces were installed in FRANCE in 1986.

4 - QUICK MELTING AND HOLDING UNIT

When a foundry needs a large and continuous quantity of a non-ferrous metal alloy, the crucible furnace described above is no longer suitable. In this case the metal is melted by heating it directly in a basin furnace with a capacity ranging between 700 kg and a few dozen tons. By means of transfer ladles the load can then be distributed among the various moulding stations, where it is stored in a holding furnace (generally a crucible, sometimes a small basin furnace).

For many years thermal engineers and manufacturers have tried to improve the heat efficiency of these basin furnaces. Because of the low thermal emissivity of liquid aluminium (limiting its radiation absorption) the furnace efficiency for light alloys is in fact rather low.

In the past, the following methods were used to recover heat lost in flue gases:

- Preheating of the load: Generally, the flue gases are forced to circulate in counter-flow with the load in a feeding hopper. This method can be improved with jet burners, which tend to facilitate convective heat transfers,

- Preheating of the combustion air by means of adapted heat exchangers.

Both methods result in a heating efficiency ranging from 40 to 50%.

Because of the competition between the various types of energy used in France, especially electricity, which, for example, allows efficiencies of 60 to 70% for an induction furnace, GAZ DE FRANCE has combined the two methods described above to propose a new type of basin furnace, the Quick Melting Unit (QMU).

4.1 DESCRIPTION OF THE QUICK MELTING UNIT

The QMU is a furnace consisting of juxtaposed cells, one for melting, the other for holding, and a recuperator, to recover heat from the combustion products.

Figure No. 8 shows a perspective of this furnace and its overall dimensions. Figure No. 9 shows cross sections of the melting cell, the recuperator, and the holding cell and its drawing troughs.

The troughs were included in the specifications of the first of these units, installed in a small workshop to provide liquid metal for 6 die stations arranged around the furnace. The troughs are covered during holding.

The melting cell, shaped like a tunnel, is heated by a burner with a rated output of 750 kW (currently set at 320 kW) and mounted at one of the ends.

The lower part of the sloping hearth (on the side of the burner) is provided with a launder enabling the molten metal to gravitate into the maintenance basin.

The holding basin has an overall length which is almost equal to the length of the melting cell. It contains two so-called "flat flame" radiant burners of 65 kW, mounted on the roof.

After the cover has been removed the furnace is loaded from above; the melting cell is completely filled with ingots, runner heads, feeder heads or scrap. As soon as the melting burner is ignited, the metal nearest to it is melted and the flue gases are used to preheat the remainder of the load. Afterwards, these flue gases are collected at the upper part of the cell's extremity; then they are sent to the recuperator below.

This single-ended recuperator preheats the combustion air of the melting burner. Consequently, the flue gases are discharged at a lower temperature, while the temperature of the combustion products rises, improving efficiency.

The combustion products discharged from the holding cell circulate in counter-flow with the molten metal in the channel connecting the holding cell with the melting cell, preheating the load for use in the recuperator. When the temperature is held for a particularly long time, the amount of heat released can be sufficient for melting the load without having to start the melting burner.

The melting burner is ignited automatically, a procedure which is triggered manually by the user. It is stopped by a regulator which compares the set temperature with the temperature measured by a thermocouple mounted in the flue at the entrance to the recuperator. The burner is only ignited for the next load when ordered by the user.

The two holding burners are also started according to an automatic procedure.

Their operation is permanently controlled by an ON-OFF control which compares the set temperature to the temperature measured by an insertion pyrometer immerged in the bath.

4.2 RESULTS

About 600 kg of ingots and about 350 kg of feeder heads, runner heads and scraps from moulding stations can be loaded in the melting cell.

The following table gives some idea of the specific heat consumption and efficiency of the furnace as compared with the net calorific value (ncv) of natural gas. These examples involve aluminium-silicon alloys containing up to 10% silicon.

The consumption indicated includes the consumption of the burners from the holding cell.

RATING	METAL TEMPERATURE	FUSION TIME	SPECIFIC CONSUMPTION	COMBUSTION EFFICIENCY	HEATING EFFICIENCY
416 kW	763°C	45 min	670 kWh/t	73%	50%
388 kW	758°C	45 min	571 kWh/t	72%	58%
334 kW	752°C	53 min	678 kWH/t	73%	52%
296 kW	724°C	61 min	538 kWh/t	76%	64%

The heating efficiency is comparable to the efficiency of induction melting.

This unit has now been in use for two years. It is used every day as follows:

- 8 hours production (uncovered troughs)

- 16 hours of holding (covered troughs), during which the hourly consumption is 23 kWh (ncv).

Under these circumstances, with a daily melting load of 5 t, which is relatively little compared with the possibilities (12 t/day including times for loading and cleaning), the mean specific operating consumption is 720 kWh(ncv)/t.

Moreover, the scale loss, the difference between the metal in the furnace and the metal which is cast, is an average of 1.7% over a period of 6 production weeks.

4.3 DEVELOPMENT

Other French foundries have decided to start using this type of energy-saving furnace, which produces high-quality cast metal. In the near future five aluminium-alloy melting units and one Zamak melting unit will be started up.

Tests with Zamak have shown that the specific consumption was 134 kWh(ncv)/t for metal heated to 409°C, with a scale loss of 1.2% and an ash rate of 0.41%.

The largest of these future units will have an aluminium-alloy melting rate of 3.2 t/h and a holding capacity of 29 t.

The user has specified this holding capacity, which is not in proportion to the melting rate, to permit him to directly receive liquid metal transported by road from various steel refineries.

This tilting unit will contain three burners, each with a maximum rating of 900 kW. They will be mounted side by side at one of the extremities of the melting cell.

Three single-ended heat exchangers installed beneath the hearth will supply the burners with preheated air.

5 - CONCLUSION

Manufacturers in the metallurgy industry, most of whose processes take place at high temperatures, are constantly concerned with saving energy, increasing the production of their installations and improving the quality of their products.

This attitude is especially found in FRANCE, where most fuels are imported (particularly natural gas).

The circumstances have induced French manufacturers of heating systems to supply their clients with the efficient gas equipment or processes they expect. Whether equipment supplier or natural gas user, all clients of GAZ DE FRANCE (a natural gas distributor) are encouraged to use gas optimally.

The three systems presented in this paper - the "MGV" metal jet burner, the "BDR" double-recuperation burner and the quick melting unit - are only a few examples of recent French developments.

The results of the various applications of these systems - in the foundry, when heating before forging or when subjecting metal to heat treatment - are the best guarantee that natural gas remains competitive in French metallurgy.

HIGH VELOCITY METAL BURNER

Fig 1

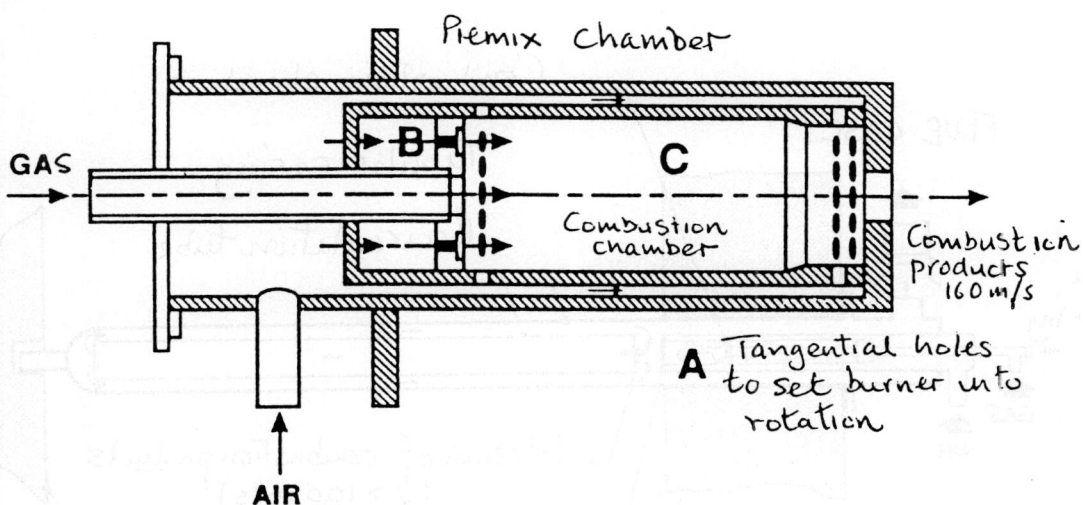

SELF RECUPERATIVE RECIRCULATION RADIANT TUBE

Fig 2.

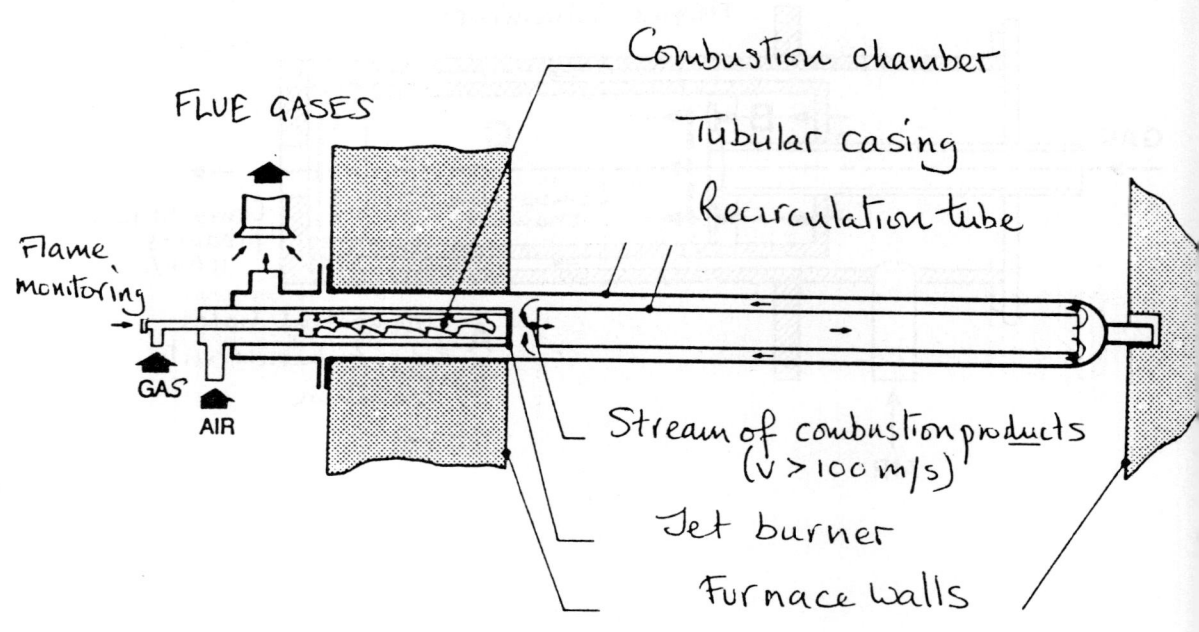

ANNEALING FURNACE EQUIPPED WITH JET BURNERS
Fig. 3

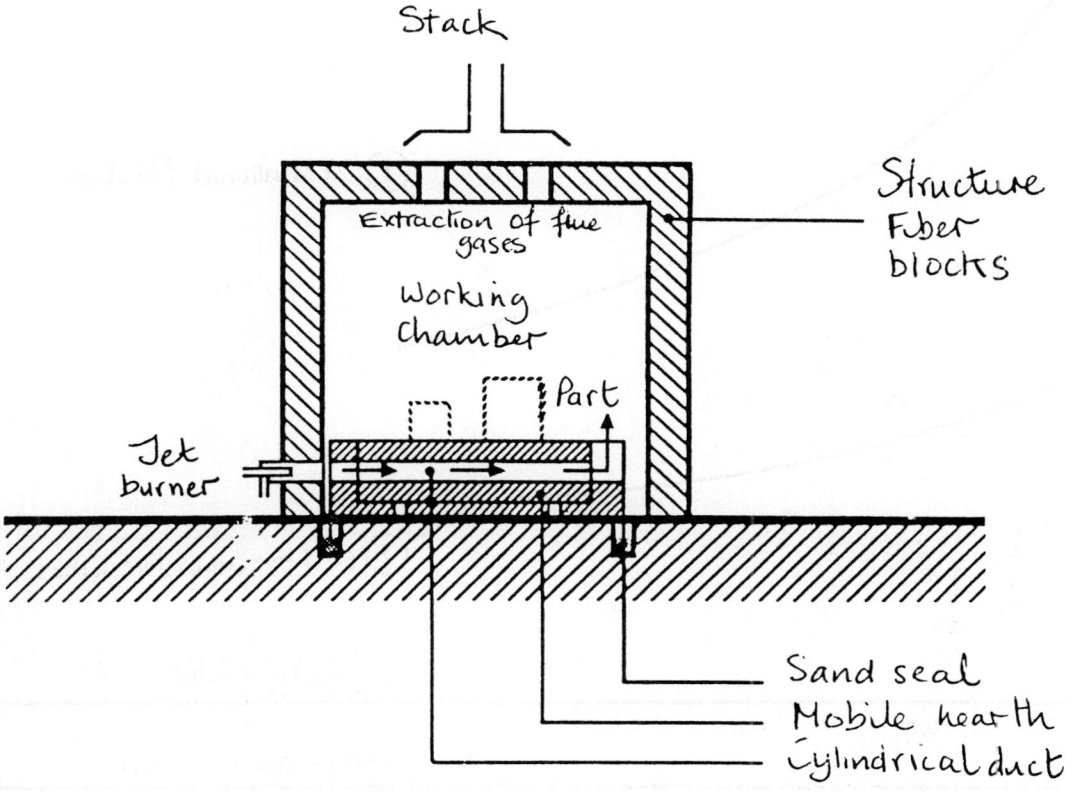

CROSS SECTION OF FURNACE

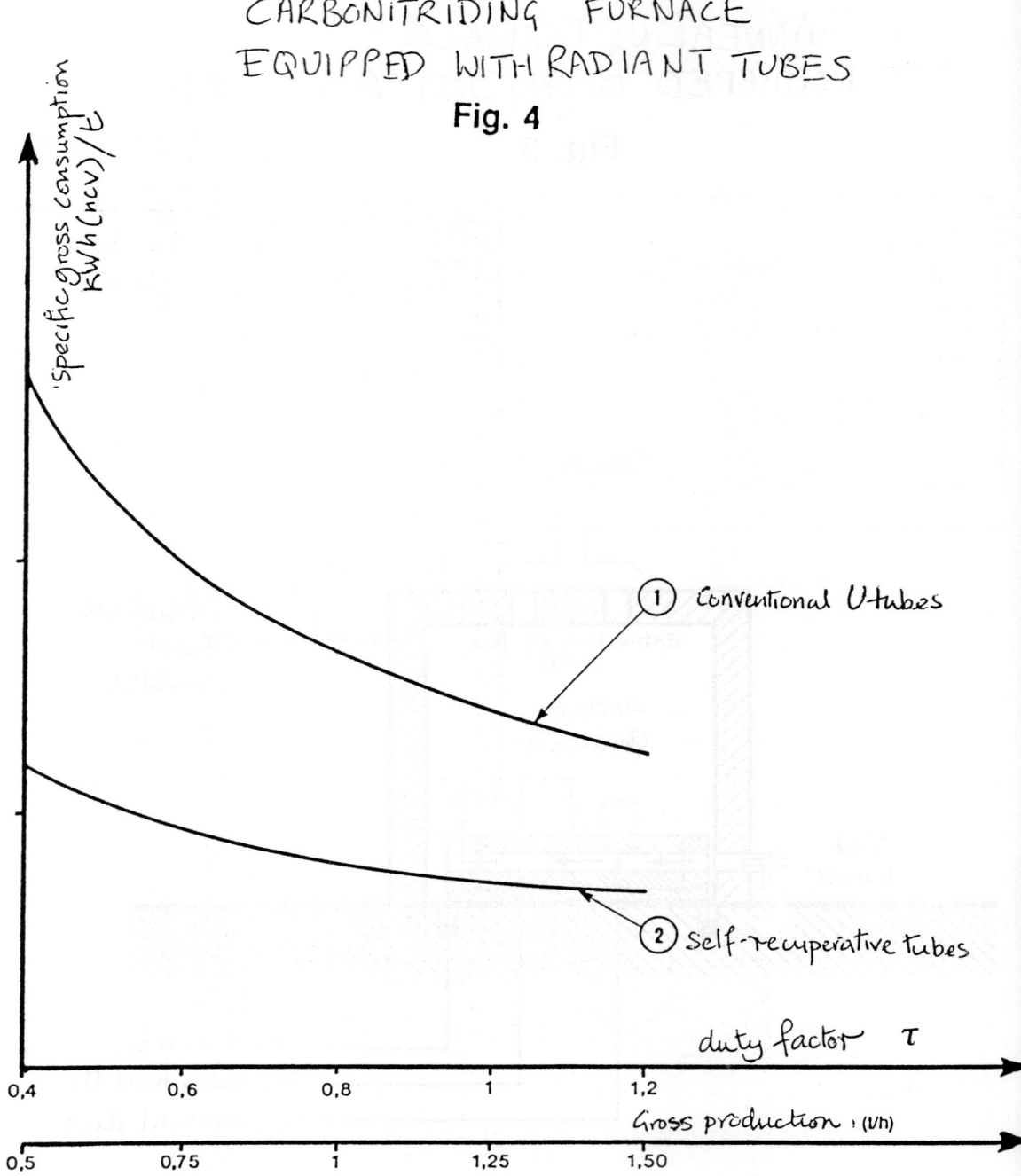

CARBONITRIDING FURNACE EQUIPPED WITH RADIANT TUBES

Fig. 4

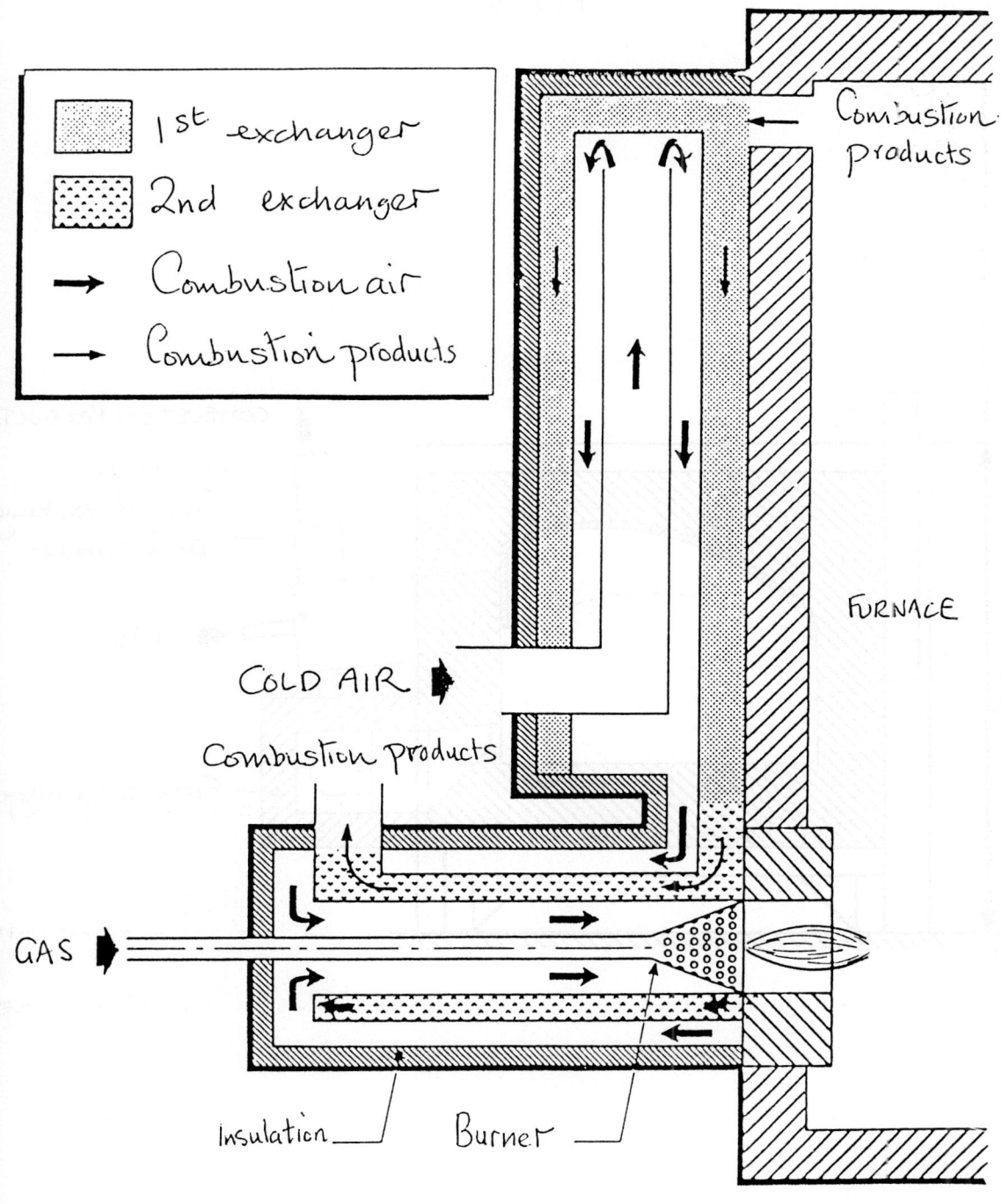

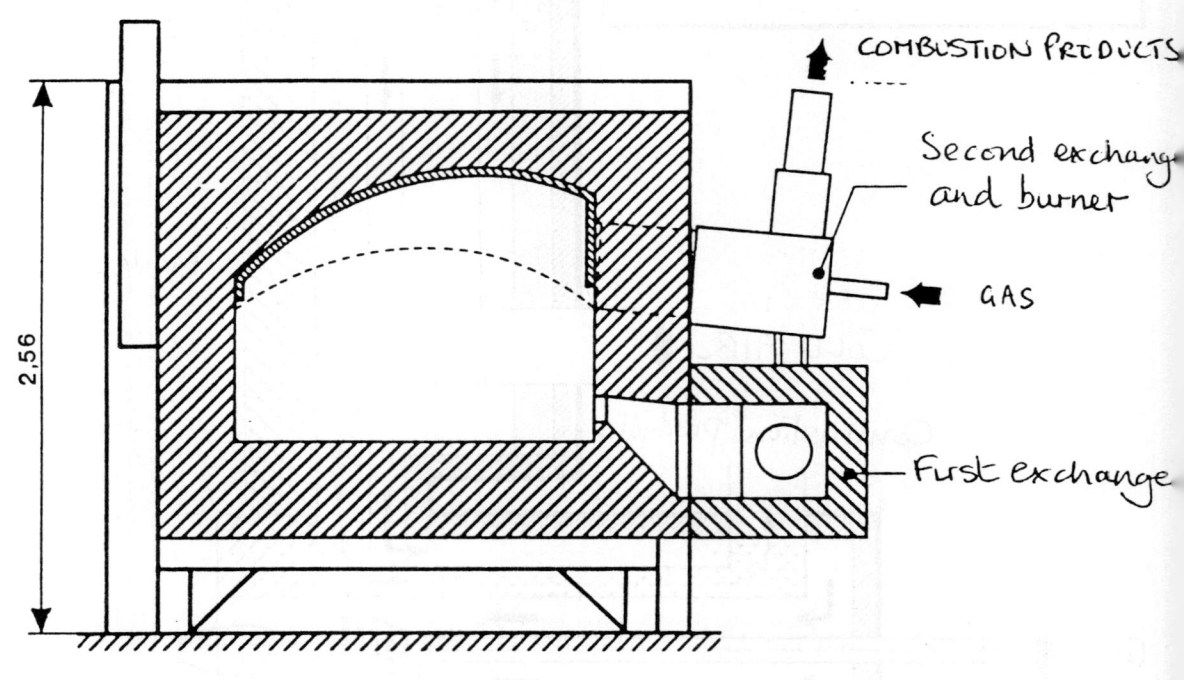

FORGE FURNACE EQUIPPED WITH A DOUBLE RECUPERATION BURNER

Fig. 6

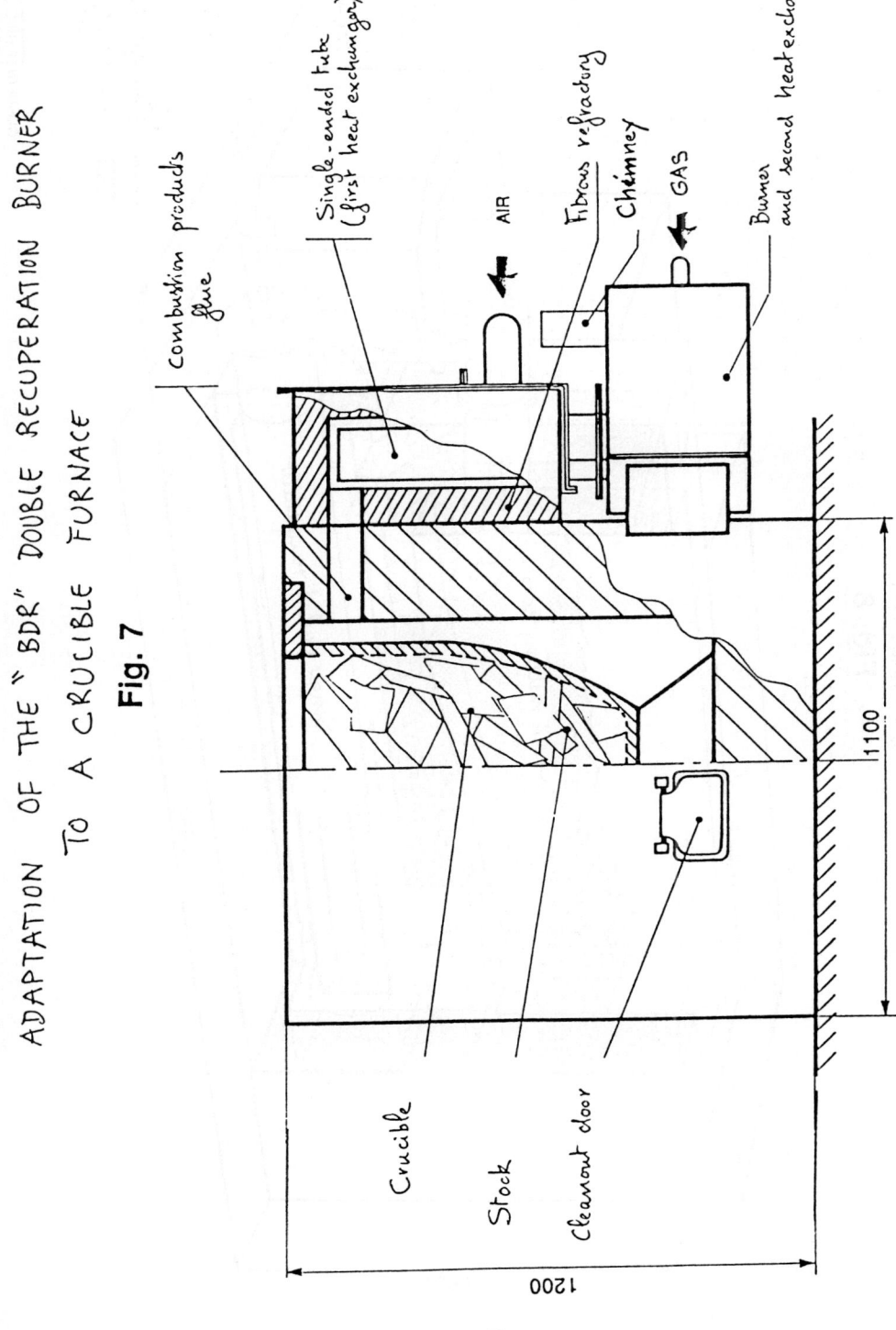

ADAPTATION OF THE "BDR" DOUBLE RECUPERATION BURNER TO A CRUCIBLE FURNACE

Fig. 7

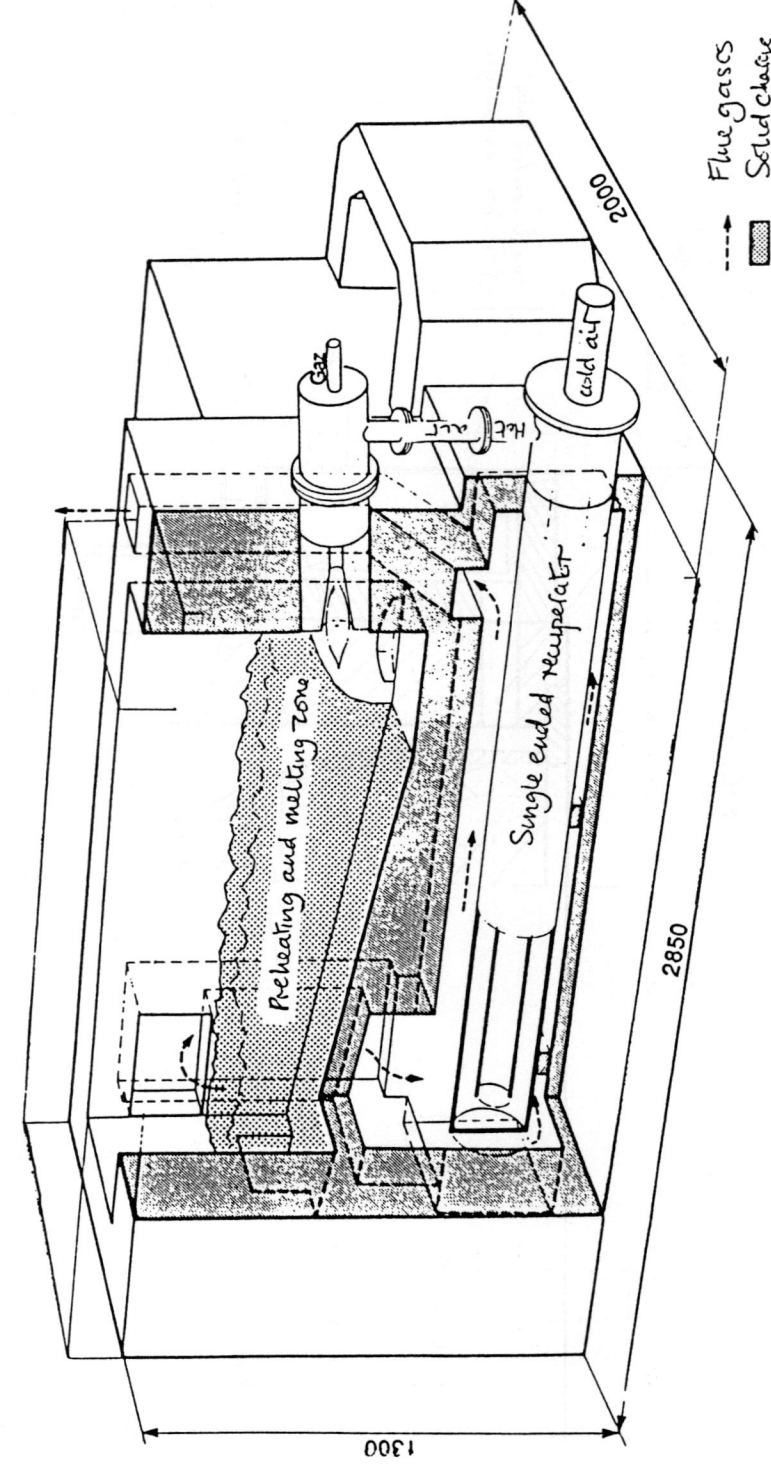

QUICK MELTING AND HOLDING UNIT (QMU) FOR ALUMINIUM

Fig. 8

CROSS SECTIONS OF THE QUICK MELTING UNIT

Fig. 9

2a Melting cell and recuperator

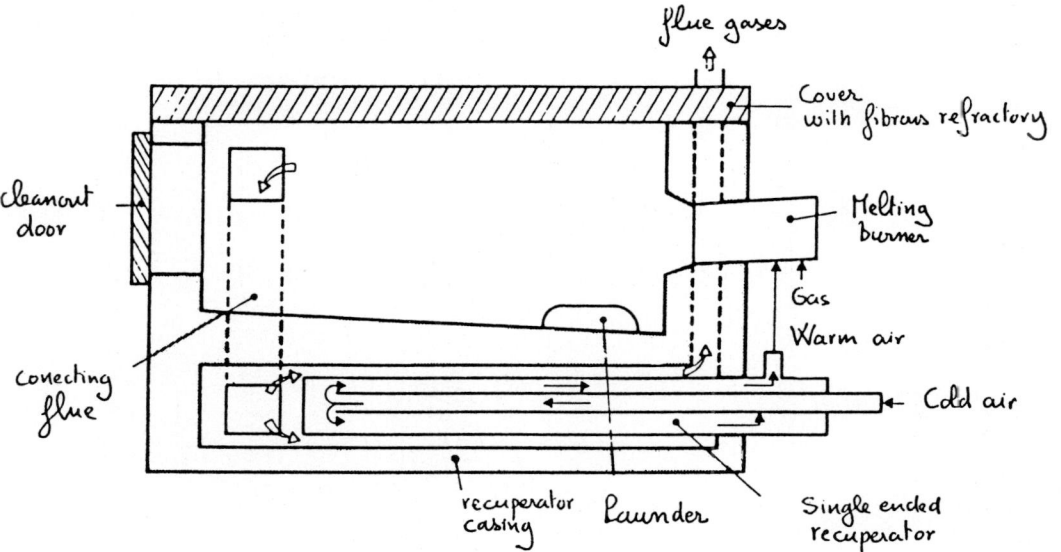

2.b Holding cell

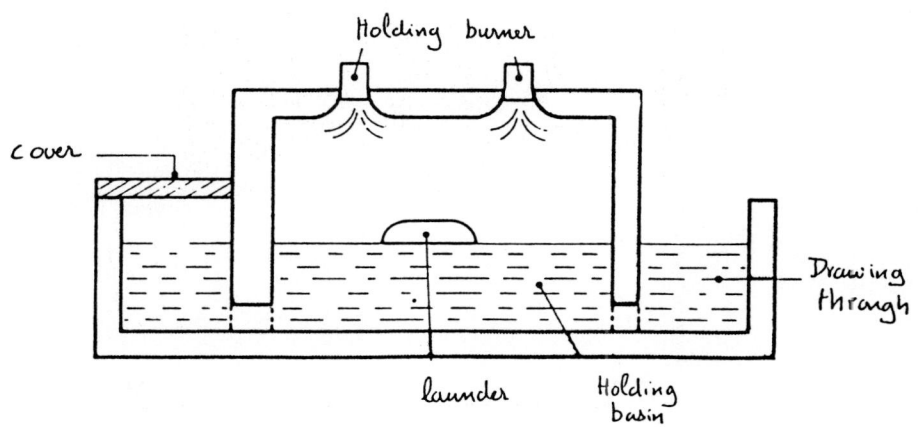

ENERGY CONSIDERATIONS OF THE GLASS INDUSTRY

by
C. W. Hibscher

of
Toledo Engineering Co., Inc.
Toledo, Ohio

I. INTRODUCTION

The glass industry, like any other industry, endeavors to operate on a least-cost basis. The glass melting process is energy intensive and, as a result, there is little choice but to utilize the least costly method of melting, i.e., a fossil fuel furnace, or an electric furnace or a combination of both types. The cost of melting is determined by both the cost of the energy and the capital cost of the furnace utilized.

This paper is presented to help utility engineers better understand the major energy considerations of the glass industry. It discusses the basics of the glass melting process and describes both fossil fuel and electric melting practices along with the associated cost factors. It attempts to approach the selection of the energy source for glass melting in an impartial manner so the utility engineer can do the necessary preliminary analysis to determine if the form of energy he represents is economically favorable before discussing possibilities with a potential glass industry client.

II. SOME HISTORY

Glass making goes back to primitive times. The first known method of commercially melting glass via fossil fuels utilized the pot type furnace, which was, and still is, typically used in conjunction with hand shop specialty glass manufacturing processes, which are inherently low-production operations. Hearth type furnaces were then utilized to manufacture glass at greater production rates, primarily for containers, tableware and flat glass. None of these early processes utilized any form of energy recovery, and, as a result, they were quite inefficient.

The first regenerative glass melting furnace dates back to 1816, when it was patented by Robert Stirling of England and was put into practical use shortly thereafter by Fredrick Siemens of Germany. During the nineteenth century, glass was melted only by means of fossil fuel. It wasn't until 1907 that Marius Sauvegeon of France received patents on a process that could melt glass electrically by means of the Joule principle.

In the 1920's Johan Raeder of Norway first melted glass electrically on a commercial basis, and, in this same period, C.E. Cornelius of Sweden was operating electric melt furnaces producing amber and green glasses.

The first commercial glass-producing, all-electric melter in the United States dates back to 1945. It was installed at Northwestern Glass in Seattle, Washington, where power rates were favorable for electric melting.

III. FOSSIL FUEL FURNACES

Most commercial glasses require 2,000,000 BTU's per ton just to melt the glass. However, this is not the total required energy since process losses are encountered. Thus the formula for computing the total energy required to melt a ton of glass is:

$$\text{Total Energy } (E_t) = \frac{\text{Energy to Glass } (E_g)}{\text{Furnace Efficiency } (\%Eff)}$$

The pot type furnace performs in the 10% or less efficiency range; thus it would require 20 million Btu's or more to melt a ton of glass with this process.

In the Stirling-Siemens type regenerative furnace, shown in Fig. No. 1, the basic furnace consists of the hearth and two (2) regenerators. The furnace is operated on a cyclical basis, and firing is from right to left for approximately 15 minutes. The left-hand regenerator stores up thermal energy while the right-hand regenerator gives up its previously recovered energy to the combustion air. After approximately 15 minutes or after a preset temperature is reached in the hot side regenerator, the reversing valve is operated and the process is reversed. This type furnace today can achieve 30% to 50% efficiency, or the actual amount of energy required to melt a ton of glass by a modern furnace is approximately 4,000,000 to 6,600,000 Btu's per ton. This is true regardless of type of fossil fuel used.

There are two basic types of regenerative furnaces used by the glass industry today: the side port, which is shown in Fig. No. 1, and the end port, which is shown in Fig. No. 2. The end port furnace is generally used for capacity ranges of 75 to 300 tons per day; it has only one set of ports at the backwall and operates in a manner similar to that just described for the side port furnace. The side port furnace is generally used for capacity ranges of 200 tons to 1000 tons per day; the upper capacity range is common in the float glass industry.

Another furnace that utilizes heat recovery is the recuperative type, which is shown in Fig. No. 3. Recuperative furnaces usually vary in capacity from 20 to 200 tons per day. Of course, this is a continuous firing process in which the combustion air is heated by the waste gas in the recuperator. Generally speaking, the recuperative furnace is not quite as efficient as the regenerative type. Typical efficiencies range from 25% to 40%. Thus the energy requirement ranges from about 5,000,000 to 8,000,000 Btu's per ton of glass.

The unit melter is another type fossil fuel furnace that was popular in days past but is rapidly being replaced by more efficient furnaces. This type furnace resembles the recuperative furnace shown in Fig. No. 3, but the recuperator is replaced by an exhaust stack. Unit melters range in capacity from 20 to 100 TPD and, obviously, have a poor efficiency factor, which ranges from 15% to 18%. Thus the energy requirement ranges from about 11,000,000 to 13,000,000 Btu's per ton of glass.

To recap, the important point to remember is that most commercial glasses require a theoretical 2,000,000 Btu's to melt a ton of glass. Fuel fired furnaces without any form of heat recovery are inherently inefficient. Recuperative furnaces can be 40% efficient, and regenerative furnaces can be 50% efficient. Fuel fired furnace performance characteristics are summarized in Fig. No. 4, and this table of information should enable one to determine the amount of energy a fuel fired glass melting process consumes.

IV. ELECTRIC BOOSTING

The practice of electric boosting fuel fired furnaces was started in the early 1950's, when glass manufacturers, encountering increased production requirements, found it economical to increase melting capacity without having to modify the physical aspects of the furnace. An electric boost system can be installed without interfering with production by inserting electrodes through the furnace sidewall blocks.

Some electrical boosts are applied for emission control rather than production purposes. Boosting will reduce the amount of fuel firing and furnace hearth temperature and, as a result, will reduce stack emissions.

A typical electrically boosted furnace is schematically illustrated in Fig. No. 5. Depending upon the amount of energy added, the furnace capacity is typically increased in the 10% to 50% range. Boost power capacities are typically in the 500 to 3000 kW range.

Assuming that all furnace losses are provided by the fuel fired operation, the boost itself would be 100% efficient at the electrode terminals. Since it takes 2,000,000 Btu's to melt a ton of glass, it can be concluded that it takes 586 kWh or 24.4 kW per boosted ton of glass. Experience has shown, however, that a figure of 25 kW to 30 kW per ton is a good rule of thumb to use for rough boost application calculations.

V. ELECTRIC MELTERS

An all-electric furnace operates on the Joule principle. (Refer to Fig. No. 6.) The melting process is started by melting cullet, which is broken glass, by conventional fuel firing. Once the glass is molten, an electrical potential is applied across the electrodes and energy is released via the Joule principle. In the case of a cold top melter, the molten glass surface is flooded with batch mixture and the cold top is formed. Then, batch is continuously fed via a traveling charger, with a feed rate in accordance with the molten glass production rate, or "pull rate", as it is called by the glass industry.

Electric melters fall into two basic classifications, i.e., cold top, shown in Fig. No. 6, and semicold top, shown in Fig. No. 7. The semicold top melter is sometimes used because its rectangular shape conforms to that of a fuel fired furnace and it can be installed in an existing plant where only that shape will fit the space available. Also, the semicold top furnace is charged from the backwall like a conventional fuel fired furnace. From outward appearances, it resembles a fuel fired furnace without regenerators or a recuperator.

The energy efficiency of the semicold top furnace varies with the pull rate. The higher the furnace pull relative to its rated capacity, the greater the batch cover that will exist, and this cover has a pronounced effect on the efficiency of the furnace. At 100% capacity, a semicold top furnace should operate close to the efficiency that is achieved by a cold top furnace. For a flint soda-lime container glass, the typical semicold top operating efficiency is 60% to 65%, or about 900 kWh per ton. However, when the semicold top furnace produces below its rated capacity, it quickly deteriorates to less than 50% efficiency (about 1400 kWh per ton).

The cold top furnace system utilizes a batch charger which travels across the backwall of the furnace, and a boom conveyor belt that travels parallel to the centerline, thus providing a complete batch cover, or blanket, as shown in Fig. No. 8. This batch cover is the key to the success of the cold top melter since it is a good thermal insulator and a self-cleansing emission control filter. The insulating capability of the batch cover is demonstrated by the fact that the molten glass temperature is approximately 2600°F (1425°C) and the temperature immediately on top of the 6" to 9" (15 cm to 23 cm) cover is less than 200°F (93°C).

Cold top melters have melted a variety of glasses throughout the world; however, in the United States and Canada, the predominant use has been the melting of sodium borate glass, the type glass used in manufacturing wool fiberglass. The emissions from a fuel fired sodium borate glass furnace are very difficult and expensive to handle from an environmental standpoint. Therefore, the majority of the wool fiberglass manufacturers in the United States and Canada prefer to use the electric cold top type furnace because it is a maintenance-free, cost-free emission control device. Only carbon dioxide and water vapor penetrate the crust to enter the atmosphere. Also, the batch crust, with its good thermal insulating characteristic, enables the unit to operate in the 65% to 80% efficiency range. See Fig. No. 9 for a table of capacities and typical energy consumptions of cold top furnaces producing sodium borate fiberglass or flint soda-lime container glass.

Some glass manufacturers have gone to cold top electric melting since, generally speaking, it is possible to obtain a more consistent glass quality than with fossil fuel melting.

The major disadvantage of the cold top furnace is that it cannot normally be used below 50% rated capacity. The exact turndown capability will vary, depending upon the design of the furnace, the type of glass melted and the glass quality requirements.

Semicold top furnaces generally have three-phase electrical loads that are unbalanced since it is physically impossible to place electrodes in the furnace sidewalls to achieve equal loading per phase. On the other hand, since cold top furnaces require uniform energy release, they usually have symmetrical electrical systems. For hexagonal shaped furnaces, direct three-phase power can be applied via one, two or four secondaries. Fig. 10 illustrates a dual three-phase secondary arrangement.

Furnaces which employ three-phase secondaries are, generally speaking, limited to 100 TPD capacity. Another furnace power scheme is the Scott-T connected transformer, as shown in Fig. 10. This connection makes it possible to have balanced three-phase primary and balanced two-phase secondary loads. Furnaces utilizing the Scott-T are either square, using one transformer, or rectangular, using two transformers. Furnaces using the Scott-T, two-phase secondary approach have achieved 240 TPD glass output. It is possible to achieve melting capacities up to 350 TPD using this arrangement.

VI. FURNACE APPLICATION BY INDUSTRY SECTOR

There is a pattern to the application of the various furnace types within the glass industry, which is as follows:

Sector	Furnace Capacity (tpd)	Type Furnace Used
Wool Fiberglass	10-250	Predominantly cold top electric
Textile Fiberglass	10-100	Predominantly recuperative
	3-15	Special cold top electric
Container Glass	100-300	Predominantly end port and side port, half of which are electrically boosted
	75-200	A few cold top and semi-cold top electrics
Float Glass	400-1000	Predominantly side-port

VII. ECONOMIC CONSIDERATIONS

Before attempting to sell a glass manufacturer on the merits of basing his process on a given method of melting and fuel type, some "homework" is required to make sure the process makes economic sense, since the glass manufacturer is interested in the most overall cost-effective approach.

A. Capital Cost

Figures 11A & 11B are graphs of approximate capital cost versus daily production capacity for the various types of glass melting furnaces. The costs are stated in a broad band manner since the price of any furnace can vary widely, depending on specifications, refractory selection, etc. Nevertheless, a capital cost should be selected and amortized according to the client's accounting practices.

The capital cost of appropriate emission control equipment in conjunction with a fuel fired furnace must also be considered. Discussion of this aspect is beyond the scope of this paper, but suffice it to say that the capital cost of an emission control system is significant and can range from $500,000 to $2,000,000, depending on capacity and types of emissions controlled.

B. Energy/Operating Cost

It is easy to compute the daily cost of operating a furnace using the following formula:

$$C_o = \frac{(Q*MR*C_e)}{Eff} + Q*C_{em}$$

Where:

C_o = Operating cost ($/day)
Q = Glass melted per day (tons/day)
MR = Theoretical energy to melt glass (Btu/ton)
C_e = Energy cost ($/Btu)
Eff = Furnace efficiency
C_{em} = Emission operating cost ($/ton)

* = Multiplication Symbol

The above formula ignores amortization and maintenance costs, as well as any other factors that make up the total operating cost.

If the fuel fired furnace requires emission control equipment for capturing particulates and SO_x, it would add about $4.00 per ton to the operating cost. NO_x control would add another $3.00 per ton. Thus, the approximate operating cost for particulate, SO_x and NO_x emission control would be about $7.00 per ton. Of course, all this environmental control is an inherent part of the cold top electric melter and, as a result, is free of further cost.

EXAMPLE NO. 1 (NO EMISSION CONTROL):

Assume the following:

- Capacity required .... 250 TPD
- Cost of Natural Gas ..... $3/MCF** = $3/MBtu***
- Furnace efficiency 40%
- Cost of Electricity .. 50 mils/kWh = $14.65/MBtu
- Electric melter efficiency 77%
- Emission control requirements ...... None

  **MCF = Thousand Cubic Feet
 ***MBtu = Million Btu

The comparison for the two methods of melting glass is as follows:

Item	Gas	Electric
- Energy Required ..	5.0 MBtu/ton	2.6 MBtu/ton
- Energy Cost	$3,750/day - or $15.00/ton	$9,500/day - or $38.00/ton

In this example, the capital cost difference between a fuel fired furnace and an electric melter is small, so there is little question that the glass manufacturer will melt glass with a fuel fired furnace.

EXAMPLE NO. 2 (EMISSION CONTROL):

Assume the same factors as stated for Example No.1, but add particulate, SO_x and NO_x emission control, which adds $7.00/ton to the operating cost of the fuel fired furnace.

The comparison to produce one ton of glass is now:

- Natural Gas $22.00/ton
- Electrical $38.00/ton

If the application calls for a furnace capacity of 300 tons per day or less, the capital amortization difference between a fuel fired furnace with emission control and an electric furnace becomes more significant and will further decrease the cost difference between fossil fuel and electric melting.

Another factor for consideration in the final decision is future energy cost projections. Obviously, the energy source that is projected to have the slowest rate of increase will have some advantage.

C. Other Considerations

There are some benefits to electric melting over fuel fired melting that the glass industry will consider in its evaluation. Some of these benefits are:

1. Since a regenerative melter requires a deep basement for its regenerators, building space requirements and costs for an electric melter are lower.

2. Glass quality is usually more consistent because the thermal history of each segment of glass is more uniform.

3. The electric melter is silent and is quite a contrast to its noisy fuel fired counterpart.

VIII. OTHER UTILITY CONSIDERATIONS

The glass melting process has some inherent characteristics that might be desirable to a utility and could possibly warrant preferential energy rates. Some of these considerations are:

A. Natural Gas

A fossil fuel furnace can be designed to operate equally well on any type fossil fuel or combination of fuels, depending on cost and/or availability. For example, interruptible gas could be attractive to a glass manufacturer if the cost savings would help justify the capital cost of the standby or alternate fuel system.

B. Electrical

In some electric melting applications, the glass melting load is approximately half the plant electrical load. The large, constant, unity power factor load of an electric melter should be attractive to electric utilities and worthy of special rate considerations.

The cold top electric melter, with its insulating batch crust, can also serve as a "peak clipping" device since it can be turned off for one or two hours per day while normal glass production is maintained. The glass manufacturer will be reluctant to become obligated to such an operation, unless a good, preferential power rate is involved, since a varying energy input to the furnace could have an adverse effect on furnace life and glass quality.

IX. CONCLUSION

The melting phase of the glass manufacturing process is energy intensive. In most applications, the decision on the type of energy used depends upon capital and operating economic factors. If emission control is required for a fossil fuel melting application, it will substantially increase the capital and operating cost factors of a fuel fired furnace system, whereas emission control has no impact on capital or operating costs for cold top electric furnaces.

Generally speaking, the glass industry will select the type of melting process which uses the form of energy that yields the most favorable balance sheet when all cost factors are considered.

****

CAPTIONS:

Fig. No. 1 - TYPICAL SIDE PORT REGENERATIVE FURNACE

Fig. No. 2 - TYPICAL END PORT REGENERATIVE FURNACE

Fig. No. 3 - TYPICAL RECUPERATIVE FURNACE

Fig. No. 4 - FOSSIL FUEL FURNACE CHARACTERISTICS

Fig. No. 5 - TYPICAL THREE-PHASE ELECTRICAL BOOST APPLIED TO A GLASS FURNACE

Fig. No. 6 - ELEVATION VIEW OF COLD TOP ELECTRIC MELTER WITH BOTTOM ROD (VERTICAL) ELECTRODES

Fig. No. 7 - PLAN AND ELEVATION VIEW OF TYPICAL SEMICOLD TOP ELECTRIC MELTER WITH VARIABLE BATCH COVER

Fig. No. 8 - COLD TOP ELECTRIC MELTER (NOTE BOOM CHARGER AND COMPLETE BATCH BLANKET ON MELTER)

Fig. No. 9 - COLD TOP ELECTRIC MELTER CHARACTERISTICS

Fig. No. 10 - SIX-POLE, THREE-PHASE SYSTEM AND SINGLE ELECTRODE SQUARE (TWO-PHASE SYSTEM)

Fig. No. 11A & B - COMPARATIVE CAPITAL COSTS

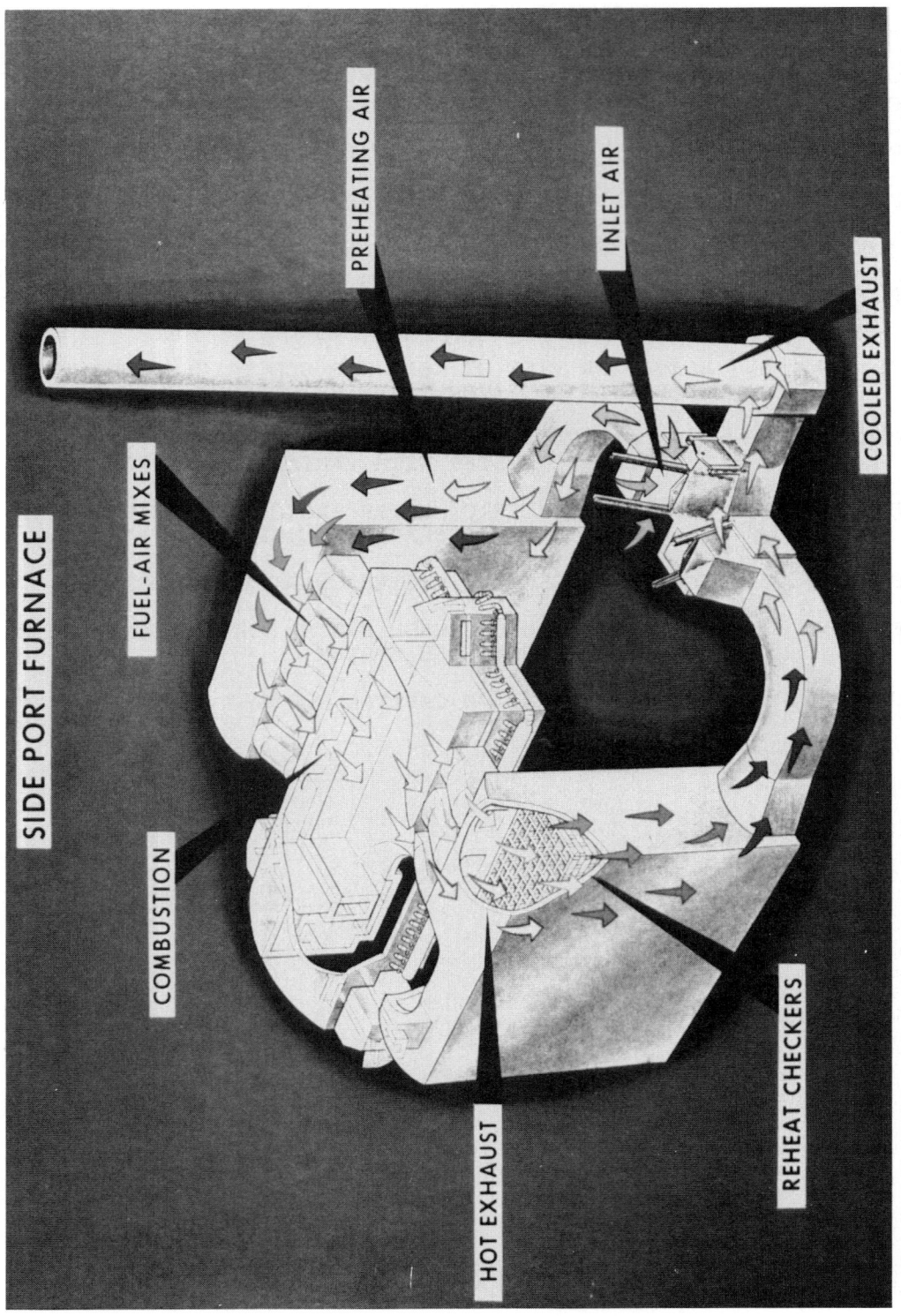

Fig. 1

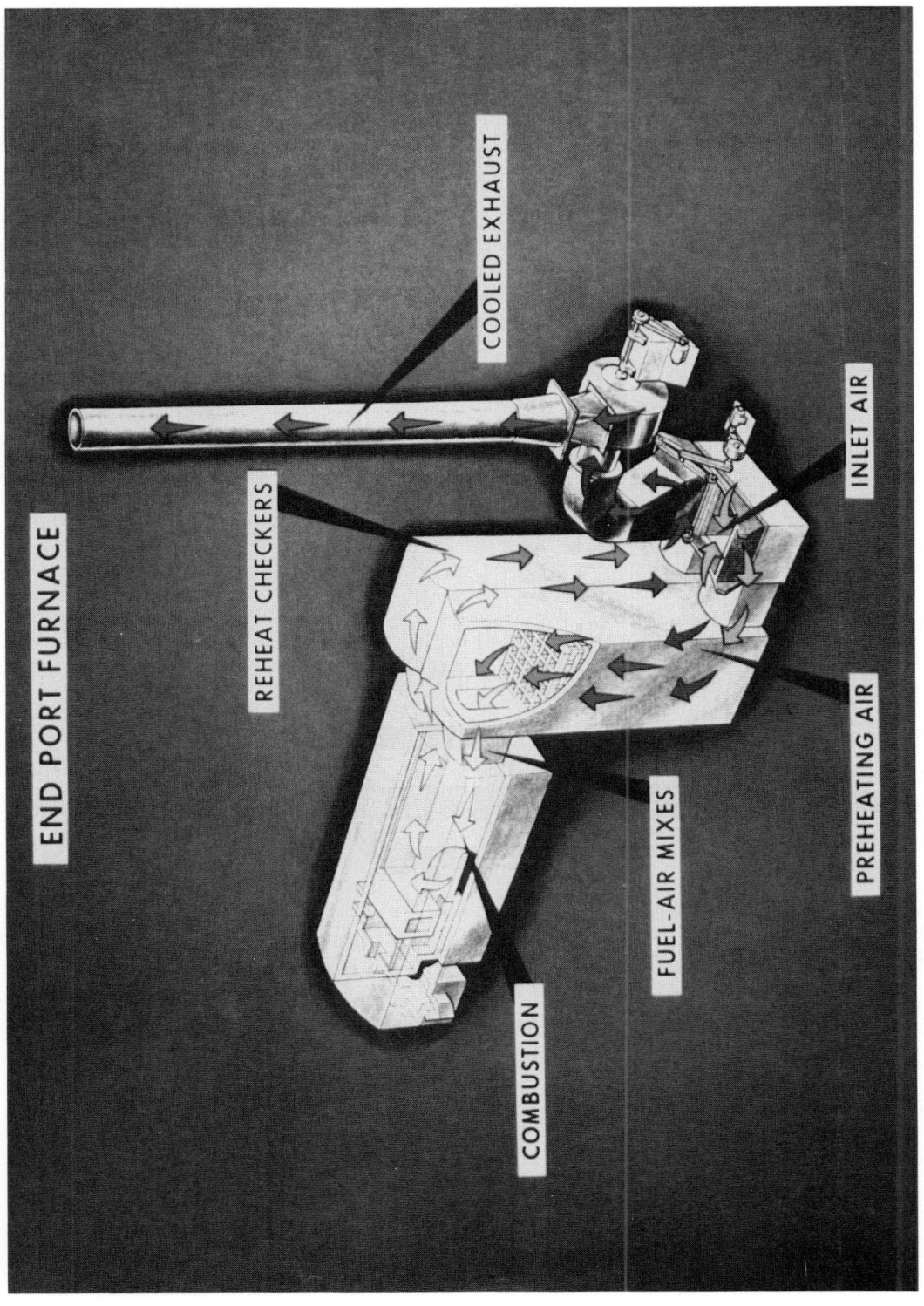

Fig. 2

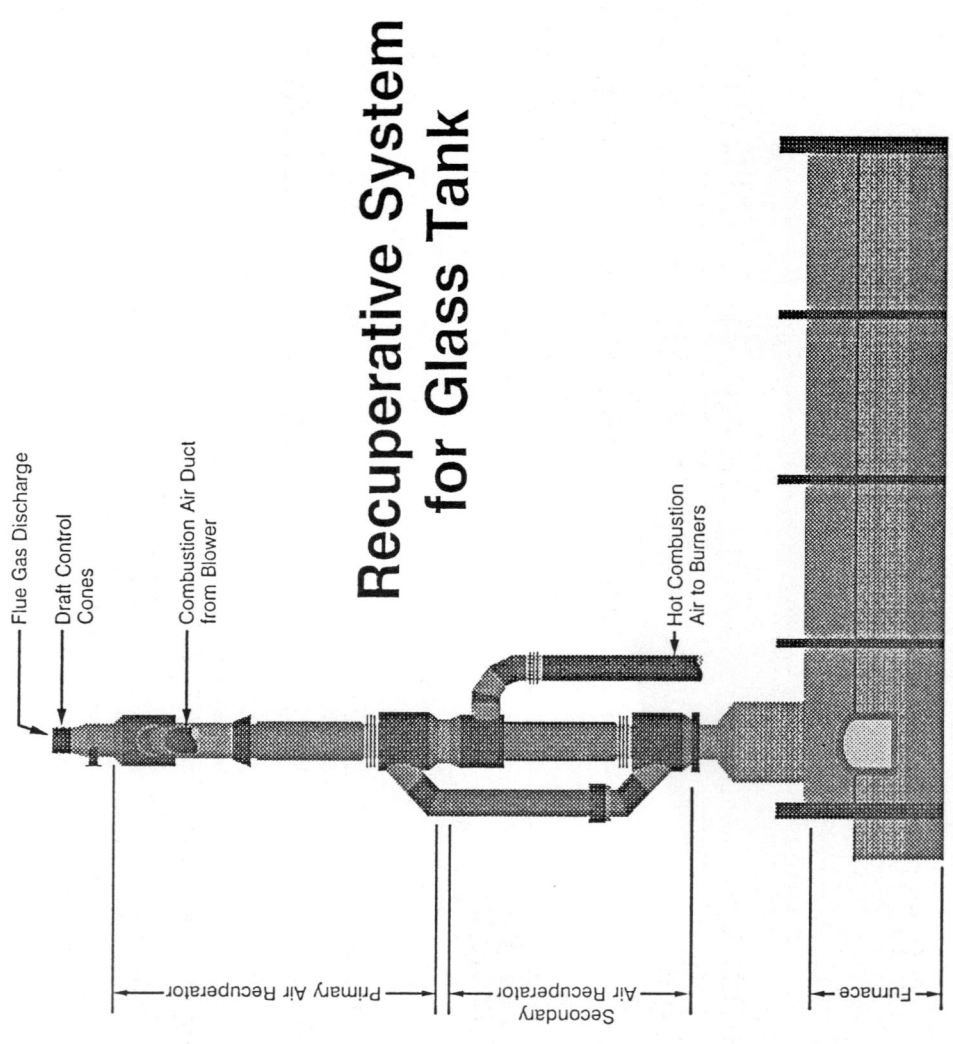

Fig. 3

Fossil Fuel Furnace Capacity & Efficiency Ranges

Type Furnace	Capacity Range (TPD)	Efficiency Range (%)	Energy Req'd (Mill BTU/TON)
Pot Furnace	Low	Very Poor	In Excess of 20
Unit Melter	20 to 100	15 - 18	11 to 13
Recuperative	20 to 200	25 - 40	5.0 to 8
Regenerative End Port	75 to 250	30 - 50	4 to 6.6
Regenerative Side Port	200 to 1000	30 - 50	4 to 6.6

Note: The Above Values are Approximate

Fig. 4

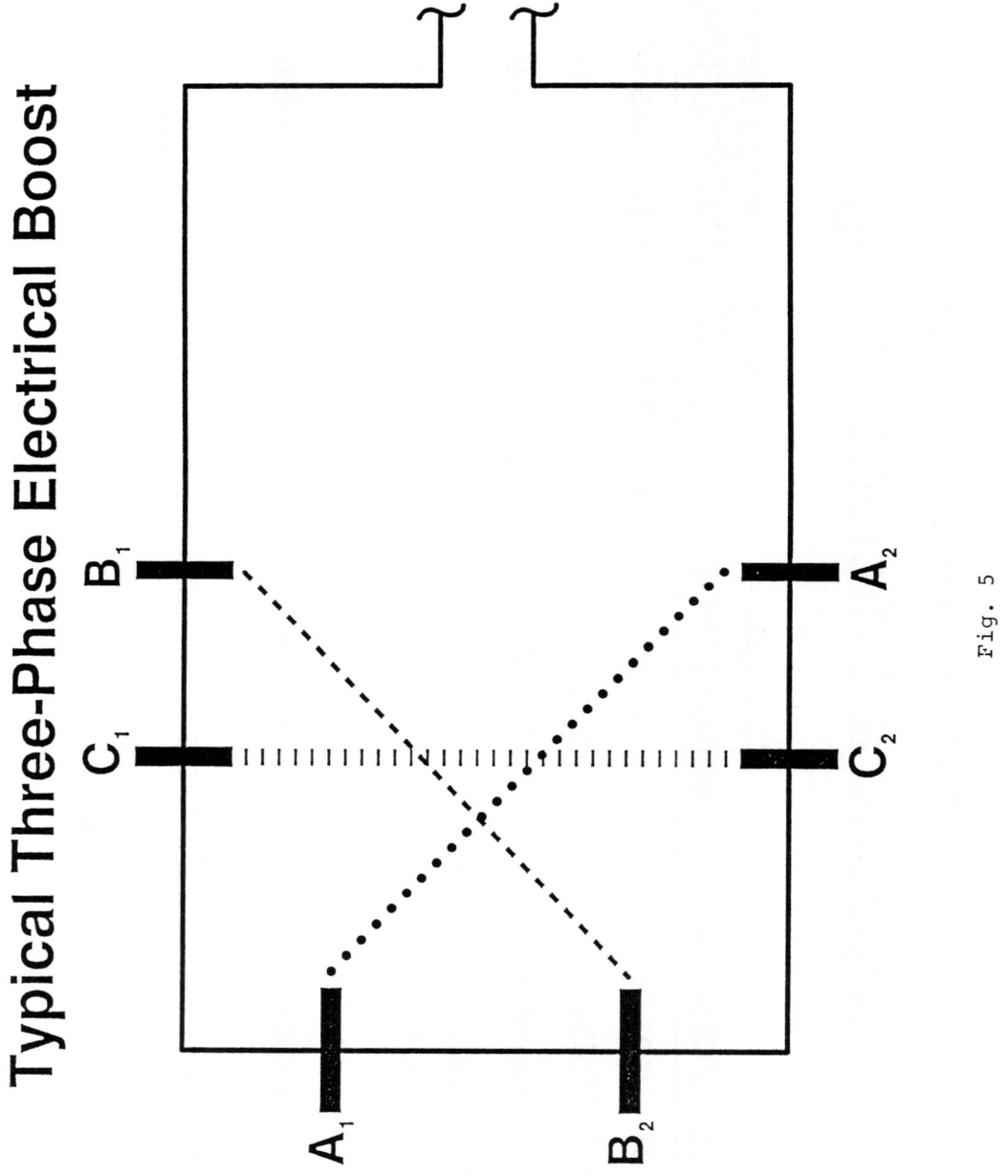

Fig. 5

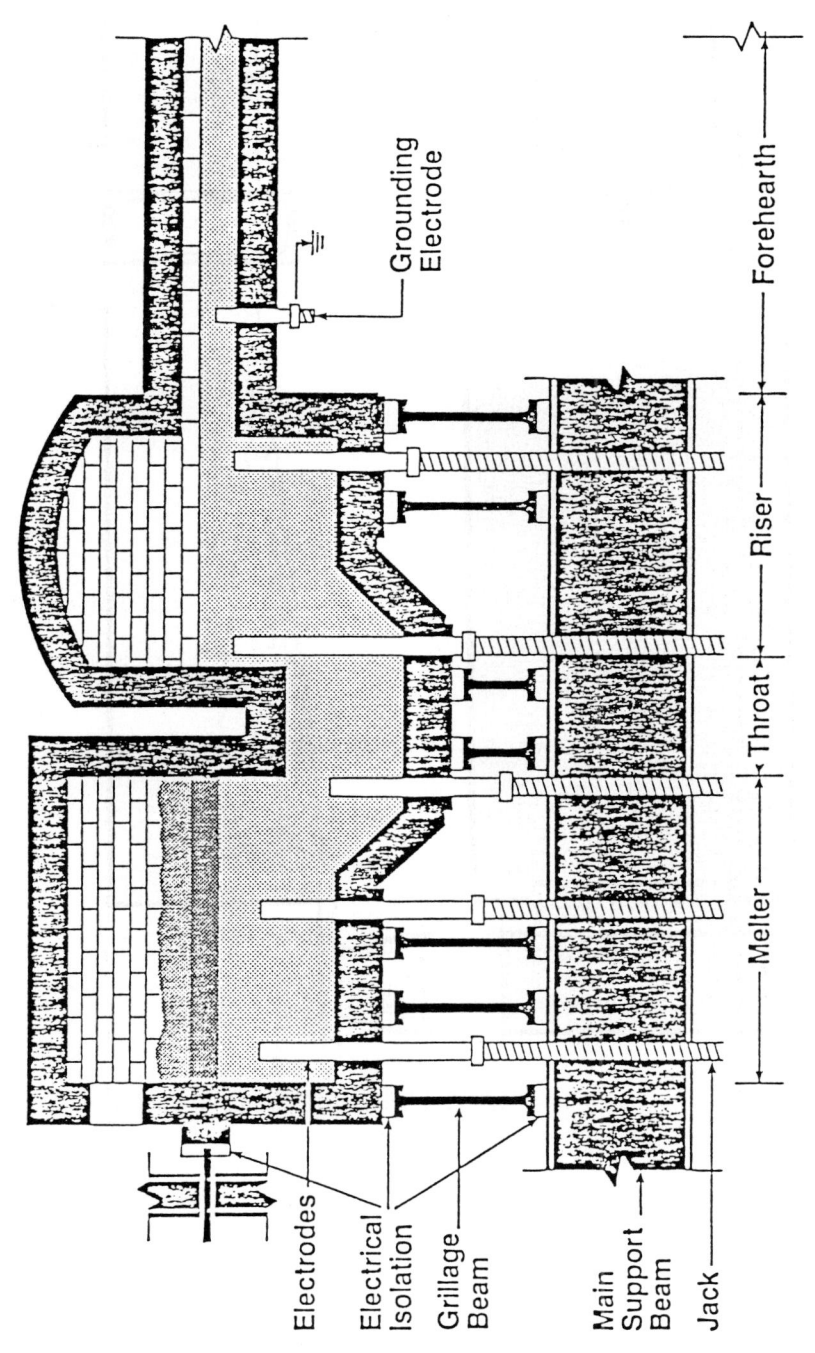

Fig. 6

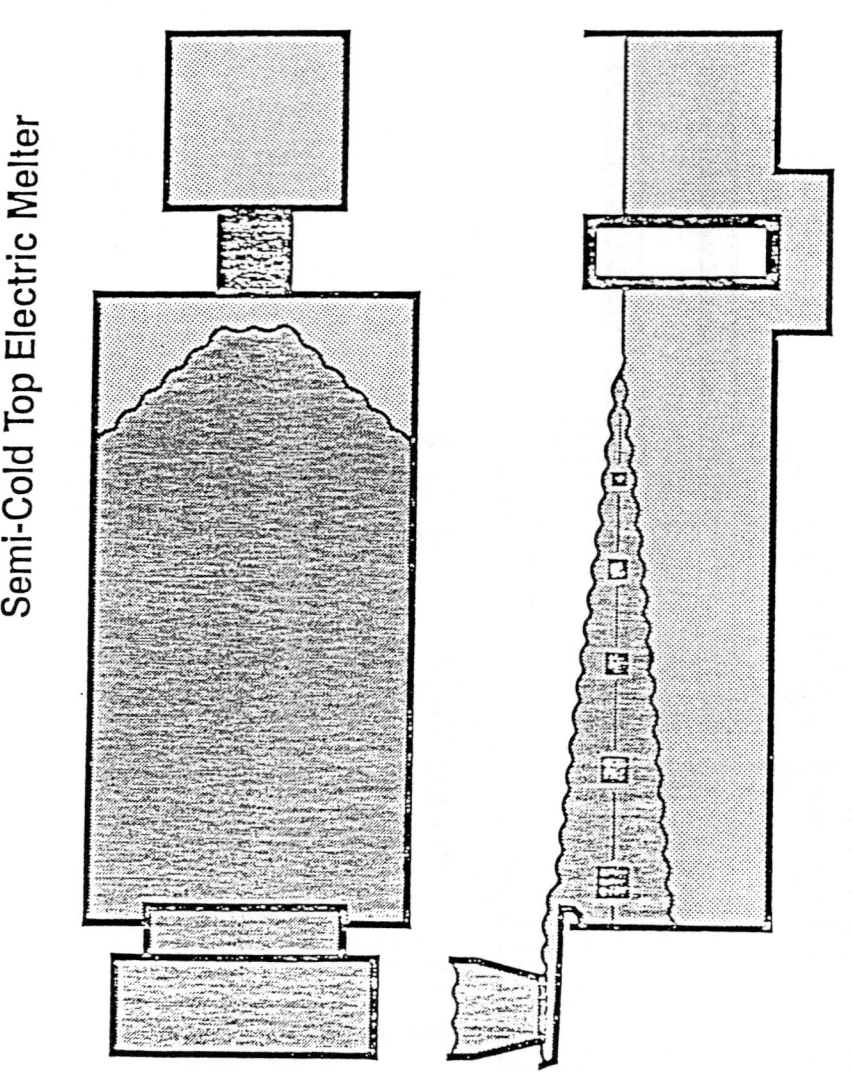

Fig. 7

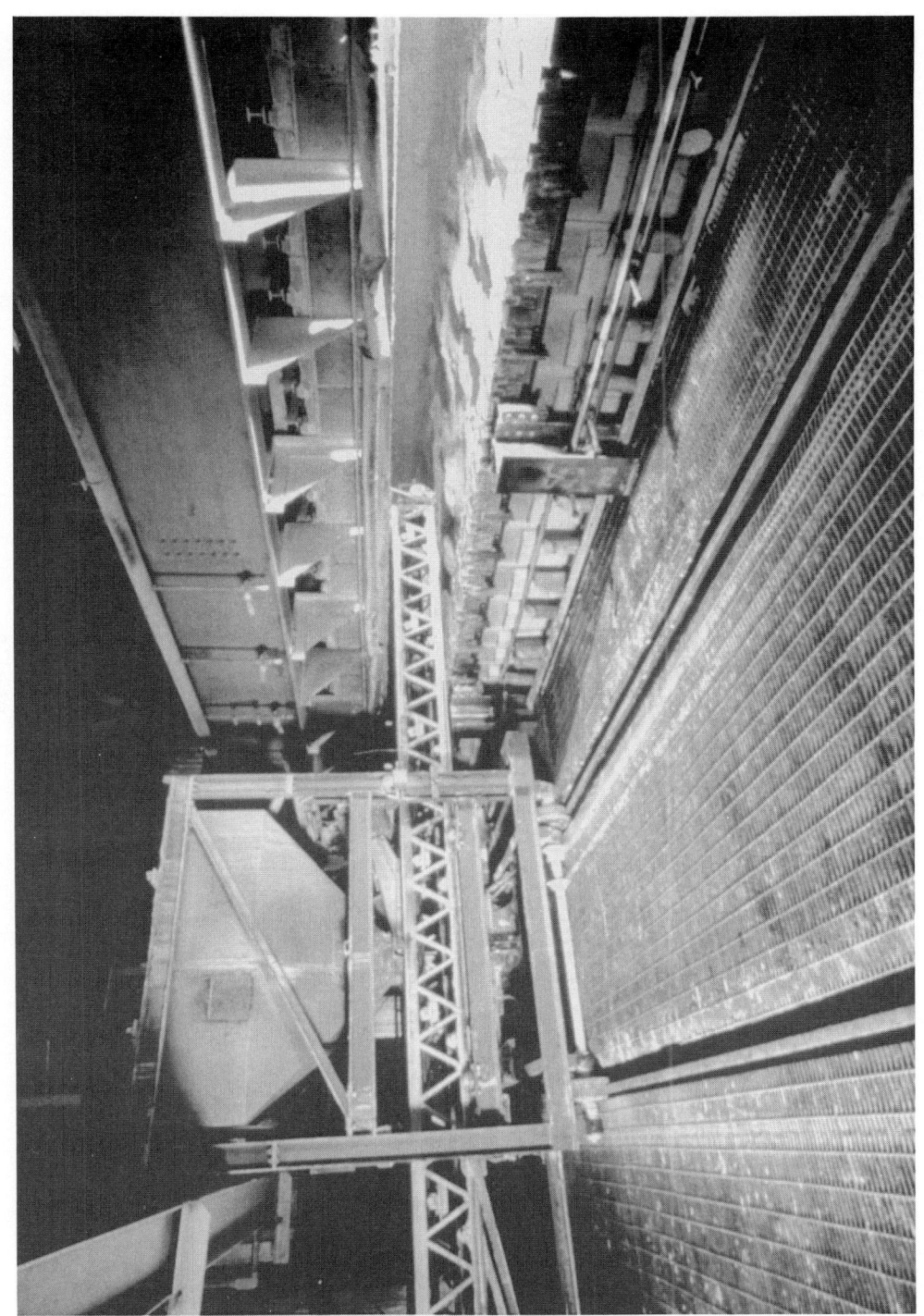

Fig. 8

Cold Top Electric Furnace - Capacity, Average Energy & Connected Load

Capacity (TPD)	Average Efficiency (%)	Average Energy (Mill BTU/TON)	Average Electrical Energy (kWh/Ton)	Connected Load (kVA)
50	68	2.95	865	2075
75	71	2.82	825	2930
100	73	2.74	805	3770
125	73	2.73	800	4675
150	74	2.69	790	5500
200	76	2.63	770	7125
250	77	2.59	760	8740

Fig. 9

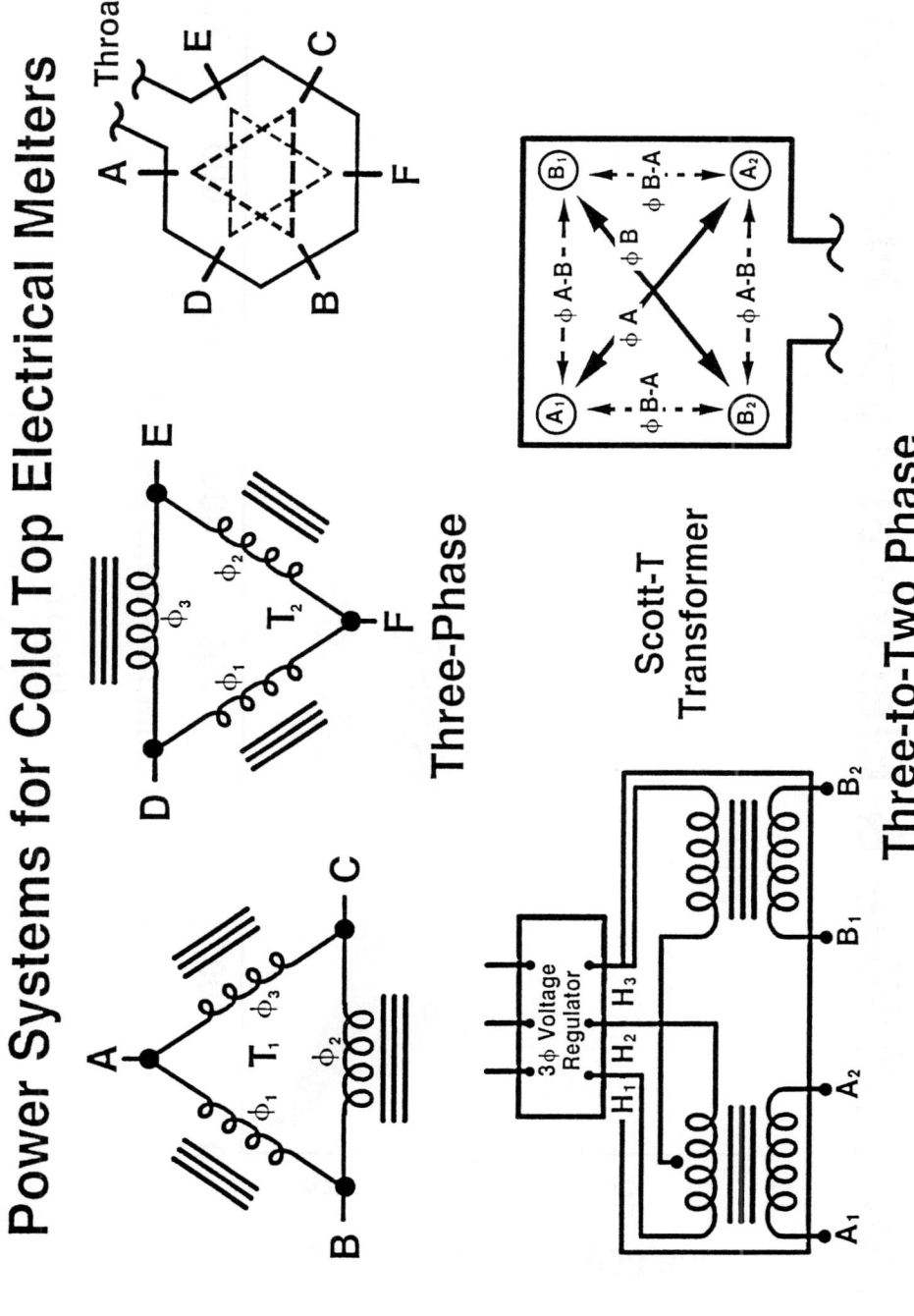

Fig. 10

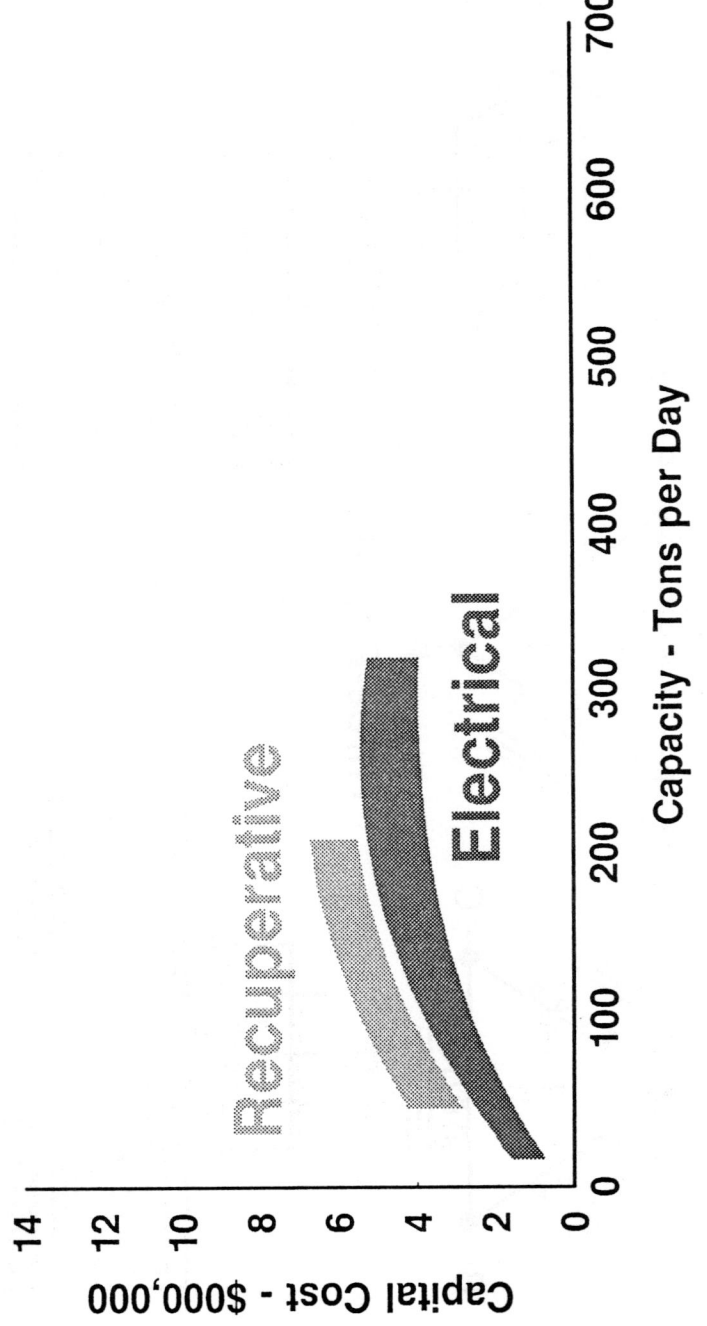

Fig. 11A

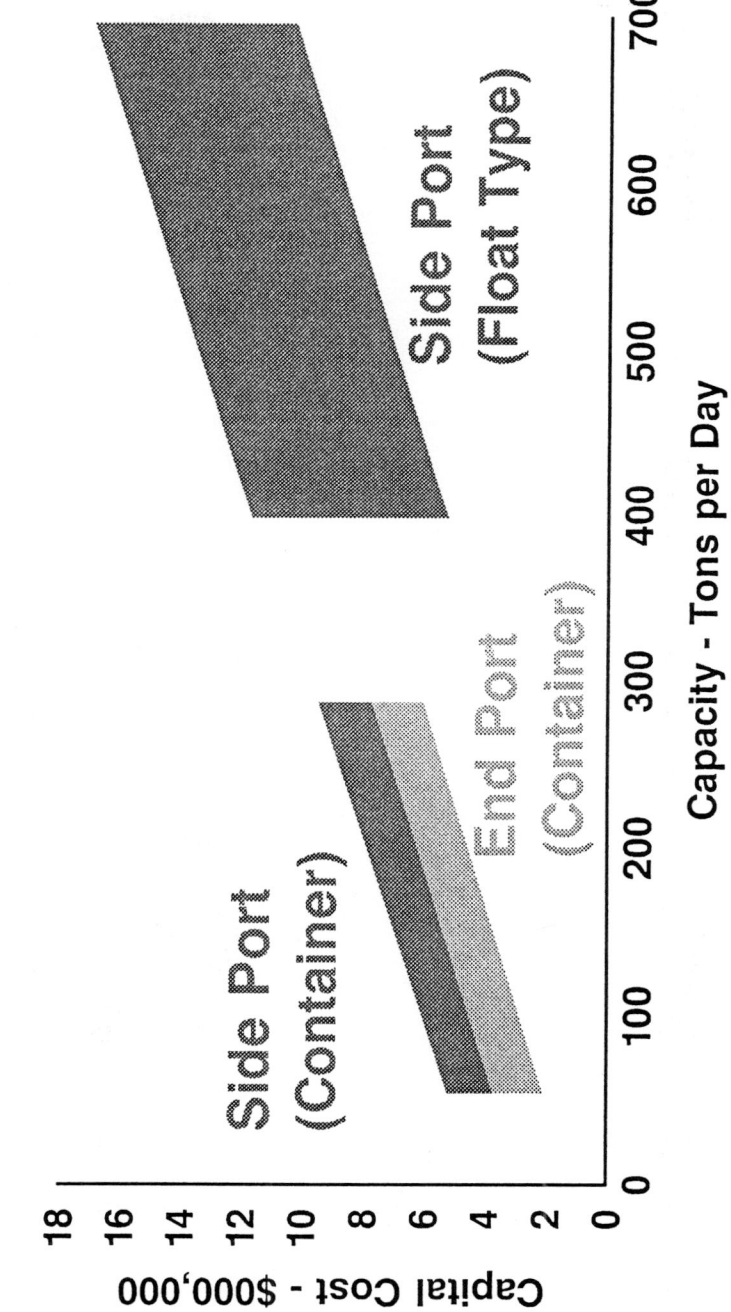

Fig. 11B

Thermal Enhanced Reciprocating Engine Cogeneration Systems

F. E. Becker, F. A. Di Bella, J. C. Balsavich
Tecogen Inc.
Waltham, MA 02254-9046

As electric rates continue to increase, there are significant economic incentives to look strongly towards cogeneration as a means for reducing overall energy costs. Today, the cogeneration market offers a number of packaged systems based on back-pressure steam turbine, combustion turbine, and reciprocating engine prime movers. However, each of these systems, and variations of them, differ significantly in their electric-to-thermal output ratios, load following capabilities and costs. Thus, in order to properly select the appropriate system, it is important to understand these differences.

This paper describes these three basic types of cogeneration systems, their unique operating characteristics, important features, and inherent limitations. It addresses mainly "packaged" cogeneration systems with electrical outputs on the order of 500 kW_e to 1.5 MW_e per unit.

In particular, it addresses the merits of a recently developed reciprocating engine cogeneration system which integrates a mechanical steam screw compressor into the system. This important feature enables low-pressure steam, normally produced in an ebullienty cooled engine, to be increased in pressure to a more useful level. A unique variation of this system, which is being investigated, utilizes the same screw compressor as an expander in a bottoming cycle. In this fashion, the screw compressor/expander can alternatively function to enhance either the thermal or electrical output to more closely match variations in load requirements.

THERMAL ENHANCED RECIPROCATING ENGINE
COGENERATION SYSTEMS

F.E. Becker, F.A. DiBella, J.C. Balsavich
Tecogen Inc.

INTRODUCTION

The cogeneration market today offers a number of packaged systems, ranging from a few kilowatts to multi-megawatts. Along with these have come the need to understand better the important operating characteristics associated with each system. For example, in the industrial sector, back-pressure steam turbine cogeneration systems have been widely used for many years. Such systems, however, typically have low electric-to-thermal-energy ratios. More recently, with the increased cost of electricity, combustion turbine and reciprocating engine cogeneration systems have found their way into the market as a result of their higher fuel-to-electric-power conversion efficiencies. For the latter systems, when thermal energy in the form of high-pressure process steam is required, gas turbines have been promoted as the system of choice. This is easily understood, since almost all the waste heat from the turbine is available for producing high-pressure steam in a waste-heat recovery boiler. However, for systems less than several megawatts in size, there has been limited market penetration. This is because the low fuel-to-electric-power conversion efficiencies (15 to 20 percent) associated with these turbines do not provide an adequate rate-of-return.

Reciprocating engines, however, have significantly improved fuel-to-electric-power conversion efficiencies, often over 30 percent. Unfortunately, the waste heat has traditionally been divided between the production of high-pressure steam in the exhaust heat recovery boiler, and hot water or low-pressure (15 psig) steam from the cooling jacket heat. Thus, the difficulty in making practical use of this low grade thermal energy has significantly limited market penetration of reciprocating engines into steam system applications.

An alternative reciprocating engine cogeneration system, which alleviates this problem by integrating a mechanical steam compressor into the system has recently been developed by Tecogen, Inc. In operation, the low-pressure steam normally produced in an ebulliently cooled engine is compressed in a screw compressor to raise the steam to a more useful process pressure level. While some power is diverted away from generating electricity to compressing steam, the fuel-to-electric-power conversion efficiency is still significantly better than that of a combustion turbine of comparable electric power output.

This paper describes the three basic types of cogeneration systems, their unique operating characteristics, important features, and inherent limitations. It addresses mainly "packaged" cogeneration systems with electrical outputs on the order of 500 kWe to 1.5 MWe. In particular, the merits of integrating a mechanical steam compressor into a reciprocating engine system to expand the market opportunities for its use are described.

COGENERATION SYSTEMS OVERVIEW

The optimization of energy utilization through cogeneration of electric power and thermal energy necessitates an understanding of the relationship between the availability of, and the need for these energy sources. Depending on the plant's requirements, the cogeneration system may emphasize either a high or low electric-power to thermal-energy ratio. To accomplish this, the three types of topping cogeneration cycles usually specified are boiler-steam turbines, combustion turbines, and reciprocating engines. Each of these systems has a particular place in the market, depending on the cost of available fuels and the value attributable to the power produced. For example, when high electric power is desired, the cycle should emphasize shaft power conversion efficiency, as would be the case with reciprocating engine drives. If the major requirement is for thermal energy, then a steam turbine topping cycle may be more appropriate. Gas turbine cycles typically fall in the middle. Following is a discussion of these cogeneration system options and the conditions that suggest their respective use.

Boiler-Steam Turbine System

The boiler-steam turbine system, as shown in Figure 1, consists of a boiler, designed to produce high-pressure steam, and a back-pressure steam turbine. The high-pressure steam is expanded through the turbine to drive the generator. The steam that is exhausted at the lower pressure is used to provide thermal energy to the process.

The electric-to-thermal ratio is mainly dependent on the boiler and process steam pressures; the greater the absolute pressure ratio across the turbine, the more power that can be produced. Whereas, in a conventional powerplant, turbine back-pressures are often reduced to very low values (1 to 2 psia) to maximize power output, typically around 33 percent, this is not possible for cogeneration systems. Instead, the steam must leave the turbine at a pressure high enough for its thermal energy output still to be of value in the process. As a result, overall fuel-to-power-conversion efficiencies are often not more than 10 percent and may be as low as 2 percent for low-pressure boilers. Thus, back-pressure steam turbines are most applicable when there is a very large thermal load compared to the electrical load.

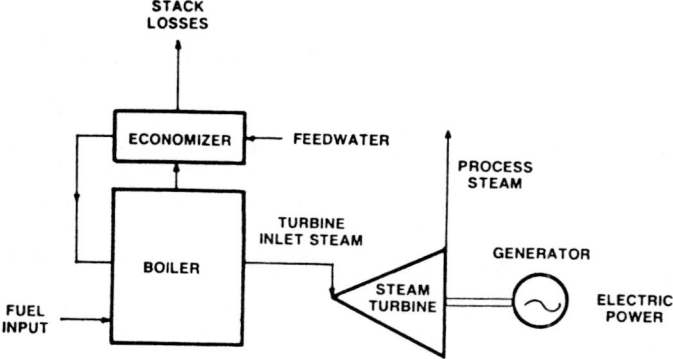

FIGURE 1. BASIC BOILER-STEAM TURBINE TOPPING CYCLE

Combustion Gas Turbines

The second basic cycle, the combustion turbine cogeneration system shown in Figure 2, consists of a gas turbine driving a generator, and a heat-recovery boiler that produces process steam from the high-temperature exhaust gases. Power conversion efficiencies typically vary from 15 to 20 percent (HHV) over a range of 400 kWe to 2 MWe, respectively. Large, 10 MWe turbines have higher efficiencies of 30 percent.

The economics of gas turbines depends very strongly on the effective use of the exhaust gas energy. For example, one way to improve the power conversion efficiency is to generate steam in a waste heat boiler at a higher pressure than required in the process and, as shown in Figure 3, expand this steam through a turbine to yield additional power. Often referred to as a combined cycle system, power conversion efficiencies can frequently be increased to over 40 percent. Although this is often considered for multi-megawatt systems, the additional complexity and cost are, however, difficult to justify for smaller packaged systems.

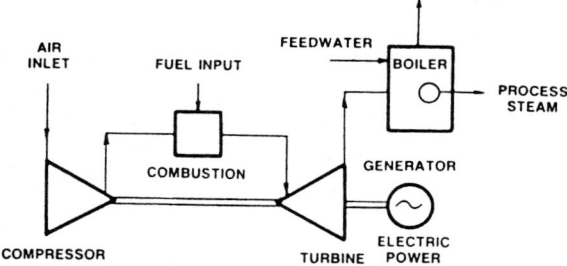

FIGURE 2. BASIC COMBUSTION TURBINE TOPPING CYCLE

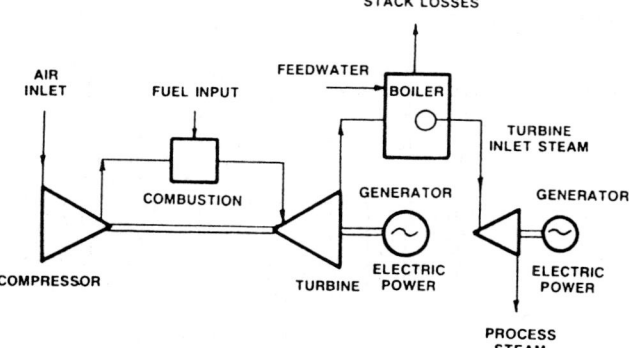

FIGURE 3. COMBUSTION TURBINE IN A COMBINED CYCLE

A variation to this cycle is to inject high-pressure steam from the waste heat boiler directly into the turbine. By varying the amount of steam injection, the electric-to-thermal ratio can be adjusted to more closely match the plant's load distribution throughout the day. This approach improves on the economics by saving on the cost of an additional steam turbine, but of course, the combustion turbine must be properly sized to handle the additional shaft power.

Most gas turbines operate with as much as 300 percent excess air. As a result, the exhaust products leave with a relatively high oxygen content of approximately 17 percent and a limiting overall thermodynamic efficiency of approximately 65 percent. If more thermal energy or steam is desired, a separate supplementary-fired burner can be installed in the exhaust gas duct to increase the turbine exhaust gas temperature from 900°F up to 2000°F. When this is done, the overall efficiency also increases to approximately 75 percent. The exhaust gas still contains approximately 10 percent oxygen, which can enable even higher exhaust gas temperatures to be reached. However, firing at these higher temperatures means adding a radiant heat section to the exhaust boiler, which is usually only practical for very large systems.

An alternative to adding a waste-heat boiler is to duct the hot exhaust gases to an existing steam boiler. The boiler must have adequate spare capacity if the total steam load is intended to increase by the heat associated with the turbine.

Reciprocating Engines

The third approach, shown in Figure 4, uses a reciprocating engine to drive the generator and a heat recovery boiler to produce steam from the hot exhaust gases. In addition, low-pressure steam or hot water can be produced from the cooling jacket heat.

For systems as low as 30 kWe, reciprocating engines have excellent power conversion efficiencies, often above 30 percent, which approach those of central station powerplants. As such, the electric-to-thermal ratio is the highest of the basic three topping cycles discussed. However, only hot water or low-pressure steam (15 psig) is directly available from the engine's cooling jacket. This represents a substantial amount of heat, approximately 30 percent of the total fuel input. Therefore, for high overall thermodynamic efficiencies, effective use of this heat must be made.

An alternative to this cycle, shown in Figure 5, is to recover the cooling jacket heat as low-pressure steam and mechanically compress it up to the desired process pressure. In this fashion, all the thermal energy is delivered to the user as high-pressure process steam. To do this, a portion of the engine's shaft power must go toward the work of compression instead of making electricity. This power requirement is a strong function of the pressure ratio, and, thus, to minimize the work input, the pressure should be increased only to the level required by the process, and not necessarily to the main steam header pressure.

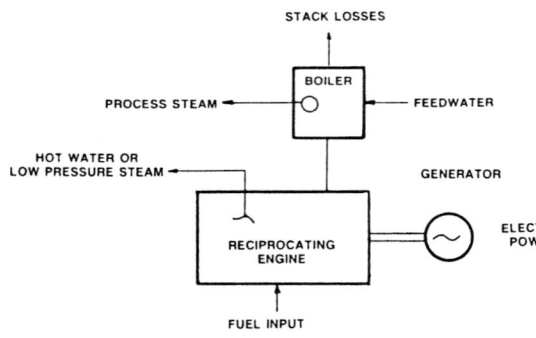

FIGURE 4. BASIC RECIPROCATING ENGINE TOPPING CYCLE

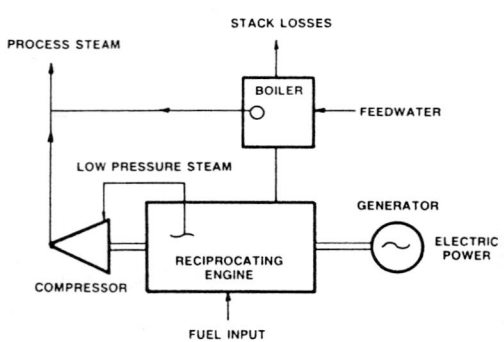

FIGURE 5. RECIPROCATING ENGINE TOPPING CYCLE WITH STEAM COMPRESSOR

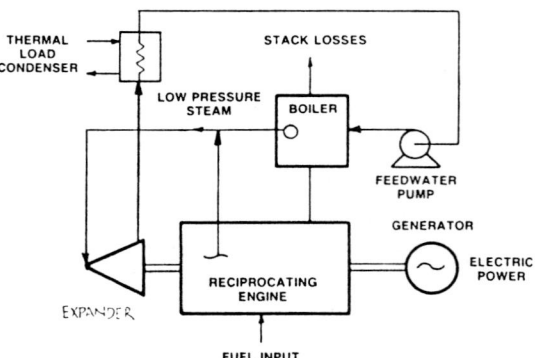

FIGURE 5a. RECIPROCATING ENGINE BOTTOMING CYCLE WITH STEAM EXPANDER

While the power requirement may seem large, with respect to the latent heat already in the steam it is relatively small. For example, 15 psig steam contains 954 Btu/lb of latent heat. Mechanically recompressing this steam to 125 psig, or a pressure ratio of 4.67, requires an additional work input of only 190 Btu/lb, or 20 percent. Of course, this energy input is not lost because it is added to the steam.

A feature of this system is that if high-pressure steam is not needed, or if there is an increased demand for electric power, the compressor can be unloaded, and the additional available engine power used to generate electricity.

A unique variation of this system, which is being investigated, utilizes the same screw compressor as an expander in a steam bottoming cycle. This arrangement is shown in Figure 5a.

The cycle works by expanding steam produced in the exhaust boiler and that in the water jacket to subatmospheric pressures. This cycle can potentially increase the power output 15 to 20 percent. Although high pressure steam is no longer available, hot water can still be made available to the user.

COGENERATION SYSTEM CYCLE SELECTION

There are many factors that influence the cogeneration cycle selection. Some of the more important are:

- Process heat and electric power demand requirements
- Present availability of process heat and power
- Modulating capability of cogeneration system
- Plant services available for operation and maintenance
- Present costs of process heat and power
- Capital availability and rate-of-return

The first factor really defines the base load size of the system and the ratio of thermal (steam) to electrical demand. If there is a large thermal-to-electric power-requirement, then the combustion or steam turbine may be the preferred system. However, the absolute size of the system is also important. For example, turbine performance drops off quickly with decreasing size, but this is not so with reciprocating engines. Also important is the in-place thermal capacity. Adding another boiler to the system to recover waste heat when the present one serves the needs simply results in unused capacity. If electric power and not thermal energy is desired, then the system selected should be one with good power conversion efficiency, for which the reciprocating engine is a good choice.

The turn-down or modulating capability in both power and thermal energy is another important factor. Cogeneration systems operate most economically at constant loads; unfortunately, in practice this rarely happens. Instead, the absolute magnitude, as well as the electric-to-thermal ratio may vary widely. For example, the power output from a steam turbine is relatively proportional to the steam mass flow rate. As a result, if there is a decrease in demand for steam, the electric power output will also decrease, unless the excess steam is simply vented or condensed. The same is true with a combustion turbine, but the loss in turbine efficiency is much more sensitive to turn-down.

Reciprocating engines retain good mechanical efficiency with turn-down, but as with any prime mover, there is also a reduction in thermal output. Because reciprocating engines have a high electric-to-thermal ratio, a separate direct-fired steam boiler may be needed to meet the thermal loads of the process. If the major thermal load is already being handled by a separate steam boiler. then obviously a new one would not be needed.

An important aspect, however, is that the engine can probably always be base-loaded without exceeding the thermal requirements of the process. Instead, any thermal load change would be handled by the boiler. In this fashion, the electrical and thermal loads can be independently modulated without affecting each other's performance.

A comparison of the performance characteristics of the three topping cycles for cogeneration systems, all producing 650 kWe plus varying amounts of 125 psig steam, is illustrated in Figure 6, with more detailed information listed in Table 1. For the reciprocating engine, direct generation of low pressure 15 psig steam from the engine jacket is included for reference purposes. For larger systems up to several megawatts, the relative values are still reasonably true.

As is most graphically illustrated in Figure 6, the reciprocating engine achieves the highest fuel-to-electric-power conversion efficiency of 28.8 percent for a basic ebullient-cooled engine, and 22.6 percent for a system that includes a steam compressor to boost the jacket steam from 15 psig to 125 psig. For this case, the steam production ratio is a fairly low 7.3 lb/hr of steam per kWe power generated. The overall thermodynamic efficiency (HHV) is 71.7 percent.

Next, if a combustion turbine is used, the electric conversion efficiency would decrease to 17.6 percent if there was no supplemental firing, and to 9.4 percent if additional fuel was burned. However, there would be an increase in the overall thermodynamic efficiency (HHV) from 61.2 percent to 72.9 percent. The increase in the overall efficiency is solely due to burning additional fuel in the waste heat boiler at close to 90 percent (HHV) efficiency. The limit of course, is that no matter how poor the turbine power conversion efficiency, by supplementary firing, the overall efficiency will approach that of a standard direct-fired boiler. With a supplementary-fired system, the steam production ratio is 21.1 lb/hr steam per kWe. This is over three times that of the reciprocating engine system.

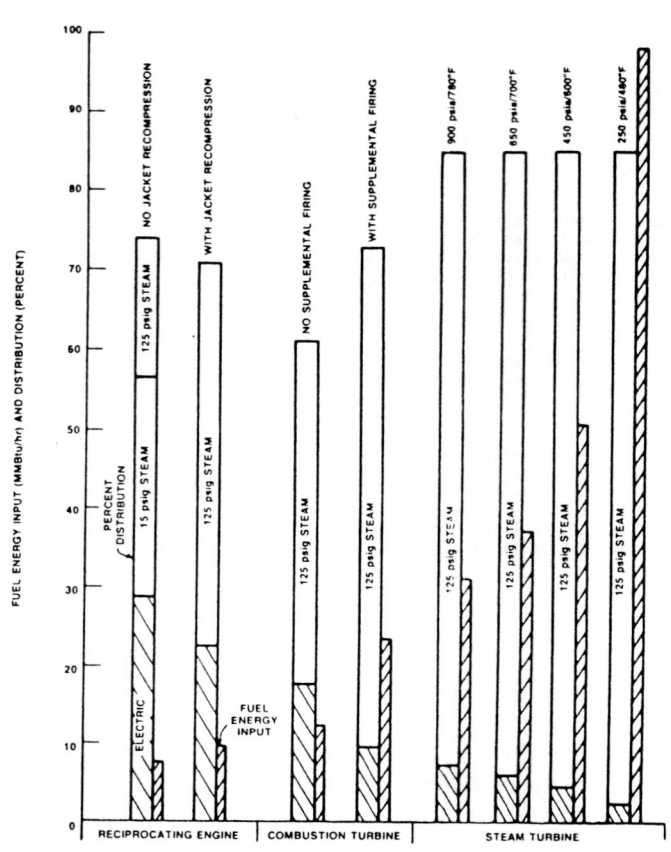

FIGURE 6. COMPARISON OF TOPPING CYCLE COGENERATION SYSTEMS - BASIS: 650 KWE, 125 PSIG PROCESS STEAM

TABLE 1
COMPARISON OF TOPPING CYCLE COGENERATION SYSTEMS

Basis 650 kW_e, 125 psig Process Steam

	Reciprocating Engine		Gas Turbine		Steam Turbine			
	No Jacket Recompression	With Jacket Recompression	No Supplemental Firing	With Supplemental Firing	Boiler Pressure (psia) Temperature (°F)			
					900/780	650/700	450/600	250/480
Fuel Input, 10^6 Btu/hr	7.7	9.8	12.6	23.6	31.5	37.3	50.5	97.9
Steam Flow, lb/hr	2100 at 15 psig 1400 at 125 psig 3500	4750	5500	15,000	23,000	28,000	39,500	80,400
Primary Fuel Conversion Efficiency* (HHV), Percent	30.2	30.2	19.0	19.0	55.0	55.0	55.0	55.0
Electric Conversion Efficiency (HHV), Percent	28.8	22.6	17.6	9.4	7.0	5.9	4.4	2.3
Overall Efficiency (HHV), Percent	74.0	71.1	61.2	72.9	85	85	85	85
Steam Production Ratio, $\frac{lb/hr\ steam}{kW_e}$	5.4	7.3	8.5	23.1	35.4	43.1	60.8	123.7

*For the reciprocating engine and gas turbine, this is the fuel-to-shaft-power conversion efficiency based on the primary fuel to the prime mover.
For the steam turbine, this is the product of the isentropic and mechanical efficiency.

The last topping cycle, the boiler steam turbine system, has the lowest fuel-to-electric-power conversion efficiency (HHV) ranging from 2.3 to 7.0 percent, depending on the boiler pressure and degrees superheat. Steam production ratios are also high, ranging from 35.4 to over 100 lb/hr steam per kWe. Since the power output, for a given turbine efficiency, increases with pressure ratio, the most direct approach to increasing the power conversion efficiency is to go to higher boiler pressures. Unfortunately, except for large megawatt plants, high-pressure boiler-steam turbine systems are difficult to justify economically.

CONCLUSIONS

The packaged cogeneration market for systems capable of producing totally high-pressure process steam has largely gone to combustion turbines. Unfortunately, their low fuel-to-electric conversion efficiency and high installed cost have limited their widespread use. Until recently, reciprocating engines, while having a better electric conversion efficiency, but not being able to make high-pressure steam from the jacket heat, did not provide a reasonable alternative. Now, however, by integrating a mechanical steam compressor into the reciprocating engine package, an improved alternative to the combustion turbine is available, and along with it new growth opportunities are now available.

Chauffage des bains industriels
Industrial water heating

'GETTING INTO HOT WATER EFFICIENTLY'

By : J.A. Davies

NORDSEA GAS TECHNOLOGY LTD.

Heating liquids for industry and commerce is a major use of energy. Steam has, until recently, always been the first choice. Steam tubes are compact, give high heat release rates and are easy to fabricate and install. Their one big disadvantage, however, is their overall energy utilisation efficiency. Sankey diagrams show point-of-use efficiencies as low as 20% with typical values of 35-45%. Fig. 1

If natural gas is piped directly to the points-of-use, however, modern gas-fired equipment will provide efficiencies of over 80% with fuel savings in excess of 50%. Several new types of equipment have been developed and their basic principles of operation are considered below.

Natural draught immersion tube burners firing into large diameter tubes immersed in liquids have been available for many years, but their firing intensity, defined as the heat input per unit cross-sectional area of the tube, is fairly low, typicall 5MW/m^2, with efficiencies of approximately 70%. This necessitates the use of large diameter tubes which can occupy a significant amount of tank space and therefore restrict their range of application. The only way to increase their application has been to substantially increase the firing intensity and thermal efficiency. This has been achieved by the development of a fully-packaged forced draught immersion tube burner system (see figure 2) in which the products of combustion are forced down a relatively small diameter tube, increasing the firing intensity to over 30 MW/m^2. The high heat transfer rates and compactness of the small bore tube design produce efficiencies of up to 85% on gross heat input.

Experience has shown that to acheive efficiencies of 80% or more the length/diameter ratio of the immersion tube should be greater than 140:1. The tube bundle can be manufactured to any practical configuration and becomes the heat exchanger, immersed in the liquid to be heated, but its length obviously raises questions of installation in some existing and new equipment. Some typical sizes and corresponding gross heat outputs are shown in table 1.

Before we can determine equipment size, we need to consider the basic process requirements. The following information is needed:

        mass of liquid to be heated
        specific heat of the liquid
        temperature rise required
        heating-up time acceptable
        heat losses from the tank

From this, the size of the tube needed can easily be determined. The heating-up time is usually of major significance.

Once the liquid has been heated and is at the desired temperature, control equipment is required to vary the thermal input to maintain the process temperature within acceptable limits. Because the burner is probably going to spend a high proportion of its time at low fire, high efficiency at all firing rates is desirable. This can only be achieved when both the gas and air are controlled at both low-fire and high-fire, requiring high/low/off with tandem butterfly valves or full proportional control using linear valves.

This additional control equipment obviously increases the cost of each assembly - and can limit the use of smaller sizes, especially. To meet this and to fill the lower capacity end of the liquid heating market, a compromise on tube size, burner design and control equipment has resulted in the development of a medium-intensity immersion tube that consists of an atmospheric-type burner with a small combustion air fan forcing the air over the burner to increase firing intensity. This design is available operating with on/off control and with an L/D ratio of about 100:1, in a size range from 50mm (2 in nb) with gross rating of 18kW (63,000 Btu/hr) to 100mm (4 in nb) with gross rating of 74kW (250,000 Btu.hr).

Multitube designs
For the standard high intensity tube design (figure 2) problems of manufacture and, in many cases, installation remain. This had led to a further development which allows the combustion of the gases to be completed in a larger diameter tube, and then return to an exhaust through a large number of small bore tubes, see figure 3. This greatly increases the velocity of the combustion products to further enhance heat transfer rates. Standard materials of construction are mild steel and 304 or 316 stainless steel but other materials can be used to suit particular process requirements.

These new developments in high intensity small-bore immersion tubes considerably increase the range of applications for the direct gas firing of existing vats, tanks, calorifiers and storage vessels. The range also opens up new markets for gas firing where, up to now, live steam and steam coils have been the only choice.

The multitube design lends itself particularly to retrofitting into existing storage and non-storage calorifiers. If a vessel is built around the immersion tube element with minimum volume storage, then it is possible to produce a packaged compact gas-fired calorifier, see figure 4. The high heat transfer rates possible using multiple small-bore tubes, coupled with minimum liquid storage, enable this design to heat large volumes of water and other liquids very quickly and efficiently.

An in-line circulation heater of this sort can eliminate the need for large stored volumes of water or solutions, and substantillay reduce the associated heat losses.

In many applications a peak water demand, which in some cases may be of only 15-20 minutes' duration, may drain existing storage units which take up valuable space and require excessive annual maintenance. In cases such as these, some buffer storage is clearly required. This, however, can be kept to a minimum by the application of a small-bore tube heater to a 600-gallon storage vessel, mounted on a frame with all the pumps, gas controls and so on, to provide a self-contained minimum storage unit specifically designed to match the process requirements.

Direct contact water heating

Typical gross efficiencies that have been measured in immersion tube installations are 85.5% at low fire and 83.5% at high fire, but the search for even higher efficiencies has led to the development of direct contact water heaters, see figure 5. These give gross efficiencies up to 98% by condensing the water vapour formed in the combustion process in order to recover its latent heat. To achieve this, the combustion products must be cooled to below 55°C, the dowpoint temperature. Conventional tubular and plate heat exchangers for such low temperatures are very large and expensive but a compact combination arrangement is possible by putting an immersion tube burner and immersion tube in its own holding (sump) tank, from which the clean products of combustion, previously flued to atmosphere, exhaust through and enclosed "cascade" tower of perforated stainless steel trays. Water "cascades" down the tower, over the perforated trays, counter current to the products of combustion from which latent heat is removed by condensation of the water vapour.

At its point of discharge from the tower, the water will have been heated to 50-60°C. Its temperature is then raised further in the holding (sump) tank, which contains the short length gas-fired immerison tube. Outlet water temperatures up to 95°C can be achieved. This increases further the range of applications now available based on the immersion tube principle Sizes range from 18kW (62,000 Btu/hr) to 2930 kW (10,000,000 Btu/hr).

The overall efficiency of the heater depends upon the cold water inlet temperature - up to 98% is possible with cold water at 15°C. A slight decrease in pH level of the water occurs, but in most applications this can be tolerated.

Typical applications where these various new developments have been applied include:

Process industries - Water heating, chemical solutions, mild acids, electro-plating, oils.

Commercial - Hot water for hotels, hospitals, schools, swimming pools offices lauderettes, vehicle washing.

Food industries - Hot water for process use and for washdown and cleaning, tray washers, pasteurisers, CIP plant.

Breweries - Water and liquor heating (including wort), plate and flat bed pasteurisers.

Textiles - Water and dye heating - Textile factories can now bleach/wash, finish and print without the use of steam.

Leisure industries - Hot water for showers and swimming pools, under-ground heating for sports field.

FIG. 1

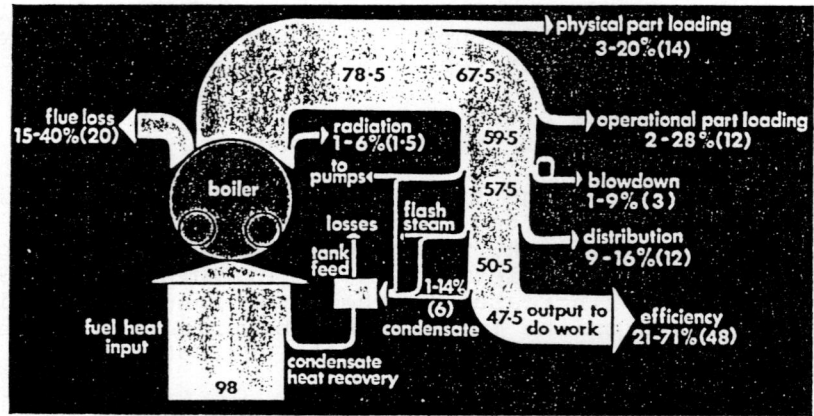

Sankey diagram for steam systems.
8

FIG. 2

Typical GT burner arrangement

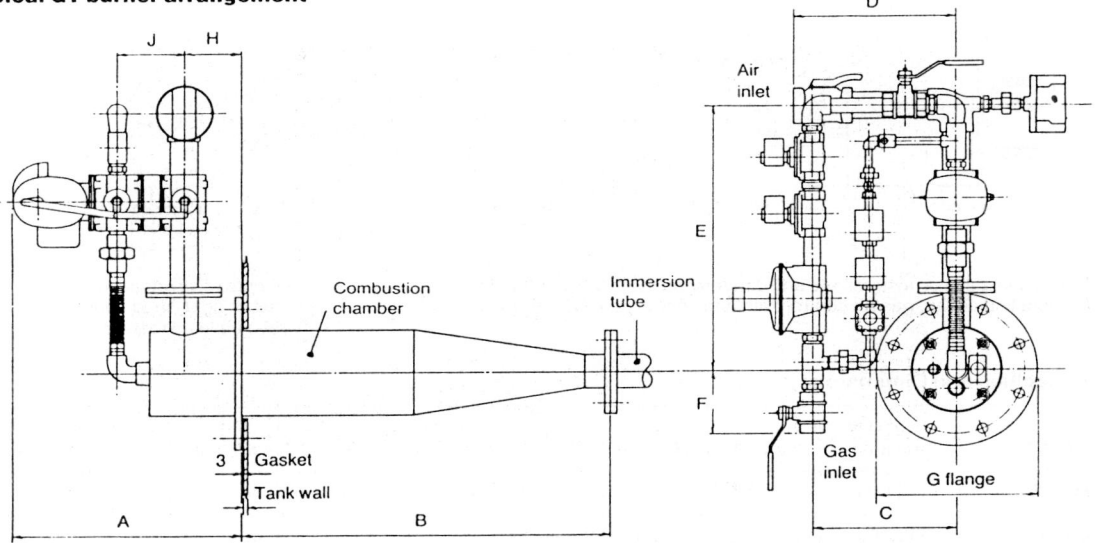

Detailed installation instructions and dimensions available. Combustion air fan, control panel and inter-connection pipework, etc not shown.

Left hand burner assembly shown. Left hand or right hand assemblies are available.

Capacities and Dimensions

Burner Type	Immersion Tube Size		Burner Gross Heat Input★		Approx – Dimensions in mm									Air Inlet BSP	Gas Inlet BSP
	in	mm	BTU/hr	kW	A	B	C	D	E	F	G	H	J	in	in
GT40	1½	40	160,000	47	400	550	250	265	425	35	254	100	118	1½	½
GT50	2	50	300,000	88	400	640	255	270	452	98	280	100	118	1½	¾
GT65	2½	65	420,000	129	420	730	280	300	490	170	305	115	124	2	1
GT80	3	80	600,000	176	420	800	300	325	590	187	336	115	124	2	1½
GT100	4	100	1,000,000	293	470	900	360	375	596	183	406	130	140	3	2
GT125	5	125	1,500,000	440	500	1040	430	485	856	236	457	148	162	4	2½
GT150	6	150	2,000,000	586	500	1150	450	485	856	236	527	148	162	4	2½

★ Burner gross heat inputs are with a 190mm.wg (7.5 in.wg) gas supply pressure. Heat releases of up to 1.8 times those given can be achieved with higher gas and air pressures. To maintain the required efficiency levels, increased immersion tube lengths will be required.

FIG. 3

General Arrangement of Multi-tube Immersion Heaters

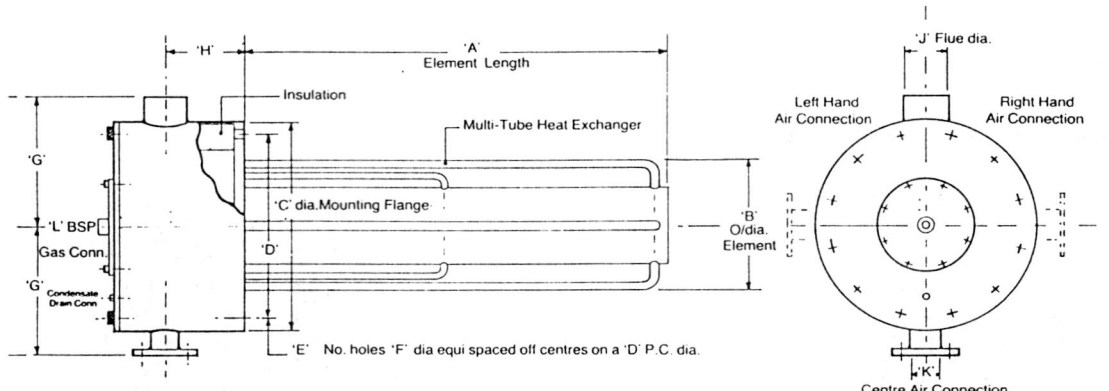

Detailed installation instructions and dimensions available on request.
Combustion air fan, gas/air control train and control panel not shown.

Centre air connection shown, left or right-hand connection available as required.

Capacities and Dimensions

Model No.	Heat Output BTU/hr	kW	A	B	C	D	E	F	G	H	J	K	L	Mounting hole size in vessel
MT128	128,000	38	1200	213	406	355,6	8	22	275	125	50	40	½"	250
MT240	240,000	70	1300	253	457	406,4	12	22	300	150	65	40	¾"	300
MT336	336,000	98	1400	313	552	495,3	12	25	350	200	80	50	1"	400
MT480	480,000	141	1600	346	552	495,3	12	25	350	200	100	65	1½"	400
MT800	800,000	234	1700	456	673	609,6	12	25	425	200	150	80	1½"	500
MT1200	1,200,000	352	1825	566	788	723,9	16	28	475	225	200	100	2"	600
MT1600	1,600,000	469	1825	566	788	723,9	16	28	475	225	200	100	2½"	600

Burner ratings are with a 190mm wg (7.8 in wg) gas supply pressure.

FIG. 4

General Arrangement of Satellite In-Line Circulation Heater

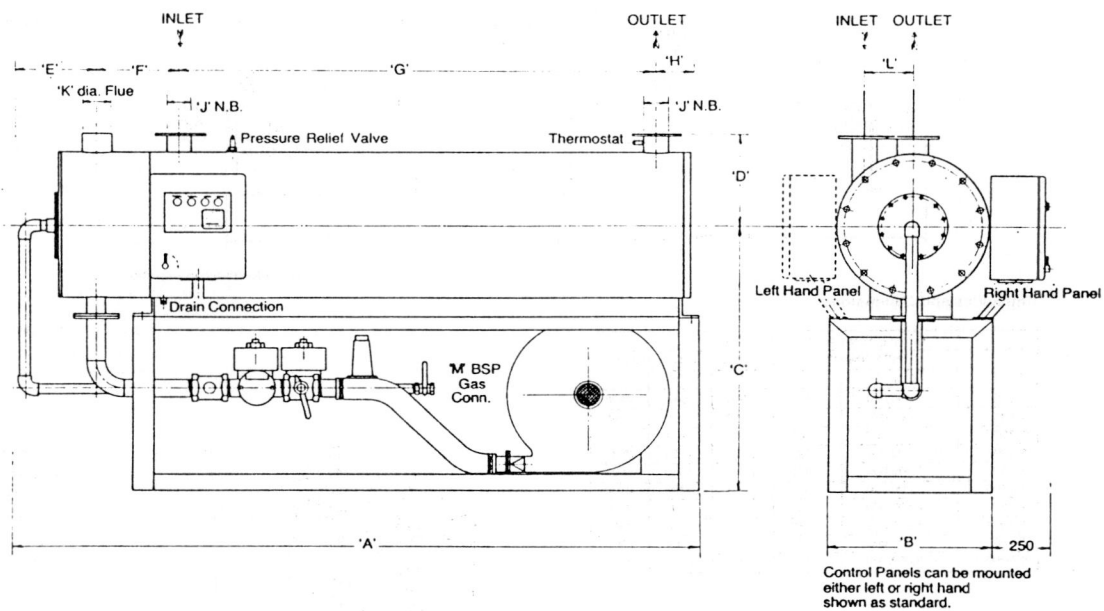

Control Panels can be mounted either left or right hand shown as standard.

Capacities and Dimensions

Model No.	Heat Output BTU/hr	kW	A	B	C	D	E	F	G	H	J	K	L	M
SA 128	128,000	38	1775	500	1000	275	225	200	1200	150	50	50	100	½"
SA 240	240,000	70	1925	500	1050	300	250	225	1300	150	50	65	125	¾"
SA 336	336,000	98	2150	600	1075	325	275	275	1400	200	80	80	135	1"
SA 480	480,000	141	2350	600	1100	350	275	300	1600	200	80	100	150	1½"
SA 800	800,000	234	2450	700	1175	425	325	300	1700	200	80	150	200	1½"
SA 1200	1,200,000	352	2680	800	1225	475	350	340	1800	225	100	200	250	2"
SA 1600	1,600,000	469	2680	800	1225	475	350	340	1800	225	100	200	250	2½"

CASCADE Gas Fired Direct Contact Water Heater

General Arrangement

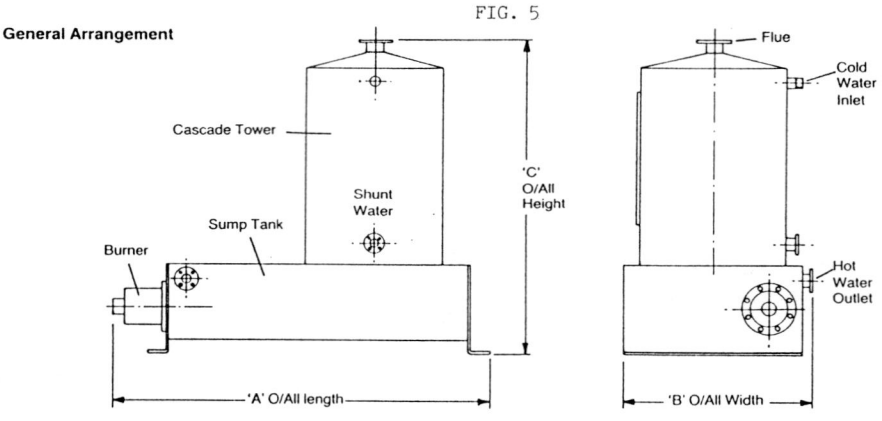

FIG. 5

* Single tower assembly shown

Capacities and Dimensions

MODEL	HEAT INPUT BTU/HR	KW	A	B	C
1-200	200,000	58.6	1500	600	2200
1-500	500,000	147	1750	850	2350
1-700	700,000	205	2000	950	2400
1-1000	1,000,000	293	2250	1100	2500
1-1500	1,500,000	440	2500	1250	2600
1-2000	2,000,000	586	2750	1400	2700
1-2500	2,500,000	733	3100	1600	2750
1-3000	3,000,000	879	3350	1700	2800
1-4000	4,000,000	1172	3600	1800	2900
1-5000	5,000,000	1465	3900	2000	3100

(SINGLE TOWER – SINGLE BURNER; DIMENSIONS approx)

Selection Chart

SINGLE TOWER – SINGLE BURNER — GALLONS PER MINUTE

REQUIRED TEMPERATURE RISE °C	1-200	1-500	1-700	1-1000	1-1500	1-2000	1-2500	1-3000	1-4000	1-5000
90	2.0	5.1	7.2	10.2	15.3	20.4	25.5	30.6	40.8	51
85	2.2	5.4	7.6	10.8	16.2	21.6	27.0	32.4	43.2	54
80	2.3	5.8	8.1	11.6	17.4	23.2	29.0	34.8	46.4	58
75	2.5	6.2	8.6	12.4	18.6	24.8	31.0	37.2	49.6	62
70	2.6	6.6	9.3	13.2	19.8	26.4	33.0	39.6	52.8	66
65	2.8	7.1	10.0	14.2	21.3	28.4	35.5	42.6	56.8	71
60	3.1	7.7	10.8	15.4	23.1	30.8	38.4	46.2	61.6	77
55	3.4	8.4	11.8	16.8	25.2	33.6	42.0	50.4	67.2	84
50	3.7	9.3	13.0	18.6	27.9	37.2	46.5	55.8	74.4	93
45	4.1	10.3	14.2	20.6	30.9	41.2	51.5	61.8	82.4	103
40	4.6	11.6	16.2	23.2	34.8	46.4	58	69.6	92.8	116
35	5.3	13.2	18.6	26.4	39.6	52.8	66	79.2	106	132
30	6.2	15.4	21.6	30.8	46.2	61.6	77	92.4	123	154
25	7.4	18.5	26.0	37.0	55.5	74.0	92.5	111	148	185
20	9.3	23.1	32.4	46.2	69.3	92.4	115	139	185	231

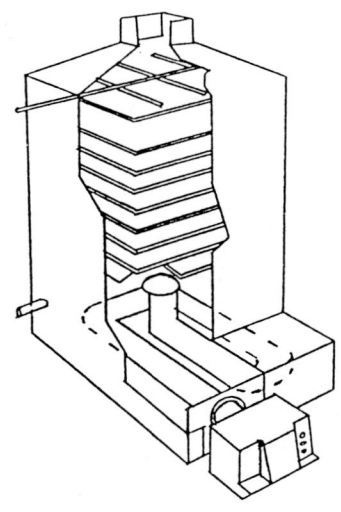

- To obtain correct size of "Cascade" Water Heater select the Temperature Rise in degrees C required in left hand column of Selection Chart and read across until the required Gallons per Minute is obtained. Select either single or twin tower assembly to suit the specific requirement.
- For temperature rises below 45 degrees Centigrade it is necessary for a proportion of the feed water to be discharged directly into the holding/sump tank via the Shunt Water Connection.
- To obtain degrees fahrenheit multiply degrees centigrade by 1.8
- To obtain litres multiply gallons by 4.546.

LE CHAUFFAGE PAR LE GAZ NATUREL EN INDUSTRIE

(cas des procédés basses et moyennes températures)

par

François LAURENT

S.N. FL ENERGIE

SOMMAIRE

INTRODUCTION

I LA COMBUSTION DU GAZ NATUREL :

    I.1 Réaction chimique
    I.2 Pouvoir calorifique supérieur et pouvoir calorifique inférieur

II CHAUFFAGE DIRECT DES LIQUIDES (ECS) :

    II.1 Principe du chauffage direct
    II.2 Action des produits de combustion sur le liquide
    II.3 Description du matériel
    II.4 Caractéristiques techniques
    II.5 Applications

III CHAUFFAGE INDIRECT DES LIQUIDES (TIC - EIC) :

    III.1 Tube Immergé Compact
        III.1.a Description
        III.2.b Caractéristiques techniques
    III.2 Echangeur Immergé Compact
        III.2.a Description
        III.2.b Coefficient de convection des produits de combustion
        III.2.c Caractéristiques techniques
    III.3 Applications

IV CONCLUSIONS SUR LE CHAUFFAGE DES LIQUIDES :

    IV.1 Installation "In Situ"
    IV.2 Installation en Annexe
    IV.3 Production en Continu

V AUTRE BRULEURS POUR LE CHAUFFAGE DE FOUR ET LE SECHAGE

    V.1 Brûleur radiant catalytique
    V.2 Brûleur veine d'air

VI CRITERES DE CHOIX POUR LES BRULEURS INDUSTRIELS :

    VI.1 Critères généraux
    VI.2 Critères particuliers.

VII TUBES RADIANTS BASSE TEMPERATURE :

    VII.1 Introduction
    VII.2 Description
    VII.3 Applications

INTRODUCTION :

Le chauffage à basse température des liquides industriels (inférieur ou égal à 100 °C) nécessite des grandes quantités d'énergie. La plupart du temps, la source de chaleur est une chaufferie centralisée vapeur, et des échangeurs sont chargés de la distribuer localement aux différents points d'utilisation.

Cependant, la nécessité d'économiser l'énergie a favorisé le développement de solutions décentralisées, qui sont particulièrement bien adaptées aux utilisations des gaz.

Il y a notamment deux procédés qui rendent possible le chauffage des bains "in situ" en Industrie par le gaz naturel :

- le chauffage direct par combustion submergée qui est caractérisé par l'absence d'échangeur. L'échange est maximum mais l'application de ce procédé est limité par le niveau de température et par la nature des produits à chauffer

- le chauffage indirect par tube immergé compact ou échangeur immergé compact qui est caractérisé par la petitesse des équipements et l'excellent coefficient de transfert de chaleur.

Les différents procédés de chauffage de liquides industriels analysés dans le présent document sont caractérisés par :

- <u>leur implantation</u> : ils sont implantés aussi près que possible du bain à chauffer et, lorsque cela est réalisable, directement dans le liquide, éliminant ainsi les pertes dûes au réseau de distribution ;

- <u>leur mode de travail</u> : ces procédés permettent de faire face rapidement à toutes demandes de chaleur pour un poste particulier dans une usine, indépendamment des autres ;

- <u>leur caractéristiques</u> : selon leur implantation et leur mode de travail, ils permettent l'obtention de très bons rendements : 85 % à 100 % sur PCI.

I LA COMBUSTION DU GAZ NATUREL :

I.1 Réaction chimique :

La combustion du gaz naturel est une réaction chimique d'oxydation dans laquelle le gaz et l'air se combinent pour donner du gaz carbonique, de la vapeur d'eau, de l'azote et de l'air en excès.

Le chauffage au gaz naturel consiste à extraire la chaleur des produits de la combustion pour la donner au fluide à réchauffer.

Pour obtenir un bon rendement thermique il faut que les fumées rejetées contiennent le moins de chaleur possible. Ceci est obtenu en réduisant la masse des produits rejetés à la cheminée par le contrôle de l'excès d'air et en abaissant la température des fumées, c'est-à-dire en poussant au maximum l'échange de chaleur.

I.2 Pouvoir calorifique supérieur et pouvoir calorifique inférieur :

En abaissant la température des fumées à moins de 60 °C, on récupère la chaleur latente que libère la condensation de l'eau formée à la combustion. Cette chaleur représente près de 11 % de l'énergie propre au gaz naturel. Le pouvoir calorifique supérieur (p.c.s.) intègre cette quantité de chaleur latente et inférieur (p.c.i.) ne la prend pas en compte.

Le chauffage des liquides par contact direct avec les fumées offre un excellent rendement car il permet justement d'abaisser au maximum la température de ces fumées et même de condenser l'eau de combustion si la température du bain est modérée.

II CHAUFFAGE DIRECT DES LIQUIDES : (ECS)

II.1 Principe du chauffage direct :

Le chauffage direct des liquides consiste à mettre le liquide à chauffer au contact intime des produits de la combustion du gaz naturel :

- soit en pulvérisant le liquide en gouttelettes dans les fumées

- soit en faisant barbotter les fumées dans le liquide lui-même (ECS).

Dans les deux cas, ce sont des surfaces d'échange considérables qui sont développées : les bulles engendrées par le barbotage d'un mètre cube de fumées offrent une surface d'échange de l'ordre de 1.000 m².

Parallèlement, le coefficient d'échange est optimal du fait du contact direct et de l'absence de toute paroi d'échange. Ces deux facteurs, joints à l'agitation des milieux en présence, conduisent à un transfert de chaleur intense vers le liquide à chauffer. Dans le cas du barbotage il suffit que les produits de combustion traversent le bain sur une hauteur de 50 cm seulement, pour que les températures des liquides et des fumées soient égalisées.

II.2 Action des produits de combustion sur le liquide :

Les produits de la combustion du gaz naturel sont propres : les effets du soufre sont inexistant. Le gaz carbonique et les traces d'oxyde d'azote entraînent à la longue une acidification faible des liquides chauffés en direct.

Dans la pratique, cette acidification n'est à prendre en compte que pour le chauffage de bain très fortement alcalin. On peut dire que dans la majorité des cas, elle reste négligeable devant la dégradation due à l'utilisation même des bains.

II.3 Description du Matériel : (Fig. 1)

Les produits de la combustion issus du brûleur sont dispersés dans le bain par des rampes de formes adaptées à la cuve.

Les fumées s'échappent du liquide à la même température que celui-ci.

La chambre de combustion est refroidie par l'air comburant pour ne pas mettre le bain en contact avec une paroi trop chaude et éviter une trempe chimique de la flamme.

La régulation peut être du type modulante ou tout ou rien : dans les deux cas elle permet d'ajuster la température du liquide au demi degré près.

Les brûleurs à barbotage s'implantent dans les cuves de travail elles-mêmes, sans aucune ouverture dans les parois de ces cuves. Ils sont aisément démontables, la vidange des cuves n'étant pas nécessaire : ceci facilite l'entretien. Il est possible également d'implanter ces brûleurs en dérivation de la cuve de travail, dans une cuve annexe.

Un atout majeur de cette technique est l'absence totale d'inertie thermique ; dès le premier kilowatt/H de gaz consommé la température du bain s'élève. Comme il est aisé, avec le gaz naturel, de mettre en oeuvre des puissances importantes, les temps de montée en température sont réduits au minimum.

Enfin, lorsque le chauffage en direct n'est pas possible, ces équipements peuvent chauffer directement un fluide caloporteur qui transmettra à son tour au liquide à chauffer sa chaleur par l'intermédiaire d'un échangeur à plaques.

II.4 Caractéristiques techniques : (Fig. 2 et 3)

Les fumées sont évacuées à la même température que les liquides

- à moins de 60 °C, il y a condensation d'une partie de l'eau de combustion et le rendement du chauffage est supérieur à 100 % sur PCI ;

- entre 60 °C et 70 °C, il oscille autour d'une valeur de 90 % sur PCI ;

- au-dessus de 70 °C, le rendement chute car l'eau de combustion ne se condense plus ; au contraire, l'eau du bain s'évapore ; cet effet peut être exploité si l'on désire concentrer le bain (industrie chimique, etc...).

Par rapport à un chauffage classique à la vapeur, le chauffage direct d'un liquide apporte un gain de rendement utile d'au moins 30 % jusqu'à une température de 60 °C et reste intéressante jusqu'à 70 °C.

II.5 Applications :

II.5.a Industrie Mécanique :

Les traitements chimiques de surfaces (dégraissage, décapage, phosphatation, etc.) sont un domaine idéal d'utilisation du chauffage direct :

- températures de bains modérées et le plus souvent inférieures à 60 °C, car les fournisseurs de bains proposent de plus en plus des produits efficaces à basse température.

- volumes importants de bains qui valorisent la puissance et la souplesse du chauffage direct,

- commodité d'emploi des brûleurs à barbotage par rapport aux autres techniques : brûleurs aisément démontables, pas de problèmes d'échangeur.

II.5.b Industrie Agro-alimentaire :

En laiterie les stations de lavage sont bien placées pour l'une ou l'autre technique : les bains d'acide à température modérée peuvent très bien s'accommoder du chauffage direct, de même que l'eau des rinçages ou lavages divers. Pour les bains de soude il faut envisager le chauffage indirect par échangeurs immergés gaz.

En abattoir des essais, suivis d'une réalisation effective, effectués sur une cuve d'échaudage de porcs ont montré que le chauffage direct est compatible avec l'utilisation.

En brasserie le chauffage direct des bains utilisés dans les pasteurisateurs et les machines à laver les bouteilles est à l'étude. La thermolisation du vin peut également être réalisée par ce moyen de chauffage.

II.5.c Industrie textile :

Le chauffage direct devrait convenir à certains bains tels que désencollage, blanchiment. Il est déjà appliqué pour la production d'eau chaude de Process.

II.5.d Autres secteurs :

Le chauffage direct intéresse bien d'autres secteurs pour la préparation d'eau chaude industrielle : eau de gâchage du béton, eaux de lavage, eaux destinées au réchauffage de produits solides ou liquides, etc...

Le chauffage direct est également utilisé en concentration de bain c'est en fait son application la plus ancienne avec la concentration d'acide sulfurique dans l'industrie chimique.

III CHAUFFAGE INDIRECT DES LIQUIDES (TIC - EIC) :

III.1 Tube Immergé Compact : (Fig. 4)

III.1.a Description :

Le tube immergé compact est constitué de trois parties : le brûleur, la chambre de combustion et le tube échangeur.

La flamme se développe dans la chambre de combustion qui est aussi compacte que possible. Ainsi, le brûleur assure une combustion intensive qui est complète malgré un faible excès d'air.

La chambre de combustion est de forme cylindrique, se terminant par un cône auquel est raccordé le tube échangeur.

Il y a plusieurs possibilités pour l'implantation de la chambre de combustion. L'une des solutions consiste à l'installer à l'extérieur de la cuve contenant le liquide à chauffer. Dans ce cas de figure, la chambre de combustion est refroidie par l'air comburant ou protégée par un matériau réfractaire. La meilleure solution possible est de l'implanter directement dans le liquide à chauffer, soit verticalement soit horizontalement.

La grande vitesse des fumées alliée au faible diamètre du tube échangeur assure un excellent coefficient de transfert de chaleur et par conséquent un très bon rendement.

Le faible diamètre du tube assure l'utilisation de la presque totalité de la chaleur contenue dans la veine de fumées. La pression du gaz et de l'air devront être suffisantes pour faire face à la perte de charge du tube échangeur.

III.1.b Caractéristiques techniques : (Fig. 5)

La plupart du temps, les rendements obtenus avec les tubes immergés compacts sont compris entre 92 % et 94 % sur PCI, pour les conditions d'utilisations suivantes : température du liquide à chauffer 70 °C, excès d'air pour brûleur 20 %.

Par sa simplicité et son faible coût, ce procédé est particulièrement bien adapté pour des installations dont la puissance est de l'ordre de 150 KW sur PCI, ou pour des cuves de dimensions particulières (grande longueur ou peu profonde).

III.2 Echangeur Immergé Compact : (Fig. 6)

III.2.a Description :

Les principales caractéristiques de ce genre d'équipement sont :

- **Compacité** : Sans augmenter la surface d'échange "produits de combustion - liquides à chauffer", on atteint un coefficient de convection des produits de combustion élevé en provoquant une forte turbulence de ceux-ci contre la paroi de l'échangeur.

ECHANGEUR IMMERGE	PUISSANCE (KW on NCV)					DIMENSION (m) l x L x H
	100	200	300	400	500	
EIC 250	———————————					0.15 x 1.3 x 0.5
EIC 450	———————————————————————					0.25 x 1.8 x 0.5

- **Bon rendement** : Grâce à une technologie simple procurant une grande fiabilité à ces équipements les rendements obtenus dépassent 92 % sur PCI.

L'échangeur compact se présente sous la forme d'un parallélépipède composé de deux parties : la première, directement raccordée au brûleur du type à mélange préalable avec grille de combustion, est appelée "chambre de combustion", elle est occupée par une série de tube verticaux ouverts parcourus par le liquide du bain. Les produits de combustion quittent donc cette zone en ayant réchauffé le liquide qui traverse les tubes de bas en haut par effet de thermosiphon. La deuxième partie de l'échangeur est conçue de telle sorte que les produits de combustion suivent un parcours déterminé autour des passages du liquide.

III.2.b Coefficient de convection des produits de combustion :

Le coefficient de convection des fumées augmente en fonction des variations locales de vitesse et donc de l'énergie cinétique. Ces variations sont obtenues à chaque fois que le flux des produits de combustion percute les parois d'échange : gauffrage.

III.2.c Caractéristiques techniques : (Fig. 7)

L'étude comparative des différents procédés pour le chauffage d'un bain à 70 °C (par exemple) montre que :

- pour les échangeurs alimentés par un fluide caloporteur à partir d'une chaufferie centralisée, la puissance surfacique est élevée mais le rendement global reste relativement faible : 70 % maximum ;

- pour les tubes immergés classiques où circulent les produits de combustion issus d'un brûleur, la puissance surfacique est faible mais le rendement est plus élevé : 70 % à 80 % sur PCI ;

- pour les tubes immergés "compacts", le rendement peut alors atteindre 90 % sur PCI ;

- pour l'échangeur compact, la puissance surfacique est élevée et le rendement reste excellent : 92 à 96 % sur PCI.

III.3 Applications :

III.3.a Traitement de surfaces :

. Galvanisation : Bain de dégraissage et fluxage.

. Galvanoplastie : Bains de dégraissage, phosphatation, acides, nickelage, cuivrage, chromage, brunissage, colmatage, etc...

. Emaillage : Bains de dégraissage, neutralisation.

. Peinture : Bains de phosphatation, passivation.

III.3.b Agro-alimentaire, agriculture :

. Agro-alimentaire : Cuves d'échaudage de porcs, eaux de trempage, bacs de blanchiment, production d'eau chaude.

. Agriculture : serres : hydroponie, distribution d'eau chaude par paillage radiant.

III.3.c Textile :

. Textile : Bacs de teinture et de blanchiment, bacs de lavage, production d'eau chaude.

IV CONCLUSIONS SUR LE CHAUFFAGE DES LIQUIDES :

Les façons d'implanter ces équipements sont nombreuses et variées, dépendant de la position de la chambre de combustion en fonction des contraintes d'exploitation, du liquide à chauffer et de la température de consigne. Néanmoins, on peut les regrouper en trois cas : l'installation "in situ", en cuve annexe, et en production en continu. Toutes les techniques de chauffe de liquide en industrie soit en direct soit en indirect peuvent être rattachées à l'un de ces cas.

IV.1 Installation "In Situ" :

L'équipement de chauffe est directement implanté dans la cuve du process. Pour ce type d'implantation, le bain n'est généralement pas sous pression (la surface libre du liquide est à pression atmosphérique) et sa température est pratiquement uniforme.

L'équipement de chauffe monte le bain en température et le maintient à une consigne constante.

C'est le mode d'implantation qui est le plus efficace.

IV.2 Implantation en cuve annexe :

Lorsqu'il n'y a pas la place suffisante pour implanter l'équipement de chauffe directement dans la cuve, on l'implante dans une cuve annexe. On confectionne alors une boucle hydraulique qui permet le transfert du liquide de la cuve du process vers la cuve où se trouve implanté l'équipement de chauffe. Il est à noter que la circulation du liquide assure une excellente homogénéité de la température du liquide dans la cuve du process. Le calcul du débit de circulation fait partie du savoir faire du constructeur.

Néanmoins lorsque le liquide travaille sous pression, la cuve annexe devra être également conçue pour travailler sous pression (dans ce cas on utilise généralement le tube immergé compact).

Lorsque la cuve du process travaille à pression atmosphérique, la cuve annexe qui comporte l'équipement de chauffe, travaille également à pression atmosphérique.

Enfin, lorsque le liquide ne peut pas être mis en contact directement avec les gaz de combustion (combustion submergée), ou au contact des parois chaudes d'un équipement indirect (les parois de l'échangeur immergé compact ou du tube immergé compact sont environ à une température supérieure de 15 °C à celle du liquide) on utilise un échangeur à plaques intermédiaires qui n'abaisse le rendement que de 1 à 3 %.

IV.3 Production en Continu : (Fig. 8)

Le générateur et son environnement constituent une boucle ouverte de circulation. Généralement, l'eau chaude, une fois utilisée n'est pas recyclée. Ainsi, le générateur est alimenté en eau froide et produit de l'eau chaude en continu. L'eau froide peut être préchauffée au travers d'un échangeur à plaques par l'eau chaude épuisée avant qu'elle ne soit rejetée à l'égout.

Afin d'avoir un rendement maximum, les fumées circulent à contre courant de l'eau à chauffer. Avant d'être évacuées, les fumées sont refroidies au contact de l'eau froide d'alimentation. L'eau chaude ainsi produite peut être mélangée avec celle provenant d'un ballon de stockage afin de faire face à d'éventuelles fluctuations importantes de débit.

Plusieurs types d'équipement peuvent être utilisés comme générateurs d'eau chaude. Parmi ceux-ci :

- La production d'eau chaude en continu par la combustion submergée qui consiste simplement en une cuve dans laquelle a été implanté un équipement de combustion submergée. Pour des températures voisines de 60 °C, le rendement dépasse 100 % sur PCI. Au delà de 60 °C, la combustion submergée est complétée par une tour de lavage de fumées qui préchauffe l'eau froide d'alimentation.

- Le générateur en continu avec un échangeur immergé compact qui est installé dans une cuve de dimensions très réduites. A des températures voisines de 90 °C, le rendement approche les 100 % sur PCI.

V AUTRES BRULEURS POUR LE CHAUFFAGE DE FOUR ET LE SECHAGE

Le développement des techniques modernes d'utilisation des gaz fait souvent appel à d'autres brûleurs pour produire des flammes très spécifiques aux usages demandés en Industrie. Le brûleur n'est pas seulement une source de chaleur, mais aussi un outil avec des fonctions bien particulières.

V.1 Brûleur radiant catalytique : (Fig. 9)

Ce système engendre une oxydation catalytique sans aucune flamme. Ceci est dû au contact avec une masse poreuse imprégnée d'un catalyseur, généralement à base de platine.

Le principe d'un tel équipement avec prémélange partiel de l'air et du gaz et mouvement de convection de l'air secondaire est décrit par la figure 9.

Le système des panneaux radiants catalytiques est intéressant, car il peut être utilisé dans des atmosphères explosives :

En effet, tant qu'il n'y a pas de matières en combustion, tels que des chiffons par exemple, la plupart des vapeurs des solvants industriels en contact avec une matière poreuse même portée à une température de près de 1000 °C, ne s'enflamme pas mais subit uniquement une réaction catalytique d'oxydation.

En d'autres termes, l'émission spectrale de ces brûleurs correspond au spectre d'absorption de la plupart des peintures habituellement utilisées. C'est pourquoi, ces systèmes sont très appropriés pour le séchage des peintures.

V.2 Brûleur veine d'air : (Fig. 10)

La pureté de la plupart des gaz, notamment l'absence de composés du soufre, rendent possible le chauffage directe de l'air par les produits de la combustion dans le but de chauffer certains process, par exemple pour des opérations de séchage.

Pour réaliser cela, un type spécial de brûleur a été développé, le brûleur veine d'air, ainsi nommé parce qu'il se place directement dans le conduit de ventilation.

Ce type de brûleur ainsi que son implantation est illustré par la figure 10.

La température des gaz chauds ainsi obtenue est voisine de 400 °C.

L'utilisation des gaz chauds résultant de la dilution des produits de combustion et de l'air est communément utilisée en séchage.

Plusieurs brûleurs veine d'air sont particulièrement adaptés pour l'incinération des effluents gazeux, sous réserve que le pourcentage d'oxygène dans les effluents soit inférieur ou égal à 18 % et que l'air de dilution soit à une température inférieure à 540 °C. Cette incinération est utilisée pour des températures de l'ordre de 800 à 850 °C.

VI CRITERES DE CHOIX POUR LES BRULEURS INDUSTRIELS :

Une fois définie la nature de l'opération de chauffage envisagée, le choix de l'équipement de chauffe à employer peut se faire en considérant des critères : d'ordre général, caractérisant le fonctionnement des brûleurs, indépendamment de son usage, d'ordre particulier, caractérisant le produit à chauffer et le four s'il existe déjà et en considérant la fonction de la flamme relativement aux critères précédents.

VI.1 Critères généraux :

Ces critères caractérisent le fonctionnement des brûleurs qui doivent être utilisés afin de répondre au cahier des charges de l'opération envisagée.

Ce sont les exigences relevées en regard de chacun de ces critères qui conditionneront un premier choix de brûleurs dans la classification des brûleurs à gaz explicitée en pose.

La température à obtenir a une grande importance aux extrêmes des gammes de températures rencontrées : à basse température, il sera souvent fait appel à des brûleurs fonctionnant en excès d'air ou avec recyclage de produits de combustion, à haute température, le préchauffage et/ou la suroxygénation de l'air de combustion seront utiles ou nécessaires.

La nature des produits de combustion exigée, indépendamment de toute autre considération, peut à elle seule fixer le choix du brûleur : combustion en défaut d'air avec utilisation complète de l'oxygène, combustion en fort excès d'air sans imbrûlés, teneur en NOx.

La souplesse de fonctionnement exigée, qui est le rapport des puissances maximales et minimales du brûleur à son réglage nominal, est un critère de choix conjoint au brûleur, à son système d'alimentation et au système de régulation. La souplesse de fonctionnement exigée sur un équipement peut être obtenue par modulation de puissance sur le ou les brûleurs, par modulation de leur temps de fonctionnement, par effacement successif de certains brûleurs ou par combinaison de ces dispositions.

Ce n'est qu'après avoir examiné ces différentes possibilités, en considération du procédé envisagé et du mode de chauffage possible que la souplesse nécessaire à chaque brûleur peut être déterminée.

La souplesse de réglage, qui est le rapport des taux d'aération extrêmes pour lesquels le fonctionnement normal du brûleur est assuré, est une grandeur importante pour des équipements multi-usages, lorsque l'on souhaite mettre en oeuvre des dispositifs de régulation simplifiés ou lorsque les perturbations influant sur le réglage des équipements sont importantes.

Le bruit engendré par le brûleur devient un critère de choix à prendre en compte dans certaines applications. Il est important de noter qu'il ne s'agit pas d'un critère absolu, mais d'un critère relatif aux associations possibles brûleur-four.

Il n'y a en effet que peu de corrélation entre le bruit engendré par un brûleur essayé à l'air libre et celui engendré par le même brûleur dans un four. Les brûleurs les plus bruyants à l'air libre s'avèrent dans certains cas plus silencieux que d'autres en fonctionnement dans une enceinte close.

VI.2 Critères particuliers :

Ces critères caractérisent le produit à chauffer et le four destiné à cet usage si la conception ou la construction de celui-ci est déjà achevée au moment du choix du brûleur.

La réceptivité thermique du produit à chauffer correspond à ses aptitudes à absorber la chaleur issue directement ou indirectement de la flamme. Il ne s'agit pas d'une grandeur physique, mais d'une notion recouvrant ce que le sens commun désigne par l'aptitude au chauffage et qui est le résultat de la composition de variables physiques indépendantes caractérisant le produit à chauffer.

La réceptivité thermique du produit à chauffer dépend notamment de :

- sa conductibilité thermique, c'est-à-dire son aptitude à diffuser vers l'intérieur la chaleur reçue en surface,

- son coefficient d'absorption du rayonnement, c'est-à-dire son aptitude à transformer en chaleur une fraction du rayonnement qui frappe la surface,

- sa surface spécifique, c'est-à-dire la surface disponible pour recevoir la chaleur par convection ou rayonnement rapportée à l'unité de masse à chauffer,

- son oxydabilité, c'est-à-dire son aptitude à développer en surface des pellicules ou des crasses faisant obstacle au transfert de chaleur.

La valeur de ces grandeurs conditionne certains procédés de chauffage.

C'est ainsi que le réchauffage de métaux peu oxydables et bons conducteurs de la chaleur tels le cuivre ou l'aluminium se réalise avec des résultats remarquables au moyen de brûleurs-jets frappant directement la surface, sans fusion locale. L'utilisation de brûleurs radiants ne convient pas car ces mêmes métaux ont un très faible coefficient d'absorption.

Certaines opérations thermiques nécessitent des solutions de compromis, en raison de la variation des grandeurs considérées au cours de l'opération elle-même. C'est le cas de la refusion de l'aluminium. En début d'opération, la masse à chauffer est divisée, sa surface est relativement propre. En fin d'opération, le produit fondu ne reçoit la chaleur que par sa surface recouverte d'une pellicule ou d'une couche de crasses isolantes.

La réceptivité du four correspond à son aptitude à servir de relais efficace au transfert entre la flamme et le produit à chauffer. La réceptivité thermique du four dépend notamment de :

- son isolation thermique, c'est-à-dire son aptitude à éviter les déperditions par les parois,

- son inertie thermique, c'est-à-dire son aptitude à emmagasiner la chaleur. Cette aptitude s'oppose à l'obtention de bons rendements en période de mise en température mais contribue à la stabilité du fonctionnement,

- la présence de parois : creusets, moufles, semi-moufles, tubes radiants, faisant obstacle au transfert de chaleur entre flamme et produit à chauffer,

- la conception du départ des produits de combustion, assurant ou non, ou mal, un préchauffage de la charge,

- la présence de récupérateurs de chaleur pour préchauffer l'air de combustion.

Les critères de choix qui viennent d'être évoqués ici, s'ils ont été volontairement orientés pour les fours, se retrouvent légèrement transposés pour le chauffage des liquides traités dans les premiers chapitres. On citera pour mémoire :

- Nature du liquide,

- Température de consigne.

Ces deux paramètres permettent de déterminer la nature du chauffage :

- Direct,

- Indirect.

VII TUBES RADIANTS BASSE TEMPERATURE :

C'est une solution pour le chauffage des locaux industriels.

VII.1 Introduction :

N'importe quel objet soumis à une température supérieure au zéro absolu émet de l'énergie sous forme d'ondes électromagnétiques. Cette émission prend sa source dans la vibration des propres atomes de cet objet, engendrée par l'excitation thermique auxquels ils sont soumis. Cette radiation se propage dans le vide à la vitesse de la lumière (300.000 km/s). Quand elle rencontre un obstacle, une partie est réfléchie, une autre partie est absorbée par l'obstacle et transformée en chaleur. Le meilleur exemple est celui du skieur qui a chaud et a une sensation de confort dans les rayons du soleil au cours d'une descente alors que la température de l'air ambiant est très basse.

Les radiations électromagnétiques donnent une sensation de confort pour les occupants d'un local, ne chauffant ni l'air ambiant ni les murs qui sont à une température plus basse qu'avec les systèmes traditionnels de chauffage.

L'énergie radiante dépend de la longueur d'onde : plus celle-ci est courte plus la radiation est grande.

Pratiquement les émissions ont des longueurs d'onde comprises entre 2 et 8 μ, ce qui correspond à des températures d'émission comprises entre 100 et 1000 °C.

Plus l'élément émetteur à une température élevée, plus le rendement de radiation sera bon.

Cependant, pour des questions de confort et de sécurité, de trop hautes températures sont inacceptables.

VII.2 Description :

Les Tubes Radiants basse température sont des émetteurs obscurs, caractérisés par une combustion se développant à l'intérieur d'un tube, porté à une température relativement basse (450 °C). Cet élément "chauffant" est un tube en forme de U, appelé couramment épingle.

Ce type d'appareil consiste donc à chauffer par les gaz de combustion d'un brûleur un tube en acier. L'émission est dirigée vers le bas par un réflecteur en acier inoxydable ou en aluminium, situé au dessus du tube.

VII.3 Applications :

Le tube radiant basse température est une solution pour le chauffage des locaux industriels :

- Construction de grande hauteur peu isolée, avec des ouvertures
- Chauffage de postes de travail
- Chauffage discontinu.

Son installation se fait à une hauteur comprise entre 3,5 m et 8 m.

Voir figures de ce chapitre à la suite du texte en version anglaise

THE HEATING BY NATURAL GAS IN INDUSTRY
(for low and medium temperatures process)

by

François LAURENT

S.N. FL ENERGIE CO

TABLE OF CONTENTS

INTRODUCTION

I NATURAL GAS COMBUSTION :

　　I.1 Chemical reaction
　　I.2 Gross calorific value and net calorific value

II DIRECT HEATING OF LIQUIDS (ECS) :

　　II.1 How direct heating works
　　II.2 Impact on liquid properties
　　II.3 Description
　　II.4 Performance data
　　II.5 Applications

III INDIRECT HEATING OF LIQUIDS (TIC - EIC) :

　　III.1 Compact Immersion Tube
　　　　III.1.a Description
　　　　III.1.b Performance data
　　III.2 Compact Immersion Exchanger
　　　　III.2.a Description
　　　　III.2.b Combustion product heat transfer
　　　　III.2.c Performance data
　　III.3 Applications

IV CONCLUSIONS ABOUT HEATING OF LIQUIDS :

　　IV.1 "In Situ" Set up
　　IV.2 Shunt Set up
　　IV.3 Hot water generator Set up

V OTHER BURNERS FOR DRYING :

　　V.1 Catalytic Combustion Radiant Burners
　　V.2 Air Duct Bar Burners

VI CRITERIA FOR CHOOSING INDUSTRIAL SYSTEMS :

　　VI.1 General Criteria
　　VI.2 Criteria of specific nature.

VII LOW TEMPERATURE RADIATING TUBE :

VII.1 Introduction
VII.2 Description
VII.3 Applications

INTRODUCTION :

The heating of low-temperature industrial baths (below 100 °C) is responsible for a substantial amount of energy consumption in industry. Most often, this heat requirement is met by centralized production of steam and the use of exchangers which are located at the points of utilization.

However, the need to save energy has given rise to the development of decentralized solutions, which are very well suited to the use of gas fuels.

There are two processes which make possible "in situ" heating of industrial baths by natural gas :

- direct heating by submerged combustion which is characterized by the absence of an exchange wall. There is maximum heating efficiency, but the application of this process is limited by the temperature and nature of the products to be heated ;

- indirect heating via compact immersion tubes or exchangers which are characterized by compactness and good heating efficiency.

The different processes of industrial liquid heating analyzed here are characterized by :

- <u>their location</u> : they are set up as close as possible to the bath to be heated, and if possible, in the liquid (thus eliminating losses due to energy distribution) ;

- <u>their operation</u> : these processes make it possible to quick meet demands for heat independently of the operation of other factory equipment ;

- <u>their performance</u> : due to their location and operation, these processes enable good heating efficiency : 85 % to 100 % on NCV.

I NATURAL GAS COMBUSTION :

I.1 Chemical reaction :

The combustion of natural gas is an oxidation reaction under which natural gas and air are combined into carbon dioxide, water vapor, nitrogen and excess air.

Heating processes using natural gas consist in extracting heat from the combustion products and transferring it to the fluid to be heated.

In order to obtain good thermal efficiency, the heat content of the combustion products vented to atmosphere must be as low as possible. To this end, the weight of flue gases is controlled through the amount of excess air and the flue gases are cooled following a maximum heat transfer.

I.2 Gross Calorific Value and Net Calorific Value :

By cooling down the flue gases below 60 °C, the heat of condensation contained in the water vapor generated during combustion is recovered. This amount of heat represents nearly 11 % of the total energy content of natural gas. The gross calorific value (g.c.v.) takes into account this amount of latent heat whereas the net calorific value (n.c.v.) does not.

Heating liquids by direct contact with the combustion products therefore has an excellent efficiency since the temperature of the flue gases can be reduced to a minimum value and the water vapor resulting from combustion can even condense where the bath temperature is not too high.

II DIRECT HEATING OF LIQUIDS : (ECS)

II.1 How Direct Heating Works :

Direct heating of liquids consists in bringing into contact the liquid to be heated and the combustion products :

- either by spraying the liquid into the combustion products

- or by bubbling the combustion products through the liquid itself (ECS).

In both cases, the heat exchange areas involved are very large since the total area of the bubbles from 1 cubic meter of combustion products is about 1.000 m^2.

In addition, the heat transfer is optimum due to direct contact and the absence of any exchanger wall. The transfer of heat to the liquid is further enhanced by the movement of both fluids. In the case of the combustion products bubbling through bath, the combustion products must travel up 50 cm only before the temperatures of the liquid and the combustion products are equal.

II.2 Impact on Liquid Properties :

Natural gas is a clean fuel and so are the combustion products since no sulfur compounds are contained. In the long run, carbon dioxide and nitrogen oxide traces slightly acidify the liquids which are directly heated.

In practice however, this acidificati should be taken into account only whe strongly alcaline bathes are heated. Most cases, acidification is negligea compared with the deterioration due to the use of the bath in a specific process.

II.3 Description : (Fig. 1)

The combustion products are sent into the liquid to be heated through a manifold of a suitable shape.

The combustion products leave the liquid surface at the same temperature as the bath. The combustion chamber is cooled by combustion air in order not to bring the liquid in contact with too hot a wall, which would have an impact on the flame property.

The control is either of the modulating or of the on-off type. In both cases, it is possible to obtain the required bath temperature with a high degree of accuracy.

This type of burner can be mounted into the tanks without any openings in the side walls. They can be easily removed so that it is not necessary to empty the tank.

This is a plus where maintenance is to be carried out. This type of burner can also be operated on a by-pass to the main tank.

One of the major advantages of this technique is that there is no thermainertia since the temperature of the bath increases as soon as the first quantity of energy is inputted. Since natural gas is a powerful source of energy, heating times are cut down a minimum.

Alternatively, this type of burner directly heat a heating fluid from which heat is transferred to the working agents through an exchanger.

II.4 Performance Data : (Fig. 2 et 3)

The combustion products leave the liquid at the same temperature as the bath :

- where the temperature is below 60 °C, part of the water vapor generated during combustion condenses and the efficiency is greater than 100 % (n.c.v.) ;

- between 60 and 70 °C, the efficiency hovers around 90 % (n.c.v.) ;

- above 70 °C, the efficiency drops since the water vapor does not condense any longer ; on the contrary, the bath water evaporates ; however, this can be used where the bath is to be concentrated.

The efficiency of direct liquid heating is at least 30 % higher than with a conventional heating system using steam where the temperature do not exceed 60 °C and this process remains viable up to 70 °C.

II.5 Applications :

II.5.a Mechanical industries :

Surface treating (degreasing, phosphatizing, etc.) are ideally suited to direct heating :

- The bath temperatures are relatively low and most often below 60 °C since suppliers more and more often offer low temperature products ;

- The quantities involved are larged and therefore enhance the flexibility of direct heating ;

– The type of burner described above is characterized by ease of service compared to other technologies since the burners are easily removable and no exchangers are necessary.

II.5.b Food Processing :

<u>Dairies</u> : washing plants can use either technique : medium temperature acid baths as well as the water used for washing can be heated directly. Soda baths should however be indirectly heated through gas fired exchangers.

<u>Slaughterhouses</u> : tests and field experiments with a hog scalding vessel have shown that direct heating is compatible.

<u>Breweries</u> : the direct heating of liquids used in pasteurizers and bottle washing machines are under study. Wine can also be heated using this technique prior to filling.

II.5.c Textile Industry :

Direct heating should be suitable for bathes like those used for bleaching. This technique is alread used for process water heating.

II.5.d Other Applications :

Direct heating can be used for many other applications where process hot water is needed eg for mixing concrete, for washing, for heating solid or liquid products.

Direct heating is also used for bath concentration. It is even the oldest application with the concentration of sulfuric acid in the chemical industry.

III INDIRECT HEATING OF LIQUIDS (TIC - EIC) :

III.1 Compact Immersion Tube : (Fig. 4)

III.1.a Description :

The compact immersion tube consists of three parts : the burner, the combustion chamber and the exchanger tube.

The flame is developed in the combustion chamber which must be as compact as possible. Thus, the burner must maintain intense combustion which must be complete with only slight excess air.

The combustion chamber is cylindrical in shape with a cone at one end for hook-up to the exchanger tube.

There are several possible configurations for combustion chamber installation. One solution is to install the combustion chamber outside the tank which contains the liquid to be heated. In this way, the combustion chamber is cooled by the air drawn in for combustion or it is insulated by refractory material. It is also possible to place the combustion chamber in the liquid to be heated. It can be mounted either vertically or horizontally.

By increasing fume flow velocity, the small diameter exchanger tube makes possible an increase in heat transfer and consequently an improvement in heating efficiency.

This reduction in diameter also noticeably increases head loss in the tube. The implementation is the result of a compromise between efficiency gains and permissible air and gas feed pressure.

III.1.b Performance data : (Fig. 5)

Generally speaking, the compact immersion tubes are designed to provide heating efficiency of between 92 % and 94 % on NCV, for the following conditions : temperature of liquid heated 70 °C, excess air in adjoining burner, 20 %.

Because of its simplicity of operation and its low cost, this type of set-up is particularly well suited to installations which require a capacity of below 150 KW on NCV or for special dimension tanks (very long or shallow).

III.2 Compact Immersion Exchanger : (Fig. 6)

III.2.a Description :

The main characteristics of equipment is :

- Compactness : High combustion product heat transfer is obtained by producing a turbulent flow along the heat exchanger walls without increasing the heat exchange surface area.

IMMERSION EXCHANGER	CAPACITY (KW on NCV)					DIMENSION (m) l x L x H
	100	200	300	400	500	
EIC 250	▬▬▬▬▬▬▬▬▬▬▬▬					0.15 x 1.3 x 0.5
EIC 450			▬▬▬▬▬▬▬▬▬▬▬▬▬▬▬			0.25 x 1.8 x 0.5

- High efficiency : This simple technology which implies improved reliability results in efficiencies greater that 92 % on n.c.v.

The compact immersion heater is roughly a rectangular parallelepipede comprising two parts : the combustion chamber directly connected to a premixed burner and containing a number of opened vertical tubes through which the liquid to be heated flows. The products of combustion leave the combustion chamber after having heated the liquid which moves from bottom to top by natural circulation. The second heat exchanger stage is designed so that combustion products follow available paths in the exchanger walls.

III.2.b Combustion Product Heat Transfer

The transfer of combustion product heat increases due to local changes in velocity and thus in kinetic energy. Theses changes occur when the flue gases impinge on the baffle plates or waffled plates of the exchanger walls.

III.2.c Performance data : (Fig. 7)

The study of various alternatives of heating a liquid to 70 °C for instance has shown that :

- heat exchangers using a heating fluid from central boiler rooms have a high output per unit area but a relatively low overall efficiency not exceeding 70 % ;

- conventional immersion tube heat exchangers have a low output per unit area but a higher efficiency of 70 to 80 % on n.c.v. ;

- compact tube heat exchangers may have efficiencies of 90 % on n.c.v.

- compact immersion heaters have a high output per unit area and an excellent efficiency of 92 to 96 % on n.c.v.

III.3 Applications :

III.3.a Surface treating :

. Galvanizing : Degreasing baths and fluxing.
. Metal plating : Degreasing baths, phosphate coating, acids, copper plating, chrome plating, burnishing, filling-up, etc.
. Enameling : Degreasing baths, neutralization.
. Painting : phosphatizing baths, passivation.

III.3.b Agriculture and food processing :

. Food processing : Hog scalding vessels, steeping, bleaching, hot water production.
. Agriculture in greenhouses : hydroponics, hot water supply by radiant systems.

III.3.c Textile Industry :

. Textile : dyebaths and bleaches, washing, hot water production.

IV CONCLUSION ABOUT HEATING OF LIQUIDS :

Various installation configurations are possible, depending upon the position of the heating equipment with respect to the liquid and upon temperature distribution. There are three installation configurations : the "in-situ" configuration, the shunt configuration and the hot water generator configuration. The heating techniques are included as examples.

IV.1 "In Situ" Set-up :

The heating unit is located in the industrial tank (or machine) itself. The available room in the tank is sufficient to mount the unit. For this type of set-up, the bath, generally, is not under pressure (the free surface is under atmospheric pressure) and its temperature is practically uniform.

The heating equipment increases and holds the bath temperature constant.

This is the configuration of maximum efficiency.

IV.2 Shunt set-up :

When there is not sufficient available space in the industrial tank to install a heating unit, a circulation loop is installed outside the bath, between the industrial tank and the heating unit. To hold heat loss to a minimum, efforts will be made to install the tank and the heating unit as close as possible to each other. The heating unit inlet/outlet temperature gradient can vary from several degrees to several tens of degrees depending upon the type of set-up.

When the industrial liquid is under pressure, the heating unit is a boiling device.

When the industrial tank is at atmospheric pressure, the heating unit is an adjoining tank in which the heating equipment (submerged combustion, compact immersion tube or exchanger) is installed.

With this type of set-up, the heating efficiency of the liquid reflects allowances for losses to fumes, losses at the walls of the heating unit and distribution losses. The latter two types of losses are on the order of 1 to 3 %.

IV.3 Hot water generator set-up : (Fig. 8)

The generator and the network which makes use of the hot water form an open circulation loop. Usually, the hot water, once used, is not recycled. Thus, the generator is fed cold water and produces hot water continuously. The cold water can be preheated via an exchanger by the spent hot water before is flows out the drain.

For maximum heating efficiency, fumes circulation will go against the current of the water which is heated. Before being evacuated, the fumes are cooled by coming into contact with the coldest water. The hot water generator can therefore be combined with a storage unit to offset fluctuations in hot water consumption.

Various types of equipment can be used as hot water generators. Among them :

- the submerged combustion hot water generator consists of a storage tank in which the heating equipment is installed. For a water temperature of less than 60 °C, heating efficiency exceeds 100 % on NCV. Beyond 60 °C, the submerged combustion tank is equipped with a fume tower scrubber which is supplied with cold water.

- the hot water generator with an immersion exchanger is installed in a small storage tank. At hot water temperatures below 90 °C, heating efficiency exceeds 100 % on NCV.

V OTHER BURNERS FOR DRYING :

The development of modern techniques in gas utilization often calls for burners producing a flame for a very specific purpose. The burner is not only a source of heat, but also a tool with a specific function.

V.1 Catalytic Combustion Radiant Burners : (Fig. 9)

These systems induce a catalytic oxydation of fuel with air without any flame. This is done through contact with porous mass impregnated by a catalyst, generally being platinum-based.

The schematic diagram of an example of a system operating with partial premixture of air and gas and forced convection is shown in figure 9.

Catalytic systems are interesting in that they can be utilized in explosible atmosphere : as long as there are no ignition relays, such as rags for example, most industrial solvent fumes when in contact with the porous mass, even when brought up to nearly 1000 °C, do not provoke ignition, but only a catalytic oxidation reaction.

On the other hand, the emission spectrum of these burners corresponds to the absorption spectrum of the most commonly used paints. Therefore, these systems are very appropriate for drying paint.

V.2 Air Duct Bar Burners : (Fig. 10)

The purity of the common high CV gaseous fuels, especially the absence of sulfur, enables direct utilization of combustion products diluted in the air in order to air out workshops or for many other drying purposes.

To do this, a special type of burner has been developed called "air duct" bar burner because it is placed directly into ventilation ducts.

This type of burner and its location in a ventilation duct is illustrated in figure 10.

The temperature of the hot gases obtained can reach 400 °C.

The utilization of the hot gases resulting from the dilution of the combustion products is common in the area of drying.

Some air duct burners are designed to provide incineration of combustible gaseous effluents, if the oxygen ratio in the effluent is at least equal to 18 % and that the attack temperature is less than 540 °C. This incineration takes place at a temperature of 800 to 850 °C.

VI CRITERIA FOR CHOOSING INDUSTRIAL SYSTEMS :

Once the industrial branch concerned with choosing a heating system is known and the nature of the heating operation considered is established, the choice of the heating system to use can be done by considering criteria of a general nature, concerning the burner's operation, independently from its specific utilization, and criteria of a specific nature concerning the product to heat and the furnace if it already exists.

VI.1 General Criteria :

These criteria concerning the operation of the burners used must be considered in order to fulfill the operation requirements.

The temperature to be obtained has great importance on the limits of the available temperature ranges : low temperatures will often call for burners operating on excess air or on recycled combustion products ; at high temperatures, preheating and/or over oxygenation of the combustion air will be useful or necessary.

The nature of combustion products required, outside of any other consideration, can determine by itself the choice of the burner : air deficiency combustion with complete oxygen utilization, excess air combustion without unburned products, absence of NO_x.

The turn down ratio required, which is the ratio of maximum to minimum burner capacity at its nominal setting, is a criterion of selection related to the burner's feeding and regulation system.

The turn down ratio required of a system may be obtained by output modulation of the burner or burners, by sucessive shut down of some burners, or by a combination of these procedures.

It is only after having examined these different possibilites with regard to the planned process and the heating technique applicable, that the flexibility of each burner can be determined.

Adjustment flexibility which is the ratio between the extreme air factor for which the burner still operates normally, is an important factor for multi-usage equipment when one wishes to put in operation simplified control systems or when the perturtations influencing the equipment settings are important.

The noise produced by the burner becomes a selection criterion to take into account in certain instances. It is important to note that it is not an absolute necessity but a criterion related to the possibility of burner furnace coupling.

There is really very little relation between the noise produced by a burner tested in open air and that produced by the same burner in a furnace. The noisiest burners in open air prove to be, in some cases, quieter than others when operating in a closed space.

VI.2 Criteria of a Specific Nature :

These criteria deal with the product to the heated and the oven designated for this purpose, provided that the design or construction of the latter has already been done at the time of the burner selection.

The thermal receptivity of the product to be heated could be defined as its capacity to absorb the produced heat directly or indirectly by the flame.

It is not a physical parameter, but a notion covering what common sense designates as heating capacity and is the result of a combination of physical variables concerning the product to be heated.

The thermal receptivity of the product to be heated depends, among other things, upon :

- its thermal conductibility, that is, its capacity to diffuse toward the inside the heat received on the surface,

- its radiant absorption coefficient, that is, its capacity to transfer into heat a fraction of the radiation hitting the surface,

- its specific surface, that is, the surface available for receiving heat through convection or radiation per mass unit to be heated,

- its oxydability, that is, its capacity to develop surface films or dross reducing heat transfer.

The value of these parameters determines some heating processes.

The **furnace receptivity** corresponds to its capacity for being an efficient heat transfer relay between the flame and the product to be heated.

The thermal receptivity of the furnace depends, among other things, upon :

- its thermal insulation, that is, its capacity to avoid heat loss through the walls,

- its thermal inertia, that is, its capacity for storing heat. This capacity opposes obtaining good heating efficiency during the temperature build up period, but contributes to the stability of the operation,

- The presence of walls : crucibles, blocks, semi-blocks, radiant tubes, being obstacles to heat transfer between the flame and the product to be heated,

- the design of the combustion products outlet, providing (or not, or badly) preheating for the product to be heated,

- the presence of heat recuperators for combustion air preheating.

VII LOW TEMPERATURE RADIATING TUBE :

VII.1 Introduction :

Any object at a temperature greater than absolute zero emits energy in the form of electromagnetic radiation. This emission originates in a body owing to the vibration of its atoms caused by the thermal excitation to which they are subjected. This radiation is propagated in a straight line with material support at a speed of 300,000 km/s in a vacuum. When it reaches a body, part of the radiation is reflected. The rest is absorbed and then converted into heat. The most striking example is that of a skier who feels warm and comfortable in the sunshine on a slope at a very low outside temperature.

Radiation therefore provides the necessary comfort for the occupants of a building while leaving the ambient air and the walls of a building at a lower temperature than is the case with conventional heating systems.

Radiated energy emitted in the form of electromagnetic waves spreads with variable intensity depending on the wave lengths. The shorter the wave length. The more intense is the radiation.

In practice, emission occurs at wave lengths of between 2 and 8 μ which corresponds to emitter temperatures of 100 to 1000 °C.

The higher the temperature of the radiating element or tube, the higher the ratio/quantity of radiated heat/total quantity of heat, known as radiation efficiency.

Moreover, too high temperatures will be inacceptable for reasons of comfort and safety.

VII.2 Description :

Low temperature radiating tubes are dark heat emitters characterised by internal combustion taking place in a heating element raised to a relatively low temperature. This U-shaped heating element is known as a "heating grip".

The operating principle of radiating tubes consists in heating a steel tube using the combustion products of the gas burner. The radiation is directed towards the ground by a stainless steel or aluminium reflector placed above the tube.

VII.3 Applications :

- Buildings of average height, poorly insulated, poorly closed
- Heating of stations or areas
- Discontinuous use of heating
- Installation height 3.50 to 8 metres from the ground.

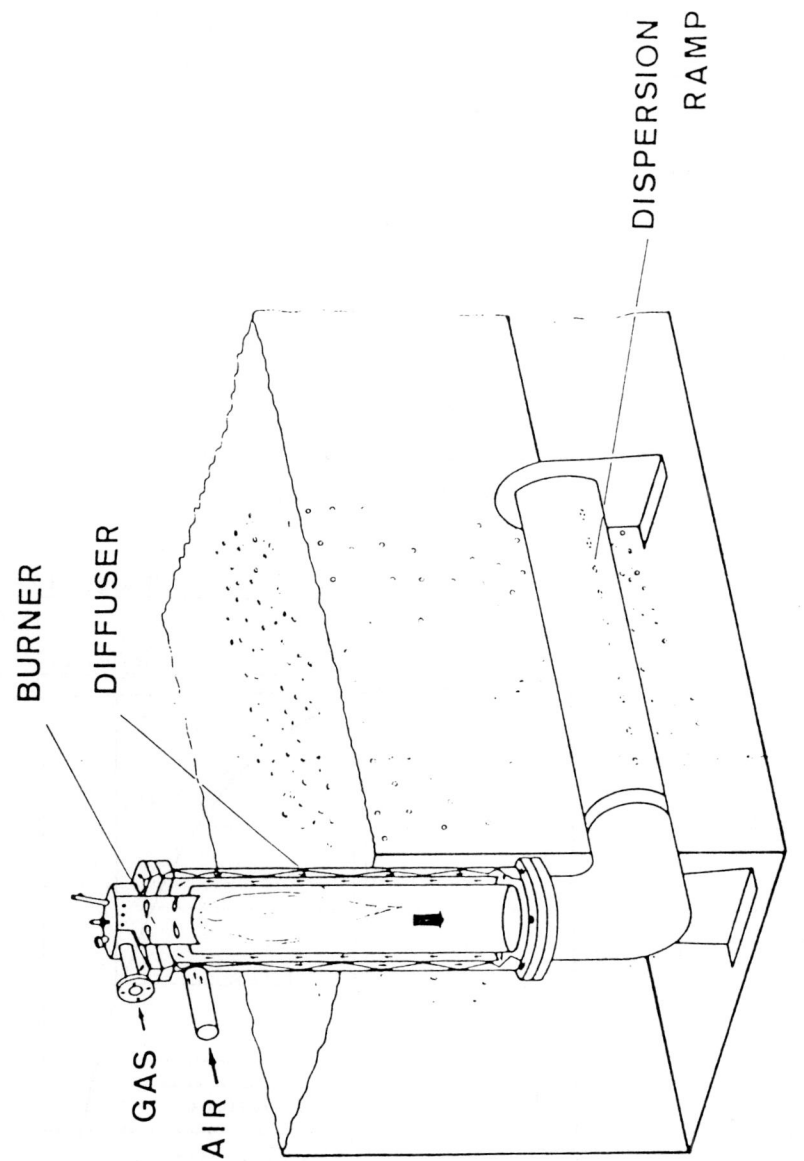

SUBMERGED COMBUSTION EQUIPMENT

FIG. 1

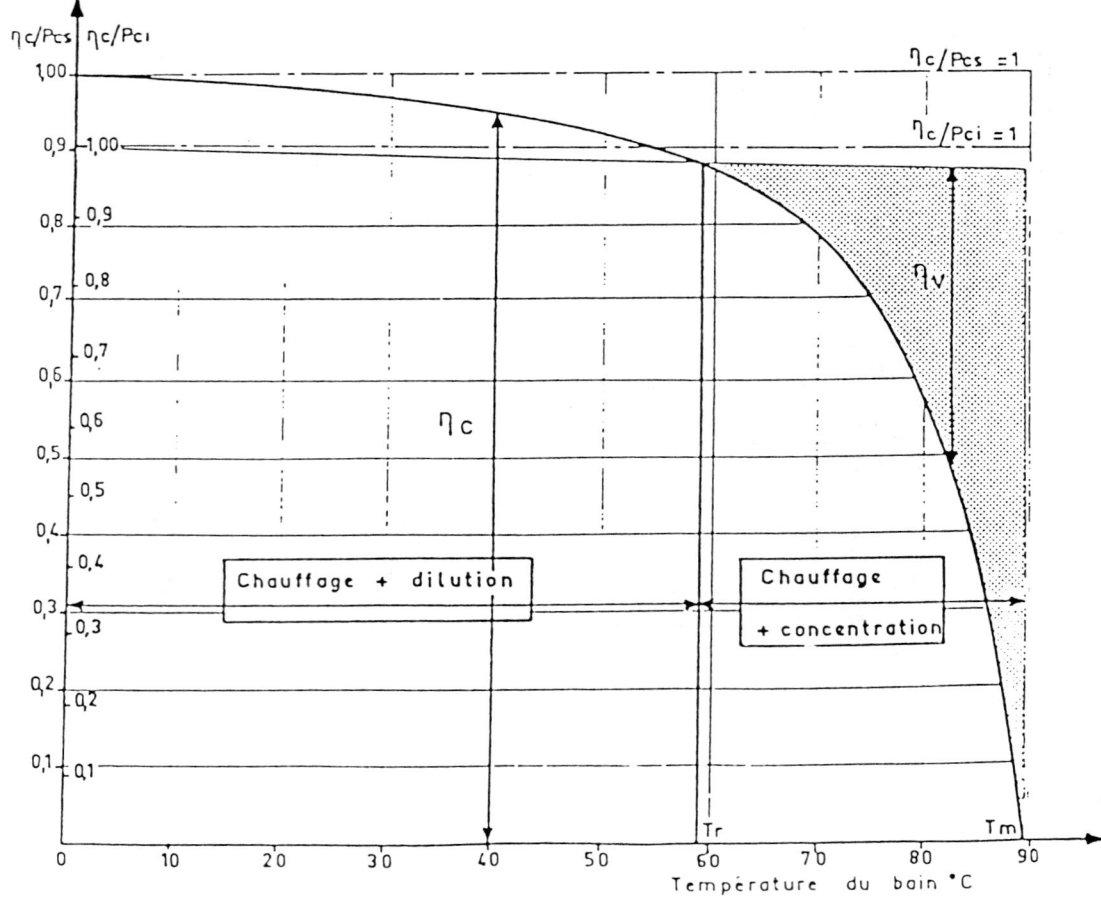

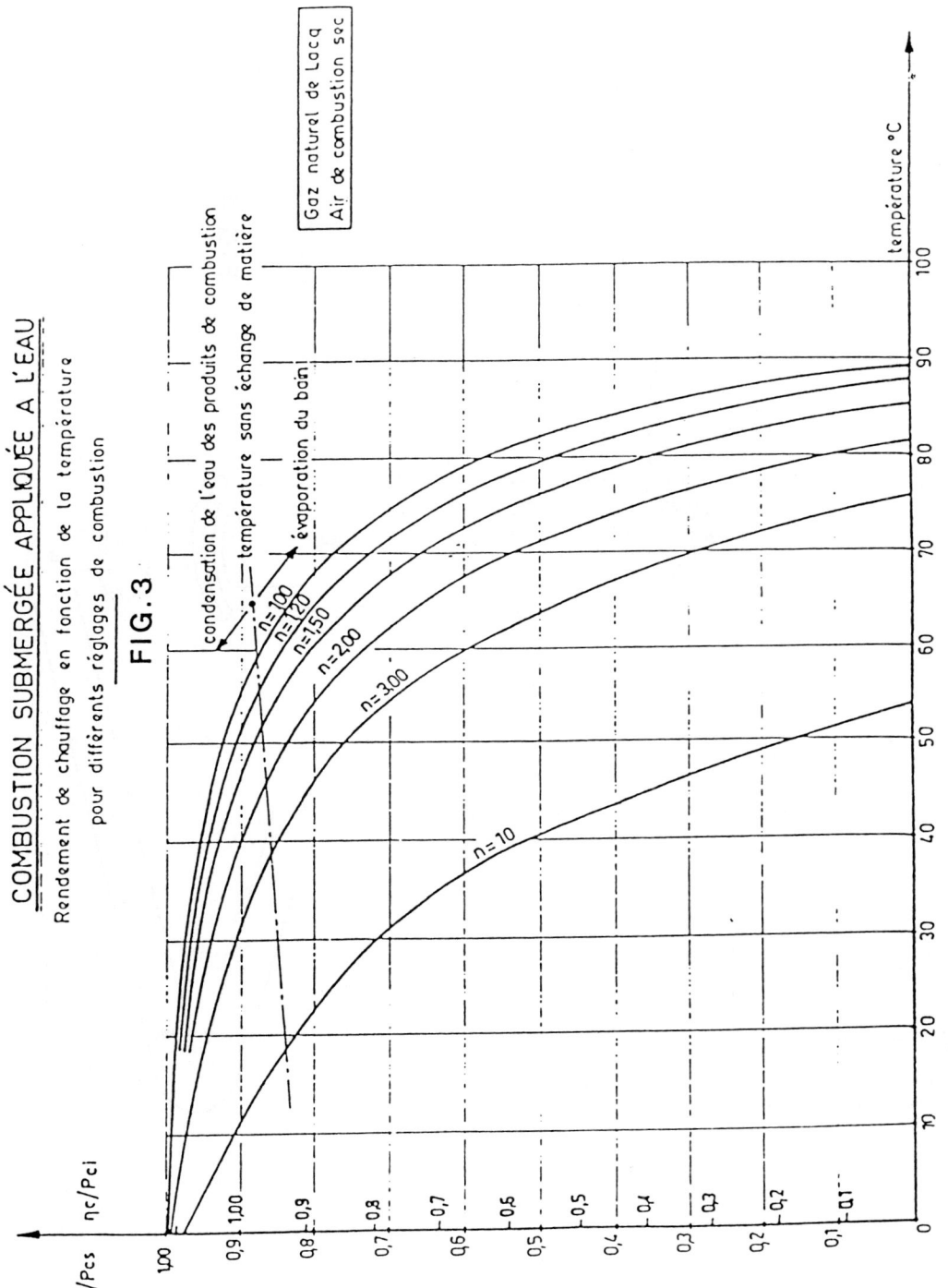

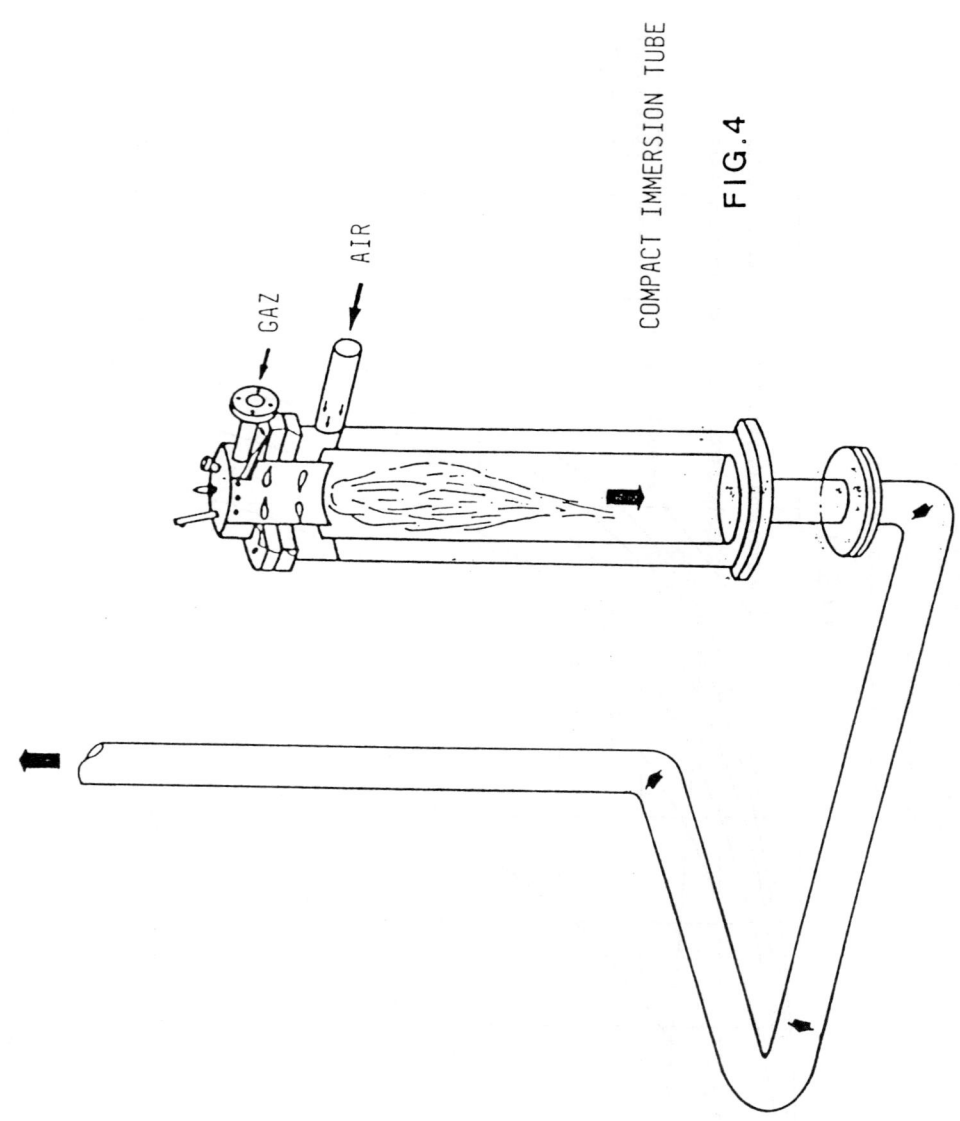

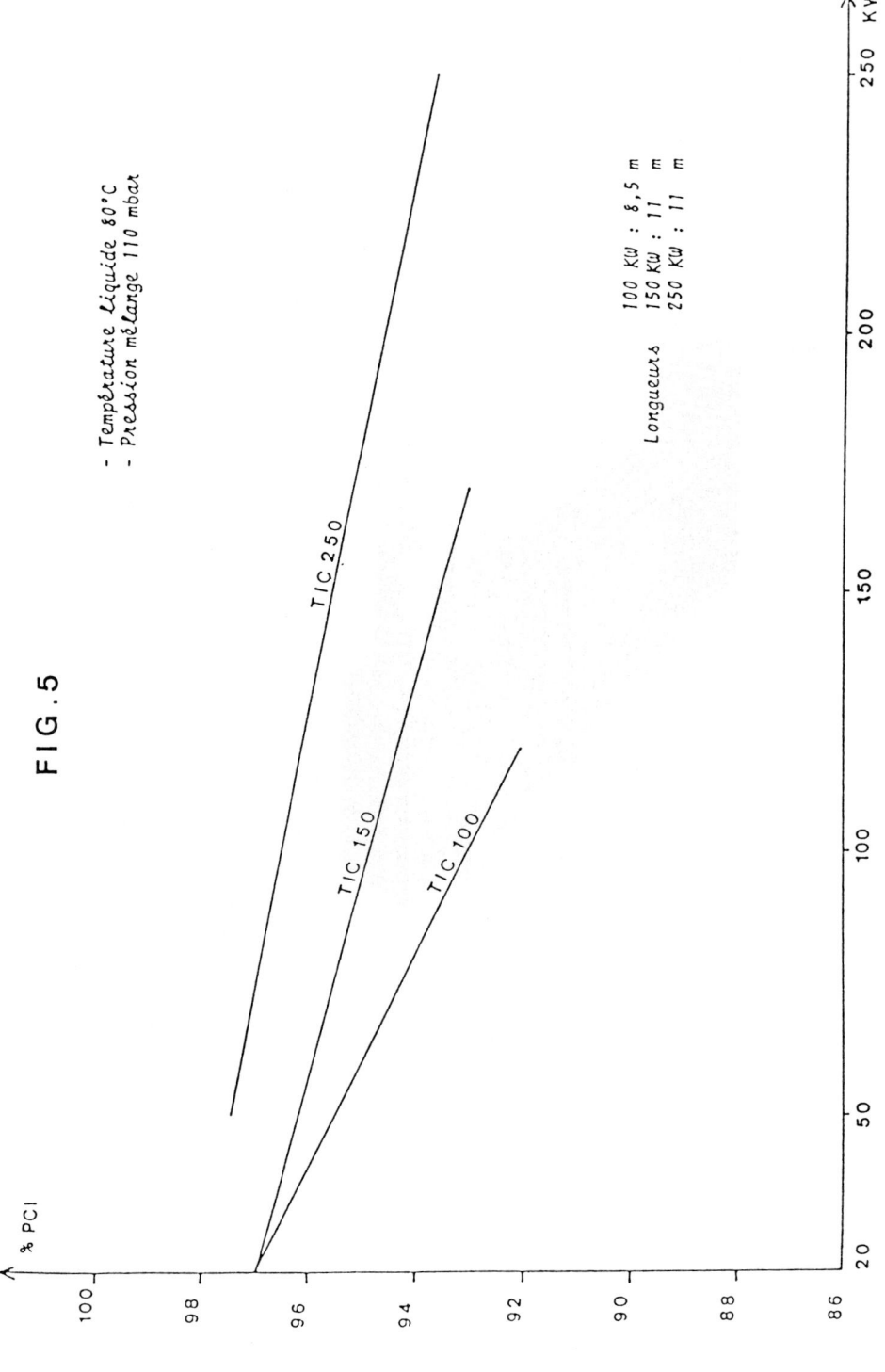

FIG. 6

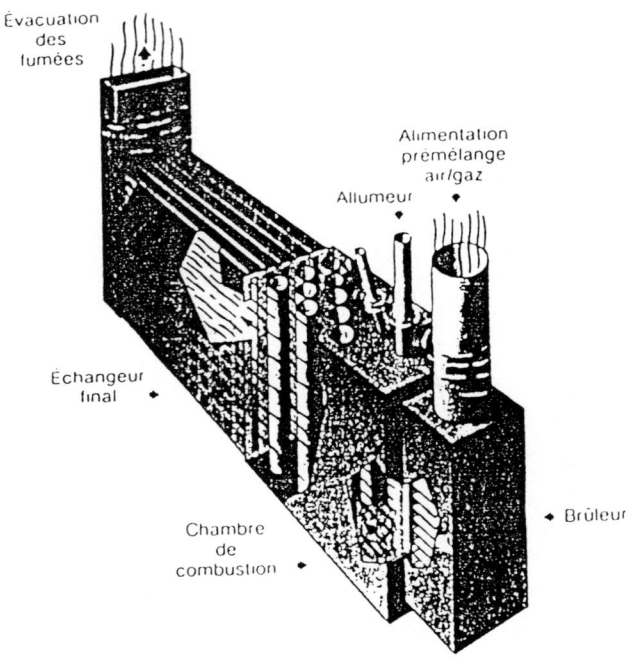

COMPACT IMMERSION EXCHANGER

FIG. 7

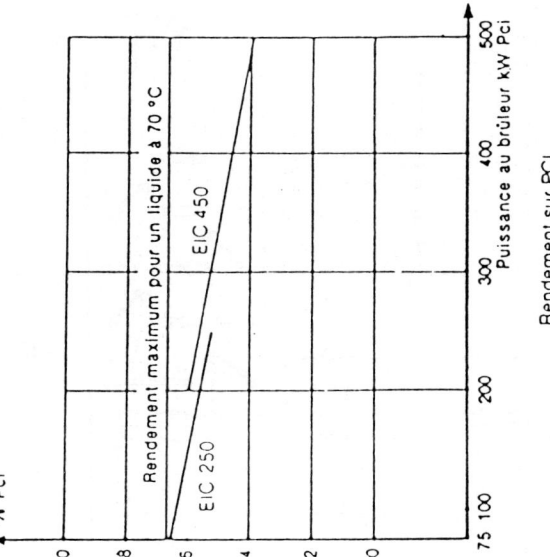

RENDEMENTS DES ECHANGEURS IMMERGES COMPACTS

HOT WATER GENERATOR SET-UP

FIG. 8

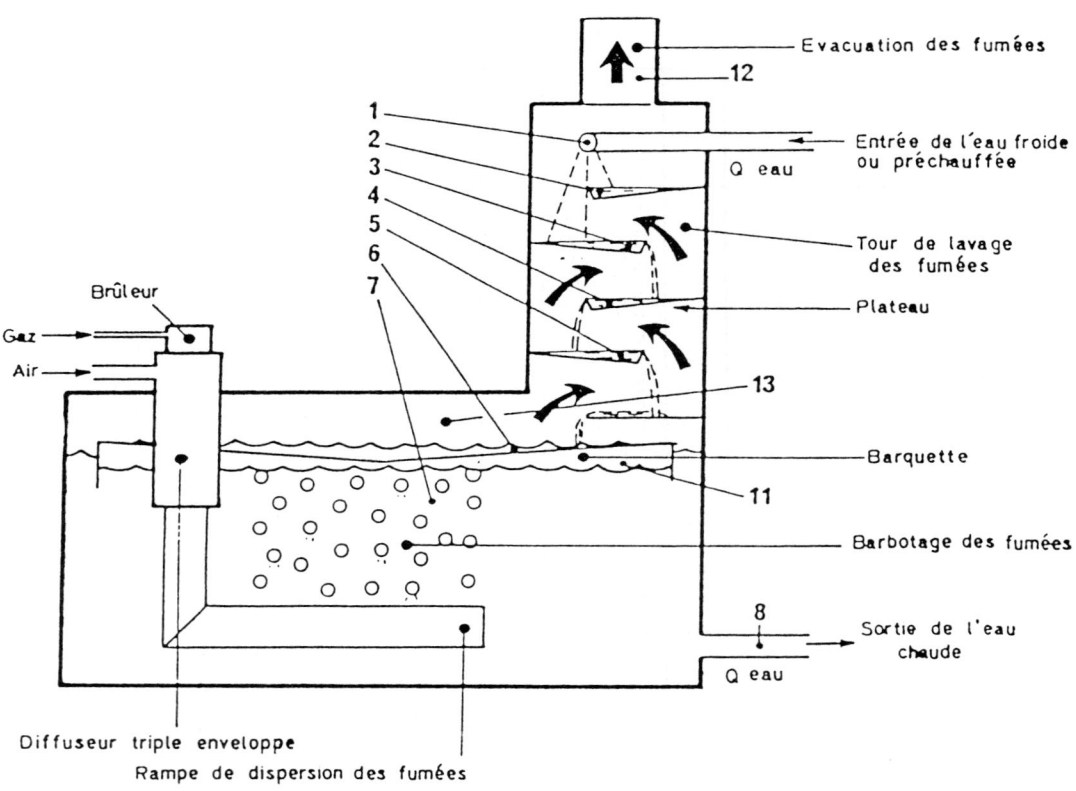

CATALYTIC RADIANT BURNER

GAS

- FIG. 9 -

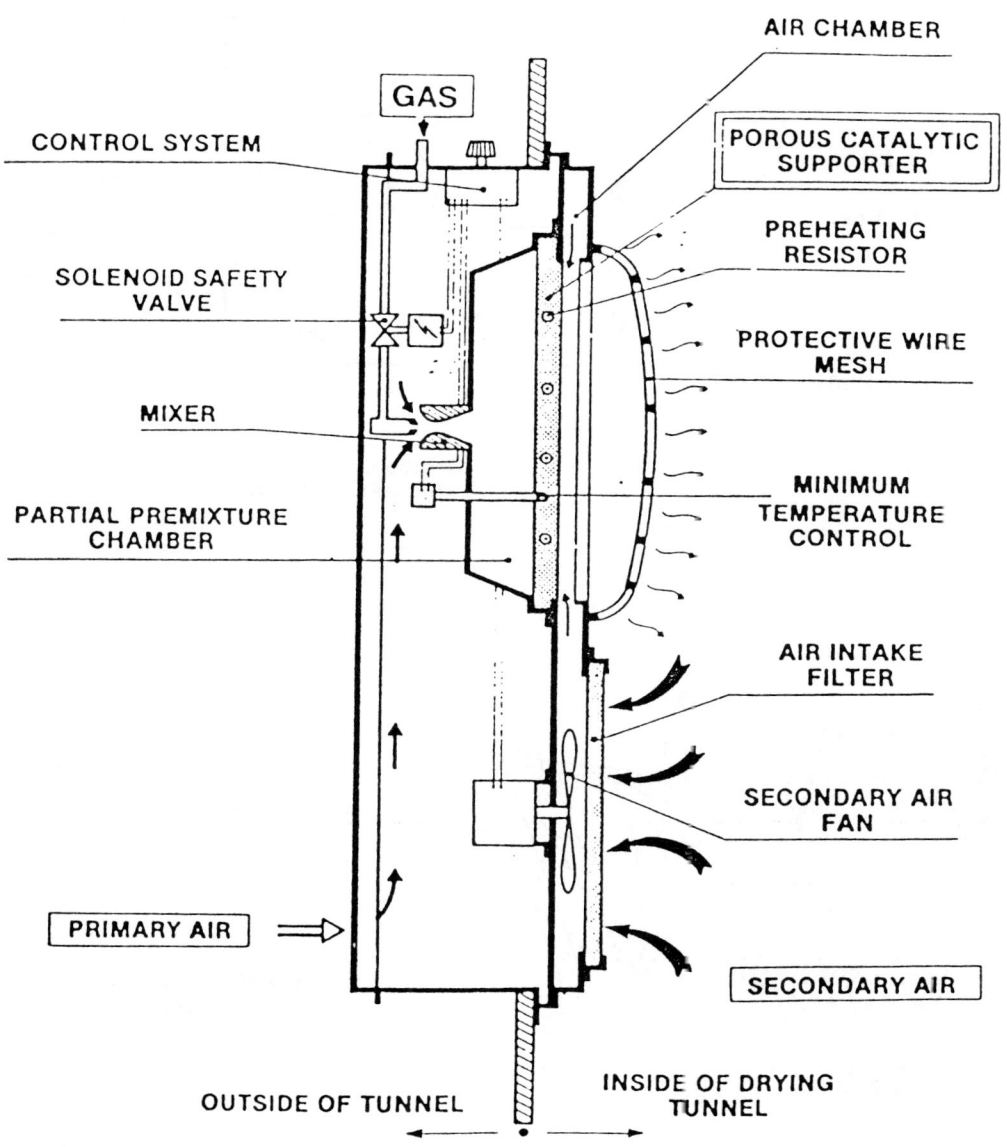

AIR HEAT BURNER
FOR INDUCT MOUNTING

FIG. 10

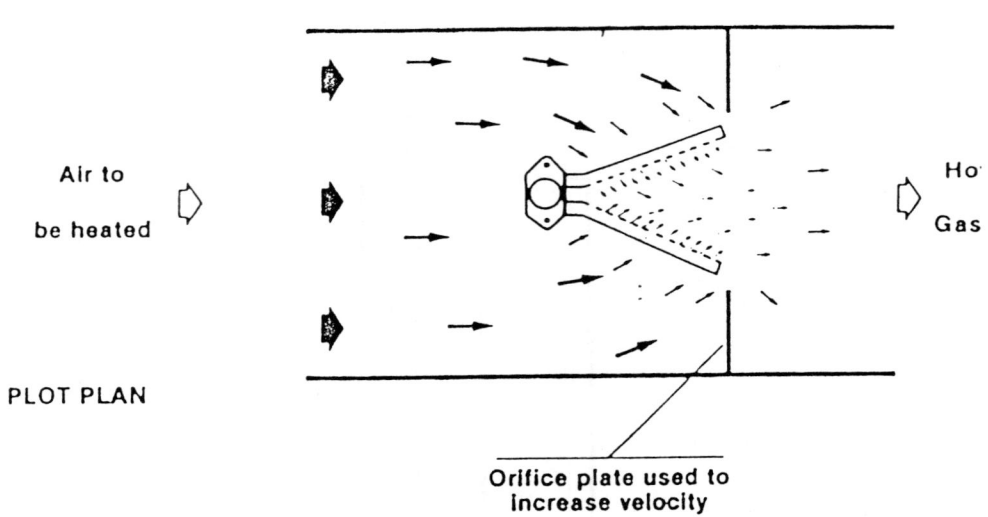

PLOT PLAN

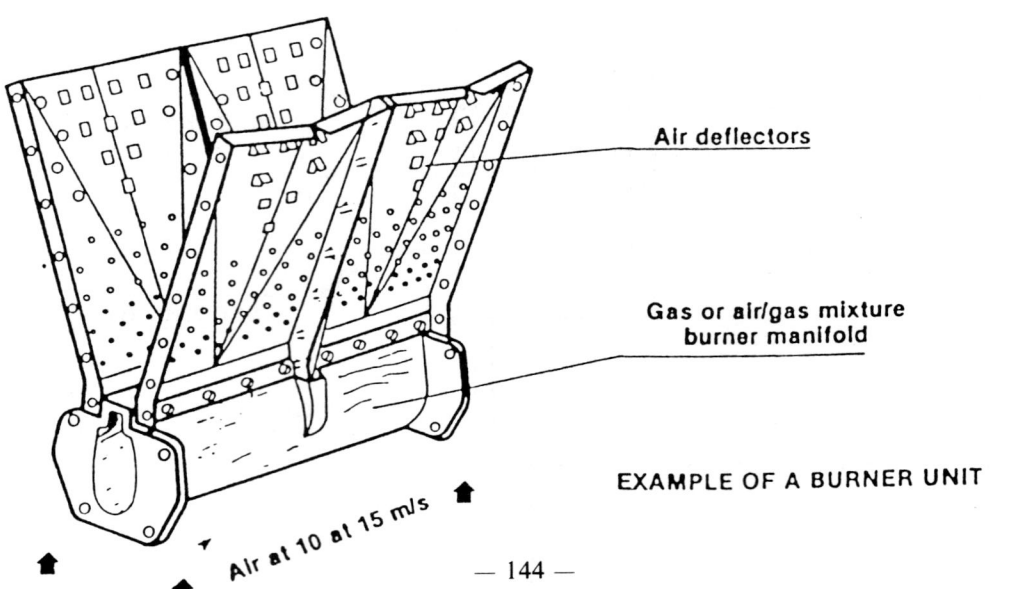

EXAMPLE OF A BURNER UNIT

Wet Catalytic Oxidation Process for Industrial Effluent Treatment

Yoshiaki Harada
Osaka Gas Co., Ltd.

Abstract

The catalytic wet oxidation process is designed to treat wastewater with the aid of a newly developed catalyst. This is a new wastewater treatment process whereby concentrated ammonia, COD (chemical oxygen demand), BOD (biochemical oxygen demand) components and suspended solids in various kinds of wastewater can be simultaneously oxidized and treated with great efficiency in a single step without dilution. The pollutants are converted into harmless N_2, CO_2 and H_2O, while the wastewater is decolored, deodorized and disinfected. Water treated in this process can be fully recycled to meet industrial requirements.

To date, the process has proven its applicability to more than 40 kinds of wastewater. These include sewage, night soil and industrial wastewater from pharmaceutical, paper, textile, dyeing, food and petrochemical plants as well as from coal gasification and liquification.

An 11,000-hour (approximately) catalyst life test on gas liquor from a coke oven, containing undecomposable components difficult to treat with conventional biochemical processes, demonstrated continuous catalytic activity.

To date, the process has been refined to commercial grade through the construction and operation of a test plant, evaluation of catalysts, confirmation of equipment materials and a chemical engineering approach to scaling-up.

Comparison of this process with conventional processes

The conventional noncatalytic wet oxidation process, called the Zimmerman Process after its inventor, has been widely applied to the treatment of wastewater containing concentrated COD components. It is now used at over 80 plants in Japan and over 300 plants abroad.

However, the Zimmerman Process has these drawbacks: the COD removal rate is not high and ammonia components can hardly be removed. This process thus requires combinations of diverse formulae for advanced treatment.

In the wet oxidation process, this limitation has been overcome by the successful development of powerfully acting catalysts. The catalytic wet oxidation process features economy and continuous, stable operation.

We hope this process will be adopted at many plants for energy efficient treatment and reuse of wastewater.

Contents

Abstract

1. Thermodynamic Treatment Process 1

2. Catalytic Wet Oxidation Process 2
   2-1 Summary 2
   2-2 Introduction 3
   2-3 Wet oxidation process (Zimmerman Process — conventional method) 6
   2-4 Catalytic wet oxidation process 7
      (1) Overview 7
      (2) Conditions of reaction 10
      (3) Treatment of wastewater (gas liquor) from coke oven .. 11
      (4) Treatment of night soil 15
      (5) Treatment of heat separated liquid from sewage sludge 17
      (6) Treatment of heat decomposed wastewater from municipal refuse 22
      (7) Treatment of wastewater containing organic chlorine compounds 24
      (8) Application to other industrial wastewaters .. 26
      (9) Features of the catalytic wet oxidation process 30
   2-5 References 31

1. Thermodynamic Treatment Process

The wet oxidation process is a standard method for thermodynamic wastewater treatment, in which components dissolved or suspended in the water are decomposed by oxidation to recover the resulting oxidation (combustion) energy as steam or other power source. The Zimmerman Process features non-catalytic wet oxidation, while the newly developed process features catalytic wet oxidation.

Oxygen (air) is used as an oxidizer at high temperature and pressure. Oxidation requires the presence of water in the reaction system (i.e. water maintained in liquid phase). A reactor is maintained below the critical temperature of water, 374°C. Unlike other combustion methods, thermodynamic processes do not require vapor condensation or dehydration. The catalytic wet oxidation process differs sharply from the wet oxidation process in its capacity for treating suspended solids in wastewater. In what follows, the catalytic wet oxidation process is compared with the wet oxidation process.

2. Catalytic Wet Oxidation Process

2-1 Summary

This process is a method for the advanced treatment of wastewater designed to subject highly concentrated pollutants contained in it to wet oxidation with the aid of a newly developed solid catalyst.

This is a new wastewater treatment process whereby concentrated ammonia, COD (chemical oxygen demand), BOD (biochemical oxygen demand) components and suspended solids in wastewater can be simultaneously oxidized and treated with great efficiency in a single step without dilution at high temperature and pressure. The process can convert these pollutants into harmless N_2, CO_2 and H_2O without forming NOx or SOx, enabling decolorization, deodorization and disinfection. Water treated in this process can be fully recycled to meet industrial requirements.

To date, the process has proven its applicability to more than forty kinds of wastewater. These include drainage, sewage and industrial wastewater from pharmaceutical, paper, textile, dyeing, food processing and petroleum chemical plants, as well as those from coal gasification and liquification. The process has virtually no limitation on applicable wastewater. It can even be applied to those containing organic chlorine compounds (trichloroethylene, etc.). With the desired reaction conditions selected, the process can be used for advanced treatment that permits direct discharge of effluent, for efficient pretreatment for biochemical processes, and also in combination with various filming processes.

An approximately 11,000-hour catalyst life test on gas liquor from a coke oven, which contains undecomposable components difficult to treat with conventional biochemical processes, demonstrated continuous catalytic activity. Our catalyst exhibits extremely stable performance, as confirmed by the short-term tests on catalytic properties. To date, the process has been refined to commercial grade through the construction and commencement of operations at our test plant, evaluation of catalysts, confirmation of equipment materials and chemical engineering approach to the scaling-up. This paper outlines the catalytic wet oxidation process and reaction mechanism, and discusses the applicability of the process to treating various types of industrial wastewater, including gas liquor from coke ovens, night soil and heat separated liquid.

2-2 Introduction

To control wastewater pollution, moves are underway to regulate COD limits in terms of total amount and permissible nitrogen and phosphorus levels to prevent closed-water eutrophication, a phenomenon becoming more prominent in recent years, as exemplified by the introduction of environmental standards for nitrogen and phosphorus levels in lakes and marshes, effective December 25, 1983. In a bid to counteract these moves for statutory regulation, the industrial circles involved are developing step-by-step wastewater treatment processes to meet specific requirements. Because gas liquor from coke ovens and gas plants is highly contaminated with undecomposable components and because the capabilities of direct biochemical and physical treatment processes are limited, conventional processes require dilution and diverse formulae, as illustrated in Fig. 1-(A), for the removal of COD and ammonia components.

In contrast, the present innovative process can both intensively degrade COD, ammonia BOD and suspended solids in a single step without diluting the wastewater, and at the same time, decolor and deodorize the wastewater. Further it does not produce sludge. As a result, the water quality obtained through this process is equivalent to or even better than that at the outlet of the active carbon treatment process shown in Fig. 1-(A). Such an approach is optimal as an effective wastewater treatment system in that it permits reuse of the water and contributes to the development of energy-efficient water treatment technology, as required in the current period of low economic growth.

This process is characterized by subjecting pollutants to wet oxidation at high temperature and pressure to convert them in a single step into harmless nitrogen, carbon dioxide, water, etc., using newly-developed solid catalysts.

Table 1 gives a breakdown of wastewater treatment processes. The Zimmerman Process, in which noncatalytic wet oxidation occurs at high temperature and pressure, boasts good industrial reference as a pretreatment for the biochemical processing of wastewater containing highly concentrated COD components and for better dehydration of sewage sludge. However, the drawbacks of the Zimmerman Process are its limited capability to decompose COD components (removal rate: 40 to 80%) in terms of the movement toward water quality control and its failure to decompose much of the ammonia in the wastewater, with the resultant need for secondary and tertiary treatment facilities as well as exhaust gas treatment.

In the wet oxidation process, this limitation has been overcome by our successful development of powerfully acting catalysts. The catalytic wet oxidation process has been successfully commercialized.

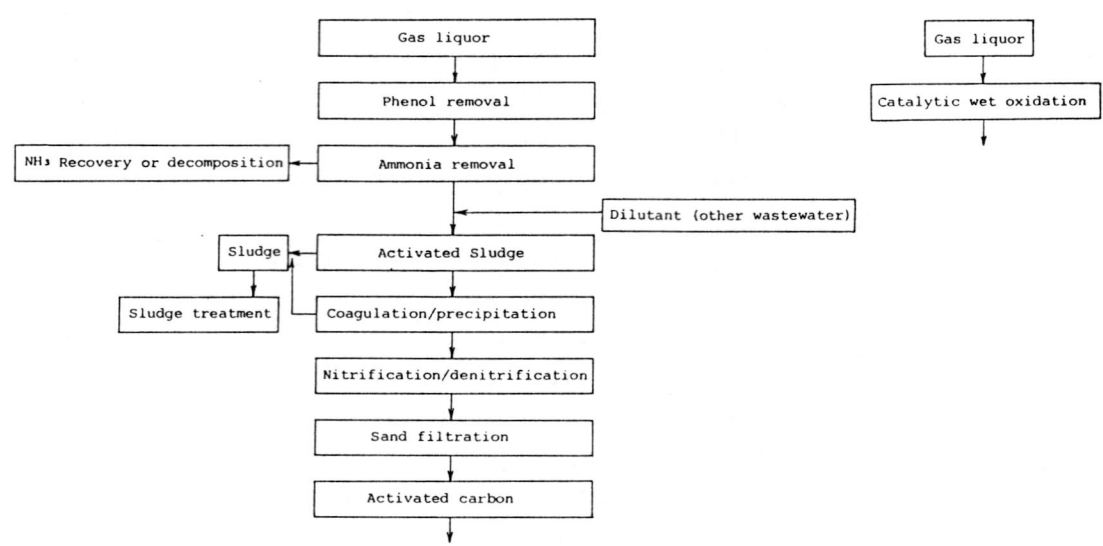

Fig. 1 Advanced treatment of gas liquor

Table 1 Wastewater treatment systems

Type	Treatment conditions	Formula			Treating time (hr)	Requirements for secondary treatment	Pollutants ability to decompose
		Oxidizer	Contact agent	Process			
Oxidation	Normal temperature (up to 50°C) and pressure	Air or O_2	Micro-organism	(Oxygen) activated sludge process	(BOD 200ppm)	Surplus sludge treatment	Undecomposable substances remain
		O_3		Ozone oxidation process	0 ~ 2	Nil	
		H_2O_2	Fe	Fenton Process	0 ~ 2	Nil	
	Intermediate Temperature (150 ~ 320°C) and high pressure	Air or O_2		Zimmerman process	0 ~ 2	Exhaust gas treatment (deodorization)	Unable to decompose ammonia, allowing organic acid to remain in the wastewater
		Air or O_2	Homogeneous catalyst		0 ~ 2	Catalytic heavy metal treatment	
		Air or O_2	Solid catalyst	OG catalytic wet oxidation process	0 ~ 2	Nil	Can thoroughly decompose, decolorize and deodorize N compounds
	High temperature (over 600°C) and Normal Pressure	Air		Incinerating process		Ash content after treatment of combustion exhaust gas	Complete combustion
Nonoxidation	Normal Temperature (up to 50°C) and Pressure		Micro-organism	Anaerobic digestion process	500 ~ 700	Surplus sludge treatment	Pretreatment
			(Absorbent)	Physical adsorption process		Adsorbent treatment	Aftertreatment
			Metallic iron	Reduction process	0 ~ 2		Dechlorination of chlorine compounds

2-3 Wet oxidation process (Zimmerman Process—conventional method)

The conventional noncatalytic wet oxidation process, called the Zimmerman Process after its inventor, was designed for the treatment of pulp mill wastewater, but its application was later expanded to the treatment of sewage sludge in Chicago and other cities in the United States. In Japan, Yokohama City uses the Zimmerman Process to treat sewage sludge, but the process is usually used for the biochemical treatment, at high temperature and pressure, of raw sludge and wastewater output from petroleum chemical plants, particularly from acrylonitrile manufacturers. The equipment is installed in over 80 plants in Japan and over 300 plants abroad, including those currently under construction.

However, the Zimmerman Process requires secondary and tertiary treatment facilities and can hardly meet current water quality standards, given its limited capability for decomposing COD and incapability of removing ammonia. Measures to deodorize waste gas at the outlet of the process are also required. Demand is growing slowly. Table 2 shows examples of treatment by the Zimmerman Process.

Table 2 Examples of treatment by Zimmerman process

		Night soil			Sewage sludge			Sewage sludge		
Temperature	℃	215 ~ 235			205 ~ 245			165		
Pressure	kg/cm²G	70			84			7.5		
Reaction time	hrs	1.3			1.0			1.0		
Process	-	Zimmerman process (non-catalytic)			Zimmerman process (non-catalytic)			Zimmerman process (non-catalytic)		
Components		Crude water	Treated water	Removal rate (%)	Crude water	Treated water *	Removal rate (%)	Crude water	Treated water*	Removal rate (%)
pH	-	7.9	8.0	-	6.7					
BOD	mg/ℓ	7,400	6,300	14.9		9.000		21,200	7,740	63.5
COD(Mn)	mg/ℓ	4,500	1,710	62.0				9,810	3,840	60.9
COD(Cr)	mg/ℓ	20,800	10,400	50.0	40,000	15,600	61.0	52,700	13,100	75.1
T - N	mg/ℓ	2,430	2,390	1.6	1,720	1,610	6.4			
NH₃-N	mg/ℓ	1,790	1,910	(Increase)	970	920	5.2			
SS	mg/ℓ	9,450	165	98.3		250		26,000	984	96.2
Sources		O city data			Satoh and Tanaka; Sewerage Association Bulletin, Vol. 15 NO.165, P. 22 (1978)			Omiya et al; Technical survey report on a small scale sludge treatment plant at Kobe city		

* Liquid liberated incidental to heat treatment

2-4 Catalytic wet oxidation process

(1) Overview

Fig. 2 shows the process flow. Raw wastewater is pressurized by a booster pump, and after pH adjustment with an alkaline solution as required, preheated by hot reactor effluent via an exchanger. After pressurization by a compressor, the air (oxygen) required for the reaction is mixed with the wastewater and fed to the furnace.

Note that if the COD concentration in the wastewater is high, the heating furnace can be by-passed except during start-up because the high temperature required for reaction can be obtained via reaction heat.

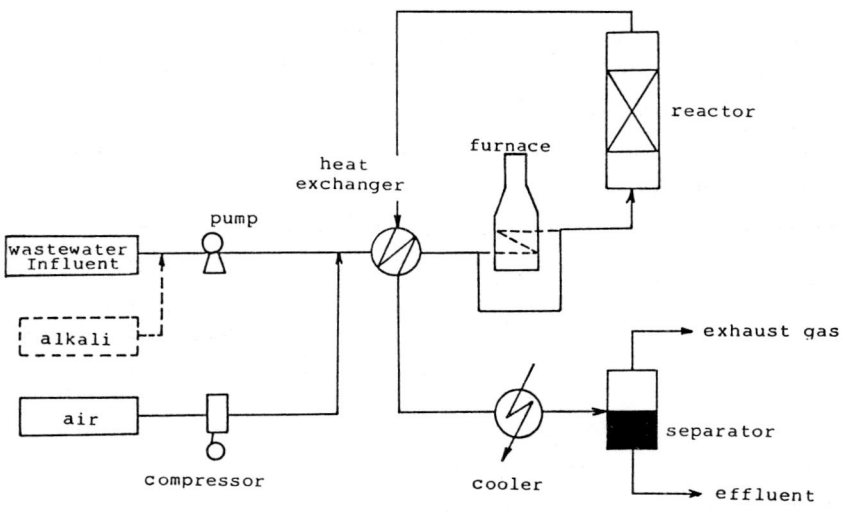

Fig. 2 Schematic process flow

Table 3 Conditions of reaction

	Range
Temperature (°C)	200 ~ 300
Pressure (kg/cm^2 G)	15 ~ 100
S V (1/hr)	0.5 ~ 10
Air ratio (vs. theoretical value)	1.05 ~ 1.2

Fig. 3 shows the interrelation between the amount of organics in the wastewater and the amount of heat required[1] (autogenous point: COD 10 g/ℓ). In this process, reaction heat derived from COD and from ammonia effectively contributes to the heat balance. Table 4 shows the heat output of various substances. The contaminants (COD, ammonia, etc.) admitted into the catalyst-packed reactor at specified temperature and pressure are decomposed under the reaction formulae specified in Table 5. As shown in Table 6, COD components are decomposed into carbonic acid gas or water via an intermediate product, which is a low molecular weight carboxylic acid. Waste gas discharged from the reactor contains neither NOx nor SOx and is odor free. The mixed gas-liquid stream output from the reactor is cooled and the heat recovered before being separated into gas and liquid as required and discharged out of the system.

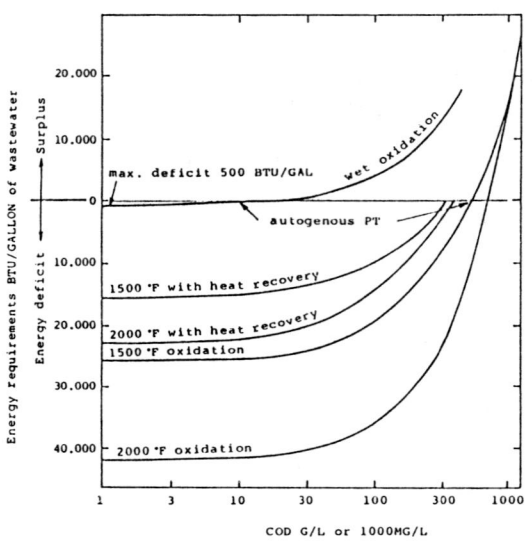

Fig. 3 Amount of organics in the wastewater; heat requirements[1] (comparison of wet oxidation and combustion processes)

Table 4 Heat output of various substances

Substance	Combustion heat	
	Kcal/kg	Kcal/kg (oxygen consumption)
Acetic acid	3,485	3,270
Oxalic acid	668	3,750
Pyridine	8,310	3,280
Phenol	7,608	3,260
Ethanol	6,806	3,400
Cellulose	3,744	3,490
Sulfite effluent	4,390	3,320
Sewage active sludge	3,635	3,040
Alanine	4,379	3,248

Table 5 Decomposition reaction

1) Nitrogen compounds (nitrogen compounds, such as of ammonia, cyanide etc.) → Decomposed into N_2, H_2O and CO_2 Ex. $NH_3 + 3/4O_2 \rightarrow 1/2N_2 + 3/2H_2O$
2) Organics (hydrocarbon, common BOD, COD components, etc.) → Decomposed into H_2O and CO_2 Ex. $C_6H_5OH + 7O_2 \rightarrow 6CO_2 + 3H_2O$
3) Sulfur compound (sulfide, rhodanate, thiosulfate, etc.) → Decomposed into SO_4 salt, H_2O and CO_2 Ex. $(NH_4)_2S_2O_3 + 7/2O_2 \rightarrow N_2 + 2H_2O + 2H_2SO_4$ $NH_4SCN + 7/2O_2 \rightarrow N_2 + H_2O + CO_2 + H_2SO_4$
(Remarks: Combustible s.s. components are decomposable as above.)

Table 6 COD reaction mechanism

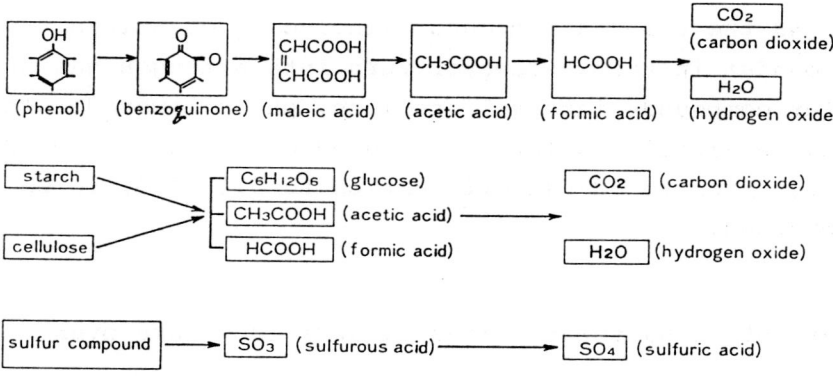

(2) Conditions of reaction

　　The conditions of reaction vary with the kind, concentration and type of contaminants in the wastewater and with the targeted water quality. Ordinarily, the requirements shown in Table 3 are applied.

2-1) Temperature and pressure

The higher the temperature and pressure, the greater the reaction rate. Sufficient pressure must be applied to keep the water in liquid phase. A reaction rate nearly proportional to partial oxygen pressure, enriching the oxygen-to-air ratio in favor of the former, or use of pure oxygen could lead to reduced temperature and pressure.

2-2) Reaction time

Prolonged reaction time (ordinarily, 0.1 to 2 hours) can enhance the decomposability of contaminants in the wastewater.

2-3) Amount of oxygen

Such contaminants can be decomposed by a volume of oxygen 1.05 ∿ 1.2 times the theoretical value derived from the decomposition reaction formula above.

2-4) pH

As the ammonia compounds (including organic nitrogen compounds) in the wastewater turn into nitrogen gas and the sulfur compounds into sulfate ions, pH is lowered. Therefore, an alkaline solution is added either before or during the reaction to adjust effluent pH to 5.8 ∿ 8.6, to be safely discharged.

(3) Treatment of wastewater (gas liquor) from coke oven

Table 7 shows gas liquor treatment performance of a test plant composed of 12 inch reactors (wastewater treatment capacity has been expanded from 6 to 60 m^3/day, as per Fig. 4). It is currently in operation at the Torishima Plant, OG. The catalytic wet oxidation process decomposes highly concentrated COD and ammonia components to 10 ppm or less after a 24-minute reaction (SV = 2.5 Hr^{-1}), and phenol and cyanide to less than the detectable limit, in addition to thoroughly removing suspended solids. Likewise, NOx and SOx concentrations in the exhaust gas were reduced below the prescribed lower limits (0.5 and 2.0 mg/Nm^3 respectively), with no signs of growth.

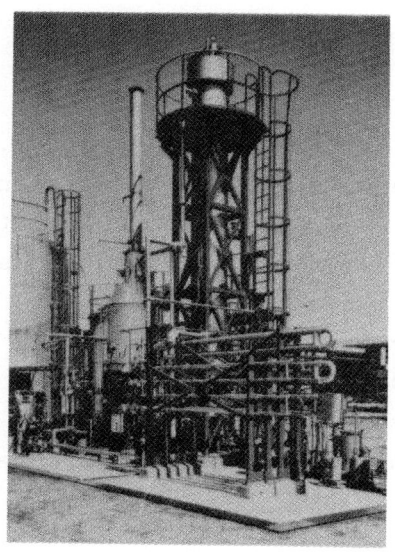

Capacity: Originally 6 m^3/d, currently scaled up to 60 m^3/d

(Successfully completed under state subsidy granted by the Agency of Industrial Science & Technology, MITI in 1979)

Fig. 4 Appearance of test plant

Table 7 Typical gas liquor treatment by OG catalytic wet oxidation process

Treatment conditions	temperature (°C)	pressure (kg/cm^{2}G)	liquor volume (ℓ/h)	air volume (Nm^3/h)	S.V. (1/h)	catalyst				
	250	70	200	14.4	2.5	Type A				
Raw wastewater and effluent	Components analyzed	PH	NH$_3$N	COD	TOD	phenol	T-N	CN$^-$	S.S.	odor
	Raw wastewater (mg/ℓ)	10.5	3,080	5,870	17,500	1,700	3,750	15	60	ammoniac and phenolic odor
	Effluent (mg/ℓ)	6.4	3	<10	N.D.	N.D.	160	N.D.	N.D.	odorless
	Decomposition rate (%)	—	99.9<	99.8<	99.9<	99.9<	95.7	99.9<	99.9<	—
Exhaust gas composition	Ingredients	N$_2$ (%)	O$_2$ (%)	CO$_2$ (%)	NO$_x$ (mg/Nm^3)	SO$_x$ (mg/Nm^3)	NH$_3$-N (mg/Nm^3)	odor		
	Composition	83.1	9.9	7.0	N.D.	N.D.	N.D.	Nil		

It is assumed that the reaction mechanism, especially the catalytic COD reaction mechanism, provides a complex, sequentially competing reaction which produces low molecular weight carbonic acid as an intermediate product. Reaction rate formulae matching the results of the experiment are as follows:

$$-d(XNH_3)/dt = K_1(CNH_3)(PO_2)$$
$$-d(XCOD)/dt = K_2(CCOD)^2(PO_2)$$

As a result of the noncatalytic treatment of gas liquor, no decomposition of ammonia is seen and the COD decomposition rate is only about one - one hundredth (1/100) that of catalytically treated gas liquor. Even after 2- to 3-fold extensions of reaction time, the residual COD value of about 1,000 ppm remained little changed in the effluent.

Our tests have confirmed that our catalyst exhibits extremely stable performance. For instance, an 11,000 hour catalyst life test on gas liquor from a coke oven demonstrated continuous catalytic activity (see Fig. 5).

Fig. 6 shows the results of case studies on material and heat balance after treatment of gas liquor at a rate of 40 m^3/hr.

The reaction rate constants of COD and ammonia components are correlated to the reaction temperature (150 ~ 280°C) in gas liquor (pH 10.5) as follows:

$$\text{LOGK COD} = 4.72 - \frac{2,020}{T(\cdot K)}$$

$$\text{LOGK NH}_3 = 22.72 - \frac{9,119}{T(\cdot K)}$$

Fig. 7 presents the relationships between COD concentrations and reaction time at 225°C, 250°C and 270°C. Ammonia components were decomposed faster than COD.

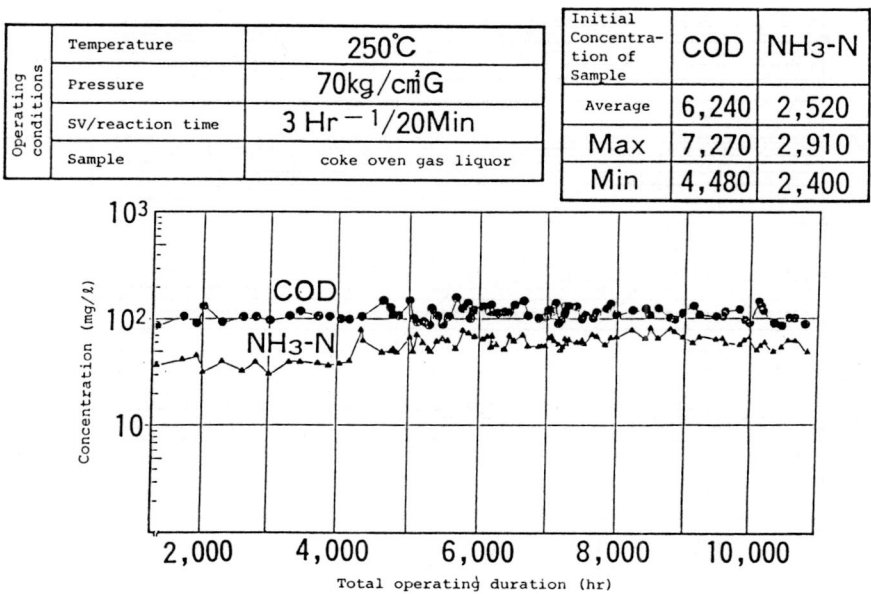

Fig. 5 Continuous activity test results: gas liquor

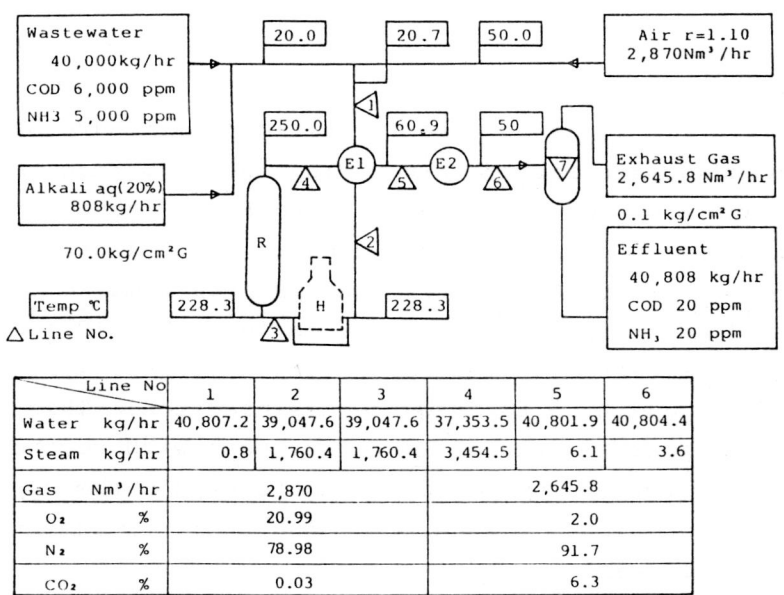

Fig. 6 Case studies on gas liquor (material and heat balances)

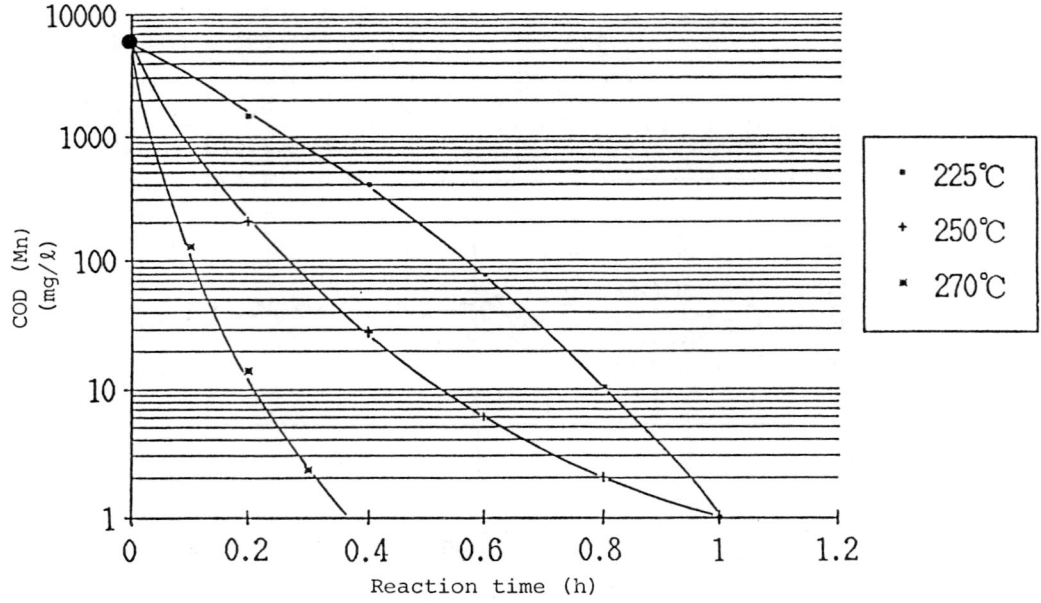

Fig. 7 Relationships between COD decomposition and reaction time

(4) Treatment of night soil

　　Several techniques to treat night soil have been developed and commercialized, including the Zimmerman and other biochemical processes. Table 8 and Fig. 8 show the results of treating night soil, collected in T city, using our new process. Specifically, this new process removed COD, ammonia and suspended solids, etc., to less than 10 ppm in a single step without dilution. Odor and color were also removed, in addition to adequate disinfection. This process does not generate sludge, and dispenses with secondary treatment facilities. We are planning to expand the application of this nondilutive process to night soil treatment on a commercial scale.

Table 8 Example test results on night soil

Operating conditions	Temperature	℃	250	250	250	280
	Pressure	kg/cm²G	70	80	90	90
	Initial pH	—	9.0	9.0	9.0	9.0
	Reaction time	Hr	1.0	1.0	1.0	1.0
Item	Raw wastewater		Effluent	Effluent	Effluent	Effluent
pH	6.85	—	7.2	6.9	7.0	7.3
COD (Mn)	4,900	mg/ℓ	34	4	3	4
NH$_3$-N	3,090	mg/ℓ	2	2	2	6
TOD	26,600	mg/ℓ	555	N.D	N.D	N.D
TC	7,100	mg/ℓ	890	730	700	520
TOC	6,200	mg/ℓ	340	50	N.D	20
BOD$_5$	15,300	mg/ℓ	518	71	24	7
P	100	mg/ℓ	1.9	3.1	1.1	0.7
SS	20,000	mg/ℓ	1.9	2	N.D	N・D

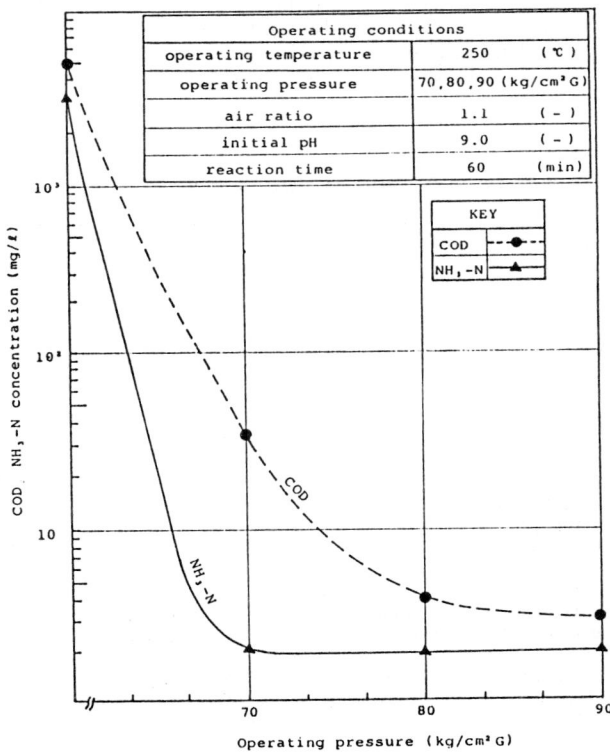

Fig. 8 Typical test results on night soil

(5) Treatment of heat separated liquid from sewage sludge

The conventional biochemical processes limit the COD removal rate to about 50%. As a result of joint research with Yokohama City, this new process offers satisfactory results[4],[5]. Table 9 lists the specifications of the test equipment, and Table 10 the items measured and analytical methods of the heat separated liquid, effluent and exhaust gas treated in this process. Figs. 9, 10, 11, and Tables 11 and 12 show the results of tests targeted to reduce COD to below 20 ppm, at which the effluent can be freely discharged.

Table 9 Specifications of test equipment

Type	Continuous flow type
Capacity	84 ℓ/d
Reactor	$1\frac{1}{2}B \times 4,100L$
Heating system	External heating by sheath heater
Maximum operating pressure	100 kg/cm^{2}G
Maximum operating temperature	300°C

Table 10 Measured items

pH	Sewage testing method (1974)
COD Hn	"
COD Cr	"
BOD	"
TK-N	"
T-N	"
NH$_2$-N	"
NO$_2$-N	"
NO$_3$-N	"
SS	"
T-P	JIS K 0102
Chromaticity	JIS K 0101
Transparency	Sewage testing method
TOD	TOC-TC C-2 (Toray)
TC	" "
TOC	" "
IC	" "
O$_2$	JIS B 7933 Magnetic power method, PHA200 (Hitachi Horiba magnetic type)
CO$_2$	Orsat gas analytical method, VIA-800 (Hitachi Horiba nondispersed infrared analyzer)
N$_2$	
NCx	JIS K 0104 Chemical emission method, ECL-77A (Yanagimoto)
SOx	JIS K 0103 Hydrogen peroxide absorption method

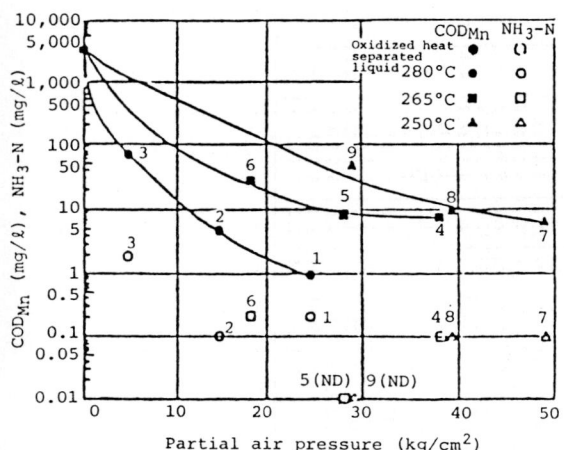

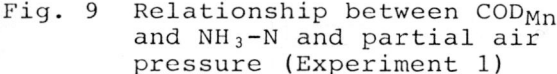

Fig. 9 Relationship between COD_{Mn} and NH_3-N and partial air pressure (Experiment 1)

Fig. 10 Relationship between COD_{Mn} and reaction time (Experiment 1)

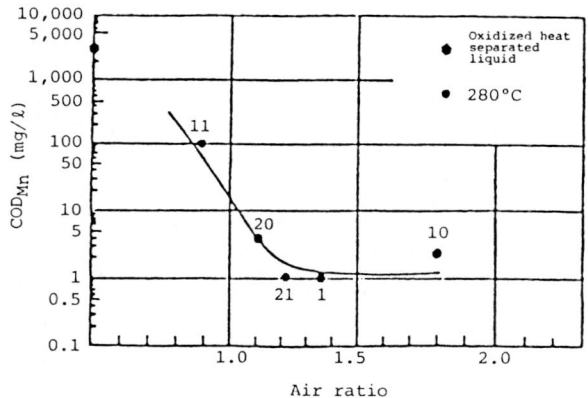

Fig. 11 Relationship between COD_{Mn} and air ratio (Experiment 1)

Table 11 Water quality test results

RUN No	operating conditions						analytical data on effluent															analytical data on exhaust gas			
	tempera-ture	pres-sure	reac-tion time	liquid air volume	air ratio	pH	pH	COD Mn	COD Cr	BOD	T-N	NH₃-N	NO₂-N	NO₃-N	T-N	SS	T-P	trans-paren-cy	chro-matic-ity	TOD	TC	TOC	IC	BOD/COD	O₂	CO₂	N₂	NOx	SOx
	℃	kg/cm²	min	ℓ/hour	-	-	-	mg/ℓ	mg/ℓ	mg/ℓ	mg/ℓ	mg/ℓ	mg/ℓ	mg/ℓ	mg/ℓ	mg/ℓ	mg/ℓ	°	°	mg/ℓ	mg/ℓ	mg/ℓ	mg/ℓ	-	Vol%	Vol%	Vol%	ppm	ppm
raw waste-water							7.4	3,100	16,000	7,300	1,700	1,000	N.D	0.8	1,700	510	49	-	7,700	18,000	5,800	5,000	800	2.4	-	-	-	-	-
I-1	230	90	82.8	2.17	1.36	9.0	6.9	1.0	24	11	N.D	0.2	0.02	180	180	1	1.3	100	51	N.D	425	8	417	11	-	-	-	-	-
I-2	230	80	87.6	2.06	1.48	9.0	6.7	5.0	130	110	0.5	0.1	N.0	190	190	2	5.5	90	35	N.D	568	40	528	22	-	-	-	-	-
I-3	230	70	87.6	2.06	1.71	9.0	6.7	71	1,500	1,200	11	1.8	2.4	130	140	2	7.1	100	20	520	755	278	477	17	-	-	-	-	-
I-4	265	90	84.0	2.14	1.37	9.0	6.6	8.1	210	130	2.0	0.1	N.D	200	200	1	26	100	35	N.0	670	95	575	22	-	-	-	-	-
I-5	265	80	85.2	2.12	1.48	9.0	6.6	8.2	220	180	1.9	0.1	N.D	190	190	1	18	100	26	N.D	608	88	520	22	11.6	5.0	83.4	-	-
I-6	265	70	87.6	2.06	1.62	9.0	6.7	26	660	450	4.2	0.2	0.04	170	170	3	16	100	19	430	670	243	427	17	7.1	6.3	86.6	-	-
I-7	250	90	82.8	2.17	1.35	9.0	7.0	6.2	170	100	1.0	0.1	0.03	210	210	1	16	50	51	N.D	550	65	485	16	8.2	6.5	85.3	-	-
I-8	250	80	87.6	2.06	1.42	9.0	7.0	9.1	250	160	0.7	0.1	0.03	210	210	3	18	18	41	N.D	630	90	540	18	15.1	3.3	81.6	-	-
I-9	250	70	82.8	2.17	1.43	9.0	7.1	43	890	740	3.1	N.D	1.3	81	81	2	18	12	110	730	910	365	545	17	8.7	6.5	84.8	-	-
I-10	230	90	68.4	2.64	1.80	9.0	6.6	2.3	46	19	0.1	0.1	N.D	310	310	0.9	13	100	42	N.D	475	25	450	8.3	8.0	8.0	90.7	N.D	N.D
I-11	230	90	54.0	3.33	0.89	9.0	6.5	98	2,200	1,600	11	0.5	4.4	220	240	0.1	21	50	37	2,130	1,180	750	430	16	7.2	6.7	86.1	-	-
I-12	230	90	52.2	3.33	1.33	9.0	7.0	16	220	240	4.1	0.2	5.2	210	210	0.1	20	16	33	N.D	530	138	392	15	12.4	4.6	83.0	-	-
I-13	230	90	33.6	1.79	1.12	9.0	6.8	8.8	140	83	1.7	0.4	0.21	310	310	5	7.5	42	18	N.D	348	70	278	9.4	9.5	6.3	84.2	-	-
I-14	230	90	52.2	1.79	1.33	9.0	6.8	37	470	360	5.0	1.2	5.4	430	440	3	6.0	10	37	N.D	435	220	215	9.7	8.7	6.4	84.9	-	-
I-15	230	90	36.0	3.34	1.33	9.0	6.9	39	1,100	950	4.3	0.6	0.3	220	220	0.5	13	30	20	760	680	370	310	24	13.1	4.1	82.8	-	-
I-16	230	90	18.0	3.35	1.32	9.0	5.9	230	3,700	2,100	14	7.4	14	180	210	28	19	19	110	3,750	1,550	1,180	370	9.1	10.0	5.5	84.8	-	-
I-17	250	70	35.0	1.66	1.21	9.0	5.7	190	3,300	2,000	11	4.9	5.3	190	190	1	20	100	46	1,200	1,400	1,330	70	12	9.4	5.5	84.1	0.1	-
I-18	250	70	73.8	1.62	1.32	9.0	6.8	11	220	130	1.6	0.4	0.92	280	280	4	9.2	55	54	N.D	610	110	500	16	11.2	5.4	83.4	-	-
I-19	250	70	111.6	1.61	1.27	9.0	6.7	2.0	66	31	0.9	N.D	0.06	90	91	2	12	100	23	N.D	523	38	485	16					

Table 12 Behavior of carboxylic acids in heat separated liquid from sewage sludge

Reaction conditions	Temperature	250°C
	Pressure	70 kg/cm^{2}G
	Reaction time	1.5 Hr
	Initial pH	9.0
	Sample solution	heat separated liquid from sewage sludge
	Raw sewage (mg/ℓ)	Effluent (mg/ℓ)
COD	3,800	5.0
BOD	8,600	57
BOD/COD	2.3	11.4
HCOOH (formic acid)	6,300	7
CH$_3$COOH (acetic acid)	460	1
CH$_3$CH$_2$COOH (propionic acid)	150	1
NH$_3$-N	1,000	N.D

Table 13 Example of treatment of heat separated liquid from sewage sludge in K city

			Heat separated liquid from sewage sludge in K city		
Testing conditions	Temperature (°C)		250		
	Pressure (kg/cm^2)		70		
	Initial pH (−)		6.9		
	SV value (1/Hr)		1.0		
	Reaction time (min)		60		
	Item	Unit	water quality		
			raw wastewater concentration	effluent concentration	removal rate (%)
Testing results	pH	−	5.45	5.85	−
	chromaticity	°	2,880	24	99.2
	transparency	"	1	30<	97<
	COD (Mn)	mg/ℓ	3,670	7.5	99.8
	BOD	"	6,900	12	99.8
	total-N	"	970	6.6	99.3
	NH$_3$-N	"	38.3	1.8	99.5
	NO$_2$-N	"	1.0	N.D	−
	NO$_3$-N	"	N.D	1.0	−
	CN$^-$	"	<0.1	N.D	−
	SCN$^-$	"	N.D	N.D	−
	phenol	"	0.9	0.1	88.9
	suspended solids	"	1,000	1.0	99.9
	oil content	"	4.1	0.5	87.8
	total residuals on evaporation	"	9,400	1,500	84.0
	TOD	"	13,000	N.D	99<
	TC	"	3,525	148	95.8
	TOC	"	3,325	<10	99<
	P	"	160	0.5	99<
	appearance and odor	−	brown, stinking odor	pale yellow, nearly odorless	−
Treated gas	NOx, SOx	mg/Nm^3	undetected		−
	odor	−	nearly odorless		−

These experiments demonstrated the following relationships between reaction conditions and effluent:

(a) A temperature of 280°C, a pressure of 90 kg/cm², a reaction time of more than 75 minutes and an air ratio of more than 1.2 are required to obtain an effluent with COD_{Mn} of less than 20 mg/ℓ and BOD of less than 20 mg/ℓ.

(b) A temperature of 250°C, a pressure of 70 kg/cm², a reaction time of more than 70 minutes and an air ratio of more than 1.3, or a temperature of 280°C, pressure of 90 kg/cm², a reaction time of more than 45 minutes and an air ratio of more than 1.1 are required to obtain an effluent with COD_{Mn} of less than 20 mg/ℓ. However, in this instance, since BOD is as high as 300 mg/ℓ, the effluent should be returned to the sewage treatment system for secondary treatment. In both (a) and (b), ammonia is reduced below 20 mg/ℓ.

(c) Various carboxylic acids contained in the heat separated liquid are decomposed in this process. (See Table 12.)

In view of the outcome, this process could be effective as a method of reducing the return rate of heat separated liquid. This process was found effective not only by itself, but in combination with a secondary process (a biochemical process) even in places where sewage sludge is concentrated to make the return rate higher than normal. Table 13 presents the results of treatment of heat separated liquid in K city, where each component was removed at a high rate similar to Yokohama City.

(6) Treatment of heat decomposed wastewater from municipal refuse

COD components were relatively well decomposed in a short time when heat decomposed wastewater from municipal refuse was treated in this process (See Fig. 12). Similarly, with the heat separated liquid the effluent was decolored and deodorized sufficiently (See Table 14).

Table 14 Treatment of heat decomposed wastewater from municipal refuse

			Wastewater from H plant			Wastewater from T plant		
Testing conditions	temperature (°C)		250			250		
	pressure (kg/cm^2)		70			70		
	initial pH (-)		9.95			10.5		
	SV value (1/Hr)		1.85			1.91		
	reaction time (min)		32			31		
	Item	Unit	raw sewage	effluent	removal ratio (%)	raw sewage	effluent	removal ratio (%)
Testing conditions	appearance	—	dark brown	closely resembles water supply	—	dark brown	closely resembles water supply	—
	chromaticity	°	4,000	30	99<			
	transparency	"	6	30<				
	pH	—	8.6	1.75		8.3	6.35	
	BOD (5)	mg/ℓ	2,600	<0.5	99.9	6,200	1,300	79
	COD (Mn)	"	3,770	20.2	99.5	5,867	60	99
	total-N	"	4,200	26.2	99.4	4,800	21	99.6
	NH$_3$-N	"	3,900	N.D	99.9<	1,717	2.9	99.8
	NO$_2$-N	"	0.2	N.D		0.8	8.9	
	NO$_3$-N	"	2.0	20		1.4	4.0	
	TOD	"	19,500	236	99.9	21,800	1,700	92.2
	TC	"	2,767	109	96.1	5,700	940	93.1
	TOC	"	2,467	73	99.8	4,800	580	87.4
	IC	"	300	36	88	900	360	62.1
	S.S	"	260	5	98.1	500	1	99<
	phenol	"	560	0.07	99.9	600	0.02	99.9<
	Cl-	"	1,300	1,300		2,400	2,400	
	CN-	"	13	<0.1	99<	120	<0.1	99.9<
	odor	—	bad odor	nearly odorless		bad odor	nearly odorless	
	exhaust gas NOx	mg/Nm^3	N.D			N.D		
	exhaust gas SOx	"	N.D			N.D		

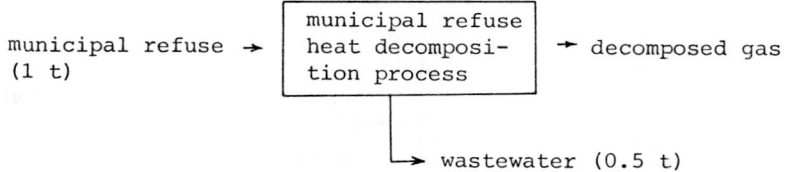

Fig. 12 Municipal refuse heat decomposition process

(7) Treatment of wastewater containing organic chlorine compounds

   Fig. 13 shows the schematic drawing for the test plant. H-1 is a tower to heat wastewater from ambient temperature up to the specified temperature, and does not contain catalysts.

   R-1, R-2 and R-3 are the catalyst-packed reactors. Wastewater flows from H-1 to R-3 via R-1 and R-2 along with air.

   Table 15 shows the GC analytical results of organic chlorine compounds.

   As the mixture passed through the catalyst-packed reactors, trichloroethylene was not detected in either the liquid or the vapor phase; chlorine ions or inorganics were found to be completely decomposed.

   When tetrachloroethylene was measured with the same equipment, more than 95% was removed in the catalyst-packed reactors, with a small amount remaining after passing through the catalytic layers. (The decomposition rate is expected to increase under optimum temperature and pressure conditions.)

   Table 16 shows the results of an autoclave test conducted on wastewater to examine the reaction of trichloroethylene. As a result, this process has been proven to decompose trichloroethylene and tetrachloroethylene. Many other organic chlorine compounds are also thought to be decomposable under appropriate conditions.

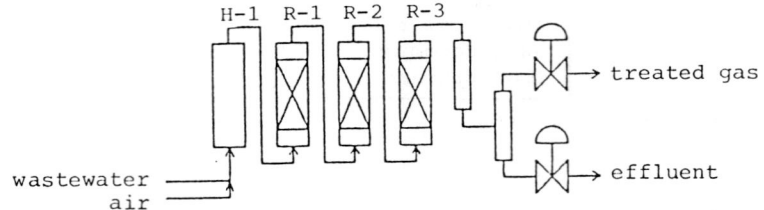

Fig. 13 Schematic drawing of test plant

Table 15 Example treatment of wastewater containing organic chlorine compounds

(250°C, 70kg/cm²G)

		raw waste-water	without catalyst (H-1)	with catalyst (R-1)	with catalyst (R-2)	with catalyst (R-3)
Reaction time/Total (hrs)			(0.51)	0.32/0.32	0.32/0.64	0.32/0.96
		raw waste-water	effluent	effluent	effluent	effluent
COD_{Mn} (ppm)		21,150	9,600	440	66	12.5
Cl^- (ppm)		2.4				130
trichloro-ethylene (ppm)	liquid phase	182	4.6×10^{-3}	0.7×10^{-3}	N.D	N.D
	vapor phase		6.1	0.5	N.D	N.D
tetrachloro-ethylene (ppm)	liquid phase	11	1.2×10^{-3}	0.7×10^{-3}	0.5×10^{-3}	0.4×10^{-3}
	vapor phase		6.6	7.3	5.9	7.7

Table 16 Autoclave test results

				raw waste-water	effluent	
					RUN1	RUN2
Reaction conditions		temperature pressure reaction time sample quantity pH catalyst amount r.p.m.	°C kg/cm^2 min ml — g rpm		280 74 60 100 11.5 10 800	250 52 60 100 11.5 10 800
Analytical results	liquid phase	pH trichloroethyl-ene	— ppm	11.5 210	9.0 2.5	9.3 2.2
	vapor phase	trichloroethyl-ene gas amount	ppm l		0.03 0.91	0.11 0.91
Trichloro-ethylene amount	liquid phase		mg	21.0	0.25	0.22
	vapor phase		mg	0	0.16	0.59
	total		mg	21.0	0.41	0.81
	recovery rate		%		98	96

(8) Application to other industrial wastewaters

　　　Table 17 shows some results of tests conducted on other kinds of industrial effluent[2],[3].

Table 17 Examples of industrial effluent treatment by OG catalytic wet oxidation process

Industrial breakdown		dyeing		alcohols		textiles		pharmaceuticals		paper mills	
Operating temperature	(°C)	250		275		250		270		250	
Operating pressure	(kg/cm²G)	46		70		70		85		70	
Intial pH	(-)	13.6		10		7.3		10.5		9.1	
Reaction time	(hr)	1.0		0.8		0.12		0.5		2.9	
Item		raw waste-water	effluent	raw waste-water	effluent	raw waste-water	effluent	raw waste-water	effluent	raw waste-water	effluent
pH	(-)	13.6	5.5	4.15	5.85	5.0	5.5	3.85	5.6	9.1	6.3
COD (Mn)	(mg/ℓ)	15,200	13	9,400	16.1	1,340	67.8	10,400	14	40,900	90
BOD	(")	33,00	28	-		5,200	3,300				
NH_3-N	(")	5	3	5.4	2.15	135.2	2.9	11	3.2		
CN-	(")										
phenol	(")					<0.1	N.D				
SS	(")										
chromaticity	(deg.)	1	0.2								
transparency	(deg.)	14	30<								

Fig. 14 shows examples of GPC measurements for dyeing wastewater, and Fig. 15 examples of FD-MASS measurements for pharmaceutical wastewater. The molecular weights of the components in the raw wastewater can be lowered by increasing the reaction conditions.

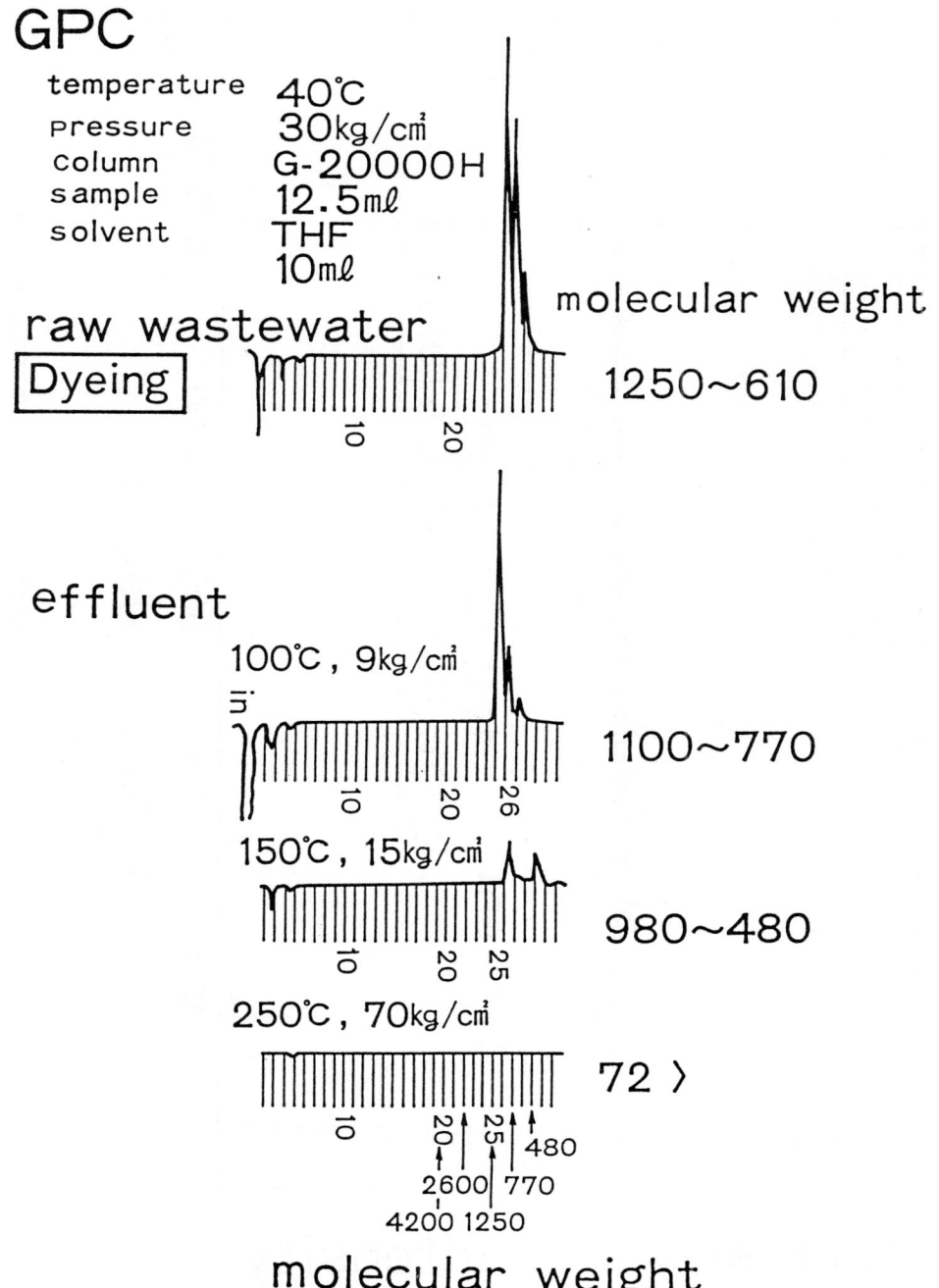

Fig. 14 Treatment conditions and example GPC measurements for wastewater from a dye plant

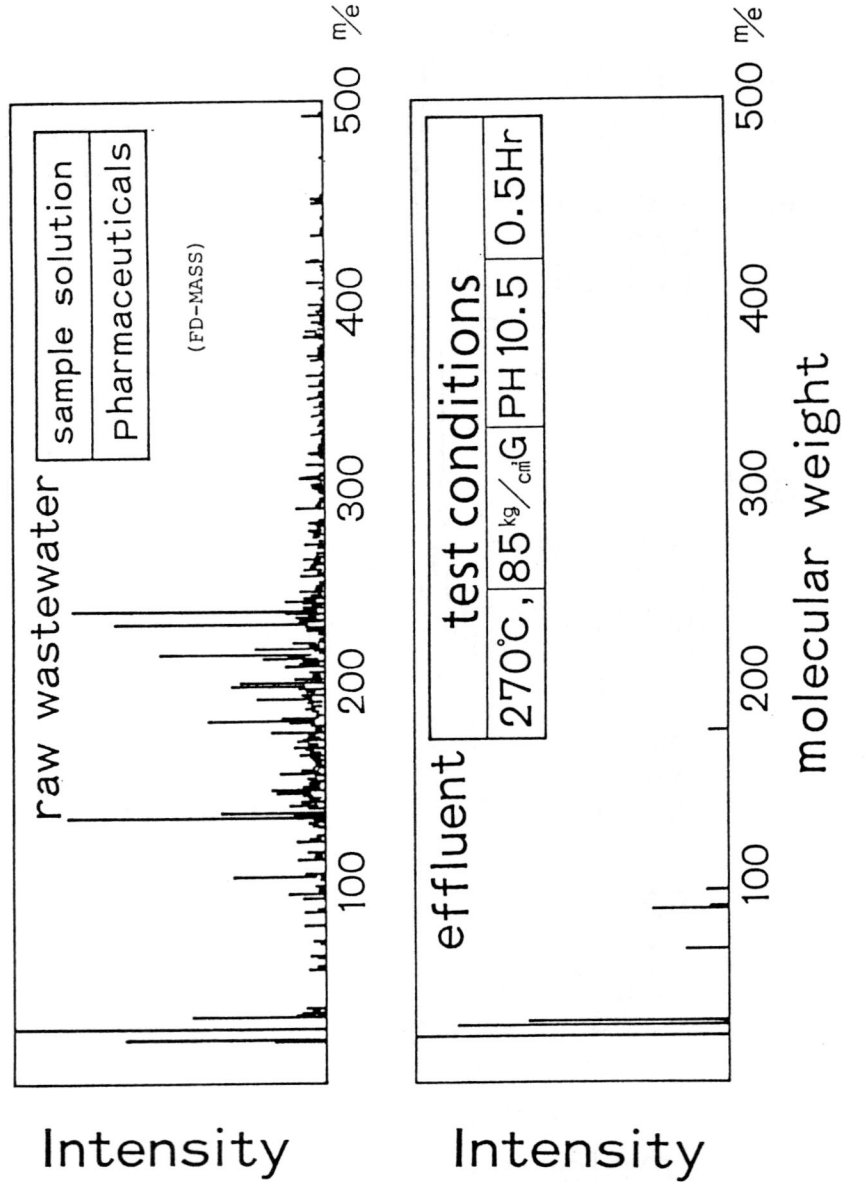

Fig. 15 Example molecular weight distribution of pharmaceutical wastewater and effluent

(9) Features of the catalytic wet oxidation process

In conclusion, the features of this process are as follows:

(1) Process
   1) Advanced single process treatment
   2) Simultaneous removal of pollutants in the wastewater, i.e., ammonia, COD, BOD, SS, etc., without dilution
   3) Simultaneous odor and color removal
   4) No NOx nor SOx, turns pollutants into harmless nitrogen gas, carbon dioxide and water
   5) No sludge generation or like byproducts

(2) Economy[2],[3],[6],[7],[8]
   The running cost is less than that of conventional processes.

(3) Operation
   Stationary state is usually reached 1 to 3 hours after start-up. Stable, continuous and automatic operation despite variations in water quality.

(4) Installation space
   The equipment is small and compact, requiring little installation space.

(5) Scope of application
   This process can be applied to various industrial effluents.

(6) Other
   1) Allows reuse of effluent.
   2) Eliminates need to treat exhaust gas.
   3) Effective utilization of reaction heat eliminates the need for heating fuel.

2-5 References

(1) A.R. Wilhelmi, C.E.P., August p.46 (1979).
(2) Y. Harada: The 28th joint study meeting on cokes (Steel Association of Japan), June 11, 1984.
(3) J. Kimoto, Y. Harada, R. Ueda and K. Katagiri: Application of catalytic wet oxidation process to various industrial wastewaters. Aromatex, Vol. 36, Nos. 7 & 8, pp. 161- 172 (1984).
(4) Nakamura and Kirihara (Yokohama City): Speeches delivered at the 21st Convention on Sewer Systems. (p. 242) (1984).
(5) Oba, Nakamura and Kirihara (Yokohama City): Sewerage Association Bulletin, Vol. 22, No. 249 (1985/2).
(6) Y. Harada et al.: Speeches delivered at the 5th Convention on Energy Sources (1986).
(7) S. Harada, K. Katagiri and Y. Harada: Chemical Apparatus, Vol. 27, No. 8, pp. 91 -95 (1985).
(8) Environmental Countermeasures Council, Pharmaceutical Association of Japan: In search for new technology III, New catalytical wet oxidation process, PA Environment News No. 6, October, 1983.
(9) H. Yamada and Y. Harada: Studies on dyeing, Vol. 28, No. 3 July, pp. 7 -19 (1982).

Moyenne température et qualité de l'air
Medium temperature and indoor air quality

THOMAS M. SMITH
MARSDEN

A NEW HIGH EMITTANCE INFRARED HEATER OFFERS OUTSTANDING CONTROL ABILITY FOR A WIDE VARIETY OF INDUSTRIAL HEAT PROCESSING APPLICATIONS AT EFFICIENCIES CLOSE TO THE THEORETICAL MAXIMUM

This paper gives a brief review of the two forms of heat transfer; conduction and radiation, followed by a comparison of the common types of gas and electric heaters used for industrial heat processing. Specifically mentioned is a new composite refractory, gas-fired infrared generator offering high powered density, outstanding fuel efficiency and unsurpassed temperature control. It is ideally suited for operations ranging from high power bulk drying to delicate curing and heatsetting. Also discussed is the combination of these unique infrared generators with mass transfer devices, material transport, and microprocessor controls into complete heat processing systems, which are compact, cost effective, and outperform conventional hot air ovens.

Conduction is the transfer of energy by physical contact. Heat transfer through a piece of metal is an example of conduction. The rate of energy transfer is directly related to the thermal conductivity (k value); the geometrical configuration of the medium; and to thermal gradient through the medium (ΔT).

In conductive heat transfer, energy flows only when the hot body is in contact with the cold body and only from the hot body to the cold body. In conductive heat transfer, for any given configuration, the higher the temperature gradient through the material and the higher the thermal conductivity of the material, the higher the rate of heat transfer.

Infrared radiation is the transfer of heat energy from one body to another via electromagnetic waves of pure energy in the wavelengths between .7 microns and 1,000 microns. The net radiant heat exchange rate between bodies varies as a function of the difference of the temperature of the bodies raised to the fourth power and of the radiative properties of the bodies (emittance, surface area, and geometry).

All substances above absolute zero temperature (0°R or 0°K) continuously emit infrared energy. Our bodies for instance continually radiate infrared energy to their surroundings and the surroundings continuously radiate infrared to our bodies. This radiation is due to the photon emission from a substance which occurs on a microscopic level. These photons, or waves, cease to be emitted when a body is at absolute zero because all molecular activity stops. All substances commonly encountered on earth are well above absolute zero. For example, water freezes at about 32°F which is equal to about 492°R or almost 500 degrees above absolute zero.

Photons, or electromagnetic waves, can be thought of as pure energy and as a continuous stream of massless "particles". The astute will recognize that this seems to violate Einstein's theory of relativity, which says that energy equals mass times the square of the speed of light or $E=mc^2$. An explanation of this apparent contradiction is beyond the scope of your speaker and the curious should consult a recent text on quantum mechanics for a detailed discussion of this topic. The type or types of radiation emitted by a body are determined by the wavelengths range of the photons being emitted.

The rate and type of emission of electromagnetic radiation is dependent on the material's microscopic nature and on its temperature. Since all bodies commonly encountered on earth continuously radiate energy, one may begin to wonder why these bodies do not fall in temperature until they reach absolute zero. This does not happen simply because bodies not only emit radiation but also absorb radiation. Unlike conduction where energy flows only from hot to cold, radiant energy flows both ways. In an exchange between two bodies (for example the sun and the earth), body 1 radiates energy to body 2 and body 2 radiates energy to body 1. The key to radiant transfer is the <u>net</u> exchange between the bodies. The earth is warmed by the sun because the energy received from the sun is greater than the energy it radiates away.

This phenomenon of radiant energy can be exploited in a well engineered system to make the net radiant energy exchange almost 100% efficient. Picture a hollow cube which has two tiny holes, one in each of two opposite walls. Let's assume for the moment that the walls of our cube are perfect insulators and opaque to infrared energy. Now, somewhere inside our cube we place a spherical, high energy state, infrared emitter sending out photons of energy in all directions. Through the tiny holes in the walls we pass a string.

The infrared energy leaving the emitter either strikes the string surface or the inside wall surfaces. Upon striking either surface, some of the energy is absorbed and converted to heat, reflected away, or transmitted through the body. Since we qualified the cube walls as being opaque and perfect insulators, they either absorb and reradiate, or reflect the incident energy.

What we have created is a system that is highly efficient in transmitting energy from one place, the sphere, to another, the string. The energy that misses the string is either absorbed by the walls and re-emitted as infrared or reflected away. In any case, the energy is not lost and eventually ends up as heat in the string. Eventually sounds like a long time, but remember that the infrared energy is bouncing around inside our cube at a speed in excess of two hundred ninety-nine million meters per second (the speed of light).

The radiative properties of a substance are determined by comparison to the ideal radiator, known as the blackbody. A blackbody absorbs and emits all energy at every wavelength, so it is both a perfect absorber and a perfect emitter. Emissivity is a measure of how well a body can radiate energy as compared with a blackbody. The radiative properties of a substance are dependent on the wavelength of the radiation and they vary somewhat as the wavelength changes. In most cases, the wavelength dependence is so small that an averaged value for the properties can be used.

As the cube example depicts, radiation hitting a surface can be absorbed by the surface, transmitted through the surface or reflected by the surface. The fraction absorbed, plus the fraction transmitted, plus the fraction reflected must equal one.

Infrared energy penetrates the surface of many substances and thermally excites the molecules within, whereas convective/conductive heating techniques deliver energy only to the surface of a substrate. This radiative ability is very desirable when heat-treating fibrous materials such as textiles, non-wovens and paper, particularly when the moisture content of the substrate is low and the heat conductivity is poor. This potential for surface penetration with infrared is particularly important when heat-treating thin, flat substrates because the heat energy is transmitted inwardly at the speed of light, rather than being slowly conducted from the outermost surface, as with conductive heat transfer.

There are two types of industrial process infrared heaters, electric and gas.

Electric heaters can be classed into three catagories. One is the evacuated glass or quartz tube with a small diameter filament in the center and filled with an inert gas to prevent the filament from oxidizing. Quartz is used for the high powered units because it absorbs less of the infrared energy emitted by the filament and it can withstand a higher operating temperature than glass.

The second kind of electric infrared heater is the flat quartz panel with its resistance wires embedded into an insulating block, which is covered by a quartz plate. The quartz plate is treated to improve its emittance, so it can radiate energy conducted and radiated to it by the hot resistance wires.

The third type of electric infrared heater is the exposed conductor. The conductor can be a metal foil or filament. The quartz lamp type heater has the advantage of heating up and cooling down very quickly. It has the disadvantage of having a very small filament surface area. In order to get any reasonable amount of power to do industrial work, the filament is driven to very high temperatures. It's not uncommon for a filament in such a quartz lamp system to operate at temperatures in excess of 4,000°F. While that may sound attactive from a power density standpoint, the wavelength unfortunately is very, very short. The very short wavelength produced does not couple well with water. Water has certain peak spectral emissive bands and most of the IR energy in these short wavelengths is outside of these bands, so coupling efficiency is poor. So much visible light is associated with these types of units, it is recommended that #6 welding glass be worn by anyone viewing these heaters operating. The quartz plate heater and the exposed element heater both operate at much lower temperatures, typically from a few hundreds degrees above ambient to about 1500 to 1600°F. As such, they emit IR energy in the desirable middle-wavelength band. Unfortunately, the quartz plates are very slow in responding to demand changes. They take minutes to change temperature, and more to cool down. They easily start fires because of their slow cool down. In addition, they have a propensity to crack when thermal cycled repeatedly.

The exposed element unit, if it's in the form of a metal foil or filament, can have relatively low mass, which means it can be changed in temperature in a matter of a few seconds. Unfortunately, it's a live element and you can get a serious electric shock by touching it. Since the elements are exposed to the atmosphere, they tend to rapidly self-destruct by oxidation at elevated temperatures. Probably the single most limiting factor for electric infrared heaters on large installations is the high relative cost of electrical power when converted to heat by resistance. Generally, electricity when converted to heat energy by resistance is 2 to 5 times the cost of heat generated by pipeline quality gas.

Gas infrared heaters also come in many types, but they can be classified pretty easily into heaters that overcome flame speed by velocity to prevent backfiring and heaters that insulate the heat of combustion, from the heating plenum. First, let me demonstrate how infrared energy is produced by combustion. If we take this kitchen match and strike it like this, I can put my finger along side of this match while the flame burns down the stalk. At first, it won't burn my finger because the heat energy is all rising. It's only when the match burns down the stalk and heats the tip red hot and produces infrared energy that I have to move my finger away.

So in order to produce infrared energy with a fuel gas, we must first combust the fuel gas, then let the hot combustion products heat something that has mass that can become hot and give off infrared energy in industrial quantities. Remember we said everything gives off infrared energy, but if we want to do things quickly we must have alot of infrared energy. Perforate, ceramic tile, gas radiant burners overcome flame speed by velocity through an orifice(s). Pre-aerated fuel gas is delivered to the back of the tile. The gas must flow through the orifices at a velocity greater than the flame speed of the fuel or flashback (backfiring) will occur, which often breaks the tile or melts the plenum. As the gas leaves the orifice(s) it expands and slows down in velocity, so that it can be ignited by the existing flame front in a chain reaction. What is produced is a series of individual little gas flames, one at each orifice. These small little flames eventually heat up the ceramic tile which emits infrared energy. It is obvious that such heaters have a number of problems. Problem one is that when they are modulated downwardly in power, the flame speed overcomes the gas velocity and the flame backfires. If the velocity is kept high enough to insure against such backfire, the flame front is pushed out, away from the tiles it is supposed to heat. Conversion to radiation efficiency is seriously comprised as most of the gross fuel energy ends up as hot gas, not infrared. Additionaly, the ceramic tile materials used have a relatively poor emissivity, typically .4 to .6.

An attempt to improve such burners led to the impingement type gas radiant burner. This impingement type was either a counter bored hole in a ceramic block where a fuel gas was ejected into the center and deflected to the outside so that it would heat the block, or a ceramic tile with a series of grooves where the fuel gas is ejected into the grooves, ignited and directed through these grooves to cause the grooves to heat up and become incandescent. The improvement which caused a much higher exit velocity of the aerated fuel gas was possible because the flame swept over the tile, marginally improving the conductive heat exchange between the hot gas and the burner block and permitting a greater turn down before backfire occurs. Unfortunately, these burners suffer from convective boundary layer problems. That is, the gas molecules that give off their energy to the tile don't self-destruct or get out of the way preventing other hotter gas molecules from coming in contact with the tile and conducting their energy to it. Conversion to radiation efficiencies of these units often is no higher than about 15% and seldom higher than 30%. They do not modulate very well and they do not offer high radiant power density. Another very troublesome problem with these old-style, perforate tile and impingement gas radiant burners is their slow cool down. If used for heat-treating flammable substrates such as paper webs, sophisticated and expensive fire prevention or extinguishing systems are required.

In 1976 a unique, gas-fired infrared generator was developed which utilizes a refractory fiber matrix. The matrix was formulated of refractory fibers, binders and fillers that gave it very desirable characteristics for use as a generator of middle-wavelength infrared energy. In operation, the matrix is clamped to a cleverly designed plenum assembly which has one or more inner compartments to receive a 100% pre-areated fuel gas and a perimeter outer compartment to receive only air. The air acts as a dynamic seal, eliminating undesirable leakage of the gas/air mixture laterally and eliminating failure prone sealants. The gas/air mixture introduced into the plenum flows through the matrix and is ignited by a spark or a pilot on the outer surface. Since the velocity of the fuel mixture through the matrix is <u>less</u> than flame speed by design, the flame settles within the outer surface of the matrix in the presence of thousands of fibers per square inch. The heat of combustion is rapidly and efficiently absorbed by refractory fibers causing them to glow and emit infrared energy. In operation, only about 1/10 of 1# of matrix per square foot of surface area is actually at radiant temperature. When the fuel source is removed, the face cools down quickly enough to be touched with the bare hand in less than 5 seconds. This is an impossibility with any other type of IR heater. Modulation of the infrared intensity, within the normal operating range of 1100 to 1600°F, can be affected in less than 1 second.

The insulating quality of the matrix prevents heat from conducting backwards, so that all the radiant energy is emitted outwardly toward the product to be heated. This very efficient generator produces infrared energy in a wavelength band that couples well with water and most other materials. It has unsurpassed modulating ability for precise temperature control and a rapid start and stop capability for safety. This infrared generator was first introduced to the textile industry where it rapidly replaced old-style ceramic tile and metal screen gas radiant burners. Customers reported a fuel gas reduction averaging 40 to 60%. Marsden's penetration into textile finishing plants is so extensive that there is a better than 50% probability that each one of you is wearing some article of clothing today that was heat processed with these new infrared generators.

In 1984, a research project was instituted that culminated in 1985's introduction of a new matrix material, which had a 50% higher emittance and was water-repellent. These two improvements have greatly increased the performance of the infrared systems which use these infrared generators, both in new equipment and as equipment that has been retrofitted in the field. As a result of the improvements made to the matrix, we now offer a limited two-year warranty on matrix failure due to flashback or burnout.

One interesting problem occurred when we started retro-fitting our new high emittance matrix firing face into existing Marsden Infrared Generator installations. Several plant engineers and maintenance men called us to complain that the new material was not hot enough! Since we had anticipated such reactions, we immediately asked them to run for a few days and carefully monitor percent dryness, or speed, or both, depending on the situation and we would call them back in about week. During the initial call we were careful not to disagree with their feeling that the new matrix was "not hot enough". In every case, when we called back about a week or so later, we were told production increased, or dryness increased, or both, and the reports from quality control were excellent. One customer who had fuel metering equipment even commented that fuel consumption remained the same with increased dryness and speed.

The point is that the quantity of infrared energy emitted is invisible to the eye. What we see when we view an infrared heater is visible light. The amount of visible light is primarily a function of temperature. Our experienced customers saw the "difference in temperature", the new matrix wasn't as hot as the old material. What they could not see was more infrared energy is being emitted by virtue of the higher emittance and the improvement to efficiency because the actual operating temperature was lower and the conversion to radiation per unit of fuel was greater.

The outstanding combination of features offered by these new, high emittance matrix infrared generators now permits their integration into compact, cost effective, heat processing systems, which outperform conventional hot air ovens in scores of industrial operations.

Integrated infrared systems can have closed-loop feedback, microprocessor-based, temperature controllers to maintain product exit temperatures within $\pm 1°C$; conditioned mass transfer airflow to effectively remove evaporated solvents, zero tension transport systems for delicate, uncured substrates, programmable tachometers which incrementally add or substract zones for start-up and shutdown, as well as a combination of infrared and conduction/convection systems where desirable.

Existing heat treatment processes can be improved by the addition of high emittance infrared generators as speed boosters or as temperature or moisture profile correctors. Many coating processes are improved in quality, as well as speed, by the non-contact, instantaneous, radiant heat transfer these units provide.

Here's a small sampling of what Marsden Systems are now doing for their users:

- Browning bagels in the Bronx
- Curing carpets in Canada
- Finishing textiles in Milan
- Drying flock in Maine
- Heating floor coverings in Chicago
- Baking biscuits in Australia
- Annealing glass in New Jersey
- Drying bookbindings in Japan
- Curing wallpaper in New Zealand
- Softening plastics in California
- Predrying clay coatings in Tasmania
- Thermosetting nonwovens in Massachusetts
- Drying printing in New York
- Sintering plastic chips in Mexico City
- Browning cottage pies in London
- Drying metal strip in Pennsylvania
- Baking flourescent tubes in Czechoslovakia

LES APPLICATIONS DU PROCEDE GAZ-CONTACT
AU TRAITEMENT DES DECHETS INDUSTRIELS

RESUME DE LA COMMUNICATION
PRESENTEE AU CONGRES TRANS TECH
du 25 au 29 Novembre 1987, à Montréal - CANADA

Par L. GAURIER
Ingénieur au Service des Techniques et Applications Industrielles
Direction des Etudes et Techniques Nouvelles du GAZ DE FRANCE

RESUME

Le procédé GAZ-CONTACT, mis au point au GAZ DE FRANCE, est une technique de traitement par voie thermique de produits divisés, dans laquelle le produit à traiter traverse la flamme d'un brûleur particulier.

Après avoir décrit le procédé et les équipements qui en découlent, la communication se propose de présenter des applications au traitement des déchets industriels :

- le traitement peut conduire à une revalorisation du produit rejeté, comme dans le cas de la régénération des sables usés de fonderie, la purification de farine de silice ou la détoxification de poussières issues des fumées de certains hauts fourneaux.

- il peut aussi n'être qu'une simple destruction, débouchant sur la récupération éventuelle de l'énergie libérée par la combustion des déchets, comme dans l'incinération des boues de peinture ou celle des déchets d'isolants électriques.

Procédé simple et d'un entretien réduit, la technique GAZ-CONTACT contribue à la protection de l'environnement tout en permettant aux industriels intéressés de réaliser des économies.

Le procédé "Gaz-contact" désigne une technique de traitement par voie thermique de produits divisés. L'originalité de la technique repose sur le fait que le produit, solide pulvérulent ou liquide pulvérisé, est injecté directement dans une flamme à haute turbulence, bénéficiant ainsi de l'effet "Gaz-contact".

1 - DESCRIPTION DU PROCEDE

1.1 - LE BRULEUR

Le brûleur, dit à "contre-rotation à ouvreau", a été mis au point et breveté par le GAZ DE FRANCE. Schématisé à la figure n° 1a, il est caractérisé par une chambre de combustion cylindrique sur laquelle sont percés les orifices d'injection des fluides :

- une rangée d'orifices radiaux de gaz,

- deux rangées d'orifices tangentiels d'air. Les sens de rotation induits par les deux rangées sont opposés, créant ainsi la "contre-rotation", qui provoque des turbulences importantes favorisant un mélange rapide de l'air et du gaz.

Cette disposition permet d'obtenir une combustion intense et une flamme courte et très stable tout en conservant l'axe du brûleur libre de toute pièce mécanique.

Les cotes principales de ce brûleur peuvent être déterminées au moyen d'abaques en fonction de la puissance désirée. Celle-ci peut varier actuellement entre 20 et 11 000 kW (PCI), pour des pressions d'alimentation en air et en gaz inférieures ou égales à 20 mbar.

Dans ses applications au procédé Gaz-Contact, l'arrière du brûleur est percé d'un orifice axial et reçoit un dispositif d'éjection du produit à traiter (figure n° 1b). Le produit est ainsi éjecté au travers de la flamme, où il est repris par les turbulences créées par la Contre-rotation. De ce fait, chaque grain du produit est soumis à un transfert thermique intense, que l'on désigne sous le nom d'effet Gaz-Contact.

.../...

1.2 - L'EFFET GAZ-CONTACT

Des essais ont été effectués sur un équipement prototype pour évaluer l'effet Gaz-Contact.

Cette évaluation a été faite par comparaison des résultats obtenus, dans les mêmes conditions de température, avec le brûleur à contre- rotation et un autre brûleur dans lequel les différentes arrivées -gaz, air et produit- sont coaxiales.

A titre d'exemple, on a considéré un traitement qui est l'élimination, sous l'action de la chaleur, d'une impureté. Les résultats comparatifs obtenus dans les mêmes conditions sont donnés à la figure n° 2. Les courbes donnent l'évolution de la teneur résiduelle en impureté en fonction de la température de traitement. Elles montrent que, à température égale, le résultat est nettement meilleur avec le procédé Gaz-contact : l'effet Gaz-Contact permet de diminuer la teneur en impureté de 40 % environ dans la zone de température considérée. On peut dire aussi qu'à teneur résiduelle égale, l'effet Gaz-Contact se traduit par une diminution de la température nécessaire, d'où un gain d'énergie.

1.3 - LES EQUIPEMENTS

Pour atteindre le temps minimal nécessaire au traitement d'un produit, il est nécessaire de monter le brûleur sur une enceinte.

Divers types d'enceintes ont été étudiés, utilisables suivant les cas. Dans les applications relatives au traitement des déchets, deux types d'enceintes ont été utilisés :

- une chambre cylindrique horizontale ou oblique, utilisée dans les applications d'incinération. Un cyclone peut être rajouté en fin de chambre pour récupérer les incombustibles ou les cendres,

- une chambre cylindrique verticale, suivie d'une chambre de détente et d'un cyclone de dépoussiérage dans le cas où les déchets peuvent être revalorisés : la partie récupérable du produit est alors récoltée au bas de la chambre de détente. L'ensemble est schématisé à la figure n° 3.

.../...

Le Centre d'Essais et de Recherches sur les Utilisations du Gaz (CERUG) du GAZ DE FRANCE, dispose d'un équipement prototype vertical à chambre de détente équipé de sondes multifonctions permettant de suivre l'évolution des températures du produit et des fumées, ainsi que la composition des fumées, le long du four. La fonction de ce prototype est la réalisation d'essais de faisabilité par produit et par type de traitement.

Parmi les nombreux essais effectués, certains portaient sur le traitement de déchets industriels. Le traitement peut être une revalorisation du rejet, soit une incinération.

2 - <u>REVALORISATION DES DECHETS</u>

Il existe dans l'industrie un certain nombre de rejets qui peuvent être revalorisés, soit pour être réintégrés dans la chaine de fabrication - comme les sables usés de fonderie ou les copeaux d'usinage de fonte, encrassés par l'huile de coupe- soit pour être commercialisés sous une forme différente -comme certaines poussières par exemple. Plutôt que d'énumérer de nombreuses applications, il est préférable d'examiner en détail quelques exemples types :

- régénération de sables usés de fonderie,

- deshuilage des copeaux d'usinage,

- détoxification de poussières.

2.1 - <u>LA REGENERATION DES SABLES DE FONDERIE</u>

2.11 - Généralités

Le sable est utilisé en fonderie pour la fabrication de moules et de noyaux, avec adjonction d'un liant, le plus souvent organique. Une fois utilisé, le sable est le plus souvent jeté en décharge agréée et remplacé par du sable neuf.

.../...

Le recyclage du sable après élimination grossière des résines peut dans certains cas s'avérer suffisant, mais seule la régénération thermique permet de récupérer un sable de mêmes caractéristiques que le sable neuf d'origine.

2.12 - Les essais - Les résultats

De nombreux essais propres à chaque type de liant organique utilisé, ont été effectués sur l'équipement prototype vertical déjà décrit.

L'ensemble de ces essais a permis d'établir une philosophie générale sur la destruction des résines, notamment un classement empirique des résines basé sur leur difficulté d'incinération, à partir de la température minimale de traitement.

Nous nous bornerons dans ce qui suit à l'examen d'un seul cas concret, qui doit déboucher prochainement sur une réalisation industrielle : il s'agit d'un sable de type "Pep-set", liant formé in-situ par combinaison d'une résine phénolique, d'un isocyanate et d'une amine.

Les essais ont dégagé deux modes opératoires possibles :

- soit un traitement en passage direct. Le sable entrant dans la zone de traitement ressort aussitôt. Dans ce cas, la température nécessaire au traitement est voisine de 750°C, valeur qui correspond, sur l'équipement prototype, à une consommation spécifique, avant récupération de chaleur, de 360 kWh(PCI)/t, le taux d'aération par rapport à l'ensemble des combustibles (gaz + résines) étant de 1,2,

- soit un traitement en sortie différée. Le sable est maintenu au contact des gaz chauds pendant 5 minutes environ au moyen d'un clapet à équilibrage pondéral réglable. Cette technologie permet un traitement à plus basse température, inférieure à 600°C, ce qui correspond à une consommation spécifique par rapport au gaz naturel, dans les conditions déjà définies, égale à 260 kWh(PCI)/t.

Les courbes donnant l'évolution des températures et de la composition des fumées dans le four, données à la figure n° 4, montrent que la majeure partie du traitement est rapidement terminée et que la réaction n'évolue déjà plus à 1 m du brûleur.

.../...

2.13 - Données économiques*

Le four, de type vertical à chambre de détente, sera équipé d'un étage de refroidissement basé sur le principe "Air-Contact".

- Coût actuel du poste sable :
    - achat de sable neuf   : 147 F/t
    - mise en décharge du sable usé : 77 F/t   224 F/t

- Coût du traitement dans l'hypothèse d'une température de 750°C :
    - gaz naturel, avec mise en chauffe journalière   : 74 F/t
    - électricité, air surpressé, estimé à   : 20 F/t   102 F/t
    - achat de sable neuf (taux de perte ~ 5 %)   : 8 F/t

- Coût d'investissement du four et de son refroidisseur (hors systèmes amont et aval) : ~ 220 000 F.

Dans l'hypothèse d'un traitement annuel de 1 500 t/an, l'économie réalisée par le traitement équilibre à franc constant l'investissement en 1,2 années.

2.2 - LE DESHUILAGE DE COPEAUX METALLIQUES

2.21 - Généralités

Le recyclage des copeaux d'usinage en refusion impose l'élimination des huiles de coupe. Actuellement, ces copeaux sont enlevés par des sociétés de services qui les stockent à l'air libre le temps nécessaire pour la disparition naturelle des huiles, puis qui les revendent.

.../...

---

* Toutes les données économiques de cette communication sont données en Francs français 1987.

Certains utilisateurs, notamment dans l'industrie de la fonte, estiment que cette procédure est peu souple et recherchent d'autres solutions. La combustion des huiles semble être une des technologies envisagées et des essais ont été effectués sur l'équipement prototype du GAZ DE FRANCE.

2.22 - Les essais - Les résultats

On a recherché au cours des essais à obtenir des copeaux deshuilés, secs et aussi peu oxydés que possible, et ce pour une température aussi basse que possible. Pour cela, le taux d'aération par rapport à l'ensemble des combustibles, gaz naturel et huiles de coupe, a été maintenu proche des conditions stoechiométriques avec des débits de gaz variables.

Les résultats ont montré :

- que des copeaux sortant à 630°C sont parfaitement propres et peu oxydés,

- que la consommation spécifique par rapport à l'ensemble des combustibles pour atteindre cette température est inférieure à 280 kWh(PCI)/t, et que la part de l'énergie fournie par les huiles peut atteindre 45 à 50 % du total,

- que la combustion des huiles est rapide : à 1,5 m du brûleur, on ne décèle plus d'évolution dans la réaction de combustion.

2.23 - Données économiques

Nous ne disposons pas des éléments sur le coût des opérations actuelles -enlèvement, stockage et rachat des copeaux. Le coût de l'incinération peut être ainsi apprécié :

- dans l'hypothèse où l'on incinère les huiles et que l'on laisse les copeaux en attente -c'est le cas le plus défavorable- il faut intégrer le coût d'un équipement complet d'incinération et les frais d'exploitation (air-gaz-électricité : ~ 40 F/t),

.../...

- par contre, si on réinjecte les copeaux chauds dans la zone de fusion, au travers d'un brûleur monté directement sur le four de fusion(*), l'investissement est nettement plus réduit et les frais d'exploitation pratiquement inéxistants : l'enthalpie des copeaux (106 kWh/t à 630°C) est totalement récupérée et l'énergie fournie par le brûleur participe au chauffage de l'enceinte.

2.3 - LA DETOXIFICATION DE POUSSIERES

2.31 - Généralités

Certains procédés industriels entraînent la formation de poussières qui se retrouvent dans les fumées et qui sont éliminées par les systèmes de filtration prévus à cet effet. La mise en décharge de ces poussières pose un certain nombre de problèmes, notamment de toxicité éventuelle.

Il est donc nécessaire d'éliminer les composés polluants avant de les rejeter, ce que le procédé Gaz-Contact a permis de faire. Un résultat secondaire a été dans certains cas de permettre d'envisager leur commercialisation.

2.32 - Essais et résultats

Deux applications de ce type (décyanuration et incinération d'hydrocarbures) ont fait l'objet de l'acquisition d'un équipement semi-industriel par les industriels concernés à la suite d'essais exploratoires sur l'équipement prototype du GAZ DE FRANCE pour l'incinération des hydrocarbures.

.../...

(*) <u>Remarque</u> : L'injection des copeaux au travers de brûleurs montés sur un four de fusion est envisagée sur un four bassin de fusion de cuivre. Cette technologie est évoquée dans une communication au Congrès de l'Association Technique de l'Industrie du Gaz en FRANCE.

Les résultats obtenus ont montré que le but recherché était largement atteint : la destruction des cyanures ou des hydrocarbures est totale. Dans le cas des poussières cyanurées, la teneur importante en alcalins des poussières influe sur l'état physique du produit traité et nécessite la mise au point d'une récupération par voie humide permettant la commercialisation des sels solubles. Pour les poussières de silice, l'élimination des hydrocarbures permet la commercialisation du produit.

Dans les deux cas, l'étude des conditions du marché permet de prévoir un bilan d'exploitation positif et un temps de retour de l'investissement réduit (environ 1 an).

3 - DESTRUCTION DE DECHETS

Lorsque la revalorisation des déchets n'est pas possible, on peut envisager leur destruction, tout en prenant les précautions nécessaires pour éviter toute pollution par les fumées issues du procédé. Cette incinération peut dans certains cas être considérée comme une revalorisation, car peut libérer une énergie plus importante que celle qui est nécessaire à l'opération.

Parmi les opérations envisagées, nous examinerons deux cas particuliers, concernant l'incinération :

- des déchets d'isolants électriques,

- des boues de peinture et de cataphorèse.

3.1 - INCINERATION D'ISOLANTS ELECTRIQUES

3.11 - Généralités

L'industrie du recyclage des métaux procède entre autres à la récupération de quantités importantes de fils électriques de toutes sortes. L'extraction du cuivre se fait de façon mécanopneumatique : les câbles et fils sont broyés et déchiquetés et le cuivre est séparé de tout ce qui l'entoure par ventilation. Si le cuivre repart en fonderie, par contre les déchets d'isolant sont irrecyclables, du fait de l'hétérogénéité de leur composition (brai, polyéthylène, feuillard d'aluminium, papier, etc ...). Ils sont donc stockés sans pouvoir se dégrader, ce qui occupe des sites relativement importants.

.../...

Un industriel a donc songé à rebrûler ces déchets. L'incinération en tas est impensable, compte-tenu de l'émission de fumées noires dues à une très mauvaise combustion. De plus, cette incinération sauvage entraîne une perte d'énergie potentielle importante, d'où l'idée d'adapter le procédé Gaz-Contact à la conception d'un brûleur mixte gaz-naturel/déchets d'isolants.

3.12 - Les essais - Les résultats

Les essais ont été effectués avec un brûleur, équipé de son système d'alimentation en produit, monté sur une chambre de combustion cylindrique assimilable à un four rotatif de fusion de métaux non-ferreux.

Après avoir déterminé le pouvoir calorifique moyen des déchets (égal à 8,5 kWh(PCI)/kg), deux types d'essais ont été entrepris : soit une substitution progressive du gaz par des déchets à puissance totale et débit d'air constant, jusqu'à l'apparition d'une combustion incomplète, soit à débit de gaz constant avec complément de puissance par adjonction de déchets jusqu'à la mauvaise combustion (on a noté que l'apparition de l'oxyde de carbone dans les fumées était simultanée avec la production de suies).

Le tableau n° 1 rassemble quelques résultats représentatifs des essais effectués, avec la symbolique suivante :

- Q_G : débit de gaz naturel — $m^3(n)/h$,
- m : débit de déchets — kg/h,
- P_c : puissance totale — $kW(PCI)$,
- τ : taux de substitution de déchets au gaz naturel — (*),
- η : rendement de combustion four vide.

.../...

(*) Le taux de substitution est le rapport entre la puissance fournie par les déchets et la puissance totale. Les valeurs du tableau sont basées sur des valeurs moyennes des pouvoirs calorifiques inférieurs de 10 kWh/m^3(n) pour le gaz naturel et de 8,5 kWh/kg pour les déchets.

Q_g	m	P_c	τ	η	$\eta\,P_c$
30	0	300	0	0,62	186
20	9,5	283	0,29	0,60	170
18	12,4	285	0,37	0,60	171
16,5	13,7	277	0,41	0,595	165
15	15,5	279	0,46	0,595	166
13	14,2	252	0,48	0,56	141
20	0	200	0	0,60	120
20	8,4	270	0,26	0,625	169
20	9,6	282	0,29	0,60	170
20	11,4	296	0,33	0,53	157
20	15,0	327	0,39	0,52	170

Le tableau montre :

- qu'il est possible de substituer jusqu'à 45 % de déchets au gaz naturel, sans altérer de manière significative la puissance fournie,

- que l'accroissement de la puissance fournie par injection de déchets ne s'accompagne d'une augmentation de puissance utilisable que pour $\tau \leqslant 0,26$. Au-delà de cette valeur, la puissance utilisable n'augmente plus : l'accroissement de la puissance fournie doit s'accompagner d'une augmentation de l'excès d'air, de façon a maintenir une combustion sans imbrûlés, et de ce fait les pertes aux fumées augmentent.

Rermarque :

La valeur limite du taux de substitution augmente si on remplace l'air de combustion par de l'oxygène : de 45 % on passe à 65 % environ. Cependant, cette technologie présente deux inconvénients :

- la flamme oxy-gaz/déchet, très courte, entraîne une cokéfaction rapide d'une partie des déchets en sortie de brûleur et son bouchage rapide,

.../...

- la consommation d'énergie primaire correspondant à la fabrication de l'oxygène nécessaire à la combustion n'est pas récupérée dans une telle opération.

3.13 - Considérations économiques

Le bilan économique de l'incinération des déchets d'isolant se situe à différents niveaux :

- sur le plan financier, la valorisation de l'énergie gratuite dépend des possibilités d'utilisation : chaudières, fours de fusion, etc ... dont les rendements utiles sont différents,

- sur le plan environnement, cela permet la remise à disposition d'aires de stockage importantes, supprime des terrils assez peu esthétiques et évite l'incinération sauvage sur tas, qui entraîne l'émission importante de suies.

3.2 - BOUES DE PEINTURE ET DE CATAPHORESE

3.21 - Généralités

La peinture en cabine aérée nécessite un lavage de l'air circulant dans la cabine par des bains particuliers qui sont recyclés. Au cours du recyclage, une décantation du bain permet d'éliminer les gouttelettes de peinture passivées, qui s'agglomèrent pour former une espèce de mastic qui est jeté en décharge agréée.

Les boues de cataphorèse proviennent du lavage des tôles après passage dans le bain de cataphorèse. Les eaux de lavage sont concentrées jusqu'à une teneur en matière sèche théorique de 10 % ; elles sont alors reprises par des sociétés de service qui les traitent avant de rejeter l'eau.

.../...

Ces divers rejets sont onéreux et il a semblé intéressant d'essayer de récupérer l'énergie potentielle en brûlant les boues sur place.

3.22 - Essais et résultats

Les essais ont été faits dans les mêmes conditions que pour les déchets d'isolant. Cependant, l'alimentation en produit nécessite un système mécanique pour diviser le produit en particules.

Le taux d'aération par rapport à l'ensemble des combustibles a été maintenu constant et voisin de 1,10, de même que la puissance totale libérée (225 kW(PCI)).

Le taux de substitution du gaz naturel par des boues de peinture atteint 60 % sans altération des conditions de combustion. Le produit a un pouvoir calorifique inférieur variant entre 9 et 11 kWh/kg du fait de vésicules d'eau incluses.

Dans le cas des boues de cataphorèse, la teneur initiale en matières sèches est trop faible (5 % mesuré) pour que le procédé soit économique sans préparation préalable du produit :

- une filtration à froid ne permet d'obtenir qu'un mélange à 17 % de matières sèches, teneur insuffisante pour assurer une incinération économique,

- une filtration à 45°C permet d'atteindre un agglomérat à 45 % de matières sèches, aisément granulable, dont le pouvoir calorifique inférieur est de l'ordre de 3,3 kWh/kg.

Les essais d'incinération ont été faits avec ce dernier produit, d'une part, et avec du produit sec d'autre part (dont le PCI se situe aux environs de 7,4 kWh/kg). Dans les deux cas, il est possible d'atteindre un taux de substitution du gaz naturel par les boues de 60 %.

.../...

3.23 - Considérations économiques

Un équipement Gaz-Contact d'incinération est en projet, dans le cas suivant : les rejets sont constitués de 200 kg/h de boues de peinture et 5 t/h de boues de cataphorèse à 5 % de matières sèches, représentant une énergie potentielle de 3 800 kW PCI environ. Cet équipement pourrait équiper une chaudière de production de vapeur, avec un apoint gaz naturel de 2 600 kW(PCI).

Si on ajoute les 300 kW(PCI) nécessaires au chauffage à 45°C des boues de cataphorèse (pour leur filtration à chaud), le bilan de l'opération est une consommation de gaz de 2 900 kW(PCI), permettant de disposer de 6 400 kW(PCI), ce qui représente un apport d'énergie gratuite de 55 % par rapport à un même équipement fonctionnant au fioul ou au gaz naturel. En réalité, l'économie réalisée est plus faible, compte tenu des consommations électriques inhérentes à la préparation des boues.

D'autre part, l'économie des frais de reprise des déchets par une société de service (~ 600 F/t pour les boues de peinture et 360 F/t de boues de cataphorèse à 5 % de matières sèches à l'époque) vient s'inscrire à l'actif du bilan.

4 - CONCLUSION

Le retraitement des rejets, industriels ou autres, en vue de les revaloriser ou de les détruire, et sa contribution à la protection de l'environnement sont un sujet d'actualité et les techniques disponibles sont nombreuses.

Parmi celles-ci, le procédé Gaz-Contact, de par les performances assez remarquables du brûleur dont il est issu et par la simplicité de sa mise en oeuvre, offre une solution séduisante à de nombreux problèmes de traitement :

- l'étendue de la gamme de puissance des brûleurs à contre-rotation permet de concevoir des unités adaptées à chaque problème posé,

.../...

- l'effet Gaz-Contact favorise un encombrement réduit,

- le passage du produit à traiter en continu évite l'engorgement de l'équipement en période d'arrêt, ce qui facilite l'entretien et raccourcit les temps de remise en route,

- l'absence de pièces en mouvement réduit les coûts d'entretien.

Le procédé Gaz-Contact offre donc aux industriels une possibilité de traitement des rejets simple, souple et peu onéreux et d'une exploitation aisée.

COMMERCIALISATION DU PROCEDE

Le procédé Gaz-contact, dont la vocation déborde le cadre du traitement des rejets industriels, est construit sous licence par deux constructeurs qui bénéficient de l'assistance technique du GAZ DE FRANCE. Il s'agit de :

- Société MEKER
  105, Boulevard de Verdun
  92400 COURBEVOIE
  Tél. : (1) 43.33.31.81

- Société SARGI
  10, Cité d'Angoulême
  75011 PARIS
  Tél. : (1) 43.57.39.43

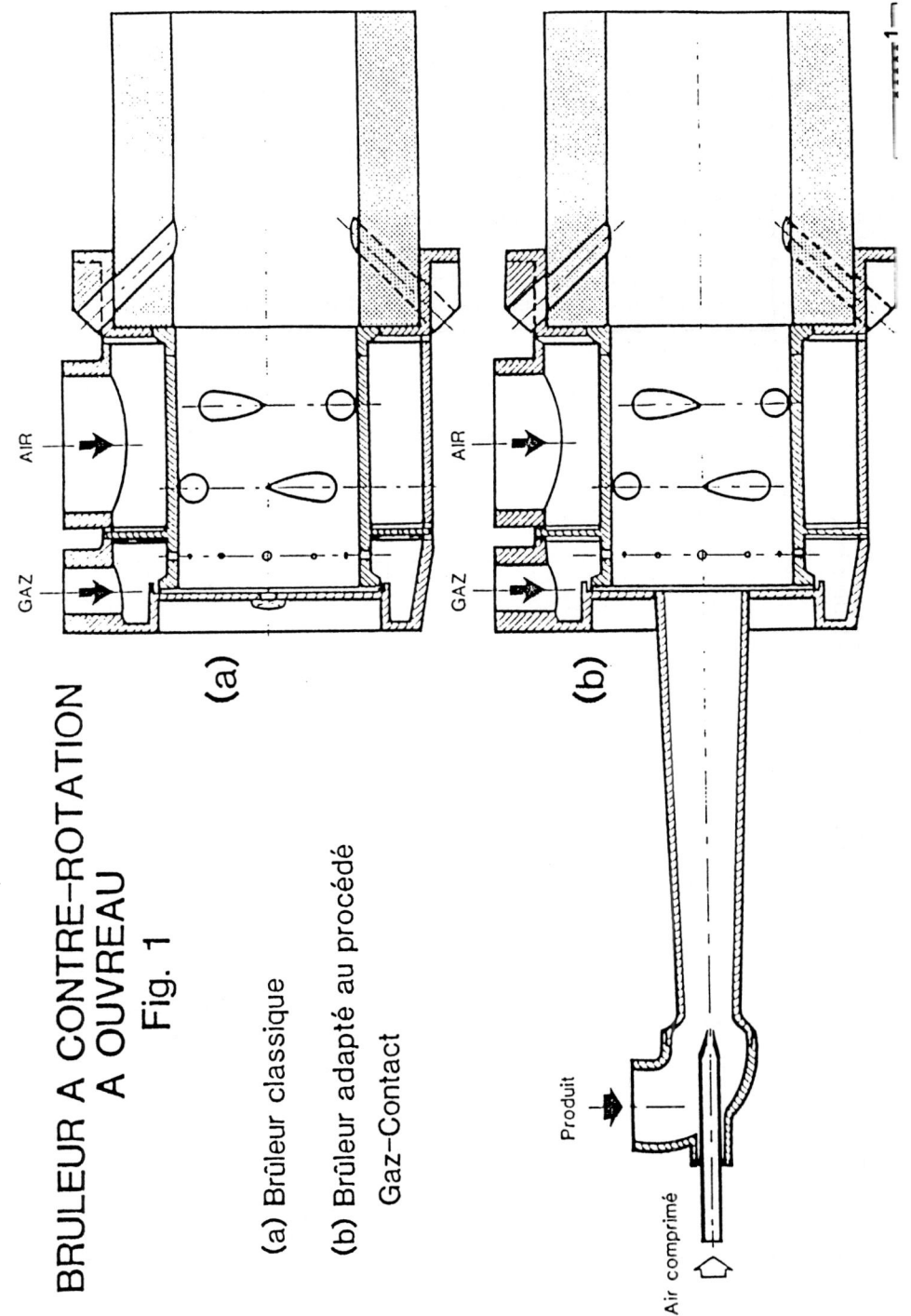

BRULEUR A CONTRE-ROTATION A OUVREAU
Fig. 1

(a) Brûleur classique
(b) Brûleur adapté au procédé Gaz-Contact

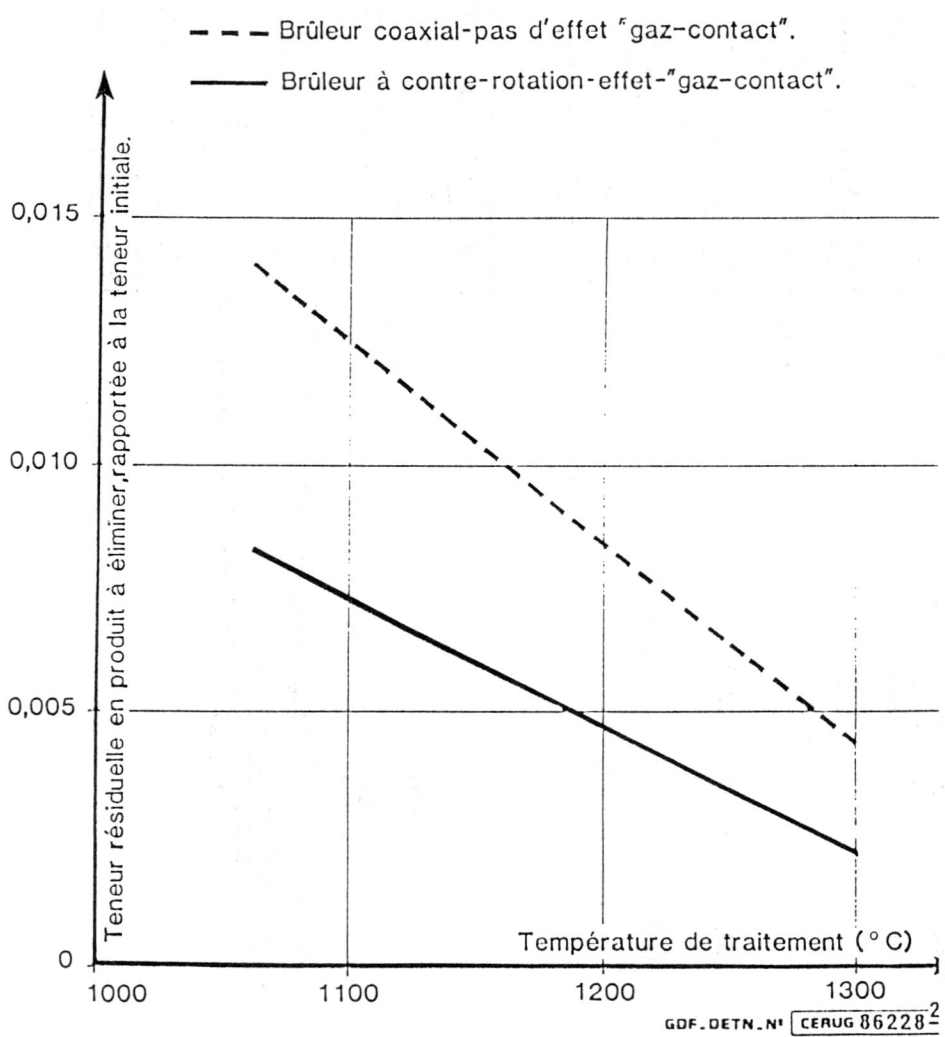

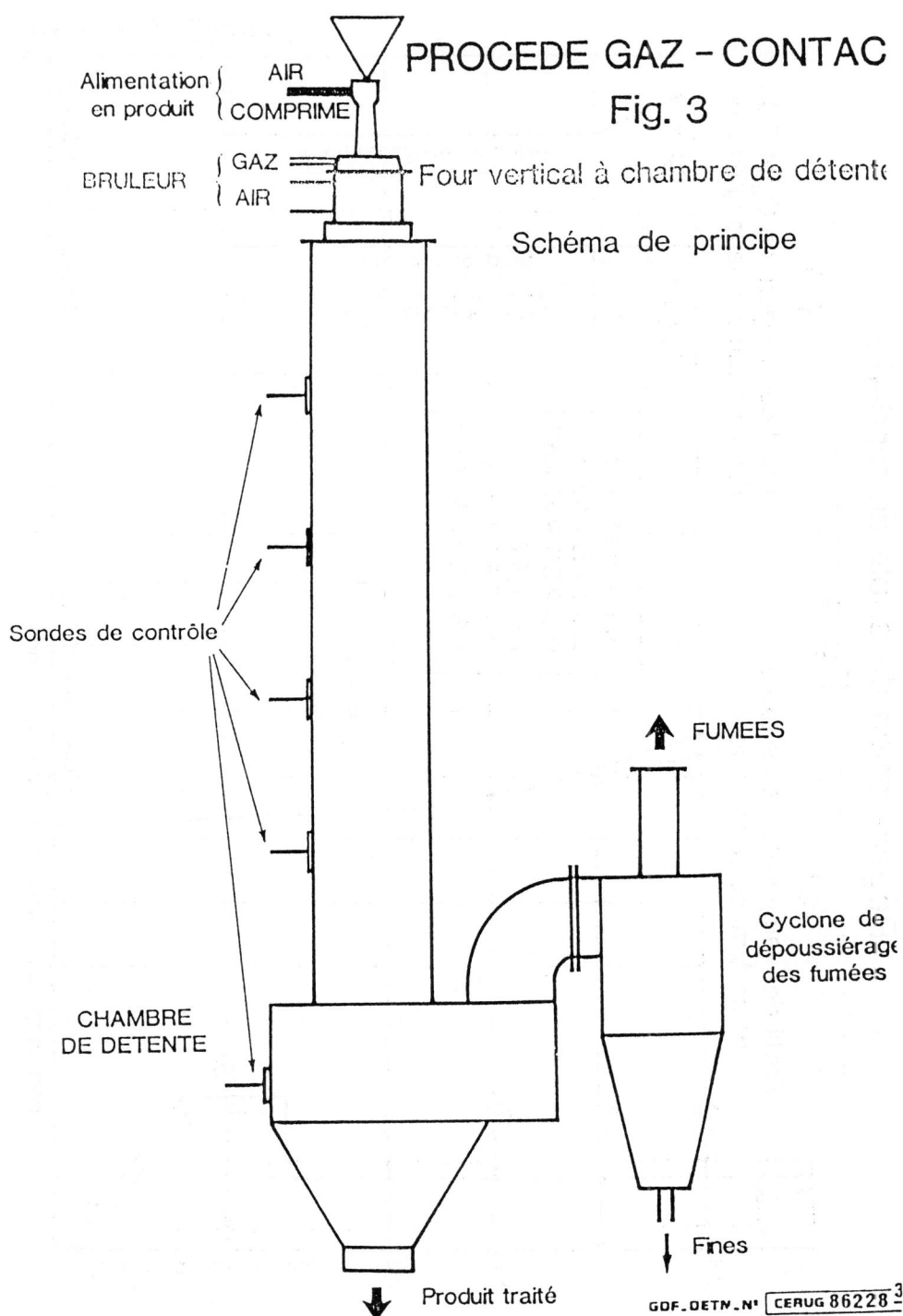

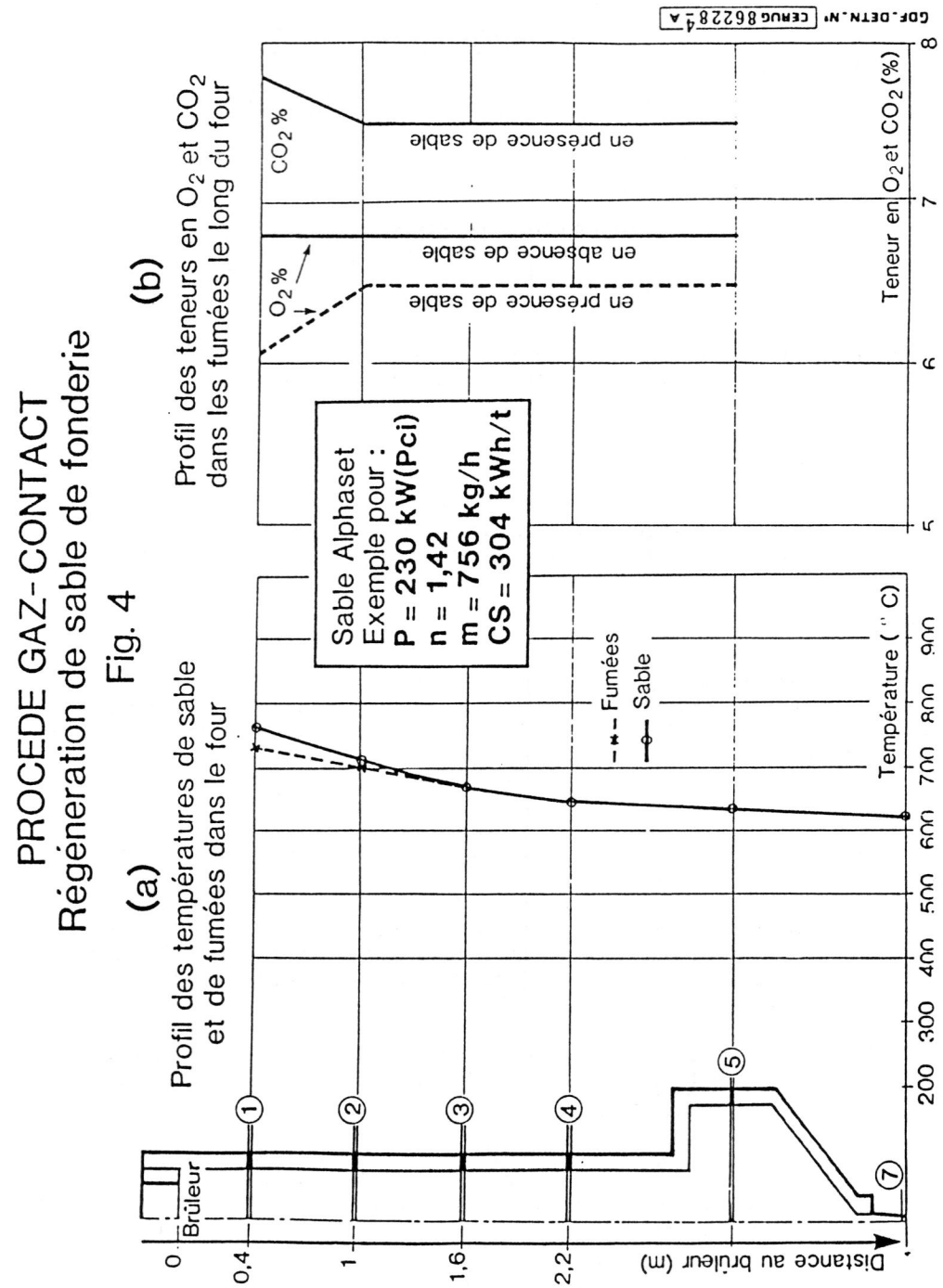

PROCEDE GAZ-CONTACT
Régéneration de sable de fonderie
Fig. 4

GAZ-CONTACT PROCESS
IN THE TREATMENT OF INDUSTRIAL WASTE

―――――

Summary of a lecture to be presented at the ....
Congress TRANS TECH in Montreal (Canada),
on the 25-29th of Nov. 87

―――――

by L. GAURIER
Engineer in the Industrial Technology Division,
Direction des Etudes et Techniques Nouvelles, GAZ de FRANCE

―――――

"Gas-contact" process, developped and patented by Gaz de France, is a technique where divided products, powdered or pulverized, undergo a treatment by heat, as they are injected through the flame of a peculiar burner, also patented by Gaz de France.

After the process ànd the subsequent equipments have been described, we will present different applications in the field of the treatment of industial waste :

- on the one hand, the treatment can lead of the recovery of a usable product, as in the heat reclaiming of used foundry sands or in the decyanidisation of dust produced by some high furnaces.

- on the other hand, the treatment can only by a combustion, leading to the recovery of heat, as in the burning of paint sludge or of wire insulators.

Plain and of low-cost maintenance, Gaz-contact process contributes in the protection of the surroundings while allowing interested industrials to save money and materials.

The "Gas-Contact process" describes a technique for heat treatment of ground products. The originality of this technique is that a pulverised product or sprayed liquid, is injected directly through a flame with a high degree of turbulence, thus benefiting from the "gas-contact" action.

1 - PROCESS DESCRIPTION

1.1 - Burner

The "counter-rotation" burner was developed and patented by Gaz de France. Shown in Fig. 1a, it has a cylindrical combustion chamber with fluid injection ports as follows:

- one row of radial gas ports,

- two rows of tangential air ports. The rotational directions imparted by these two rows are opposite, thus creating opposite swirls which cause a high degree of turbulence, favoring quick air and gas mixing.

This configuration results in intense combustion and a short, very stable flame while maintaining the burner centerline free from mechanical parts.

The overall dimensions of this burner may be determined by means of graphs depending on the desired output. Rating may vary between 20 and 11 000 kW (n.c.v.) for air and gas supply pressures less than or equal to 20 mbar.

In its applications to the Gas-Contact process, the rear of the burner features an axial port and is fitted with a device for ejecting the product to be processed (see Fig. 1b). The product is thus ejected through the flame, where it is caught in the turbulence created by the opposite swirls. Therefore, each grain of the product is subjected to an intense heat transfer, known as the Gas-Contact action.

1.2 - Gas-contact action

An evaluation of the Gas-Contact action has been done during prototype tests.

The results obtained under the same conditions of temperature using the counter rotation burner and another burner in which the different inlets, i.e. gas, air and product, are coaxial were compared.

As an example, we studied a method of eliminating impurities under the action of heat. The comparative results obtained under the same conditions are given in Fig. 2. The curves show the change in the residual amount of impurity after treatment. For equal temperature, they show that the result improves with the Gas-Contact process since it reduces the impurity content by approximately 40% in the temperature zone considered. With an equal residual content, the gas-contact action could mean a decrease in the required temperature, resulting in energy savings.

1.3 - <u>Equipment</u>

The burner must be mounted in a furnace in order to reach the minimum product treatment time.

Various types of furnaces have been studied, to be used selectively. For waste treatment applications, two types of furnaces have been used:

-a horizontal or inclined unit used for incineration applications. A cyclone may be added at the chamber end to recover unburned matter or ashes,

-an upright unit, followed by a decelerating chamber and a dust-removing cyclone in the case where waste may be reused. The recovered portion of the product is collected at the bottom of the decelerating chamber. The assembly is shown in Fig. 3.

The Gas Utilization Research Center (CERUG) at Gaz de France has a vertical prototype equipment with a decelerating chamber. It features multipurpose probes to monitor the temperature of the product and flue gases as well as the composition of the flue gases, along the furnace. This prototype is used for product and treatment feasibility studies.

Among the numerous tests performed, the treatment of industrial waste was tested. Treatment could result in reuse of the waste, or incineration.

2 - REUSE OF WASTE

A certain number of waste products may be reused, either for reintegration into the chain of manufacture - such as foundry sand or metal shavings fouled with oil from cutting - or be sold in a different form, such as certain types of dust, for example. Rather than enumerate the various applications, it is preferable to examine in detail a few typical examples:

- regeneration of used foundry sand,

- cleansing of metal shavings,

- decyanidization of dust.

2.1 - Regeneration of foundry sand

2.1.1 - General

Foundry sand is used in mold and core manufacturing, with the addition of a bonding agent, usually organic. Used sand is most often thrown away and replaced by clean sand.

In certain cases, sand recycling after coarse elimination of resins may be sufficient. However, only thermal regeneration allows recovery of sand with the same properties as clean, new sand.

2.1.2 - Tests - Results

Numerous tests have been conducted for each type of organic bonding agent used on the vertical prototype equipment described above.

All tests lead to a general knowledge of the destruction of resins, notably an empirical classification of resins based on their incineration difficulty, beginning from the minimum treatment temperature.

The paper will examine a single concrete case, which should lead to industrial scale development. This is "Pep-set" sand, with an *in situ* bonding agent formed by combination of a phenolic resin, an isocyanate and an amine.

The tests showed two possible procedures:

-Either direct-pass treatment, i.e., the sand entering the treatment zone exits immediately. In this case, the required treatment temperature is close to 750° C, a value which corresponds on the prototype equipment to specific consumption before heat recovery of 360 kWh(n.c.v.)/t, with the fuels (gas + resins) air factor being 1.2.

-Or, delayed output treatment. The sand is maintained in contact with hot gases for approximately 5 minutes by means of a valve with adjustable, weighted balance. This technology enables treatment at a lower temperature, under 600° C, which corresponds to a specific consumption equal to 260 kWh(n.c.v.)/t with respect to natural gas, under the conditions already defined.

The curves showing the change in temperature and the composition of flue gases in the furnace are given in Fig. 4. They show that the major portion of the treatment is rapidly terminated and that the reaction no longer occurs further than 1 m from the burner.

2.1.3 - Economic data*

The upright type unit with an expansion chamber shall be equipped with a cooling stage based upon the "Air-Contact" principle.

- Present cost of sand:

  . Purchase of new sand: 147 FRF/t
                                                    224 FRF/t
  . Disposal of used sand: 77 FRF/t

- Treatment cost at temperature of 750° C:

  . Natural gas, with daily heating: 74 FRF/t

  . Electicity, pressure-boosted air,
    estimated at: 20 FRF/t 102 FRF/t

  . Purchase of new sand: 8 FRF/t

- Investment cost of furnace and cooler
  (excluding upstream and downstream
  systems):   Approx. 220 000 FRF

For annual treatment of 1500 t/year, the savings would equal the costs of the investment in 1.2 years at constant monetary values.

2.2 - De-oiling of metal shavings

2.2.1 - General

Recycling of factory metal shavings by remelting requires the elimination of cutting oil. At present, these shavings are collected by vendors who store them in the open air for evaporation of oils, then resell them.

* All economic data are given in 1987 French francs.

Certain users, notably in the melting industry, feel that this procedure is somewhat rigid and are looking for other solutions. Combustion of oils is one of the technologies considered and tests have ben conducted on Gaz de France prototype equipment.

2.2.2 - <u>Tests - Results</u>

Tests have been conducted to obtain dry, de-oiled shavings with as little oxidation as possible. For this, the air factor with respect to all fuels, i.e., natural gas and cutting oils, was maintained close to stoichiometric combustion conditions with variable gas flow rates.

The results show:

- shavings exiting at 650° C are perfectly clean and show little signs of oxidation,

- specific fuel consumption to reach this temperature is under 280 kWh(n.c.v.)/t, and the amount of energy supplied by the oils may reach 45% to 50% of the total,

- the oils burn rapidly: at 1.5 m from the burner no more change in the combustion reaction is detected.

2.2.3 - <u>Economic data</u>

Elements concerning the cost of present operations: removal, storage and repurchase of shavings are not available. The cost of incineration may be estimated as follows :

- if oils are incinerated and the shavings are stored - the most unfavorable case - the cost of complete incineration equipment and the operating costs (air, gas, electricity: approx. 40 FRF/t) must be taken into account.

- however, if hot shavings are reinjected into the melt-down zone through a burner mounted directly on the melting furnace*, the investment is clearly further reduced and operating costs practically inexistent: the enthalpy of the shavings (106 kWh/t at 630° C) is fully recovered and the energy supplied by the burner contributes to the heating of the furnace.

---

* REMARK: Injection of shavings through burners mounted on a melting furnace is planned on a copper-melting basin furnace. This technology is mentioned in a paper at the ATG (French Gas Association) conference (1984).

2.3 - Detoxification of dust

2.3.1 - General

Certain industrial processes lead to the formation of dust which is found in the flue-gases from blast furnaces and eliminated by filtration systems designed for this purpose. Discharge of this dust poses a certain number of problems, notably toxicity.

It is thus necessary to eliminate the pollutant components before rejecting the dust. This is possible with the Gas-Contact process. In certain cases, a secondary result has been the possible sale of by-products.

2.3.2 - Tests - Results

Two applications of this type (decyanidization and incineration of hydrocarbons) have led to the purchase of semi-industrial equipment by companies concerned, following exploratory tests on Gaz de France prototype equipment for incineration of hydrocarbons.

The results obtained have shown that the desired goal was largely attained: destruction of cyanides or hydrocarbons was total. In the case of cyanized dust, the high alkaline content of the dust influences the physical state of the product treated and necessitates the development of a wet recovery process so that the soluble salts can be marketed. After elimination of hydrocarbon dust, silica dust can be marketed.

In both cases, market surveys predicted profits and a fast return on investment (approx. 1 year).

3 - WASTE DESTRUCTION

When waste is not reused it may be destroyed, while taking the steps necessary to prevent pollution by the combustion products released by the process. This incineration may in certain cases be considered as energy recovery because it may release a greater amount of energy than that required by the process.

Among possible operations two particular cases will be examined:

- incineration of electrical insulation waste products.

- incineration of paint and cataphoresis sludge.

3.1 - Incineration of electrical insulation waste products

3.1.1 - General

The metals recycling industry recovers important quantities of electrical wire of all types. Copper is extracted mechano-pneumatically: the wire and cable are sectioned and ground, and the copper is separated from the surrounding materials by air dispersion. The copper may be remelted; however, the insulation waste materials cannot be recycled because of the lack of uniformity in their composition (tar, polyethylene, aluminium strip, paper, etc.). They are thus stored without being destroyed, which takes up a relatively large amount of storage space.

One company has considered burning this waste. Bulk incineration is not possible because of the large amount of black smoke due to poor combustion. In addition, this type of informal burning leads to a signigicant loss of potential energy. Hence the idea of adapting the Gas-Contact process to the design of a mixed natural-gas/insulation waste burner was put forward.

3.1.2 - Test - Results

Tests were conducted with a burner fitted with its product feed system, mounted on a cylindrical combustion chamber similar to a rotary melting furnace for non-ferrous metals.

After determining the mean calorific value of the waste (equal to 8.5 kWh(n.c.v.)/kg), two types of tests were carried out: either gradual substitution of waste for gas at constant energy output and air rate, until incomplete combustion occurred; or at constant gas rate and with an increase in output due to additional waste until poor combustion occurred (the appearance of carbon monoxide in the flue-gas was simultaneous with production of soot).

Table No. 1 shows a few results which are representative of the tests conducted, with the following symbols:

- Q_g: natural-gas flow rate (m3(n)/h),

- m: rate of waste feed (kg/h),

- P_c: total output (kW(n.c.v.)),

- τ: substitution ratio for natural gas (*),

- η: combustion efficiency with furnace empty.

The table shows:

-that it is possible to substitute up to 45% waste for natural gas without significantly altering the useful ouput,

-that the increase in the useful output due to injection of waste is accompanied by an increase in useful output for $\tau \leq 0.26$. Beyond this value, total output does not increase further: the increase in the useful output due to waste must be accompanied by an increase in excess air to maintain combustion without unburned matter. Because of this, flue-gas losses increase.

---

* The substitution ratio is the ratio between the energy supplied by the waste and the total energy output. The values in the table are based on the mean values of net calorific values : 10 kWh/m3(n) for natural gas, and 8.5 kWh/kg for waste.

Remark: The limit value on the substitution ratio increases if combustion air is replaced by oxygen: from 45% to approx. 65%. However, this technique has two disadvantages:

-the very short oxygas/waste flame leads to rapid coking of a part of the waste at the burner outlet causing it to become quickly plugged,

-the consumption of primary energy corresponding to the production of the combustion oxygen is not recovered in this type of operation.

Qg	m	Pc	τ	η	Pc
30	0	300	0	0.62	186
20	9.5	283	0.29	0.60	170
18	12.4	285	0.37	0.60	171
16.5	13.7	277	0.41	0.595	165
15	15.5	279	0.46	0.595	166
13	14.2	252	0.48	0.56	141
20	0	200	0	0.60	120
20	8.4	270	0.26	0.625	169
20	9.6	282	0.29	0.60	170
20	11.4	296	0.33	0.53	157
20	15.0	327	0.39	0.52	170

3.1.3 - Economic considerations

The economic results of incineration of insulation waste materials can be examined at different levels :

-financially, the use of free energy depends upon the possibilities available: boilers, melting furnaces, etc., each having different output productivity,

-environmentally, this enables quick reuse of large storage areas, eliminates ugly dumps, and avoids the need for bulk incineration which causes a large output of soot.

3.2 - Paint and cataphoresis sludge

3.2.1 - General

Painting in a ventilated booth necessitates washing of the air circulated in the booth by means of special baths which are recycled. During recycling, the bath is decanted to eliminate drops of passivated paint, which combine to form a compound which is normally discarded or removed.

Cataphoresis sludge results from automotive body washing after it has gone through the cataphoresis bath. Washwater is concentrated up to a theoretical content of dry matter of 10%; it is then removed by contractors which treat it before discarding the water.

These various types of waste are costly and it may be profitable to try to recover their potential energy by burning the sludge on site.

3.2.2 - Tests - Results

Tests were conducted under the same conditions as for insulation waste materials. However, product feed requires a mechanical system in order to break the product down into particles.

The air factor with respect to all fuels has been maintained constant and close to 1.10, the same as for total output (225 kW(n.c.v.)).

The substitution ratio of paint sludge for natural gas reaches 60% without alteration of the combustion conditions. The product has a net calorific value varying between 9 and 11 kWh/kg because of the water bubbles contained in the material.

In the case of sludge from cataphoresis, the initial content of dry matter is too low (5% measured) for the process to be economical without prior preparation of the product:

- cold filtering yields a mixture with only 17% dry matter, which is insufficient to make incineration economical,

- filtering at 45° C enables an aggregate of 45% dry matter to be obtained, which may be easily granulated and whose net calorific value is approx. 3.3 kWh/kg.

Incineration tests were carried out with this latter product, and with the dry product (whose n.c.v. is approx. 7.4 kWh/kg). In both cases a natural gas substitution ratio of 60% is achievable.

3.2.3 - Economic considerations

A project is underway for Gas-Contact incineration equipment for waste made up of 200 kg/h of paint sludge and 5 t/h of cataphoresis sludge with 5% dry matter, representing a potential energy of approx. 3800 kW n.c.v.. This equipment may be fitted on a steam generator, with additional natural-gas firing of 2600 kW(n.c.v.).

If the 300 kW(n.c.v.) necessary for heating cataphoresis sludge to 45° C (for hot filtering) are added, the operating costs reveal gas consumption of 2900 kW(n.c.v.), yielding 6400 kW(n.c.v.), which represents additional free energy of 55% V/g the same equipment operating on fuel-oil or natural gas. Actually, the savings are less, taking into consideration the electrical consumption needed for sludge preparation.

The savings in disposal costs paid to a contractor (approx. 600 FRF/t for paint sludge and 360 FRF/t for cataphoresis sludge with 5% dry matter, at the time of the study) may be added to the positive side of the operating costs sheet.

4 - CONCLUSION

Waste treatment, whether it concerns waste produced industrially or by other means, for the purpose of reusing it or destroying it, and the contribution this makes to environmental protection, are topics of concern today and there are many available techniques.

Among these, the Gas-Contact process offers an attractive solution to many treatment problems, due to the remarkable performance of its burner and its simplicity of use. These advantages are:

- the extent of the rating range of counter rotation burners enables design of units adapted to each problem confronted,

- the Gas-Contact effect favors size reduction,

- the continuous passage of the product to be treated avoids equipment clogging during shutdowns, facilitates maintenance and reduces restart time,

- the absence of moving parts reduces maintenance time.

The Gas-Contact process offers a simple, easy-to-use, flexible and low-cost method of treating waste products.

SALES INFORMATION

The Gas-Contact Process, with applications that go beyond industrial waste treatment, is manufactured under license by two companies with the technical assistance of Gaz de France:

- Société MEKER
  105, boulevard de Verdun
  92400 COURBEVOIE
  Tel.: (1) 43.33.31.81

- Société SARGI
  10, Cité d'Angoulême
  75011 PARIS
  Tel.: (1) 43.57.39.43

Systèmes de combustion industriels
Industrial combustion systems

TRANSTECH 1987

TITLE: "NEW TECHNOLOGIES TO INCREASE COMBUSTION EFFIENCY AND REDUCE NOx"

AUTHOR: Normand Brais, Ing., M.Sc.A.
Technical Director, TODD COMBUSTION LTD.

INTERNATIONAL SYMPOSIUM ON MEASUREMENTS, PROPERTIES AND UTILIZATION OF NATURAL GAS, MONTREAL, QC., CANADA. NOVEMBER 25-27, 1987.

Date: November 1987

ABSTRACT

To meet tomorrow's environmental challenge, combustion equipment designers must seek for new methods and approach the problems in a more comprehensive manner. The semi-empirical methods actually in use have long reached their limits as far as the flame structure prediction is concerned.

A new technology which uses mathematical models applied on a discrete grid to simulate a flame in its environment is presented here. The flame structure is thus predicted and a two-step approach is used to model the formation of thermal NOx. The first step involves the main exothermal reation of methane in air, and the second involves the solution of the Zeldovich reaction scheme for the generation of nitrogen oxides.

A single step reaction scheme is used for the methane combustion calculation which is kinetically controlled. The limiting control of turbulence is taken into account by using a reaction rate which is the minimum to that given by the Arrhenius and Eddy-Break-Up models. A flux model is used to calculate radiative heat transfer.

In the second step, a chemical equilibrium analysis is performed to determine the concentration of radicals (O, OH, and H) in the product stream and conservation equations are then solved for N and NO which utilise the convective and diffusive transport terms calculated in the first step.

The method is applied to a large industrial burner featuring an axial and a swirling recirculating flow region into which fuel is injected either tangentially or axially. Parametric variations on the burner geometry and operational variables are then studied in terms of their impact on NOx emission.

CONTENTS

I- Introduction

II- NOx reduction methods

III- Description of the model

IV- Application to burner design

V- Discussion of results

VI- Conclusion

- Nomenclature
- References

I- INTRODUCTION

Combustion generated pollution is now recognised as a threat to the environment. The most obvious air pollutant is smoke, being visible to the naked eye. Other pollutants of importance are, carbon monoxide (CO), unburned hydrocarbons, sulfur oxides (SOx) and finally nitrogen oxides (NOx). Virtually all of these pollutants have a harmful effect on the ecosystem [1]. Emotive phrases have evolved over the years which described these effects, as in the "greenhouse effect", "acid rain", "city smog", and the "ozone layer hole".

In this work we concentrate on the last pollutant mentioned, NOx which is responsible amongst other things for the apparent depletion of the earth's ozone layer through a chain reaction mechanism. The quantitative influence of this chain mechanism in the stratosphere is uncertain. However, this gap in knowledge and the fact that a hole in the ozone layer above the antarctic has increased alarmingly in size in recent years, has led to a worldwide tightening of legislation governing the sources of NOx emission.

The term NOx usually implies two major oxides, nitrogen oxide (NO) and nitrogen dioxide (NO2). In combustion, NO is the dominant of the two components, NO2 being mainly derived from NO. It is the prediction of NO we are concerned with in this paper, loosely referred to as NOx. The following passages lead to NO production.

* From reaction of N_2 with oxygen, "thermal NO",

* from N existing in the fuel, "fuel NO", and,

* from reaction of fuel derived radicals with N_2 ultimately leading to NO, the "prompt NO".

It is the first of these three mechanisms we are concerned with here, since it is the one that can be most affected by burner design.

Since, air borne pollution is no observer of human boundaries, world wide concern over the issue has come under the UN/ECE convention on "Long Range Trans-Boundary Air Pollution", which is negotiating an international standard on NOx emissions. Similar activities have been undertaken in the EEC, where particularly stiff controls already exist in power stations operating in Germany and the Netherlands. Typically, Dutch legislation requires limits of 200 ppm NOx for liquid fuel and 120 ppm NOx for gas fuel industrial burners [3]. In the near future these figures are expected to be halved.

It is under this climate of tightening legislation that new improved methods of design are called for to replace existing burners/combustors, and improved methods of operation required to prolong the use of existing units.

II- NOx REDUCTION METHODS

The main factor controlling thermal NOx is temperature. In fact, NOx formation is insignificant at temperature below 1800K. In has been observed [4] that:

$$NOx \propto e^{.009T}$$

where T=reaction temperature in Kelvin. All other factors can be viewed as means of affecting temperature. Therefore, the burner designer needs to avoid hot spots and also keep the time available for NOx formation to a minimum. Both these factors are affected by an increase in the flow of air into the combustion zone. However, care needs to be exercised if CO and unburned hydrocarbon levels are to be kept to a minimum. Practical means of control include:

* Low excess air combustion since O_2 concentration is reduced.

* Exhaust, or flue gas recirculation effective if the recirculation gas is cooled before being injected into the combustion zone.

* Water injection into the primary combustion zone of a burner as used in industrial turbines; utilizes the latent heat of water droplets to reduce temperature.

* Staged combustion, which introduces primary, secondary or even tertiary combustion zones and hence allows tighter control on temperature limits. In order to be effective, both air and fuel delivery needs to be staged. Desing complexities result.

In order to be able to evaluate the influence of these factors, a mathematical model which represents correctly the physico-chemical aspects of the problem is needed. The object of this paper is to report the development of such a model and present preliminary calculations.

III - DESRIPTION OF THE MODEL

The problem of simulating a real burner accurately still remains a formidable one. Not only has one to contend with complex flow fields which often include swirl and regions of flow reversal and are highly turbulent, but also one has to tackle complex chemical kinetics which govern the combustion and subsequent formation of trace chemicals.

It is clear that the combustion and NOx reactions in a burner are inseparable, and the latter is a direct consequence of the former. However, it has been observed in experiments [1] that the main oxidising reaction between fuel and aire is not affected by the formation of trace species which lead to NOx. Hence, although the NOx reactions tend to be endothermic, the radicals involved occur in minute concentrations and they do not affect the exothermic reaction occurring in the bulk of the burner. On the other hand, as pointed out earlier, the temperatures generated by the combustion are the determining factor in NOx formation. With these observations in mind, one can treat the combustion and NOx formation steps as separate.

Conservation Equations Solved

Flow and reaction in a burner is defined in terms of a set of elliptic partial differential equations that express the conservation of mass, momentum, energy and other fluid variables in three-dimensional recirculating flow. With the primitive variable representing velocity, chemical species, temperature and turbulence variables the equations can be written in a generalised form:

$$\frac{\partial}{\partial t}(\rho \varphi) + \mathrm{div}(\rho \vec{V} \varphi - \Gamma_\varphi \,\mathrm{grad}\, \varphi) = S_\varphi \qquad (1)$$

where ρ, V, Γ_φ, and S_φ are density, velocity vector, turbulent exchange coefficient and source rate per unit volume respectively. The sources and exchange coefficients for velocities and turbulence have been discussed in detail elsewhere [12, 13] together with the effects of buoyancy. The $K-\varepsilon$ model of turbulence is used to calculate the effective viscosity [13] in all regions of the flow, except where strong swirl exists. In these regions a mixing length model is used instead.

The numerical analogue of equations (1) was solved using PHOENICS on a cylindrical polar finite difference grid.

Combustion Model

Calculations were performed using a single step combustion model which could be either diffusion controlled or kinetically controlled. In both cases the equation for a mixture fraction [14] is solved; in the first case the mass fraction of fuel at any point is determined from it, while in the second, an additional conservation equation is solved for the mass fraction of fuel. The mass fractions of products and oxidant are then derived from these quantities [15].

The disappearance rate of fuel (CH4) was calculated in the kinetically controlled model as being the minimum of that given by an Arrhenius expression and eddy-break-up expression [16].

$$R_{fu} = -C_R \rho \frac{\varepsilon}{k} \min\left[m_{fu}, \frac{m_{ox}}{s}, \frac{m_{pr}}{1+s}\right] \quad (2)$$

where, C_R either takes a constant value of 4 or is calculated locally as a function of k and ε ie.

$$C_R = 23.6 \left[\frac{\mu}{\rho} \cdot \frac{\varepsilon}{k^2}\right]^{0.25} \quad (3)$$

The effect of radiation was included using a flux model [15, 17] which solves ordinary differential equations for radiation fluxes along each coordinate direction.

The ideal gas law was used to calculate density variations and the specific heat was allowed to vary as a function of temperature and composition.

The combustion calculation yielded field values of all the dependent variables, which were stored on disc for use in the NOx prediction.

NOx Calculations

The chemistry involved in the formation of NOx will now be described. The model employed incorporates one of the simplest and most widely used mechanisms for calculations involved nitric oxide formation, namely the Zeldovich mechanism:

$$N_2 + O = NO + N, \qquad (4)$$

$$O_2 + N = NO + O, \qquad (5)$$

$$OH + N = NO + H, \qquad (6)$$

As mentioned earlier, the basic assumption in this work is that reaction (4)-(6) can be considered as decoupled from the main fuel-burning reaction. In addition, the species appearing in these reactions are assumed to form part of the product stream of the single combustion reaction which in the first step of the calculation was assumed to be a single entity.

The species O, O_2, OH, H, H_2, CO and CO_2 are assumed to exist as chemical equilibrium. Their concentration is determined from a minimisation of Gibbs free energy subject to the following constraints: (a) mass balance of the elements present in the system. (b) specified enthalpy and, (c) specified pressure. The polynominal equations for species concentrations are solved in a single pass by calling the code CREK [18] in the ground station of PHOENICS. The mass fractions of N and NO are determined by solving conservation equations (equation (1)) which have as convection and diffusion fluxes the ones determined in the combustion step. It is assumed that the concentrations of the other species remain invariant, with the justification that they are produced by reactions which are considerably faster than those involving nitrogen.

The source term for the two conservation equations comes from a summation of the reaction rate for all reactions in which each species participates; ie. the Zeldovich reactions. The forward and backward reactions are given by Arrhenius expressions of the form:

$$R = K \rho^2 F_1 F_2 \qquad (7)$$

where F_1 and F_2 are the concentrations of participating species and K the reaction rate coefficient, given by

$$K = 10^B \, T^N \, e^{-T_{act}/T} \qquad (8)$$

with $10^B \, T^N$ being the pre-exponential factor, and T_{act} the activation temperature. The values of these quantities are given in Table 1.

REACTION	FORWARD			REVERSE		
	10^B	T_{act}	N	10^B	T_{act}	N
$N_2 + O = NO + N$	7.6×10^{10}	3.8×10^4	0	1.6×10^{10}	0.0	0
$O_2 + N = NO + O$	6.4×10^6	3.15×10^3	1	1.5×10^6	1.95×10	1
$OH + N = NO + H$	6.3×10^8	0.0		2.5×10^9	2.45×10	0.5

Table 1: Constants used for the forward and reverse reactions (Equations 7, 8)

IV- **APPLICATION TO BURNER DESIGN**

The above described model was derived to predict the NOx emissions of a typical burner used in large steam generators.

It widely recognised [19], [20] that significant NOx emission reduction can be achieved through burner design. However, better understanding of the flame structure produced by a given burner is necessary in order to identify and apply successful design modifications.

Such modifications involve fuel injection distribution and pressure, air flow characteristics, and swirl stabilisation. Furnace geometry also needs to be considered since it conditions the heat transfer rate and the combustion products flow pattern [21].

The burner under investigation is the Todd axial air flow type using a blade swirler to impart a tangential velocity component to a portion (15%) of the total air flow. The latter principle is commonly used to stabilize high intensity industrial flame [22].

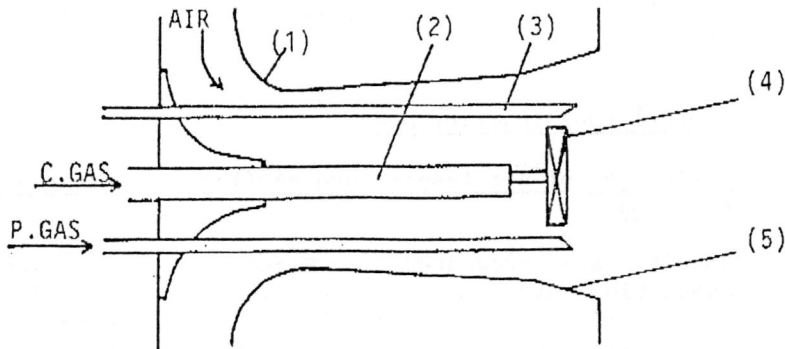

Figure 6: Typical Burner Investigated

As shown in Figure 6, the burner major components include a venturi air register (1), a central fuel injector (2), six peripheral fuel injectors (3), a swirler (4), and an exit quarl (5).

The characteristics of the burner being simulated were:

* Maximum heat output: 100 MMBTU/hr
* Combustion air temperature: 500 degrees F.
* Burner air side pressure drop: 10" WG
* Fuel: Natural gas (100% CH4)

A grid was defined using a polar coordinate referential which simulates a cylindrical combustion chamber 9 ft. in diameter by 20 ft. long.

At the upstream end of this combustion chamber, inlet boundary conditions were set, thus allowing for the burner outflow to be specified. A constant pressure boundary was assumed downstream, at the exit.

The cylindrical combustion chamber was selected initially to reduce computing cost. However, in the course of our parametric study, rectangular furnaces were also simulated.

This parametric study covered the influence of furnace size, combustion air temperature, fuel injection mode, burner pressure drop, burner heat input, and number of burners on thermal NOx emission tendencies. Some highlights of the most significant results are presented here.

4.1 Central Fuel Injetion Mode

4.1.1 Influence of air temperature on flame structure and NOx emissions

Results are presented in Figures 7 to 9 where the combustion air temperature is increased from 70 degrees F. to 300 degrees F. and finally to 500 degrees F. The flame temperature contours reveal the evidence that flame length is decreasing as combustion air temperature increases. NOx concentration contours in the flame are shown in Figures 10 to 12 and display a significant increase when air temperature is increased. A synopsis of these results is presented in Table 2.

COMBUSTION AIR TEMP. (F.)	70	300	500
Primary Air ratio %	15.5	13.3	12.03
Adiabatic Flame temp. (K)	2162	2226	2283
Maximum Field Temp (K)	1557	1591	1650
Maximum NOx conc. (PPM)	214	396	587
Exit NOx conc. (PPM)	138	285	482

Table 2: Summary of NOx Parametric Study 1

Another point worth noting concerns the flame aerodynamics in the furnace as depicted in Figures 13 to 15. As the air temperature is increased, the extent of both internal and external recirculation zones is enhanced significantly. Internal recirculation is generated by the swirler and is responsible for the stabilisation of the flame, thus suggesting a better flame stability as air temperature is increased.

Although these are well known practical facts, the simulations were able to reflect their implications on the flame structure.

4.1.2 Influence of furnace geometry on flame structure

The same burner is now simulated in a rectangular furnace 9 ft. wide, 14 ft. wide and 26 ft. long, which is considerably larger than in the previous simulation.

The streamlines in Figures 16 and 17 show an increase in the radial expansion of the external recirculation region in the vertical direction of the furnace and causes significant departure from symmetry. However, the ignition zone structure (internal recirculation) remains almost unchanged. Temperature profiles across the furnace setion show clearly the flame asymmetry generated by the furnace confinement. (Figure 18)

The NOx contour plot given in Figure 19 shows a different structure from previous predictions for the cylindrical furnace. The maximum concentration is now well away from the burner and the mean NOx emissions at the exit, as a result, are reduced by 27%.

These tendencies were known from experimental evidence however no satisfatory explanations can be given at this stage.

4.1.3 Influence of dual-burner firing on flame aerodynamics

This study has great practical implications since most of the large industrial steam generators use an array of burners, from 2 to 10 in the mid-size, up to 32 burners for the 750 MW utility boilers.

The velocity vectors in a cross-section located 4.76 m downstream are shown in Figure 20 and provide information on the interaction between adjacent burners.

The interaction affects the fuel consumption rate where the flames overlap as can be seen from Figure 21.

Unfortunately, NOx emission runs were not completed when this paper was written. However, it is obvious from the early results that the number of burners and burner arrangement in a given furnace will strongly influence NOx emission predictions.

4.2 Peripheral Fuel Injection Mode

In this case, the burner uses six axial spuds located on a radius immediately outside the swirler to inject the fuel. The spud geometry allows the gas to be injected with a variable tangential and radial velocity component, while the axial component is maintained constant. This design along with its multitude of variations is used in practice when shorter flames are desired to satisfy furnace depth limitations. Amongst the design variations, the annular injector or "gas ring" falls into this category.

As shown in Figure 22, the flame structure is significantly altered. The fuel concentration is much lower (near stoichiometry) in the stabilization zone than with the central injector mode. This will have major consequences on temperature and NOx concentrations. In addition, the fuel depletion rate is faster and results, as expected, in a shorter flame.

Temperature contours (Figure 23) show higher maxima in the stabilization zone and in the flame periphery. This actually explains the fact that this flame is usually more stable at high firing rates. It also indicates that thermal NOx emissions will be higher than with the central fuel injection mode. This was also experienced during field tests where an approximate 30% NOx emission increase was observed.

Although this design is easier to deal with for flame stability and length considerations, low NOx burner designers would be advised to treat it with caution.

V- **DISCUSSION OF RESULTS**

The partial results of this study show that the design of low NOx combustion equipment must take into consideration the combustion chamber geometry. It also demonstrates that NOx emission is intimately related to the flame structure.

The flame structure was seen to be governed mainly by the fuel injection mode and the aerodynamics prevailing inside the furnace.

The partial results obtained so far in this investigation suggest that the central fuel injection where a fuel rich core is created in the flame front is well adapted for low NOx operation. However, some stability problems may arise when fuel concentration in the internal recirculation becomes too high to sustain combustion. This phenomenon was experienced in the field and was solved by the introduction of a small quantity of air flowing through the co-axial inner conduit of the gas injector. This model derived design alteration has proved to be very effective in the field in improving the flame stability, while leaving NOx emissions unchanged.

VI- CONCLUSIONS

The present mathematical model is a powerful design tool to assist the burner designer in predicting NOx emission trends. It allows comparative evaluations to be successfully performed on a series of burner design variations.

However, more experimental work in conjunction with the present model is required in order to predict absolute values of NOx emissions on specific applications. Particularly, a fuel-NOx model and an oil droplet combustion model must be incorporated to widen the application range of the present work.

Nonetheless, the preliminary results partially presented here were sufficient, with the help of some empirical burner design guide rules, to accomplish major improvements in the NOx emission performances of recent burner installations. For instance, the modelling results have suggested the effectiveness of a selective flue gas recirculation concept through the burner. Such a flue gas recirculation system was designed accordingly and implemented in a refinery early in July 1987. Impressive NOx reduction levels (80%) were achieved with a relatively small amount of the gas being recirculated (less than 16% of total). This was already a significant contribution to better burner design.

Empirical burner design methods have long reached their limits. But in the light of mathematical modelling work, new audacious burner designs are merging to meet todays and future environmental constraints.

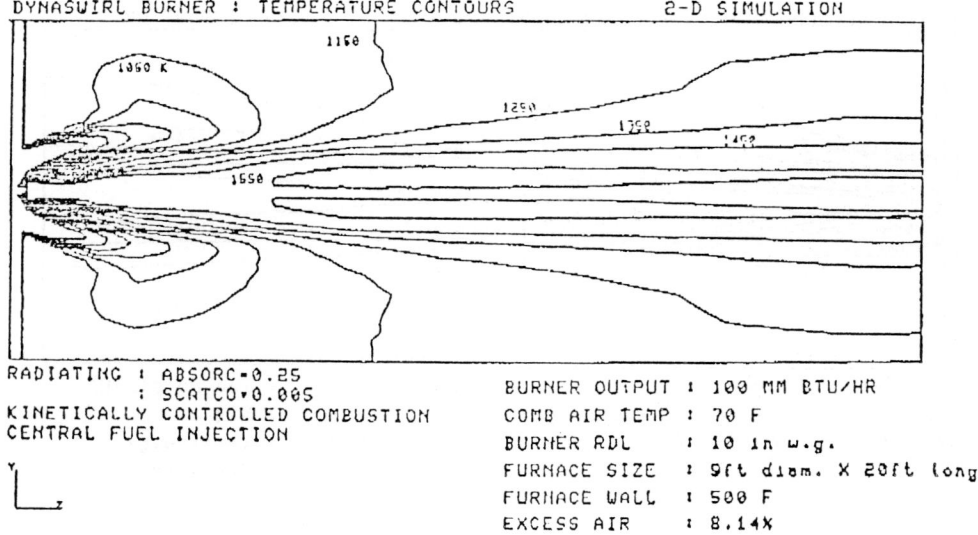

Figure 7

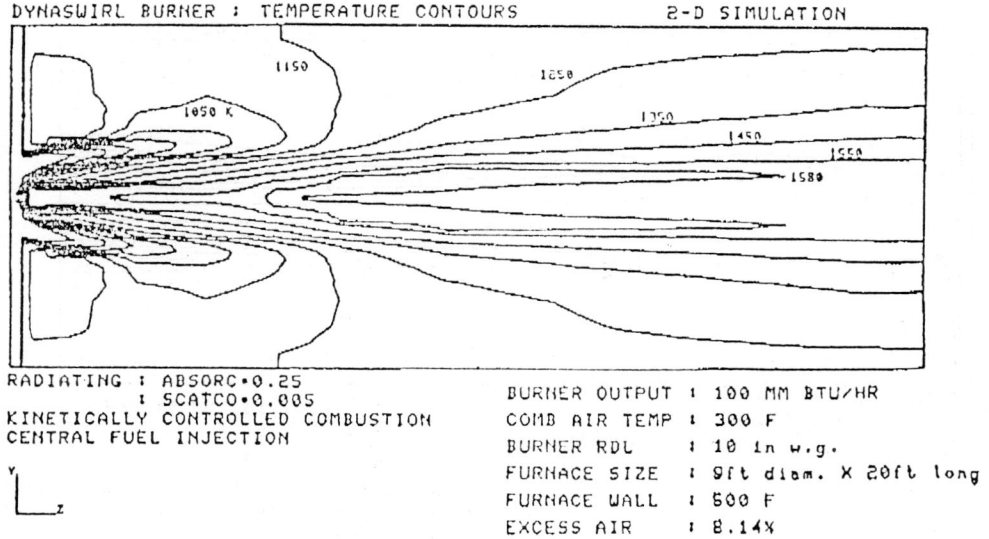

Figure 8

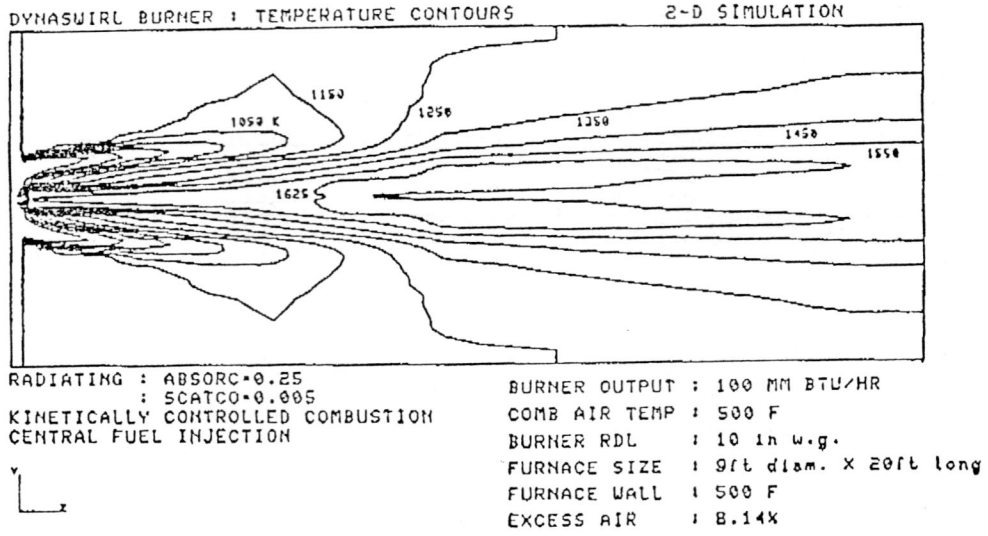

Figure 9

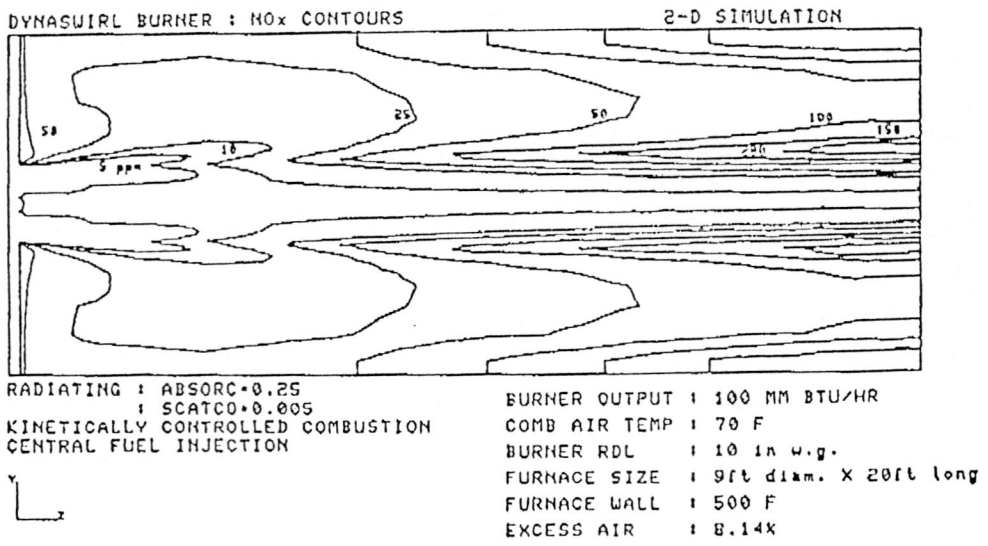

Figure 10

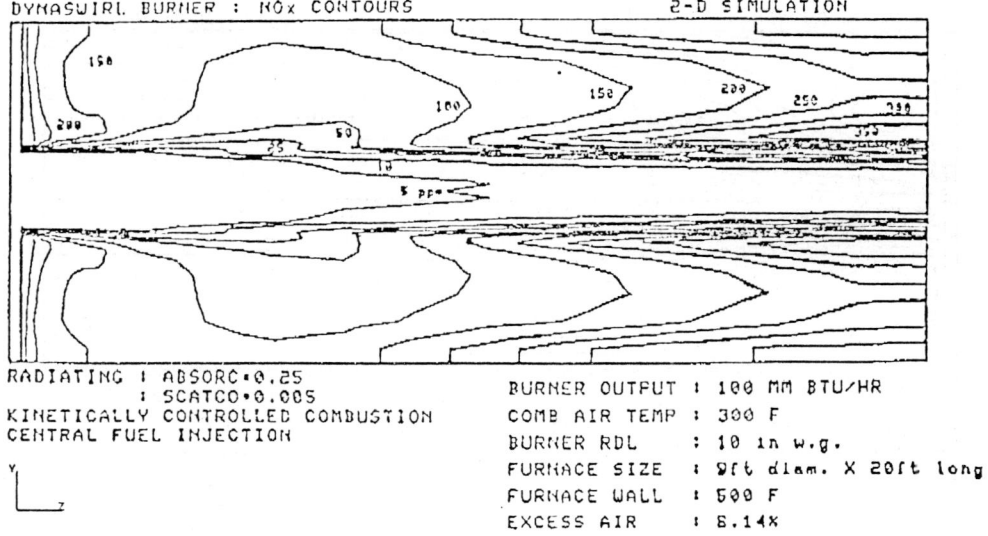

Figure 11

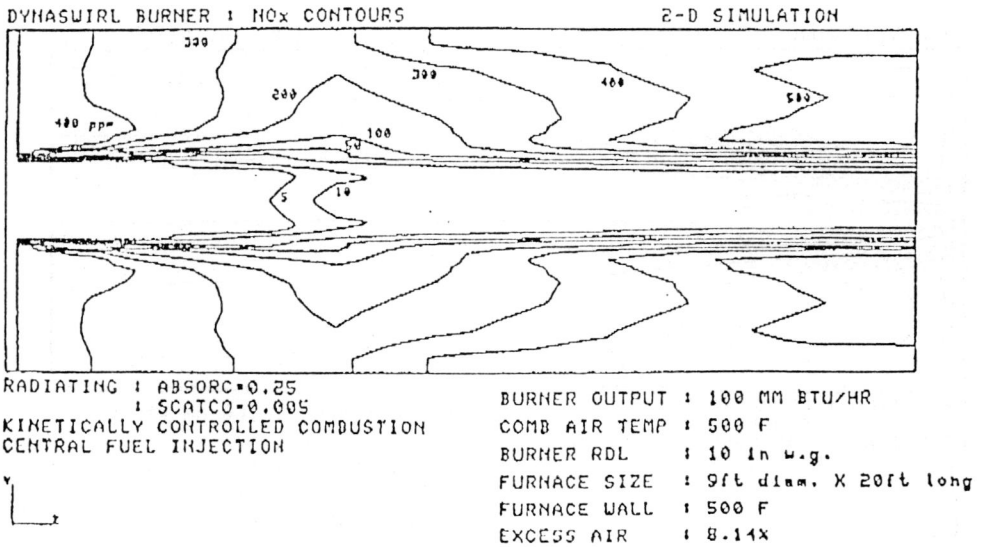

Figure 12

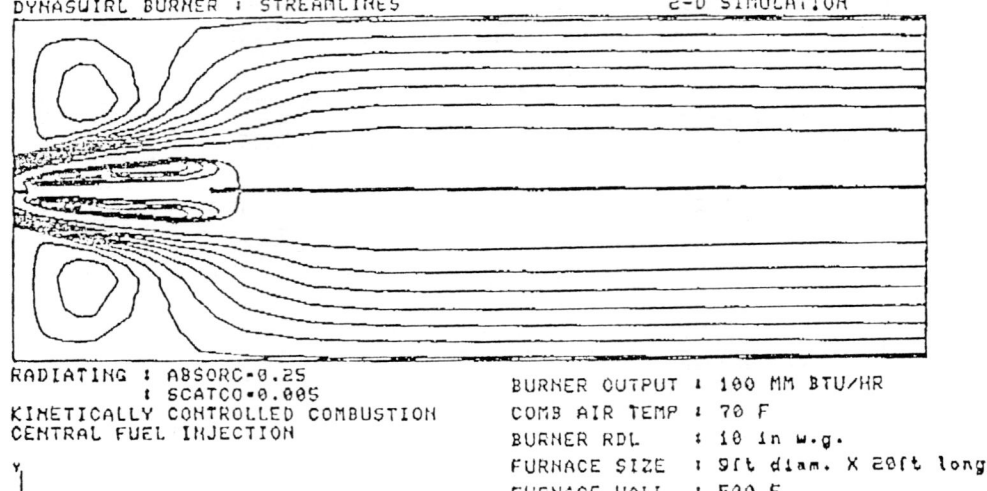

Figure 13

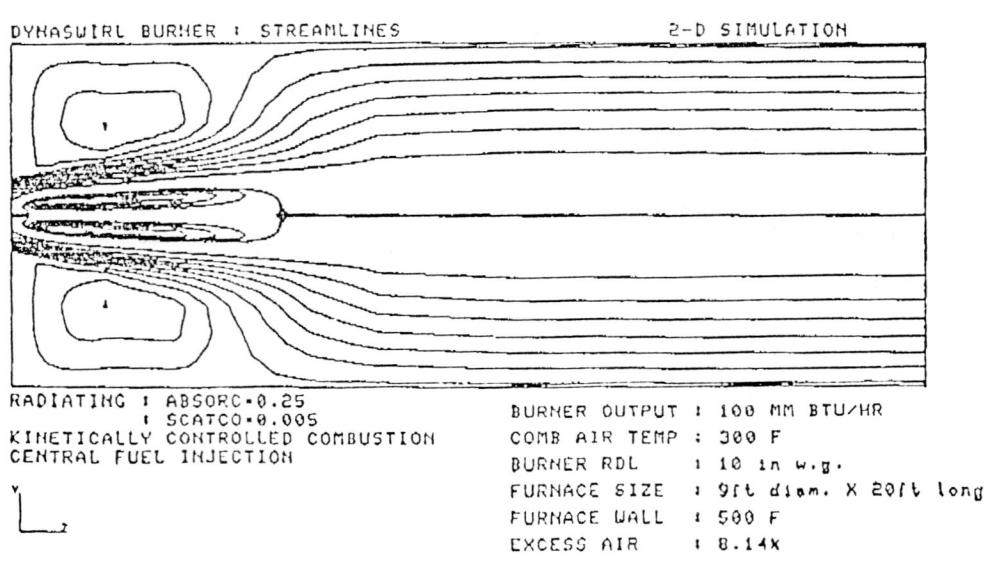

Figure 14

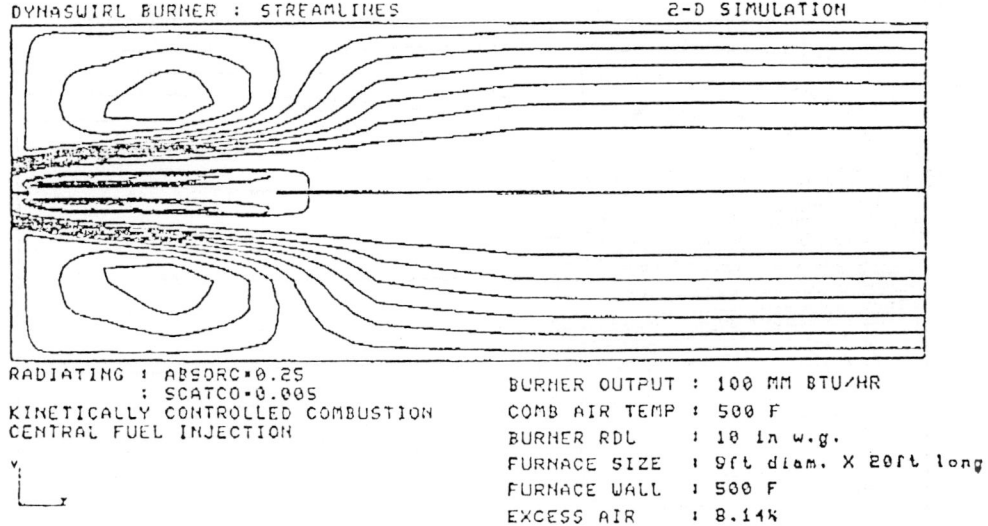

Figure 15

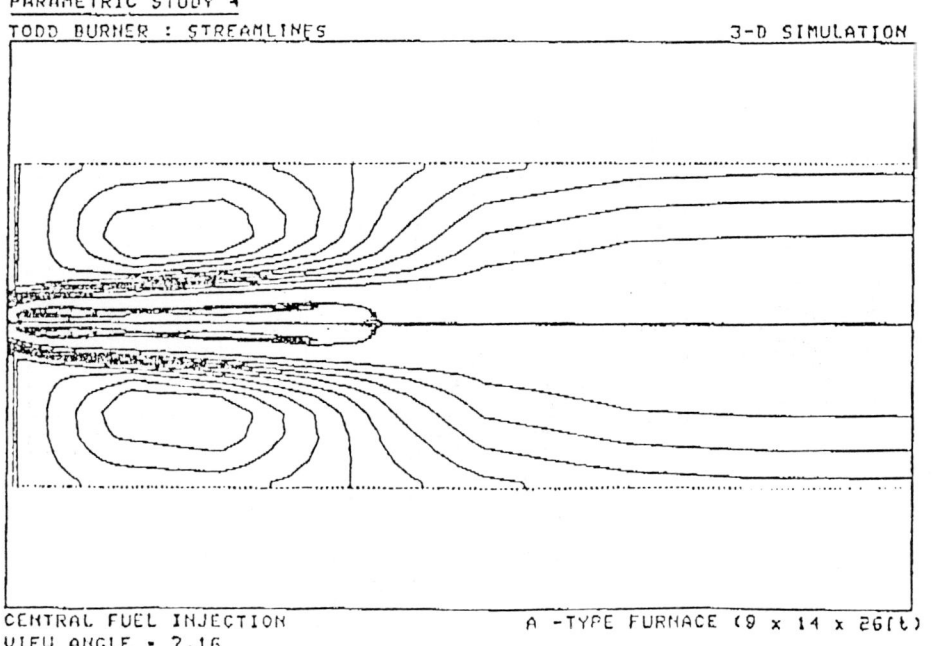

Figure 16

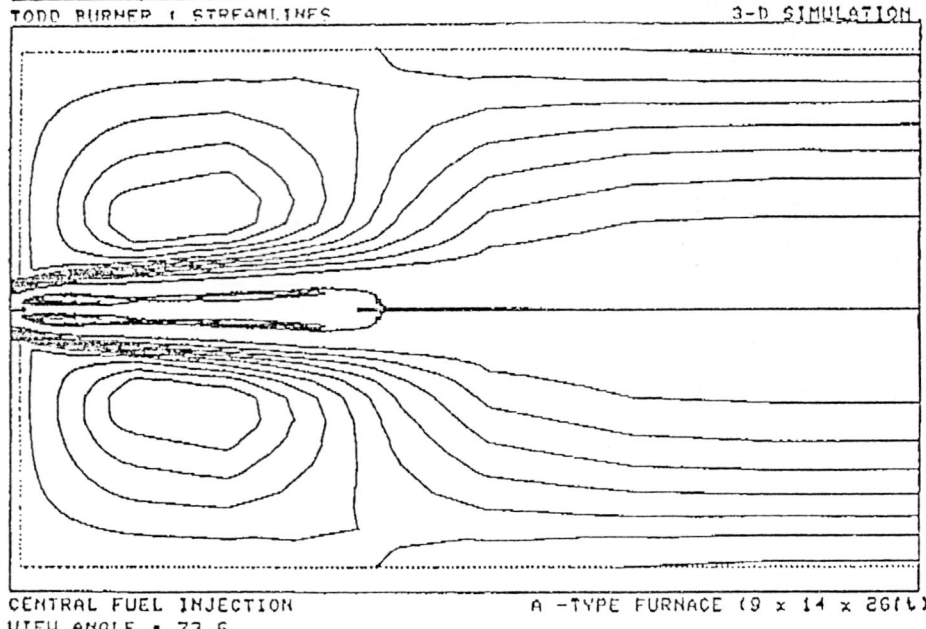

Figure 17

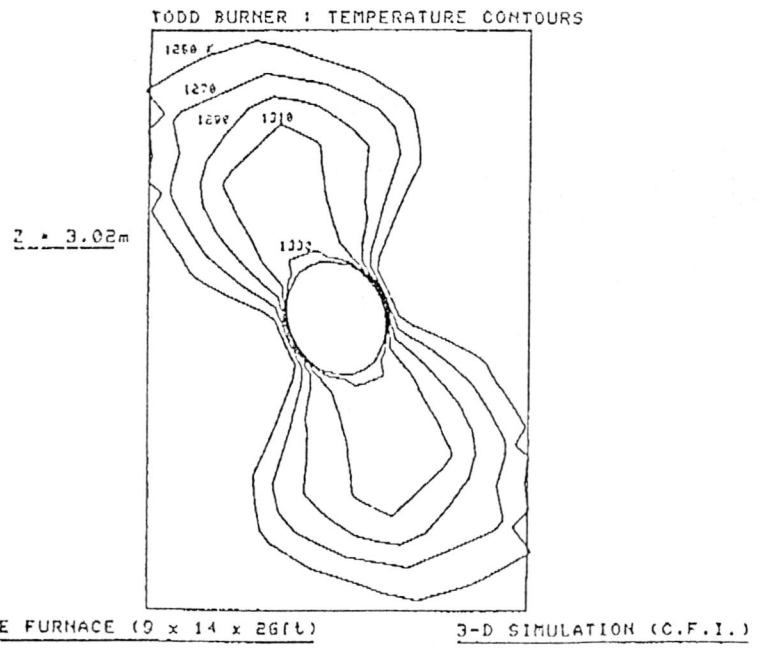

Figure 18

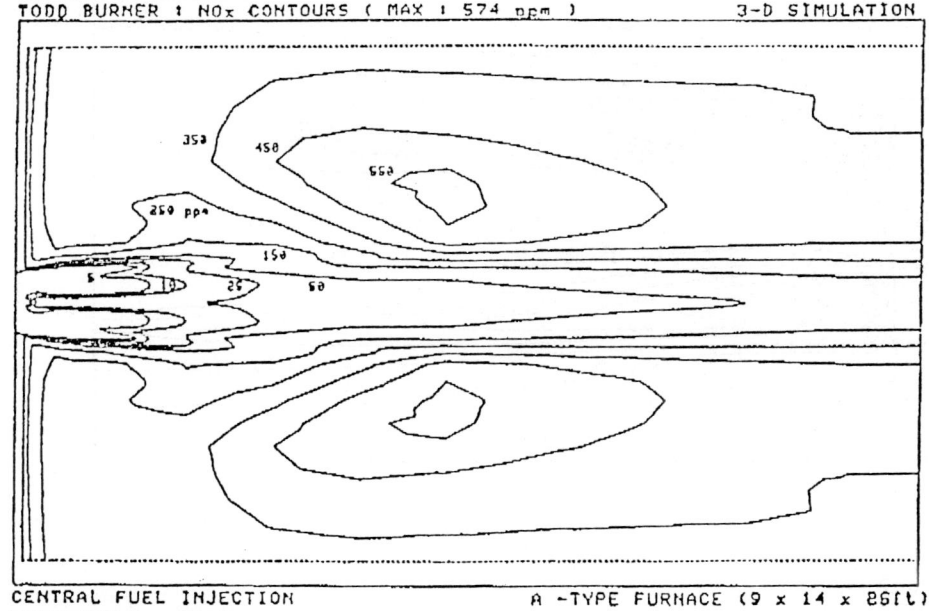

Figure 19

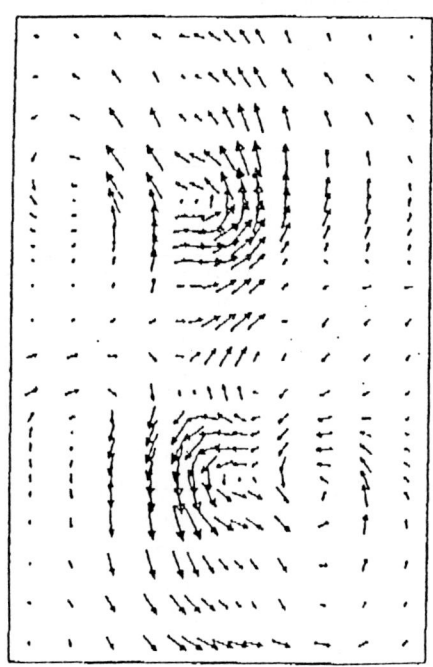

Figure 20

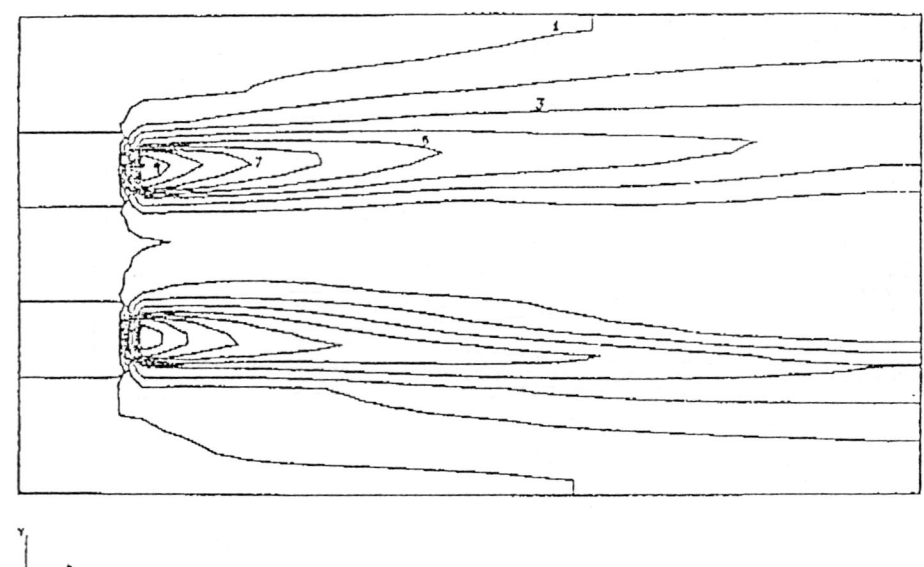

Figure 21

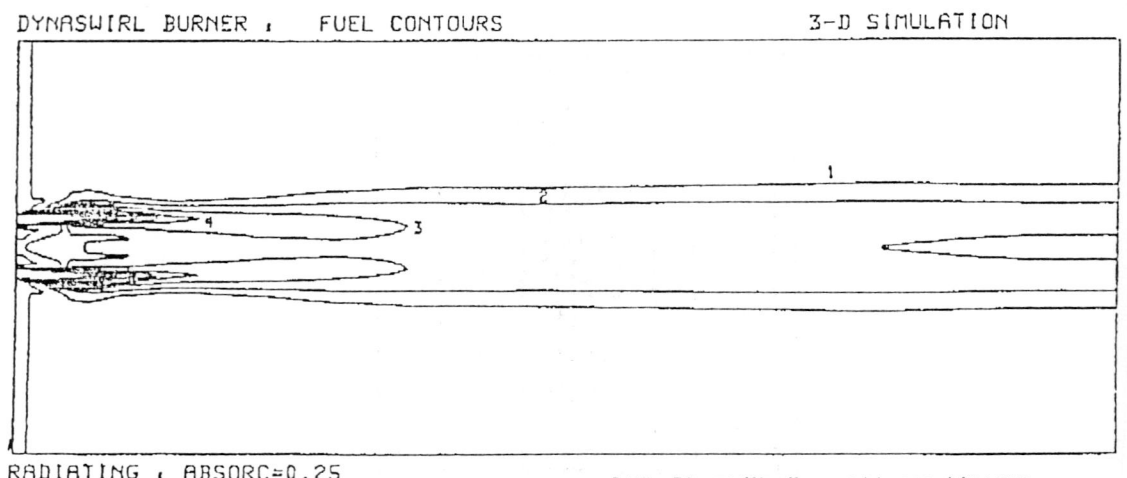

RADIATING , ABSORC=0.25
, SCATCO=0.005
KINETICALLY CONTROLLED COMBUSTION
CONTOUR RANGE , 0.005,(10),0.205

BURNER OUTPUT , 100 MM BTU/HR
COMB AIR TEMP , 500 F
BURNER RDL , 10 in w.g.
FURNACE SIZE , 9ft diam. X 20ft long
FURNACE WALL , 500 F
EXCESS AIR , 5 %

Figure 22

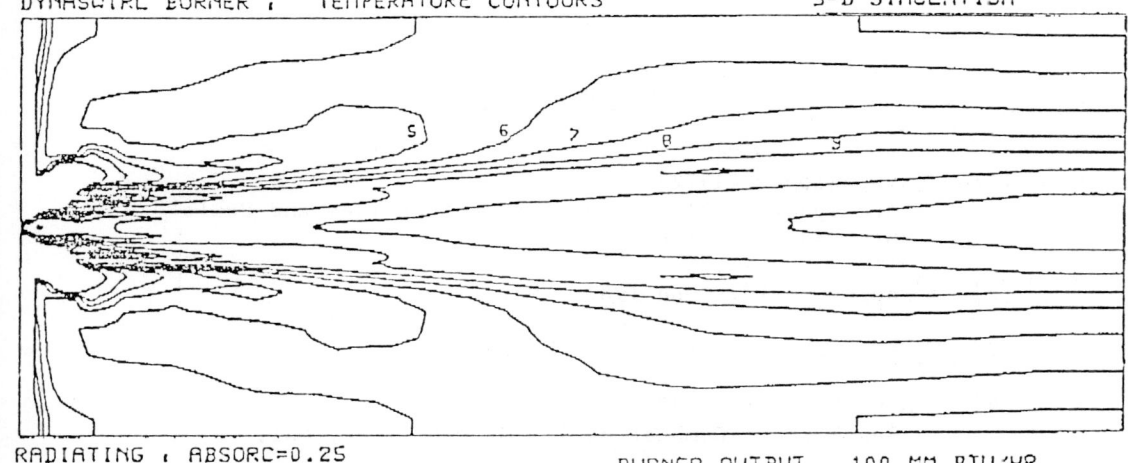

Figure 23

REFERENCES

[1] R.F. Sawyer (1972)
'Atmosphere Pollution by Aircraft Engines and Fuels'
AGARD Advisory report 40.

[2] Energy World, June 1987: No. 148.

[3] Process Engineering, March 1987p. 41.

[4] A.H. Lefebvre (1983)
'Gas Turbine Combustions' McGraw Hill, p. 481.

[5] Shefer R.W. and Sawyer R.F. (1976)
'Lean Premixed Recirculating Flow Combustion for Control of Oxides of Nitrogen'

[6] Quan V, Kliegel J.R. and Peters R.L. (1975)
'Predicted Effects of Fluid Dynamic Parameters on Nitric Oxide Formation in Turbulent Jet Diffusion Flames'
Combustion and Flame 25, p. 67.

[7] Mizutani Y and Katsuki M. (1976)
'Emissions from Gas Turbine Combustors' Bulletin of JSME 19, p. 1360

[8] Khalil E.E. (1981)
'Numerical Computation of Combustion Generated Pollutants'
Proc. Italian Flames Days (La Rivista du Combustibili).

[9] Hutchinson P. Khalil E.E. and Whitelaw J.H. (1977)
'Measurement and Calculation of Furnace Flow Properties'
AIAA Journal of Energy 1, p. 212.

[10] Hung W. (1975)
'An Experimentally Verified Nox Emission Model for Gas Turbine Combustors, ASME 75-GT-71

[11] Zeldovich Y.B., Sadovinkov P.Y. and Frank-Kamenctskii D.A. (1974)
'Oxidation of Nitrogen in Combustion'
Academy of Sciences of USSR, Moscow

[12] Markatos N.C. Malin M.R. and Cox G. (1982)
'Mathematical Modelling of Buoyancy-IOnduced Smoke Flow in Enclosures'
Int.J. Heat and Mass Transfer 25, pp. 63-75.

[13] Rodi W. (1978)
'Turbulence Models and their Applications in Hydraulics - a State of the Art Review'
SFB 80/T/127, Univ. of Karlsruhe

[14] Spalding, D.B. (1977)
'GENMIX: A General Computer Program for Two-Dimensional Parabolic Phenomena'
Pergamon Press.

[15] Markatos N.C. and Pericleous K.A. (1983)
'An Investigation of Three-Dimensional Fires in Enclosures'
ASME - MTD 25, pp. 115-124.

[16] Magnussen B.F. and Hjertager B.H. (1976)
'On Mathematical Modelling of Turbulent Combustion with Special Emphasis on Soot Formation and Combustion'
Proc. 16th Int. Symposium on Combustion. The Comb. Inst., pp. 719-729.

[17] Hamaker H.C. (1947)
'Radiation and heat Conduction in Light Scattering Material',
Philips Res. Rep. 2, pp. 103-111

[18] Gordon S. and McBride B. (1971)
'CREK: A Computer Program for Calculations of Complex Chemical Equilibrium Compositions' NASA SP-273.

[19] Siegmunc C.W. and Turner D.W. (1974)
'NOx Emissions from Industrial Boilers: Potential Control Methods',
Journal of Engineering for Power, Jan., p. 1

[20] Lisauskas R.A. and Snodgrass R.J. et al (1985)
'Experimental Investigation of Retrofit Low NOx Combustion Systems' Joint Symposium on Stationery Combustion NOx Control, May 6-9, Boston, 1985.

[21] DeSoete G. (1977)
'Etude Parametrique des Effets de la Stratification de la Flamme Sur les Emissions d'Oxydes d'Azote' Revue de l'Institut Français de Pétrole 32(3), p. 427.

[22] Gupta A.K. Liley D.G. and Syred N. (1984)
'Swirl Flows' Abacus Press.

NEW TECHNIQUES IN THERMAL PROCESSING

JIM WHITE

ECLIPSE, INC.

INTRODUCTION

LADIES AND GENTLEMEN:

GOOD MORNING AND THANKS FOR ATTENDING THIS SESSION ON "NEW TECHNIQUES IN THERMAL PROCESSING." IN ADDITION TO DISCUSSING NEW TECHNOLOGIES, I WOULD ALSO LIKE TO DISCUSS SEVERAL NEW AND UNIQUE APPLICATIONS OF EXISTING BURNER TECHNOLOGIES THAT HAVE DRAMATIC "NEW LOAD" POTENTIAL FOR THE GAS INDUSTRY AND SEVERAL ENLIGHTENING "ELECTRIC TO GAS" CONVERSION APPLICATION TECHNIQUES WHICH ALSO SHOW THE POTENTIAL FOR SIGNIFICANT NEW GAS LOAD. I WILL BE DISCUSSING NEW TECHNOLOGIES WITH HIGH TEMPERATURE FURNACES, LOW TEMPERATURE AIR HEATING AND INFRA RED HEATING, LIQUID IMMERSION HEATING, AS WELL AS THE LATEST IN CONTROL TECHNOLOGIES WHICH PROVIDE THE ULTIMATE IN SYSTEM CONTROL AND EFFICIENCY FOR TODAY'S HIGH PERFORMANCE BURNERS.

OVER THE PAST SEVERAL YEARS, THERE HAS BEEN A COMPLETE RESTRUCTURING OF THE THERMAL PROCESSING INDUSTRY, AROUND THE WORLD. THE CONVERSION OF PARTS FROM PRIMARY METALS TO PLASTICS, THE REPLACEMENT OF MANY HEAT TREATED PARTS WITH PLASTICS, THE CHANGE FROM HOT FORGINGS TO COLD FORGINGS, THE OUTSOURCING FORGINGS FROM AND TO THIRD WORLD COUNTRIES, THE EMERGENCE OF POWDERED SINTERED METAL PRODUCTS, THE DECLINE OF INTEGRATED STEEL MILLS AND THE EMERGENCE OF SMALLER, MORE EFFICIENT SPECIALTY MILLS AND THE RESULTING SHIFT OF PRIMARY METALS TO THIRD WORLD COUNTRIES, TOGETHER WITH THE EMERGENCE OF SEVERAL NEW ELECTRICAL TECHNOLOGIES IN THERMAL PROCESSING, HAVE ALL COMBINED TO DRASTICALLY CHANGE THE STRUCTURE OF THE GAS-FIRED INDUSTRIAL THERMAL PROCESSING INDUSTRY. THERE ARE APPROXIMATELY 40% FEWER MANUFACTURERS TODAY THAN THERE WERE 5-7 YEARS AGO AND THE CONSOLIDATION IS CONTINUING AS THE MANUFACTURING CAPACITY CONTINUES TO DECLINE TO MATCH THE CORRESPONDING REDUCTION IN MARKET SIZE.

ADD TO THIS, THE "GLOBALIZATION" OF MANY BASIC INDUSTRIES, WHICH NOW MAKES MOST MARKETS "WORLD MARKETS" AND THE FACT THAT MANY EUROPEAN MANUFACTURERS ARE LOOKING TO THE U.S. AND CANADA FOR THEIR FUTURE GROWTH, YOU HAVE A MARKET UNDERGOING CONSIDERABLE CHANGE AND STRESSS, WITH MANY NEW TECHNOLOGIES FIGHTING FOR A SHARE OF A SHRINKING MARKET. YOU ALSO HAVE THE NEW GAS TECHNOLOGIES, COMPETING DIRECTLY WITH NEW ELECTRICAL TECHNOLOGIES ALL OF WHICH HAVE SPECIFIC APPLICATION ADVANTAGES. THIS IS ALL FURTHER COMPLICATED BY THE RAPID CONVERSION OF NORTH AMERICAN INDUSTRY TO JIT OR CELLULAR MANUFACTURING CONCEPTS, WHICH INTRODUCES A WHOLE NEW SET OF VARIABLES TO THE MANUFACTURER, WHO IS TRYING TO PROVIDE THE BEST SOLUTION TO HIS CUSTOMER'S PROBLEMS. INTERTWINED AROUND ALL OF THE ABOVE IS THE INCREASING DEMAND AND INSISTENCE BY THE CUSTOMER FOR SIGNIFICANTLY HIGHER QUALITY FINISHED PRODUCTS. OLDER TECHNOLOGIES, PROCESSES, AND SOLUTIONS ARE NO LONGER ACCEPTABLE. SIMPLE FUEL REDUCTION AND SIMPLE PAYBACKS ARE NO LONGER THE ONLY

PURCHASE CRITERIA. PROCESS CONTROL, VASTLY IMPROVED QUALITY, AND SIGNIFICANTLY INCREASED PRODUCT THROUGHPUT, ARE ALL BECOMING INCREASINGLY MORE IMPORTANT IN THE ULTIMATE EQUIPMENT SELECTION PROCESS, AND ALL ARE NECESSARY TO ENSURE SURVIVAL. PROVIDING THE OPTIMUM COMBUSTION, BURNER AND CONTROL TECHNOLOGY, TO SOLVE THIS NEW SET OF MANUFACTURING PROBLEMS AND VARIABLES, IS THE KEY TO BEING SUCCESSFUL, IN TODAY'S HIGHLY DEMANDING AND CHANGING COMPETITIVE MARKET. THE SOLUTION TO THE CUSTOMER'S PROBLEM MUST ALLOW THE CUSTOMER TO COMPETE, <u>ON A GLOBAL BASIS</u>, WITH GLOBAL COMPETITORS AS WELL AS ON A DOMESTIC BASIS WITH BOTH DOMESTIC AND GLOBAL COMPETITORS, SINCE MOST INDUSTRIES ARE RAPIDLY BECOMING GLOBAL INDUSTRIES, AND WE ALL MUST BE THINKING ON A GLOBAL BASIS.

THIS PAPER WILL NOT DISCUSS ANY OF THE NEWER TECHNOLOGIES IN BASIC OVEN AND FURNACE DESIGN BECAUSE THESE INNOVATIONS TRULY BELONG TO THE DESIGNERS OF THAT EQUIPMENT. THIS PAPER WILL CONCENTRATE ON THOSE NEWER, HIGHLY INNOVATIVE

TECHNOLOGIES RELATING TO THE COMBUSTION AND CONTROL OF TODAY'S GAS FIRED EQUIPMENT.

REACTION BONDED SILICON CARBIDE SER'S FOR RADIANT TUBE FURNACES

HISTORICALLY, GAS FIRED, RADIANT TUBE ATMOSPHERE FURNACES (SLIDE 1) UTILIZING NI CR RADIATION TUBES HAVE BEEN LIMITED TO METAL TUBE OPERATING TEMPERATURES OF $1750°F$-$1850°F$. AS TUBE TEMPERATURES INCREASE, TUBE LIFE DECREASES, AS DOES THE NET HEAT FLUX ACROSS THE TUBE OR AMOUNT OF HEAT AVAILABLE TO DO USEFUL WORK. BECAUSE OF THESE METAL TEMPERATURE LIMITATIONS, GAS FIRED ATMOSPHERE FURNACES HAVE BEEN LIMITED TO OPERATING TEMPS OF $1650°F$-$1750°F$ AND IF THE PROCESS REQUIRES HIGHER TEMPS, THEN THE ONLY ALTERNATIVE HAS BEEN THE USE OF ELECTRICALLY HEATED FURNACES, A MARKET COMPLETELY LOST TO THE GAS INDUSTRY. THE ADVENT OF REACTION BONDED, SILICON CARBIDE CERAMIC TUBING HAS OPENED THE HIGH TEMPERATURE ATMOSPHERE FURNACE MARKET TO THE GAS INDUSTRY. THE PHYSICAL CHARACTERISTICS OF REACTION BONDED SILICON

CARBIDE, ARE SUCH THAT THE MATERIAL CAN CONTINUALLY WITHSTAND TUBE TEMPERATURES OF $2600°F$. HOWEVER, THE DESIGN OF A SER (SLIDE 2, 3, 4) INDIRECT SYSTEM IS SUCH THAT YOU MUST HAVE AN INNER AND OUTER TUBE AND IF THE INNER TUBE IS LIMITED TO $2600°F$, THE OUTER TUBE WILL BE APPROXIMATELY $2400°F$ AND THE FURNACE OPERATING TEMP LIMITED TO APPROXIMATELY $2300°F$.

THESE HIGHER TUBE TEMPERATURES WILL ALLOW EITHER MUCH HIGHER FURNACE OPERATING TEMPERATURES WITH SOMEWHAT HIGHER HEAT FLUXES, OR LOWER CONVENTIONAL FURNACE TEMPERATURES WITH MUCH HIGHER HEAT FLUX RATES. (UP TO 200 BTU/HR./IN.^{2} FROM 50 BUT/HR.IN.^{2}) (SLIDE #5) THESE ULTRA HIGH FLUX RATES WILL ALLOW EITHER MUCH HEAVIER LOADS TO BE HEATED IN A FURNACE OR WILL SIGNIFICANTLY DECREASE, THE HEAT-UP TIME IN BATCH TYPE FURANCES. IN BOTH CASES, FURNACE THROUGHPUT IS SIGNIFICANTLY INCREASED WHICH ULTIMATELY LOWERS OPERATING COSTS. TUBE LIFE (DUE TO THERMAL CORROSION) SHOULD BE SIGNIFICANTLY INCREASED ALTHOUGH WE DON'T KNOW EXACTLY BY

HOW MUCH YET, BECAUSE OF TOTAL ELAPSED INSTALLELD TIME ON A VARIETY OF UNITS. THERMAL SHOCK HAS BEEN PROVEN NOT TO BE A PROBLEM. THE TECHNOLOGY OF THE COMPLETE SYSTEM HAS BEEN PROVEN IN THE LABORATORY AND IN THE FIELD FOR UP TO 15 MONTHS, AND IS IN THE PROCESS OF BEING COMMERCIALIZED ON A LARGER SCALE. (SLIDES 6 & 7) WHILE THERE IS SIGNIFICANT NEW GAS POTENTIAL IN THE HIGHER TEMP MARKET, THERE IS SIGNIFICANTLY HIGHER POTENTIAL IN THE HIGHER HEAT FLUX RATE LOWER OPERATING TEMP MARKET, WHERE THE CUSTOMER CAN SIGNIFICANTLY INCREASE HIS THROUGHPUT AND QUALITY WITH EXISTING EQUIPMENT.

THE ULTIMATE SUCCESS OF THIS TECHNOLOGY WILL BE TOTALLY DEPENDENT UPON THE FINAL SILICON CARBIDE TUBE COSTS. TODAY, ITS PRICE IS NOT COMMERCIALLY ATTRACTIVE. SEVERAL COMPANIES ARE ACTIVELY WORKING ON LOW COST PRODUCTION TECHNIQUES AND IT APPEARS ONE OR MORE WILL BE SUCCESSFUL WITHIN ONE YEAR. IF THIS LOW COST TUBE PRODUCTION BECOMES A COMMERCIAL REALITY, THIS TECHNOLOGY, WHICH IS NOW PROVEN AND AVAILABLE,

CAN RAPIDLY START PENETRATING THE MARKET WITHIN 12-18 MONTHS, AND THUS NOT ONLY OPEN UP A SIGNIFICANT NEW MARKET BUT MAKE GAS INCREASINGLY MORE COMPETITIVE AND DESIRABLE IN EXISTING MARKETS.

REACTION BONDED SIC RADIATION SER'S FOR ALUMINUM/ZINC HOLDING FURNACES

MANY GAS AND ELECTRIC TECHNOLOGIES HAVE BEEN UTILIZED OVER THE YEARS FOR ALUMINUM HOLDING FURNACES FOR DIE CASTING AND SIMILAR APPLICATIONS. WHILE THERE HAVE BEEN MANY APPLICATIONS USING GAS, THE INDUSTRY TREND HAS BEEN TO USE EITHER A VARIETY OF ELECTRICAL ELEMENTS OR ELECTRICAL ELEMENTS IN A SIC TUBE. THE HIGH COST OF ELECTRICITY AND THE VERY HIGH MAINTENANCE AND OPERATIONAL COSTS HAVE MADE ELECTRICITY A VERY EXPENSIVE FUEL OPTION.

IN MANY APPLICATIONS, WHERE IT IS STRICTLY A "HOLDING" OPERATION, WITH NO MELTING REQUIRED, GAS FIRED REACTION BONDED SIC SER'S, MOUNTED HORIZONTALLY ABOVE THE MOLTEN

ALUMINUM BATH, HAVE PROVEN TO BE VERY SUCCESSFUL (SLIDE 8). NOT ONLY ARE THE FUEL OPERATING COSTS MUCH LOWER, BUT ALSO ARE THE VERY SIGNIFICANT MAINTENANCE COSTS AND ELECTRICAL ELEMENT REPLACEMENT COSTS. BECAUSE THE GAS IS FIRING INSIDE A SIC TUBE, THERE IS "0" ALUMINUM CARRYOVER IN THE PRODUCTS OF COMBUSTION, WHICH IS A SIGNIFICANT IMPROVEMENT OVER DIRECT GAS FIRED METHODS AND THIS ADVANTAGE WILL RESULT IN VERY SIGNIFICANT SAVINGS BY NOT LOSING METAL IN THE FLUE GAS.

TUBE LIFE HAS BEEN GOOD WITH AVERAGE TUBE LIVES OF APPROXIMATELY 5+ YEARS ANTICIIPATED. TUBE LIFE OF TWO YEARS HAS BEEN OBTAINED WITH NI CM TUBES. AS WITH THE RADIANT TUBE APPLICATION DISCUSSED ABOVE, THE MAIN DETERMINANT TO THE ULTIMATE COMMERCIAL SUCCESS OF THIS TECHNOLOGY WILL BE A LOW COST SIC R.B. TUBE WHICH, AS DISCUSSED PREVIOUSLY, SHOULD BE AVAILABLE IN APPROXIMATELY 12 MONTHS' TIME.

NITRIDE BONDED SIC IMMERSION SER'S FOR ALUMINUM/ZINC "REMELT"

AS WITH ALUMINUM/ZINC HOLDING FURNACES, THE DESIGN OF ALUMINUM/ZINC "REMELT" FURNACES FOR DIECASTING AND SIMILAR APPLICATIONS HAS PRIMARILY BEEN ELECTRIC, ALTHOUGH DIRECT FIRED GAS WITHOUT RECUPERATION, AND WITH CERAMIC TUBE RECUPERATION, HAVE BEEN SUCCESSFULLY APPLIED. DIRECT FIRING HAS HISTORICALLY BEEN "LESS THAN SUCCESSFUL" BECAUSE OF THE LARGE "CARRYOVER LOSS OF ALUMINUM" AND VERY EXPENSIVE AND TROUBLESOME RECUPERATORS.

REMELT FURNACES, WITH NO FLUXING AGENTS, ARE A GOOD APPLICATION FOR DIRECT IMMERSION SIC - <u>NITRIDE BONDED</u> SER'S. (SLIDE 9, 10, 11, 12). SEVERAL RESEARCH ORGANIZATIONS ARE TESTING THESE MATERIALS AROUND THE WORLD AND THERE ARE MANY UNITS IN AND OPERATING, WITH VARYING DEGREES OF SUCCESS. THE MAIN OPERATIONAL PROBLEM HAS BEEN INCONSISTENT TUBE LIFE, DUE TO INCONSISTENT TUBE QUALITY. RECENT FIELD TEST RESULTS OF A NEW MANUFACTURER'S TUBES HAVE INDICATED THAT

SIGNIFICANT IMPROVEMENT HAS BEEN MADE IN TUBE QUALITY. IF THE ONGOING FIELD TESTS AND PARALLEL LABORATORY TESTS CONFIRM THE IMPROVED TUBE MANUFACTURING QUALITY, THIS TECHNOLOGY CAN BE COMMERCIALIZED IN 6-12 MONTHS. CONSISTENT TUBE LIVES OF 3 MONTHS HAVE PROVEN PRACTICAL AND IF THIS CAN BE IMPROVED TO SIX MONTHS, THROUGH BETTER TUBE QUALITY AND IMPROVED THERMAL HEAT TRANSFER ACROSS THE TUBE, THEN IT IS LIKELY THIS TECHNOLOGY WILL BE MAKING VERY SIGNIFICANT INROADS WITHIN 12 MONTHS. (SLIDES 13, 14, & 15)

NITRIDE BONDED SIC SER'S FOR ALUMINUM MELTING

MOST LARGE ALUMINUM MELTERS - "REVERB FURNACES" HAVE TRADITIONALLY USED EITHER HEAVY OIL BURNERS OR GAS BURNERS, WITH OR WITHOUT SOME FORM OF RECUPERATION, OR ADVANCED HEAT RECOVERY. BECAUSE PRIMARY MELTING NORMALLY REQUIRES SIGNIFICANT AMOUNTS OF "FLUXING AND DEMAGGING" USING HEAVY CONCENTRATIONS OF ALKALAI SALTS AND CHLORINE/FLOURINE CRYSTALS, THE USE OF RECUPERATION, OVER THE PAST SEVERAL YEARS, HAS BEEN LESS THAN IDEAL, AND THE VERY HIGH

INSTALLED COSTS AND OPERATIONAL COSTS OF NEWER TECHNOLOGIES, MAY VERY WELL LIMIT THEIR GROWTH, ONCE THERE HAS BEEN MORE OPERATIONAL DATA OBTAINED AND REPORTED ON THEIR OPERATIONAL EXPERIENCE.

HIGH PERFORMANCE NB SIC SER'S, CURRENTLY UNDER DEVELOPMENT, MAY PROVIDE THE ULTIMATE SOLUTION TO THIS APPLICATION. THE COMBUSTION AND RECUPERATION TECHNOLOGY HAVE BEEN PROVEN. TUBE LIFE, TUBE QUALITY AND TUBE COSTS, ARE THE KEY, TO THIS TECHNOLOGY'S SUCCESS. THIS TECHNOLOGY IS APPROXIMATELY TWO YEARS AWAY FROM SUCCESSFUL COMMERCIALIZATION.

ULTRA EFFICIENT AIR TO AIR RECUEPRATORS ON ALUMINUM MELTING FURNACES

ULTRA EFFICIENT AIR TO AIR HEAT EXCHANGERS (S-16), WITH EFFICIENCIES OF 80-90% POSSIBLE, ALSO PROVIDE A VERY PRACTICAL AND EFFICIENT ALTERNATIVE ON ALUMINUM MELTING FURNACES USING DIRECT FIRED BURNERS, WHERE NO FLUXING OR DEMAGGING OPERATIONS ARE USED. (S-17)

THE APPLICATION ON THE NEXT SLIDES (#18, 19, 20) WHICH WAS AN AGA COOP AD, THE FURNACE ACHIEVED A 55% PRODUCTIVITY INCREASE AND ACHIEVED A 65% FUEL REDUCTION AT THIS INCREASED MELT RATE! THE AIR QUALITY WAS ALSO IMPROVED BY INCINERATING THE OIL VAPORS FROM THE PARTS BEING MELTED. THE AVERAGE FUEL COST HAS BEEN REDUCED TO APPROXIIMATELY 1-1/4 CENTS/LB. OF ALUMINUM MELTED. THIS PARTICULAR OEM NOW HAS APPROXIMATELY 10 OF THESE FURNACES IN OPERATION, SEVERAL FOR UP TO THREE YEARS.

<u>ELECTRIC TO GAS CONVERSION OF HEAT TREATING FURNACES</u>

THE RAPIDLY ESCALATING COST OF ELECTRICITY IN MANY PARTS OF NORTH AMERICA, TOGETHER WITH THE RECENT "PLUNGE" OF INDUSTRIAL GAS COSTS, HAS SIGNIFICANTLY INCREASED THE RATIO OF ELECTRIC/GAS COSTS TO AT LEAST 3-4/1 AND IN SOMES AREAS UP TO 6/1. THIS HUGE COST DIFFERENTIAL HAS MADE IT VERY ATTRACTIVE TO CONVERT EXISTING ELECTRIC FURNACES (SLIDE 21, 22) TO GAS, AND TO ENSURE THAT "NEW" FURNACES USE GAS RATHER THAN ELECTRICITY. THESE APPLICATIONS OFFER HUGE NEW

POTENTIAL LOAD TO THE GAS INDUSTRY. ALTHOUGH THERE ARE MANY APPLICATION CONVERSIONS TO REPORT, THIS PAPER WILL DISCUSS ONLY ONE.

THE APPLICATION SHOWN IN THE ATTACHED SLIDES 23, 24, 25) IS A VERY LARGE STEEL STAMPING PLANT IN THE U.S. MIDWEST, USING 7 GE CONTINUOUS FURNACES, TO HEAT TREAT STEEL LAMINATIONS FOR ELECTRICAL TRANSFORMERS, MOTORS AND SIMILAR PRODUCTS. AFTER HEATING, THE LAMINATIONS ARE COOLED SLOWLY TO PROVIDE THE EXACT METALURGICAL AND ELECTRICAL CHARACTERISTICS REQUIRED. THESE HUGE FURNACES (196' LONG) OPERATE 24 HOURS/DAY, 7 DAYS/WEEK, 50 WEEKS PER YEAR. .

THESE 7 FURNACES WERE CONVERTED FROM ELECTRICITY TO GAS USING ECLIPSE NI CR SER'S. THE ONLY OTHER MAJOR FURNACE REDESIGN COMPONENT REQUIRED WAS THE ROOF WHICH WAS MODIFIED FOR THE SER'S.

THE RESULTS OR "NET DELIVERABLES" TO THIS CUSTOMER WERE DRAMATIC AND WERE AS FOLLOWS, FOR EACH OF THE 7 FURNACES:

$6,000.00/WK. IN ENERGY SAVINGS

PAYBACK OF 14 WEEKS.

200#/TRAY OF INCREASED CAPACITY OR

1000#/HR. CAPACITY INCREASE OR

20% CAPACITY INCREASE OR

8,400,000# PRODUCTION INCREASE/YEAR/FURNACE WITH AN OVERALL FUEL SAVINGS OF 20%, INCLUDING THIS ADDITIONAL CAPACITY!

ON A YEAR BASIS, THESE RESULTS TRANSLATE TO 58,000,000#/YEAR INCREASE AND A FUEL SAVINGS OF $2,100,000 ANNUALLY!

THE RESULTS SPEAK FOR THEMSELVES. THE CUSTOMER RECEIVED A 20% PRODUCTION INCREASE, A FUEL SAVINGS OF 20% AND A PAYBACK OF 14 WEEKS/FURNACE. THE LOCAL GAS UTILITY RECEIVED A HUGE NEW LOAD INCREASE. WHERE ELSE CAN YOU GET 5.8 MILLION# OF INCREASED PRODUCTION AND SAVE OVER $2 MILLION AT THE SAME TIME?

GAS FIRED INFRA RED BURNERS IN THE PULP AND PAPER INDUSTRY

PROCESS HEAT IN THE PULP AND PAPER INDUSTRY, HAS TRADITIONALLY BEEN PROVIDED BY LARGE STEAM DRIERS WITH THE STEAM BEING SUPPLIED FROM LARGE REMOTE CENTRAL STEAM BOILERS, FIRED BY EITHER HEAVY OIL, COAL, WOOD BY-PRODUCTS OR SOMETIMES GAS. SPOT HEATING THROUGHOUT THE PROCESS, HAS PRIMARILY BEEN SUPPLIED BY ELECTRIC RESISTANCE HEATING AND MORE RECENTLY BY MICROWAVE AND OTHER ELECTRIC TECHNOLOGIES. HIGH PERFORMANCE, GAS FIRED INFRA RED BURNERS, STRATEGICALLY AND EXPERTLY APPLIED, HAVE BEEN VERY SUCCESSFUL IN PROVIDING VERY SIGNIFICANT PRODUCTION INCREASES OF HIGH QUALITY PRODUCTS AND ADDITIONAL LOAD FOR THE GAS INDUSTRY. THE MAJOR OPPORTUNITY FOR ADDITIONAL GAS LOAD IN THE PULP AND PAPER, INDUSTRY COMES FROM THE ABILITY OF HIGH PERFORMANCE GAS INFRA RED BURNERS, STRATEGICALLY LOCATED AND APPLIED TO INCREASE THE THROUGHPUT OF THE MILL BY 10-15% WITHOUT REQUIRING ANY ADDITIONAL CAPITAL OUTLAY, OTHER THAN THAT FOR

THE COMBUSTION SYSTEM. THE FOLLOWING EXAMPLES ILLUSTRATE THE HUGE POTENTIAL OF THIS TECHNOLOGY.

A) ALABAMA KRAFT - EUFALA, ALABAMA (SLIDE 26)

   WORLD'S LARGEST AIR KNIFE COATER

   BURNERS ARE 264" LONG OR 22'

   OUTPUT OF MILL INCREASED BY 12%

B) ALABAMA KRAFT - 2ND INSTALLATION (SLIDE 27)

   ORIGINAL EQUIPMENT COULD NOT PROVIDE SUFFICIENT DRYING, AND POOR QUALITY AND LOW PRODUCTION RATES WERE EVIDENT.

   IR BURNERS IMPROVED DRYING SIGNIFICANTY AND INCREASED PRODUCTION BY 9%.

C) DOMTAR - MISSISSAUGA, ONTARIO - BOARD DRYER (SLIDE 28)

   FOUR ROWS OF IR BURNERS BETWEEN 2ND AND 3RD PRESSES OF HOT PRESS SECTION

PRODUCTION WAS INCREASED BY 128% WITH SAVINGS OF 3.36% STEAM/TONNE; OR USING FORMER SPEED, A SAVINGS OF 19.3% STEAM/TONNE.

ELECTRIC TO GAS CONVERSIONS USING GAS FIRED I/R BURNERS

HIGH PERFORMANCE GAS FIRED I/R BURNERS HAVE ALSO BEEN SUCCESSFULLY APPLIED IN MANY OTHER INDUSTRIES AND AT THE SAME TIME, REPLACING THE PREVIOUS ELECTRIC HEATING EQUIPMENT. SEVERAL OF THESE ELECTRIC TO GAS CONVERSIONS ARE HIGHLIGHTED BELOW USING HIGH PERFORMANCE IR BURNERS. IT SHOULD BE NOTED THERE ARE SEVERAL EMERGING ELECTRIC TECHNOLOGIES WHICH CAN BE SUCCESSFULLY COMPETED AGAINST WITH SIMILAR IR GAS EQUIPMENT.

A)   VACUUM FORMED SHEET PLASTIC (SLIDE 29, 30)

HEATING FOR VACUUM FORMED SHEET PLASTIC AND SIMILAR PLASTIC FORMING TECHNOLOGIES HAS ALWAYS BEEN SUPPLIED BY ELECTRIC HEATERS. THE APPLICATION IN THE SLIDE IS AT THE SNOW CORP. IN DALLAS, TEXAS AND IS VACUUM

FORMING 4' X 8' SHEETS OF PLASTIC. THE RESULTS OF THE CONVERSION ARE AS FOLLOWS:

- PRODUCTION INCREASED BY 35%

- MANPOWER REDUCED FROM 3/SHIFT TO 1/SHIFT

- TOTAL ENERGY REDUCED BY 60% @ 35% PRODUCTION INCREASE.

B) <u>MANUFACTURING FIBERGLASS PIPE (SLIDE 317)</u>

- PREVIOUS ELECTRIC HEATING SYSTEM HAD EXPERIENCED LONG CURING TIMES, LOW QUALITY AND POOR PRODUCTION RATES.

- 42' LONG IR BURNER UTILIZED.

- PRODUCTION INCREASED BY 16%, BETTER QUALITY AND CONSISTENT PRODUCTION RATES WERE PROVIDED TO THE CUSTOMER.

C) **CURING EPOXY COATING OF GAS TRANSMISSION PIPELINE (SLIDE 32)**

REPLACED AN ELECTRIC INDUCTION SYSTEM.

INCREASED CAPACITY BY 18%

IMPROVED QUALITY (FROM 80% CURE TO 95% CURE).

REDUCED TOTAL ENERGY COST BY 17%, WITH 18% INCREASE IN CAPACITY.

D) **PREHEATING REINFORCING STEEL RODS PRIOR TO EPOXY COATING (SLIDE 33)**

- MOST REINFORCING RODS FOR HIGHWAYS AND BRIDGES ARE NOW COATED WITH EPOXY TO PREVENT COROSION FROM SALT ATTACK ON THE STEEL RODS.

- THE APPLICATION WAS PREVIOUSLY DONE WITH INDUCTION BUT THE EPOXY ADHESION WAS POOR (POOR QUALITY) AND THE PRODUCTION RATE WAS LOW AND THUS INEFFICIENT.

- IR BURNERS COMPLETELY RESOLVED THE EPOXY ADHESION PROBLEMS. PRODUCTION WAS INCREASED BY OVER 20% AND THE TOTAL FUEL COSTS WERE REDUCED BY 15%.

SMALL BORE LIQUID HEATING SYSTEMS

ON THURSDAY, JOHN DAVIES FROM NORDSEA DISCUSSED THE BRITISH GAS SMALL BORE HEATING SYSTEM IN THE U.K. ECLIPSE IS THE BRITISH GAS LICENSEE OF THIS TECHNOLOGY (SLIDE 34) IN NORTH AMERICA AND RECENTLY HAS SUCCESSFULLY APPLIED THIS TECHNOLOGY IN THE U.S., CANADA, AND THE U.K. IN FACT, SEVERAL U.S. OEMS ARE CURRENTLY USING THIS TECHNOLOGY ON MOST OF THEIR NEW SYSTEMS AND ITS USE IS ACCELERATING VERY RAPIDLY. (SLIDE 35) IT RECEIVED TREMENDOUS RECEPTION AT THE RECENT FINISHING SHOW IN CINCINNATI.

THE MAJOR ADVANTAGES OF THIS TECHNOLOGY OVER THE PREVIOUS TECHNOLOGY SUPPLIED BY ECLIPSE AND OTHERS FOR IMMERSION HEATING, ARE ITS HIGHER EFFICIENCY AND HEAT TRANSFER RATES. HOWEVER, THE MAJOR BENEFIT TO THE CUSTOMER, IS NOT THE FUEL

SAVINGS, BUT EITHER THE REDUCTION IN TUBE LENGTH AND DIAMETER FOR A GIVEN INPUT (SLIDE 36), OR MORE HEAT RELEASE PER A GIVEN LENGTH AND DIAMETER OF PIPE (SLIDE 37); I.E., HE CAN NOW INSTALL THE AMOUNT OF TUBE HE REQUIRES - IN THE LIMITED SPACE AVAILABLE. THEY ARE ALSO USING THIS TECHNOLOGY AS A STRATEGIC MARKETING PLOY - IT IS NEW AND DIFFERENT AND THE FIRST REAL TECHNOLOGICAL CHANGE IN THIS INDUSTRY IN 25 YEARS! (SLIDE 38)

IN ADDITION TO SOLVING THE OEM'S PROBLEMS, REGARDING INSUFFICIENT TANK SPACE, TO LOCATE THE REQUIRED AMOUNT OF TUBING, THERE ARE ALSO MANY EXCELLENT OPPORTUNITIES TO REPLACE ELECTRIC IMMERSION HEATERS AND TO REPLACE STEAM COILS FROM INEFFICIENT STEAM BOILER APPLICATIONS. IN ALL SITUATIONS, THIS TECHNOLOGY WILL INCREASE GAS LOAD, WILL PROVIDE AN EXCELLENT COMPETITIVE WEAPON AGAINST ELECTRIC IMMERSION HEATING, AND WILL IMPRESS THE CUSTOMER WITH THIS NEW TECHNOLOGY IN AN INDUSTRY THAT HASN'T HAD ANY SIGNIFICANT NEW SUCCESSFUL TECHNOLOGY IN OVER 25 YEARS!

EXHAUST STREAM AS A RESULT OF "DRIVING OFF" THESE VOLATILES, DURING THE APPLICATION OF HEAT IN "THE CURING" OF THESE PRODUCTS.

ANOTHER EMERGING APPLICATION IS TURBINE EXHAUST REHEAT CYCLES, UTILIZED TO PROVIDE HIGHER QUALITY STEAM FROM THE LOW QUALITY STEAM AVAILABLE FROM TURBINE EXHAUSTS IN COGENERATION SYSTEMS.

THESE TECHNOLOGIES REQUIRE A COMBUSTION SYSTEM WHICH CAN TAKE HIGH TEMPERATURE EXHAUST STREAMS (TO $1100^{O}F$) WITH OXYGEN CONTENT AS LOW AS 11% AND SOMEWHAT LADEN WITH FLUE GAS SYSTEM CONTAMINANTS AND VOLATILES.

THESE HIGH ENERGY EXHAUST SYSTEMS ARE NORMALLY APPLIED WITH THE ULTRA HIGH EFFICIENT AIR TO AIR EXCHANGERS, DISCUSSED EARLIER.

AIR HEATING

THE MOST INNOVATIVE TRENDS IN PROCESS AIR HEATING ARE TO PROVIDE BURNERS THAT WILL FIRE "ON RATIO" (SLIDE 40) ACROSS the complete firing range of the burner, and again the use of highly efficient air-to-air exchangers, to recuperate a major portion of the energy that would normally exhaust from the system. In addition, many segments of the food industry, are switching to indirect systems, from direct systems to prevent the products of combustion from coming into contact with the food. Ultra high efficient heat exchangers have proven to be the successful technology for this application.

The advantage of the on-ratio firing, (slide 41) is energy savings, as is, the use of recuperators. Because of the large volumes being exhausted and energy being consumed, large energy savings have been proven possible.

CONTROLS

The advent of the microprocessor and its adoption to "smart" industrial controls, has led to the utilization of several new families of industrial process controls. The purpose of

THIS PAPER IS NOT TO PROVIDE DETAILS ON THESE CONTROLS, OTHER THAN TO BRIEFLY MENTION THOSE CONTROLS HAVING THE GREATEST EFFECT ON INDUSTRIAL THERMAL PROCESSING.

A) TEMPERATURE CONTROLLERS AND RECORDERS (SLIDE 42). - 3 MODE CONTROLLERS AND PROGRAMMERS, CAN PROVIDE TEMP CONTROL, WITH PLUS OR MINUS .1% ACCURACY; AUTOMATIC SELF TUNING CAPABILITY AND ABILITY TO COMMUNICATE DIRECTLY WITH COMPUTERS. THIS TRANSLATES TO PLUS OR MINUS $1^{\circ}F$ CONTROL WITH CORRECTLY DESIGNED AND LOCATED BURNERS AND CORRECTLY SIZED GAS CONTROL VALVES.

B) <u>GAS CONTROL VALVES (SLIDE 36)</u>

ELECTRONIC GAS FLOW CONTROL VALVES WHICH WILL PROVIDE THE CONTROL ACCURACY TO MATCH THAT OF THE TEMPERATURE CONTROLLER DISCUSSED ABOVE ARE NOW AVAILABLE.

C) <u>AIR FUEL RATIO CONTROLLERS (SLIDE 43)</u>

THESE CONTROLS WILL AUTOMATICALLY MATCH THE AIR FLOW TO THE GAS FLOW TO MAINTAIN A PRECISE AIR TO FUEL RATIO.

D) OXYGEN CONTROLLERS

THESE CONTROLS WILL SEPARATELY MAINTAIN A PRECISE AMOUNT OF OXYGEN IN THE FLUE GAS STREAM.

THE ABOVE SUMMARY TOUCHES ON SEVERAL OF THE NEWER TECHNOLOGIES EITHER CURRENTLY BEING APPLIED IN THE THERMAL PROCESSING INDUSTRY OR ARE CLOSE TO BECOMING COMMERCIALLY AVAILABLE. ALL OF THESE INNOVATIVE TECHNOLOGIES WILL PROVIDE THE GAS INDUSTRY WITH A WHOLE ARRAY OF NEW EQUIPMENT TO OBTAIN ADDITIONAL GAS LOAD AND INCREASED MARKET SHARE AND CAN BE USED AS A COMPETITIVE STRATEGIC WEAPON IN COMPETING WITH ELECTRICITY!.

THANK YOU.

REGENERATIVE BURNER SYSTEMS
Case histories on industrial furnaces

Russell T. Chapman

North American Mfg. (Canada) Inc.

Bolton, Ontario

Efficiency of a fuel fired furnace varies with exhaust temperature and fuel/air ratio. Even with proper burner adjustment, conventional high temperature furnaces have considerable flue losses. As an example 52% of the heat from combustion goes out the flue in an 1800 F furnace--only 48 % is available to heat the work, balance wall and opening losses, etc. Higher operating temperatures mean hotter flue gases and greater flue losses. 2400 F waste gas temperature means 69% heat loss from flue gases. Efficiency can be improved by preheating combustion air with waste gases.

There are two basic types of heat exchangers for waste heat recovery: Recuperators and Regenerators. Recuperators have metallic or ceramic walls that separate two gas streams. Heat from flue gases is transferred through the partition to combustion air. As a result recuperators must be constructed of materials that do not leak and can withstand high temperatures. Usually construction materials are expensive and good for one but not both requirements, making recuperators susceptible to catastrophic failure.

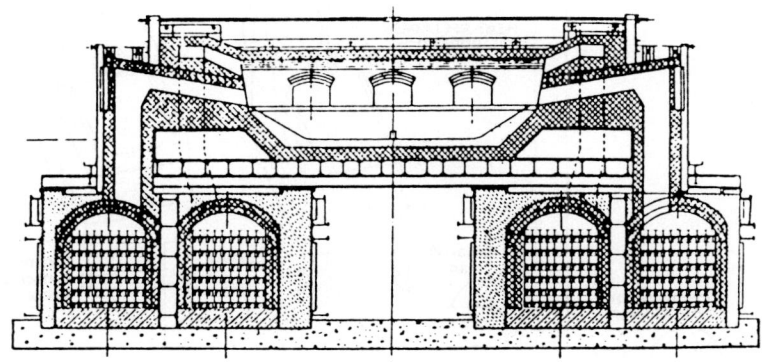

Figure 1: Furnace with traditional regenerator.

Regenerators consist of two chambers, each containing a permeable storage bed of ceramic or metal. Flue gas flows through one chamber giving up heat, while combustion air flows through the other absorbing heat. After a period of time, flows are switched, and air flows through the heated bed while flue gas heats the other chamber in preparation for the next cycle. These flow reversals occur at regular intervals of 15 to 20 minutes.

Regenerators have been used in steel and glass industries since the 1850's. Although highly efficient, their usage has been restricted due to high initial cost and large size. They are often larger than the furnace they serve and require large exhaust fans. Regenerators have far higher heat recovery efficiency than recuperators. There is no worry about leakage since no barrier is needed between combustion air and flue gases.

NEW DIRECT FIRED BURNER

Compact burners have been developed for industrial process furnaces that surmount regenerator size and cost problems. Developed in a joint venture with the Gas Research institute, the burners are described as heat reclaiming burners since they are radically different in design and operation from traditional regenerators. Their bed material has a much larger surface-to-weight ratio. Cycle times have been shortened drastically from 20 minutes to 20 seconds, permitting a radical reduction in physical size. Burners operate in pairs, with one firing while the other acts as flue and heat absorber.

Because of the large surface area in the heat storage bed, combustion air preheats are within 150 F of flue gas temperature. So much heat is extracted from exhaust gases that, they are cool enough to be handled with ordinary steel pipe and rubber flexible couplings on a 2400 F furnace. Exhaust temperatures are lowered to just above the dew point, which not only signifies superior fuel efficiency but also permits use of induced draft fans or venturi eductors of standard low cost materials.

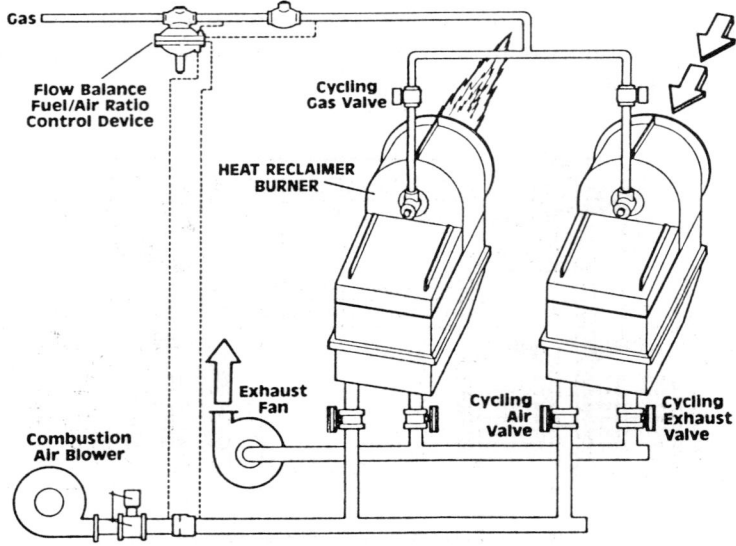

Figure 2: Direct fired burner piping schematic.

Air preheat temperatures frequently in the 2000 F+ range, produce very high flame temperatures. Because flame radiation varies as the fourth power of the absolute temperature, resultant heat transfer is increased. The very high air temperature causes most gaseous fuels to undergo thermal cracking, which turns the flame luminous and further enhances radiation.

The direct fired burner system uses an exhaust fan to draw flue products through the bed of the non-firing burner. Every 20-30 seconds, the cycling air, exhaust, and gas valves reverse. During the second half of the cycle in the illustration, the right hand burner would be firing and the left burner exhausting.

Responding to signals from a furnace temperature controller, control is achieved in one of three ways:

1. On-off--All three cycling valves (air, exhaust, and gas) operate or are off.

2. Modulating--A motorized valve controls combustion air input, and fuel follows via cross-connection to the mass flow ratioing device.

3. Fuel only--That cross-connection is "bled" by a motorized control valve in the impulse line.

In both #2 and #3, the cycling valves continue reversing burner input and exhaust every 20-30 seconds.

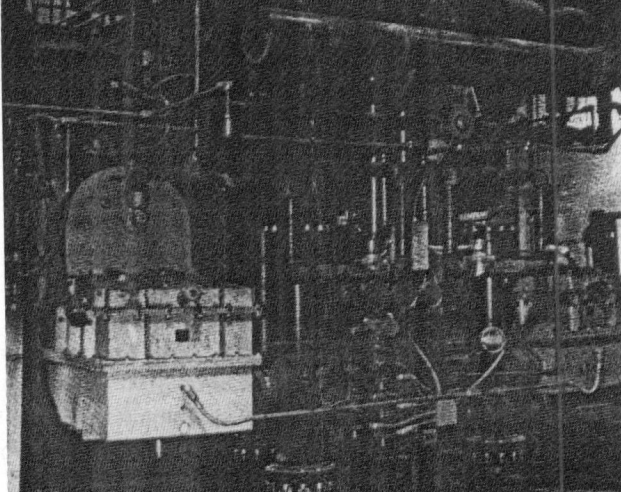

Photo 1: Direct fired burner on aluminum melter.

To illustrate the improvement in efficiency, compare three systems: 1) a conventional burner system with no waste heat recovery (cold air burner); 2) burner system with a ceramic matrix recuperator; and 3) a heat reclamation burner system. The comparison is made on a furnace with 2300 F exhaust gases firing natural gas. Performance is based on equipment operating at 80 % of maximum. Although higher preheats can be obtained at lower flows, dollar return on investment shrinks. Thus 80 % was felt to represent a typical selection for optimizing pay-back.

The cold air system is the least efficient with an available heat (best possible efficiency) of 29 %. The ceramic matrix recuperator improves available heat to 55 % because it preheats combustion air to 1200 F. The heat reclaimer type burner has the highest available heat of 77 % because it heats combustion air to over 2000 F. The ceramic matrix system saves 47 % over the cold air system while the heat reclaimer burner system saves 63 %. Comparing the heat recovery systems, the heat reclaimer burner saves 28 % over the ceramic matrix recuperator.

Savings for a particular furnace should be based on actual equipment sizing, usage, temperature, firing rates, and resultant air preheats delivered to the burner.

FURNACE MODERNIZATION

A comparison of car bottom furnaces at a Pennsylvania forge shop illustrates the application of a heat reclamation system. A load of 164,000 lbs (1 or 2 ingots) must be heated in 72 hours to forging temperature (2150 F).

The previous furnace had conventional burners located near the roof, because there was inadequate space to fire beneath the load. The bottom of the ingots were not heated adequately unless they were removed from furnace, rolled over, and turned end to end.

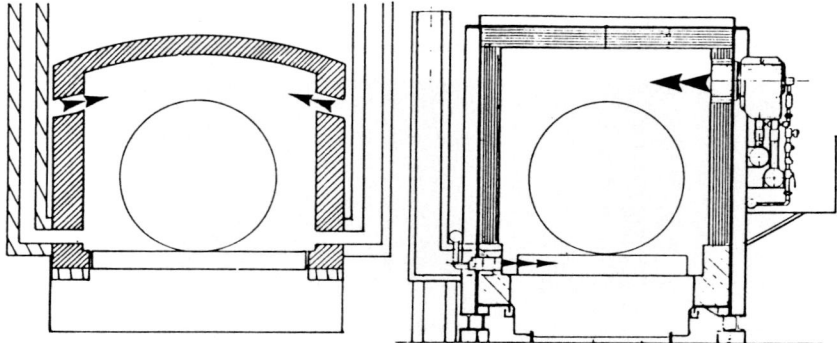

Figure 3: Old furnace on left. New furnace on right.

A new furnace uses six pairs of heat reclaimer burners, all on one side, near the roof. There are eight high velocity burners on the opposite side near the hearth. The heat reclaimer burners provide high efficiency heating capacity, while the high velocity burners contribute stirring energy for uniformity of temperature and even heating. Stirring burners' input is 10% of the total.

Fuel savings are 40 to 45 percent depending on the heating cycle. The cost of modernization was paid back in one year. In addition, more uniform heating improves product quality.

GLASS TANK

A unit melter producing soda glass for bottles and containers measures 36' X 10' and has two zones, without physical partition: a 2500 F melting zone and a 2700 F fining zone. 16 gas premix burners were replaced with seven pair of regenerative burners located on opposite side walls of the tank.

Fuel consumption has been lowered from 26 to under 12 MM BTU/hr while production has risen from 40 to 55 tons/day. The result is a 58% reduction in BTU/ton. The tank was actually run at higher production rates with regenerative burners but the glass feeder mechanism choked.

Melting glass can produce particulate (or other) carry over in the flue gases which tends to plug the heat storage bed. Special burner construction is used which permits easy bed removal and replacement with clean material. Once removed the bed material is cleaned by tumbling in a cement mixer. Beds are cleaned every two to three weeks.

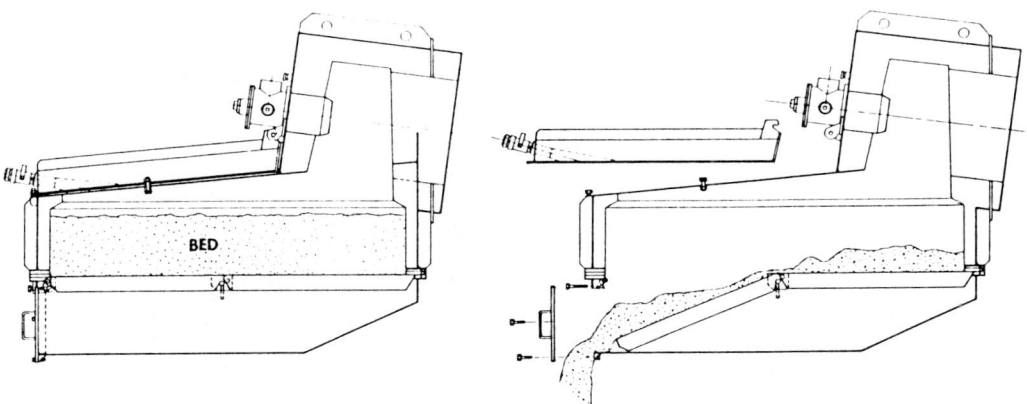

Figure 4: Burner designed for quick bed removal and cleaning.

Aluminum reverberatory melting furnaces also can have carry over of particulate. The amount varies with charge type. Furnaces melting clean ingot have almost no carry over while furnaces melting contaminated scrap can have significant amounts. Bed replacement and cleaning can vary from once a week to every other month. Bed material is cleaned by washing with water.

RADIANT TUBE BURNER

Heat reclaiming burners have been developed for radiant tubes, which heat furnaces with protective atmospheres.

The radiant tube burner system uses eductors (rather than an exhaust fan) to maintain a negative pressure in the radiant tube. Air flows to both burners all the time: When the cycling exhaust valve is closed, combustion air is forced through that burner's bed and is preheated to near tube temperature before it is mixed with gas; during the other half of the cycle, the valve opens and the exhausting air flowing through the eductor creates a suction.

Control is realized simply by turning off both cycling gas and main air valves in response to signals from the furnace temperature controller.

APPLICATION TO CONTINUOUS FURNACE

A continuous radiant tube galvanizing furnace is heated with 208 "U" shaped radiant tubes. Furnace temperature is 1800 F with an atmosphere of hydrogen and nitrogen. Conversion to heat reclamation resulted in the following:

1) Fuel savings are 47%.

2) Better tube life and more uniform tube temperatures are obtained with heat reclamation's alternate firing. Conventional burners produced hot spots that tend to cause early tube failures.

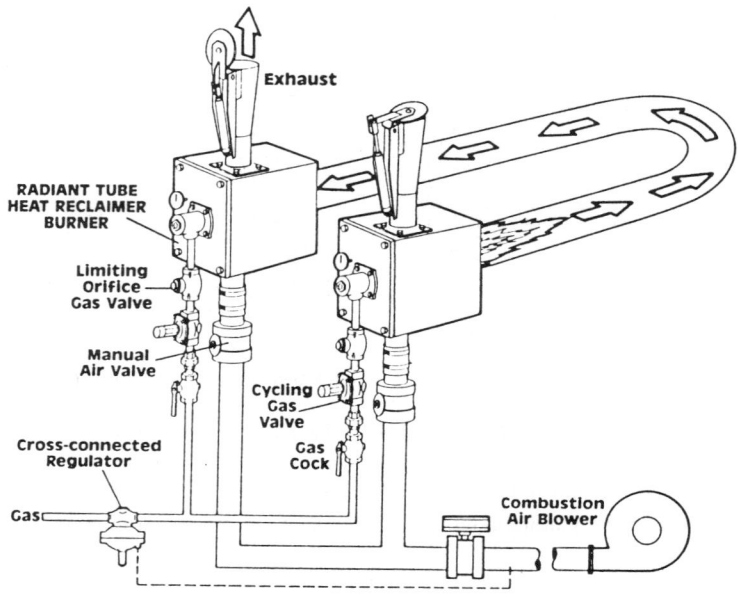

Figure 5: Radiant tube burner piping schematic.

3) Lower ambient temperatures around the furnace result from reducing tube exhaust temperatures from 2000 F to 375 F. Extra pay for hot furnace work is eliminated. Better maintenance is expected because of the cooler working environment.

4) With the conventional burner, the tube operates under positive pressure. If a tube breaks, combustion gases leak into the furnace, contaminating the atmosphere. When contamination increases to a certain level, steel surface quality is ruined. The heat reclaiming burner operates with a negative tube pressure; So if a tube leaks, furnace atmosphere is not contaminated.

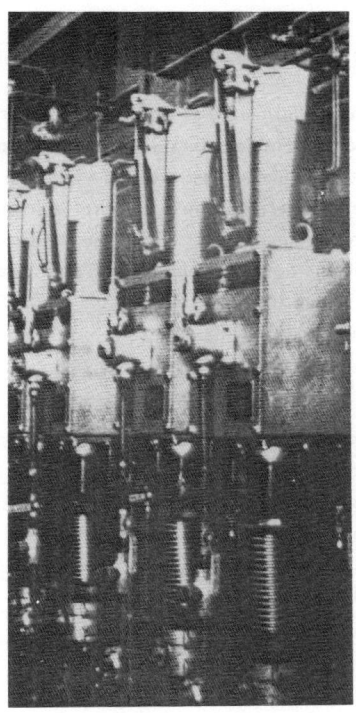

Photo 2: Radiant tube burners on continuous galvanizing furnace.

FUTURE APPLICATIONS

The application of compact regenerative burners to furnaces permits new approaches to the design of process heating equipment. Traditional designs try to maximize fuel efficiency by attempting to scrub as much heat as possible from the combustion gases. The equipment is generally expensive, large and elaborate because of the extended surface area necessary for low temperature convection heat transfer. The following are examples of such equipment.

FIRED TUBULAR HEATERS

Fired tubular heaters, such as steam boilers or petrochemical heaters consist of a radiant section (combustion chamber) and a convection section with an economizer or air preheater. Regenerative burners provide equal efficiencies without the capital cost of convection banks and preheaters. In addition, firing the radiant section with regenerative burners on both ends can produce a more even temperature profile and a greater heat flux on the radiant tubes.

CONTINUOUS GLASS FURNACES

Many conventional continuous furnaces use traditional regenerators which are often larger than the furnace and represent considerable capital investment. Compact regenerative burners can exceed the efficiencies of traditional regenerators at a fraction of the equipment cost. In addition, flames from the regenerative burners can profile heat input to locate a "hot spot" within the furnace to produce superior quality glass. The new compact regenerative burners can be cleaned of particulate while the tank is in operation. Traditional regenerators can only be cleaned by shutting down the tank which involves considerable work. Thus high efficiencies are maintained during the entire furnace campaign.

STEEL REHEAT FURNACE

Conventional reheat furnace design incorporates long unfired sections to allow exhaust gases to preheat incoming steel. There is a significant dollar investment in refractory bricks, steel structure, foundation, and space. Regenerative burners can produce the same production in a shorter furnace or increased production in the same length furnace by maintaining elevated temperatures to the charge door. This is accomplished while improving efficiency over conventional furnaces. A new reheat furnace has been constructed in the Midwest US which has no unfired zone. It has just been started up.

POLLUTION CONTROL

NOx is an air pollutant produced in the combustion process. Natural gas produces less than other fuels but minimizing NOx is desirable. Research is under way to enable the regenerative burner bed to reduce NOX to N_2.

Since the bed has a temperature gradiation from top to bottom, an elevation can be selected that is maintained at temperatures compatible with the required reactions.

In addition, since the volume of exhaust gases is reduced, any other pollution abatement equipment that might be located downstream of the burners can be smaller.

CONCLUSION

High temperature gas fired furnaces have always suffered from low fuel efficiencies. Heat reclamation burners offer state of the art heat recovery for direct fired and radiant tube high temperature industrial furnaces such as forge furnaces, glass day tanks, metal melting furnaces and ceramic kilns.

Pulse Firing: How & What
Tony Martin
HAUCK MANUFACTURING COMPANY

The majority of modern, industrial gas burners are designed to provide specific flame shapes or nozzle exit velocities; for example, Flat Flame, Radiant Tube, High/Medium Velocity, Radiant Cone, etc. All do a specific job and enhance furnace efficiency by creating suitable conditions within the furnace chamber. To illustrate this, let us take an example of High Velocity Burners fitted to a car bottom, heat treatment furnace.

High Velocity Burners would be selected for a number of reasons:

1) The velocity of the jet stream of combustion products re-entrains existing furnace atmosphere back into the circulating stream thus maximizing the fuels available heat.

2) The HV burner develops a short flame profile, enabling more work load to be charged into the furnace with less risk of flame impingment.

3) The high velocity combustion products create a stirring and turbulent atmosphere in the furnace chamber maintaining temperature uniformity.

4) This stirring action scrubs against the charge load surfaces, introducing convection as a heating source. Some materials accept heat more readily from convection than from a radiant source, so heat up times can be reduced for the same amount of fuel.

All of these benefits are created by the burners firing at high fire which, in addition to all of the above, is when a burner is most efficient. Unfortunately this condition cannot be maintained throughout the total heating cycle. During a ramp-up control program or when the set temperature of the furnace is achieved, the controlling instrument will drive the burners to a low or intermediate firing rate. This virtually destroys all of the benefits that HV burners were fitted for in the first place. The stirring action ceases and thermal buoyancy takes over, allowing the hotter, less dense products to rise, creating a temperature differential between the roof and hearth. The flue effect can also create temperature imbalance. Convective heat transfer is lost, as is product re-entrainment. Where uniformity is of vital importance, burners have to be controlled on excess air to maintain velocity. This, of course, is grossly inefficient and can create other problems such as surface oxidization of the charge and thermal shock to the refractory lining.

Fortunately technology offers us a way out: a method by which furnace heat input can be reduced without the loss of any of the benefits of high velocity.

Some 15 years ago a burner control system was devised in Europe which in effect turned burners *off* rather than turning them *down*. Instead of having zone air and gas control valves, each individual burner has its own air solenoid valve and gas regulator (see Figure 1) cross-connected as for any regular ratio system except that these valves do not modulate. They are either open or shut. No special piping arrangements are necessary for zone control; this is all taken care of by wiring at the control panel. An optional internal bleed bypass arrangement allows for sufficient air and gas flow to maintain a low fire flame if required. These are extremely low flows giving 50 or 60:1 on-ratio turndowns, which are repeatable and reliable because no moving parts are involved.

So, how does pulse firing work? Figure 2 shows a typical setup of control modules. The standard temperature control instrument provides a 4-20mA signal to the converter. This analogue signal is changed to a sawtooth voltage and is supplied to the various pulse control modules. A power supply module converts the standard 120 volts A.C. supply to 10 volt D.C.

The sawtooth has a peak of 10 volts and a trough of 0 volts. Each burner is assigned a specific, freely selectable ignition or trigger voltage between 0 and 10 volts. Consequently when that particular trigger voltage is reached, the burner with the relevant assigned voltage will fire for a set period of time, generally six seconds. If we have a 4-burner control zone, the burner trigger voltages could well be 2 1/2, 5, 7 1/2 & 10 volts. The angle of the sawtooth varies depending on demand. The greater the angle from the horizontal, the higher the input and the smaller the angle, the lower the demand. As can be seen from the diagram, for an input of 50% of demand only two burners out of the four are firing at any one time. As the demand falls off the sawtooth angle lays down, extending the time between trigger points so that at 25% demand only one burner out of four is firing. However, over a 24 second period all of the four burners have fired at high fire and at maximum efficiency. The system also embodies as an option a controlled cooling mode where the fuel is isolated and just air is pulsed. This system will generally only be used with radiant or immersion tubes. Figure 3 through Figure 10 shows a typical firing pattern of an eight burner, single zone furnace at 25% and at 50% demand.

At the heart of the pulse firing system are the solenoid operated control valves. These valves must be designed to operate at a frequency of up to 10 cycles a minute. Over a twelve month period, assuming a 12 hour day, 5 day week, this equates to almost 2 million cycles. Regular valves designed for 1 million cycles-to-failure will last less than six months in this environment. Valves designed for 20 million cycles-to-failure or up to ten years life are available for this arduous duty. Figure 11 shows a direct acting air solenoid valve for pulse firing. Each valve has a built-in flow control adjustment to balance burner air pressures. Flow control is adjusted with a screw in the base of the valve, which raises or lowers a throttling disc below the valve seat. On the top of the valve is an adjustable dashpot, to throttle the opening and closing times of the valve. The opening time of the valve can be extended from instantaneous to 3 seconds, ensuring a smooth transition from burner off to high fire. Closing time can also be regulated up to 2 seconds.

The gas flow is controlled by a ratio regulator which is opened by pressurizing the impulse line downstream from the air valve. To effect fast actuation the ratio regulator contains no spring and the diaphragm is weighted to ensure fast closing and effective shut off. Figure 12 shows a cross section of the ratio regulator valve with the removable low fire insert clearly defined.

A gas solenoid is also available, designed to much the same specification as the air valve, but this valve's function is generally that of a regular safety shutoff or blocking valve. The only time that the gas valve would provide any pulse control would be to shut off the gas flow for a cooling cycle.

Burners can be operated in several different modes, the most common of which is with a direct spark igniter and preset low fire pilot flame burning on the main burner nozzle. This system, using the internal bleed bypasses in the air and gas valves, was covered earlier in this article. Another option that may become available is to use the air and gas valves without the bypass inserts and run the burner with a separate permanent pilot. At present this system does not conform to codes of practice and in many cases would not give as effective a turndown as the bypass method. The final system which could be used very effectively on radiant or immersion tubes would again be to eliminate the bypass inserts from the air and gas valves and relight the main burner from a direct spark igniter. This gives infinite turndown and eliminates the excessive heating of the tube at the burner end during low fire periods. The burner only fires in the manner in which it was designed to fire - at high fire.

The electronic modules are divided into two sections: Pulse and Burner Management. All of the modules are of similar appearance and designed on the card or plug-in principle see Figure 13. These cards are built up to provide an infinite variety of burner numbers and zones. Very often the original configuration can be altered simply by wiring charges in the control panel. Burners can be added or taken out of zones in seconds without any costly piping modifications. The control modules are 5" high and vary in width from 1" to 2 1/2" making the electronics very compact.

Pulse firing allows the operator to realize the full benefit from his modern burner system. One company whose heat treatment furnace was retrofitted with a pulse fired system during the summer of 1985, has already reported a significant productivity increase, plus improved product quality as a result. The productivity increase has, by itself, provided a fuel saving, but combined with the reduction in excess air required for uniformity has contributed to a larger than expected saving.

The flexibility that pulse firing provides due to greater turn-down potential allows an increased number of temperature processes to be carried out in the same furnace, allowing a wider variety of services to be offered to customers without the loss of uniformity control.

Microprocessors are now being applied to furnaces in order to achieve better control and improved performance. However, without a direct connection to each burner, the full advantage of the computer to achieve better control cannot be realized. Pulse firing is the system concept that now takes individual firing control to each burner. Through its combination of high performance valves and analogue to digital control philosophy, the pulse firing technique provides excellent burner and furnace control. In fact pulse firing - now being introduced into the U. S. but proven in Europe - promises to provide a lot of answers to previously unanswered control problems.

Tony Martin

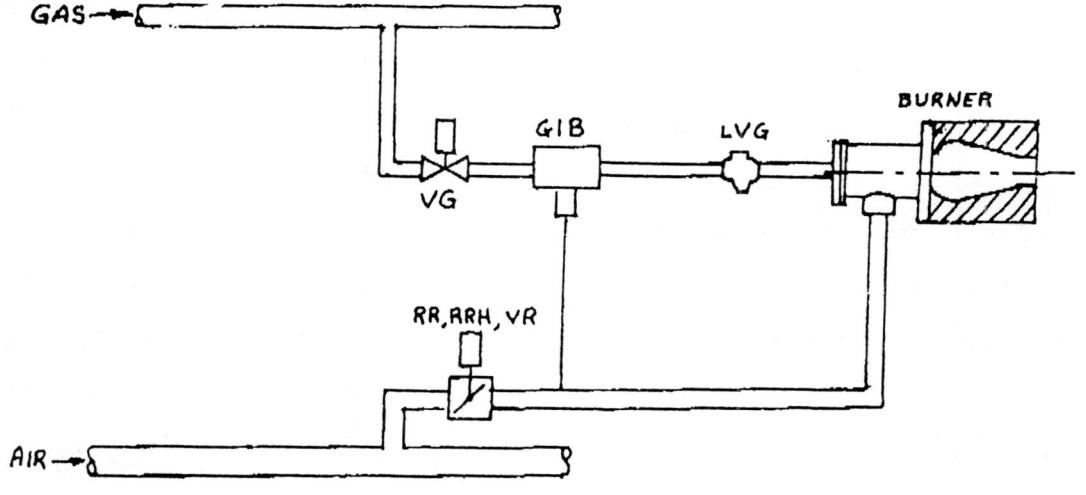

Figure 1

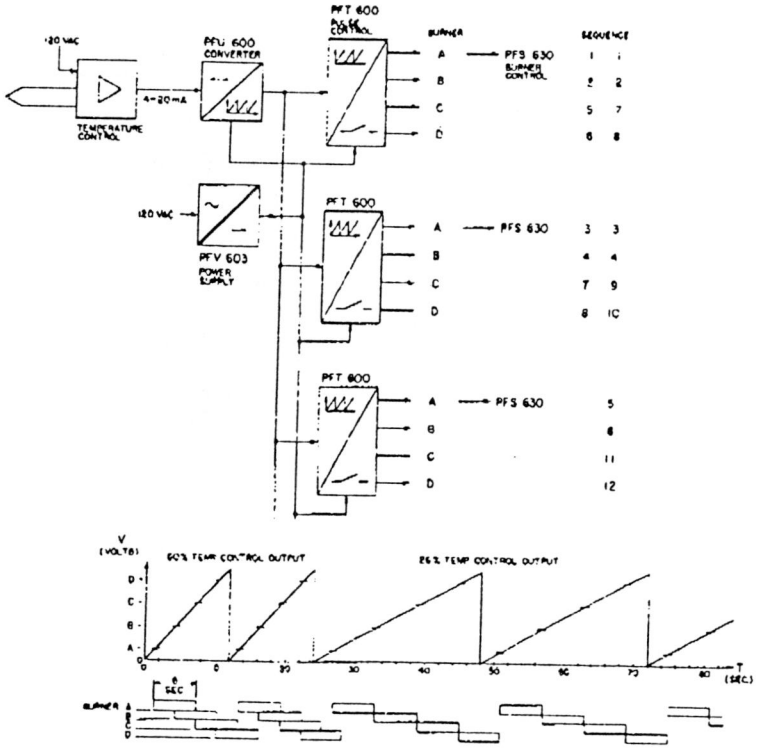

Figure 2 - The control schematic for pulse firing system.

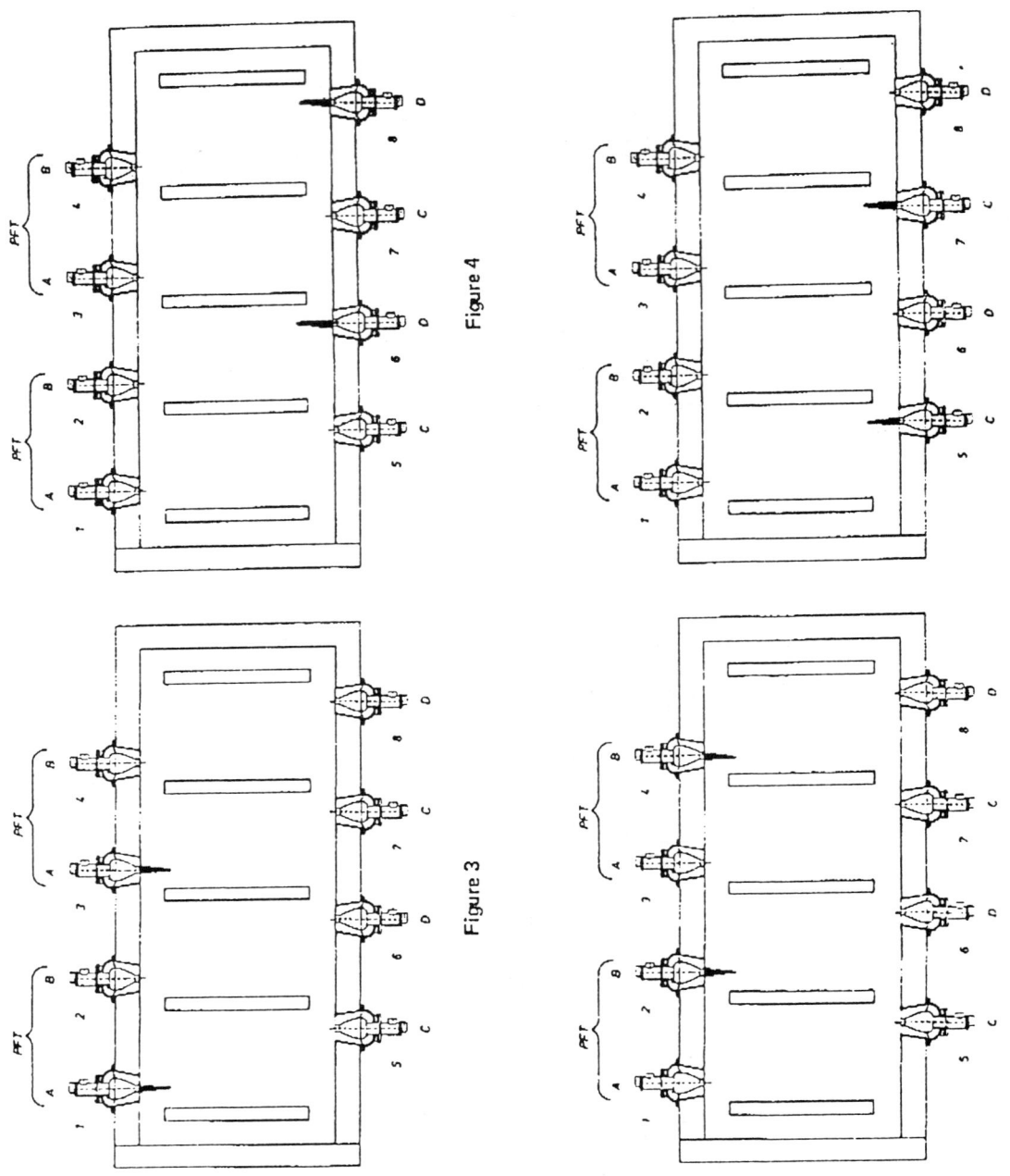

Figure 3

Figure 4

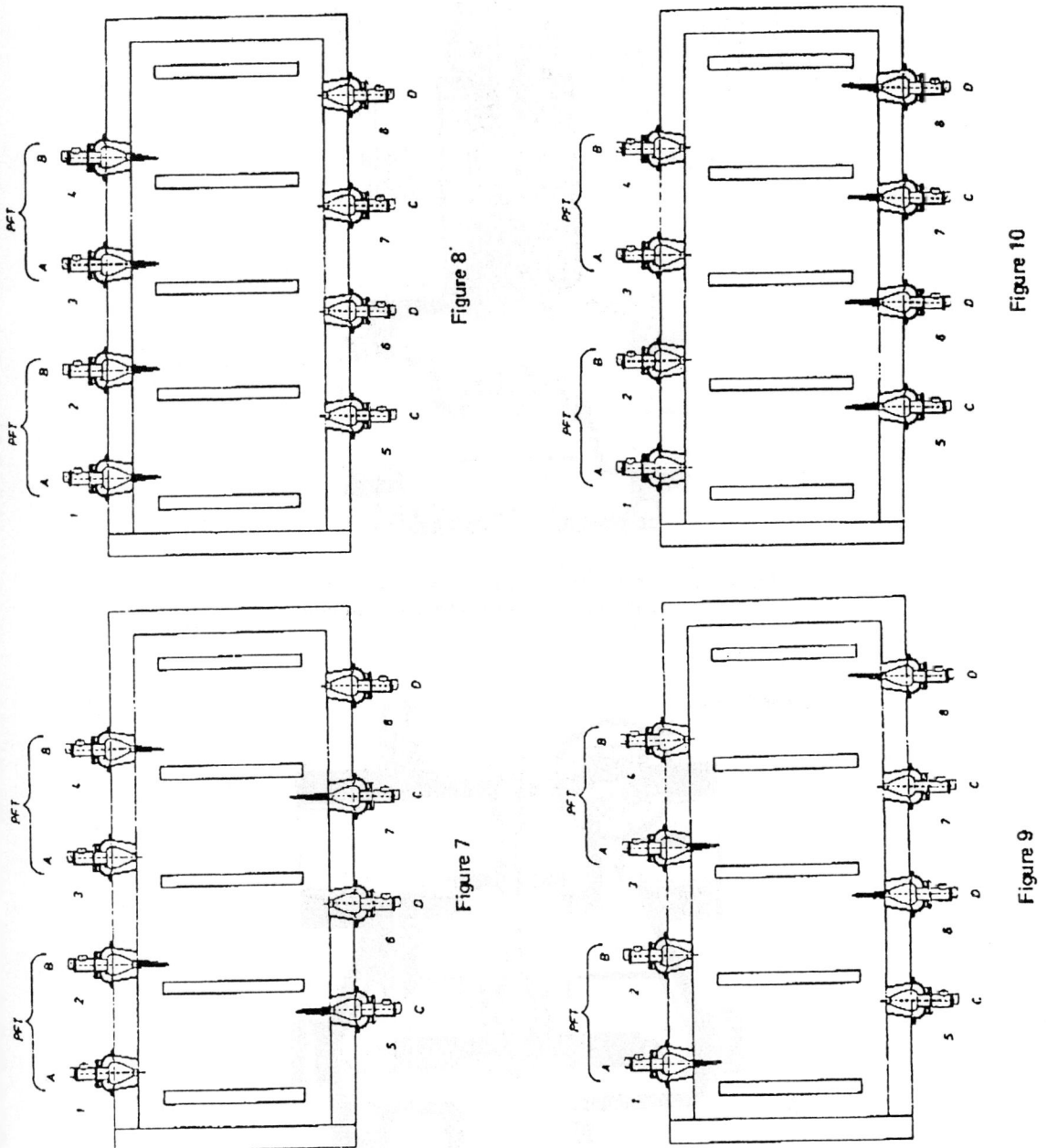

Figure 7
Figure 8
Figure 9
Figure 10

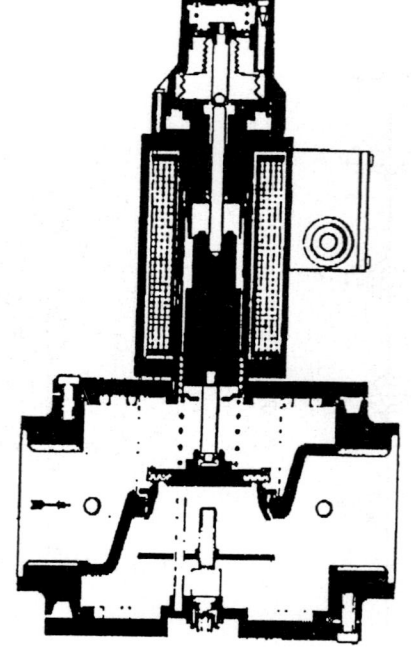

Figure 11 - Cross-sectional view of a typical VR air solenoid valve with attached damping unit.

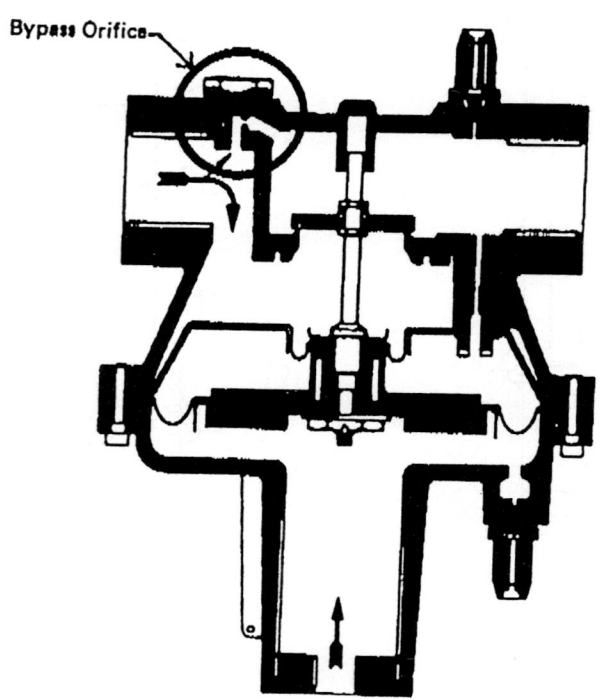

Figure 12

Figure 13 - Individual burner flame monitoring and control cards.

MESURAGE DU GAZ NATUREL
NATURAL GAS MEASUREMENTS

Mesure du débit

Flowrate measurements

Mot de bienvenue
présenté par
Dr Tapan K. Bose, Directeur
Groupe de recherche sur les diélectriques,
Département de Physique
Université du Québec à Trois-Rivières
C.P. 500, Trois-Rivières
Québec, Canada / G9A 5H7

Distingués invités,
Mesdames, Messieurs,
Chers collègues,

Il me fait plaisir de vous souhaiter, à tous, la bienvenue à ce symposium international portant sur le mesurage, les propriétés et l'utilisation du gaz naturel.

La réalisation de ce symposium a été rendue possible grâce à l'initiative et au dynamisme de monsieur Pierre Gauthier et de ses collaborateurs de Gaz Métropolitain. Nous tenons aussi à souligner l'aide précieuse, que nous ont apporté le Dr Manfred Jaeschke, de Ruhr Gas, et le Dr James Holste, de Texas A & M University, dans l'organisation scientifique de ce symposium.

J'espère que cette conférence vous permettra d'échanger des idées et d'établir des collaborations fructueuses. En plus, il est toujours intéressant de se retrouver dans la belle ville de Montréal.

Il y a un petit changement au programme de la session B. Dr. Gerard Van Rossum a été dans l'impossibilité de se joindre à nous dans le cadre de ce symposium. Le programme corrigé n'affectera que la session de jeudi.

Le jeudi matin nous aurons trois conférenciers soit le **Prof. Kenneth Hall** de Texas A & M, le **Dr. Manfred Jaeschke** de Ruhr Gas (Allemagne) et **Dr. Edouard J. Farkas** de Canadian Gas Research.

Dr. Hall parlera de l'importance des mesures de la densité en fonction de la température, de la pression et de la composition du gaz pour obtenir une mesure précise du débit du gaz naturel.

Dr. Jaeschke nous entretiendra d'une recherche thermodynamique destinée à l'amélioration de la précision des mesures de la densité et du facteur de compressibilité.

Dr. Edward Farkas donnera un exposé sur le développement d'une distributrice pour le gaz naturel utilisé comme carburant par les véhicules automobiles.

Le **jeudi après-midi** les trois conférenciers seront le **Dr. Donald Robinson** de Robinson Associates (Alberta), **M. Jean-Paul Coquand** de Gaz de France et le **Prof. James Holste** de Texas A & M University.

Dr. Ronald Robinson parlera de l'importance des hydrates gazeux dans le développement et l'opération de sites de production ainsi que de pipelines souterrains et sous-marins.

L'odorisation du gaz naturel est étroitement liée à la sécurité du public. **M. Coquand** nous expliquera comment, à Gaz de France, ils ont réussi à développer une technique où convergent de nombreuses disciplines comme: la physique, la chimie, la technologie et la science des procédés, la physiologie, la psychologie et la psychophysique.

Dr. Holste a bien voulu, à la dernière minute, remplacer Dr. Van Rossum. Son exposé sera une revue des méthodes actuelles de la mesure précise de la compressibilité. Je le remplacerai comme président de la session durant son exposé.

Cet après-midi, les conférenciers de la session B seront **Dr. Georges Mattingly** du NBS (Etats-Unis), **Dr. Richard A. Furness** du Cranfield Institute of Technology (Angleterre) et **Mr. Carl Griffis** du Gas Research Institute (Etats-Unis).

Dr. Mattingly parlera de l'importance des étalons primaires pour les mesures des gaz. Il donnera plus de détails sur les approches et techniques employées pour établir des programmes de mesures certifiées pour les mesures de débit.

Dr. Furness discutera de la théorie des compteurs à turbine ainsi que des récents progrès de la recherche expérimentale et de la modélisation par odinateur.

Monsieur Griffis parlera des recherches menées au NBS au Colorado sur le compteur à orifice. Il discutera aussi des nouvelles idées dans le développement des débit-mètres.

C'est avec grand plaisir que je vous présente **Monsieur Richard Miller** qui sera notre conférencier pour la session commune de ce matin.

Richard W. Miller a gradué de l'Université Northeastern et détient un baccalauréat et une maîtrise en génie mécanique. Il est un conseiller sénior pour les problèmes associés au debit avec la compagnie Foxboro et un Fellow de la compagnie Foxboro et de l'Association américaine des ingénieurs mécaniques (ASME). A Foxboro, il est activement associé à la recherche sur les débit-mètres, le développement et le programme d'ingénierie.

Monsieur Miller est l'auteur de "Flow Measurement Engineering Handbook" paru chez McGraw-Hill. Il a aussi écrit vingt-six articles techniques, détient cinq brevets sur les débit-mètres et est président ou membre de nombreux comités techniques nationaux ou internationaux élaborant des étalons pour la mesure du débit.

Récemment, M. Miller fut élu vice-président de l'ASME et a reçu la distinction pour service dévoué de cette association. Le titre de la conférence de Monsieur Miller sera "An overview of the field of gas flowrate measurements". Il nous donnera un historique de la mesure du débit axé sur la mesure du débit des gaz.

Je demande maintenant à Monsieur Miller d'adresser cette session commune.

Distingnished guests,

Ladies and gentleman,

It gives me great pleasure to welcome you to the international symposium on measurement, properties and use of natural gas.

The initiative and dynamism of Mr. Pierre Gauthier and his collaborators at Gaz Metropolitan have made this symposium possible. We would also like to thank Dr. Manfred Jaeschke of Ruhr Gaz, Germany, and Prof. James Holste of Texas A & M university for their help in the scientific organisation of this symposium.

I hope this conference will enable you to exchange ideas and develop useful collaboration. Besides, it is always interesting to be in the beautiful city of Montreal.

There is a slight change of program in session B. Dr. Gerard Van Rossum from Holland could not join the symposium. As a result the program for session B on Thursday morning session will be **Prof. Kenneth Hall** of Texas A & M university, **Dr. Manfred Jaeschke** of Ruhr Gaz, Germany and **Dr. Edward J. Farkas** of Canadian Gas Research Institute.

Dr. Hall will talk on the importance of density measurement as a function of temperature, pressure and composition for accurate metering of natural gas flow.

Dr. Jaeschke will talk about thermodynamic research related to the improvement in the accuracy of density and compressibility factor measurements.

Dr. Farkas will speak on the development of a dispenser for natural gas as a fuel for motor vehicules.

For the Thursday afternoon session the speakers are **Dr. Donald Robinson** of Robinson Associates (Alberta), **Mr Jean-Paul Coquand** of Gaz de France and **Prof. James Holste** of Texas A & M university.

Dr. Robinson will speak on the importance of gas hydrates in the design and operation of production facilities and of underground and sub-sea pipelines.

Odorisation of natural gas very closely related to the public security. **Mr Coquand** will explain how Gaz de France has solved the problem of odorisation by resorting to several disciplines of science such as physics, chemistry, psychology and physiology.

Prof. Holste is very kind to agree at the last minute to replace Dr. Van Rossum. His talk will be a review of the existing methods for the accurate determination of the compressibility factor. I shall replace him as chairman of the session during his talk.

This afternoon, the speakers in session "B" will be **Dr. Georges Mattingly** of NBS (United States), **Dr. Richard A. Furness** of Cranfield institute of technology (England) and **Mr. Carl Griffis**, Gas research institute (Chicago).

Dr. **Mattingly** will talk on the importance of primary standards for gas measurements. He will elaborate on strategies and techniques for establishing measurement assurance programs for flow measurements.

Dr. **Furness** will discuss about the theory of turbine meters and cover the recent advances in experimental research and computational modelling.

Mr. **Griffis** will talk on Orifice meter research carried out at NBS, Colorado. He will also discuss about new concepts in meter design.

It gives me great pleasure to introduce **Mr. Richard Miller** who will address a joint session this morning.

Richard W. Miller is a graduate of Northeastern University with a BS and MS in Mechanical Engineering.

He is a Senior Flow Consultant with The Foxboro Company, and a Fellow of The Foxboro Company and of the American Society of Mechanical Engineers. At Foxboro he is actively associated with their flowmeter research, development, and engineering program.

Mr. Miller is the author of the McGraw-Hill book FLOW MEASUREMENT ENGINEERING HANDBOOK. He has written twenty six technical papers, holds five flowmeter patents, and is the chairman, or a member, of various national and international flow measurement standards and technical committees.

Recently he was elected an ASME vice-president and received the ASME DEDICATED SERVICE AWARD.

Dr. Miller's talk this morning will be on "JAn overview of the field of gas flowrate measurements". He will cover the history of flow measurement as it relates to gas flow measurement.

I will now ask Mr. Miller to address the joint session.

THE HISTORY OF FLOW MEASUREMENT— PAST, PRESENT AND FUTURE

by
Richard W. Miller
The Foxboro Company
Foxboro, Massachusetts

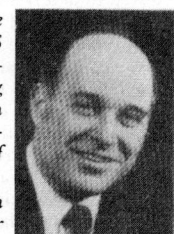

Richard W. Miller is a graduate of Northeastern University with BS and MS degrees in Mechanical Engineering. He received an outstanding alumni award from Northeastern and lectures there in its evening program. Also, he is a member of Northeastern's advisory board.

He is a Flow Consultant with The Foxboro Company, his employer for the past 23 years. At Foxboro he has been associated with their flowmeter research, development, and engineering programs.

He has conducted several flow measurement courses for the Instrument Society of America (ISA), the American Society of Mechanical Engineers (ASME), Foxboro and at several petro-chemical and natural gas producing companies.

Mr. Miller is the author of the McGraw-Hill book, The Flow Measurement Engineering Handbook. He has written numerous technical papers, holds several patents, and is the chairman, or a member, of the national and international flow measurement standards and technical committees of ASME, the American National Standards Institute (ANSI), the American Gas Association (AGA), the International Standards Organization (ISO), and the International Organization of Legal Metrology (OIML).

INTRODUCTION

The history of flow measurement is not a single history, but that of four distinctly different user groups, each developing their own vocabulary, standards, and practices. Not unlike using the QWERTY typewriter keyboard, some groups are highly reluctant to change because of economic considerations, familiarity with existing procedures, and because it "works." Each, then, has its own QWERTY keyboard with which to write standards, buyer and seller contracts, and to communicate among themselves. It is an interesting experience for a member of one group to be discussing a measurement problem with a member of another group and find that little can be agreed upon, except that the metric and SI systems, at least in the United States (U.S.), are not acceptable. The four user groups are conveniently categorized as:

- *Water and Waste*
- *Custody Transfer*
- *Process Measurement and Control*
- *Laboratory Users*

Each group occupies a unique time frame in the overall history of flow measurement, with the *Water and Waste* user group being the oldest, dating back to Roman times when the free discharge orifice flowmeter was used to meter the water used in the household. The economic issues, regarding the price of water, were no less critical than metering fuel oils today; one of the first recorded lawsuits involved a user who had filed the edge of the orifice. In the United States, the American Water Works Association (AWWA) was formed to write recommendations for the water and waste community. Because of the divergence of this group, each serving a different municipality located within a different state, truly national standards are difficult to produce. Each municipality essentially writes its own procedures using AWWA recommendations as a guide.

The *Custody Transfer* users began their historical development in the early 1900's. This group of users needed to transfer large quantities of liquids or gaseous hydrocarbons and then receive payment or pay a bill. They had the unique problems of writing contracts, maintaining the flame, and transporting large quantities of expensive products between states and, after World War II, between countries. The safety aspects associated with the products and the requirement to fuel the nation give this group unique measurement and legal problems; 0.1% change in any of the numbers used in making the flow calculation literally means millions of dollars in profit or loss, depending on whether you are the buyer or seller. Since thousands of metering installations exist, and changes in numbers means changes in dollars, this user group changes measurement practice slowly and surely. In the U.S., two trade associations, the American Petroleum Institute (API) and the American Gas Association (AGA), were formed to write metering practice recommendations. Although used as standards in writing contracts, these practices were never referred to as standards. Only recently have these groups been interested in promoting standardization in the U.S. or internationally.

The major users of flow metering equipment are the *Process Measurement and Control* (PMC) group. The products metered by the first two user groups are usually well defined; natural gas, hydrocarbon gases, and water usually have well-defined fluid properties. The PMC users have to measure and control ammonia, steam, ethylene, oxides, and fluids with names too difficult to pronounce, let alone measure. This user group had its beginnings in the early 1900's, but its growth really began after World War II, when the world economy demanded more and more consumer goods, food, and products affecting the quality of life. The Instrument Society of America (ISA), the Scientific Apparatus and Manufacturers Association (SAMA), and Process Measurement and Control (PMC) are all well recognized names to this user group. The terminology of measurement is rooted in the recommendations and practices of these organizations. Of the four user groups, this is the group that accepts newer metering technology quickly, provided it is reliable. The reason is clear—existing meters may not be well suited for the application and something has to work better. Until recently, the main concern of this group was for control. Although measurement always precedes control, repeatability, rather than absolute accuracy, was the most important consideration. This thinking changed dramatically after the 1974 oil embargo, when the cost of energy and feedstocks skyrocketed. Plant balances in error by 5-20% became intolerable, and both accurate measurement and repeatability for control became equally important.

The fourth user group comprises the *Laboratory Users*. This group has always consisted of users who consider accuracy, the closeness to the truth, as their sole measurement objective. The American Society of Mechanical Engineers (ASME) Fluid Meters Research Committee was formed in the early 1900's to meet their needs. The early interest of this group was in the metering of steam or water and in the acceptance tests of steam engines and later of steam turbines. The ASME Performance Test Code (PTC) committee was formed to produce very detailed standards. In the age of rockets and jet aircraft, the accurate metering of fluids other than steam became critical, and this user group expanded to include users at Pratt and Whitney, General Electric, Rocketdyne, etc. and numerous national laboratories. The vocabulary of this group is steeped in statistical jargon that is generally foreign to the other groups. Also, many of the meters considered by the first two user groups as "the meters of choice" are seldom, if ever, used.

THE DEVELOPMENT OF METERS

Although flow was metered as early as the time of the Romans, the first flow laboratory was not developed until the late 1880's when Herchel began his experiments to optimize the Venturi for the measurement of water. A diagram of a typical Venturi meter is shown by Figure 1. Herchel's objective was simple; namely, determine the design dimensions to give a predictable flow coefficient and a minimum overall pressure loss. The Herchel laboratory was the forerunner of today's modern laboratory, and the first Herchel Venturi metered the inlet water flow into the 1898 New York World's Fair. This meter is still in use at the Alden Hydraulic Laboratory.

Fifteen years later, in 1913, E. O. Hickstein presented the first data on pipe tap orifice flowmeters. This work, and that of others, led to several other tap locations. In 1912, T. R. Weymouth of the United Natural Gas Company conducted experimental test work using flange taps, and in Europe, corner taps were being tested to determine the flow coefficient. In 1916, E. G. Bailey presented data on the measurement of steam flows with orifice flowmeters. Although the orifice was being used for many different fluids, it wasn't until 1930 that an organized test program was formulated to obtain data to write a coefficient prediction equation. This program was conducted at Ohio State University under the direction of Prof. S. R. Bietler and jointly sponsored by AGA, ASME and the National Bureau of Standards (NBS). The Buckingham fitting equation, based on the 1935 Ohio State data, has been used in the United States ever since to predict the discharge coefficient for flange tap installations.

In 1975, J. Stolz proposed a universal orifice discharge coefficient equation for flanged, corner, and radius taps. This equation was adopted by the International Standards Organization (ISO) in that organization's standard ISO 5167. The publication of this document, and the high cost of energy-related fluids being metered by orifices, has led to numerous test programs sponsored by the European Economic Community (EEC), American Petroleum Institute (API), and the Gas Research Institute (GRI), to obtain new data on orifice flowmeters as they are manufactured today.

The orifice flowmeter continues to be the meter most widely selected and far outnumbers all other flowmeter installations. They are produced in all sizes from 0.01 to 30 inch bores. Typical present-day concen-

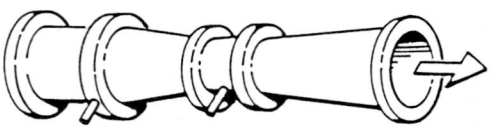

Figure 1—Venturi flowmeter.

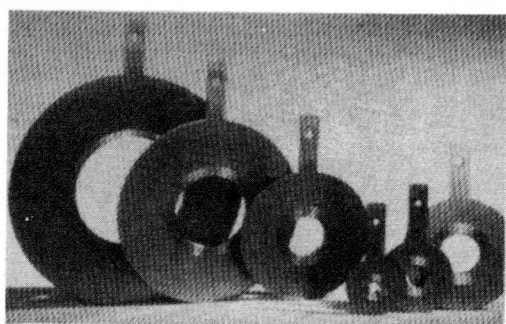

Figure 2—Typical concentric orifice plates.

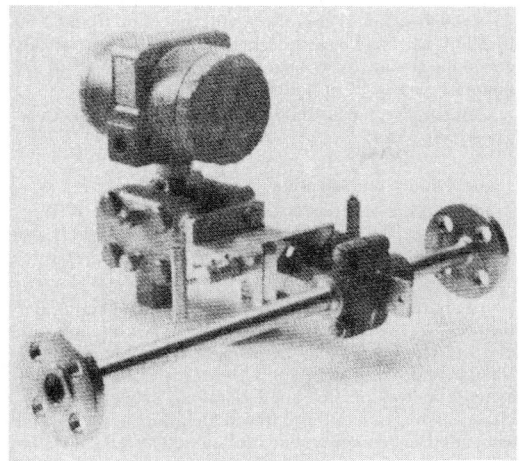

Figure 3—Integral orifice flowmeter assembly.

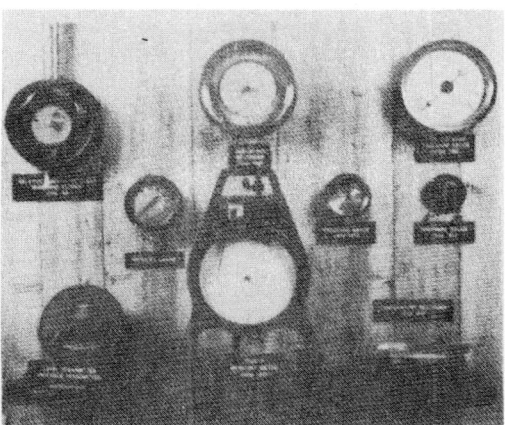

Figure 4—Early Instrumentation.

tric orifice plates for pipe flange mounting are shown in Figure 2. A complete meter "run" with an attached transmitter for differential pressure measurement across the orifice is shown by Figure 3. The orifice is not well suited to high pressure, high temperature steam applications, and the Venturi was regarded as too expensive. For these reasons, the early work of Froude (1847) on flow nozzles, a Venturi without a divergent cone, led to the development of the ISA flow nozzle in Europe and the ASME wall tap nozzle and throat tap nozzles (1950's).

The commercial success of the orifice, Venturi, and flow nozzle led to development of industrial instrumentation. Some of these *early* instruments are shown in Figure 4. Improvements in differential producer designs continue to this day, as indicated by the target flowmeter in Figure 5. Different primary elements, combined with a wide variety of available secondary elements, are used to indicate, record, compute, and control the majority of flow measurements today.

In the same time frame, another group of meters was being developed for other applications. These meters are conveniently thought of as linear meters, since the readout is linear with flow as opposed to the differential producers where the square root of the differential is proportional to flow rate. The variable area meter (Rotameter) was first used to meter fuel oil in the early 1900's. The positive displacement meters were introduced in the same time frame for metering water to households, and for general fueling applications. Today they are still used predominantly in these applications as well as for those requiring accurate measurements over a wide range.

Other linear meters include the turbine and vortex meters. The need for improved accuracy, wider range, and higher pressure capabilities led to the development of the turbine flowmeter by the aerospace industry. Industrial turbine meter designs for the measurement of natural gas and for liquids made their appearance in the 1950's, with newer designs being continually introduced. The vortex flowmeter, a "bladeless" turbine meter, was first commercially introduced in 1970. A "cut-away" view of one is shown in Figure 6. Today they are increasingly being accepted as a general purpose meter for all liquids, gases, and vapor flow.

The magnetic flowmeter was introduced in the early 1950's as the first "obstructionless" flowmeter. An example is shown by Figure 7. It is today widely used in the pulp and paper industry and in the chemical industry

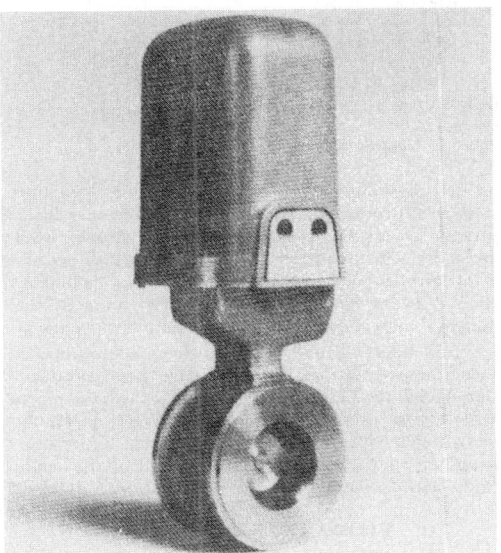

Figure 5—Target flowmeter.

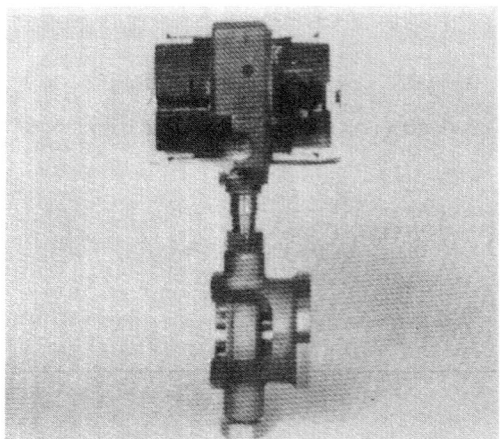

Figure 6—Vortex flowmeter "cut-away".

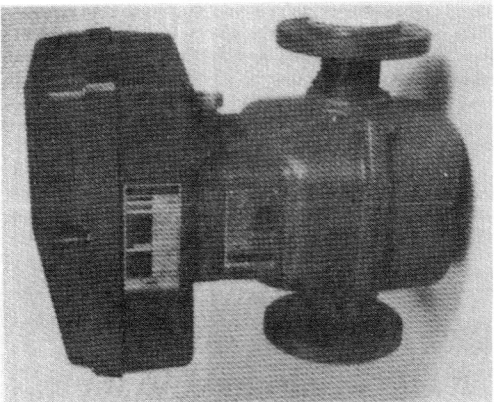

Figure 7—Magnetic flowmeter.

for metering difficult fluids. The ultrasonic flowmeter, another obstructionless flowmeter, has recently had a resurgence with the lower cost of the electronics available today. This meter has not had wide appeal because of the growth pains experienced by newer technology when it is brought into the harsh environment that industrial meters are expected to continuously work in.

True mass flowmeter concepts have been proposed since the early 1900's, but few have been produced commercially and even fewer have been used, the recent advent of the Micro-Motion "coriolis" mass flowmeter being the notable exception. This meter is presently being tried by many companies on difficult to handle fluids, and its history is now being written.

FLOWMETER ACCURACY

In the 1970's, the price of steam went from $1.50 to $15.00/1000 pounds, natural gas from $0.06 to $3.60/1000 standard cubic feet, and that of oil from $2.50 to $30.0/barrel. Each user group had to address this economic change by looking at the *in-situ* accuracy of the meters being used to meter these fluids.

Accuracy may be thought of in four different ways. These ways are:

- Laboratory Accuracy
- In-Situ Accuracy
- Agreed Upon Accuracy
- Ca'vaet Emptor Accuracy

Laboratory accuracy is the accuracy achieved under the best of conditions in which all measurements are corrected for known bias errors using traceable reference standards. In-situ accuracy is the transfer of the coefficients obtained in the flow laboratory, as well as influences of environment and installation on the meter and associated instrumentation, into an actual field installation. Agreed upon accuracy is the agreement between parties as to the meter to be used in a custody transfer application and the calculation procedure established in accordance with a contract; absolute accuracy is, until recently, of secondary importance. Ca'vaet emptor accuracy, meaning "buyer beware," is most prevalent when a new meter or instrumentation is first introduced. The buyer is often faced with unjustified claims that often exceed laboratory accuracy. Accuracy, then, is based on the mutual trust between the user and the vendor.

Each user group accepted one of the above accuracy definitions because of their specific requirements: the *Laboratory Users* apply all corrections necessary to properly test a steam turbine, rocket, or jet engine; the *Custody Transfer* and *Water and Waste* users had to agree upon methodology and metering systems; the *Process Measurement and Control* users, being mainly concerned with repeatability, seldom attempt to achieve laboratory accuracy but rely heavily on manufacturers claims and, as a result, select their suppliers cautiously.

On critical applications, laboratory accuracy can only be approximated by installing a calibrated flowmeter in series with the meter (transfer proving), a calibration system in series with meter (such as the ball prover), or to calibrate the meter prior to installation.

In order to estimate in-situ accuracy, it is important to recognize that flow is seldom measured directly but is a calculated value using a suitable equation that contains terms for the many measured and unmeasured variables. The accuracy of each instrument that measures the variable, and that of an ancillary equation of state to calculate fluid properties from measured variables (pressure, temperature, specific gravity, etc.), contributes to the overall accuracy, or, in today's jargon, the *overall uncertainty*.

Excluding the so-called true mass flowmeters, there are two basic equations for calculating flow rate. The first is for the differential producers (orifice, nozzle, Venturi, etc.) in the form:

$$q = \left[\frac{\pi d^2}{4} \frac{2}{1-\beta^4}\right] YC\sqrt{\rho \Delta P}, \quad (1)$$

where $\beta = d/D$. For this equation, q is the mass flow rate (nominally, per hour), d is the diamter of the orifice bore or Venturi throat, D is the inside pipe diameter, C is the (calibrated) *discharge* coefficient, Y is the gas expansion factor with $Y = 1.0$ for liquids, ρ is the density and ΔP is the differential pressure measured across the differential producer.

The flow equation for the linear flowmeters such as vortex, turbine and positive displacement meters can be expressed in the form:

$$q = [60\rho f_{Hz}]/K_{F,P}. \quad (2)$$

Here, q is again the mass flow rate (per hour), ρ is the density, f_{Hz} is the measured frequency in Hertz (pulses per second) and the meter's (calibrated) *K-factor* is $K_{F,P}$. This K-factor is taken in units of pulses per unit of cubic length; for example, per cubic meter or foot of length. It is understood that consistent units are to be used in these flow rate equations with metric units being preferred.

These fundamental flow rate equations (kg, m, s) are then rewritten in flow rate units peculiar to a particular user group in accordance with his QWERTY keyboard. Gas being calculated in standard cubic feet, that of liquids in gallons, and that of steam (or vapors like ammonia, ethylene, etc.) in pounds. This equation rearrangement introduces other variables into the equation, such as base gravity, base pressure, base temperature, etc. These auxiliary equations further complicate the uncertainty calculation by introducing additional uncertainty terms.

Uncertainty calculations are complex and well covered in recent US and ISO standards. The approach is to consider each equation variable to determine its random and bias error. Since the flow rate is calculated from an equation, it is important to ascertain how sensitive the calculation is to each measured variable. For example, the differential pressure appears under a radical sign and, therefore, a 1% error contributes a ½% error to the calculation. These "sensitivity factors" (X_v) are then multiplied by the estimated bias (B_v) and precision error (S_v) to arrive at a *root sum squared* accuracy statement for the flow rate at a point. An example uncertainty calculation is given in Table 1 for the calibration data shown in Figure 8 for a vortex flowmeter compared to a flow nozzle. Refer to the standards for the variable designations. The example vortex meter has an overall uncertainty at the 95% confidence evel of $\pm 0.34\%$.

TABLE 1.

Example Uncertainty Calculation for the Vortex Flowmeter Data of Figure 8

Variable	Bias	Std. Dev.	Sensitivity
V	B_v	S_v	X_v
VORTEX METER			
f_{Hz}	Nil	Nil	1.0
ρ_f	±0.03	±0.07	1.0
G	±0.1	±0.05	0.5
Z_f	±0.1	±0.001	1.0
T_f	±0.002	±0.005	1.0
CRITICAL FLOW NOZZLE			
Cd^2	±0.15	±0.08	1.0
Y_{CR}	±0.07	±0.04	1.0
T_f	±0.002	±0.005	0.5
ρ_f	±0.03	±0.07	1.0
Flow Constant	±0.003	±0.003	1.0

$B = \sqrt{\Sigma(X_v B_v)^2} = \pm 0.204\%$ $S = \sqrt{\Sigma(X_v S_v)^2} = \pm 0.136\%$

Overall Uncertainty @ 95% is
$U_{95} = \sqrt{B^2 + (tS)^2} = \pm 0.34\%$

The in-situ uncertainty is based upon two considerations; first are the meter and instrument performances under reference conditions; and second are there possible *influence* quantities that add additional bias error and imprecision (random error). The flowmeter and the instruments used to measure differential pressure, flowing pressure, and temperature perform differently when subjected to the in-situ installation. The swirl and dis-

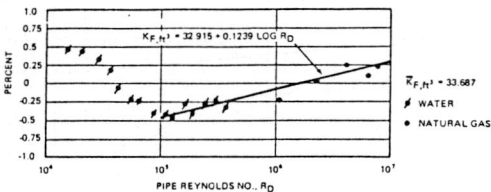

Figure 8—Example vortex flowmeter calibration results.
[The *percent* designation on the ordinate means percent deviation from the mean K-factor of 33.687 here.]

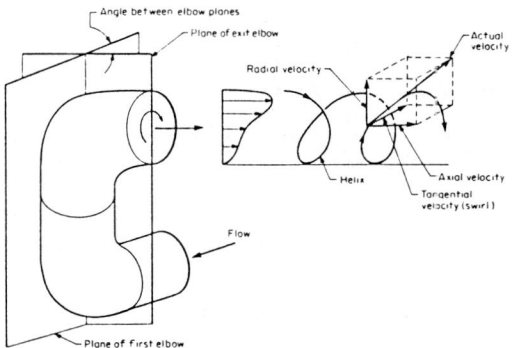

Figure 9—Illustration of the flow profile and swirl resulting from flow through elbows.

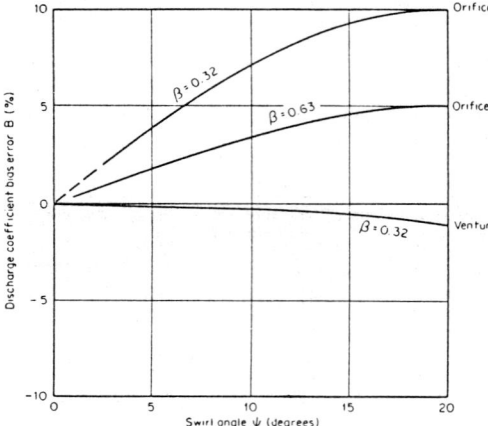

Figure 10—Bias error effects due to swirl.

torted velocity profile emanating from reverse bend upstream elbows, as indicated in Figure 9, result in the additional bias errors shown in Figure 10 where β is the diameter ratio, d/D, again. Other flowmeter *influence* quantities are pulsating flow and cavitation. Bias errors for pulsating flow are typically correllated as shown in Figure 11.

Three fluid properties are usually required in order to solve the flow rate equation:

- Flowing density
- Flowing viscosity
- The isentropic exponent

For differential producers (orifice, nozzle, Venturi, etc.) the calculated flow is proportional to the square root of density, and for linear meters (vortex, turbine, etc.) the flow rate is directly proportional to density. The viscosity of the fluid is used to calculate the pipe Reynolds number, R_D, which is a dimensionless value (number) used to predict the effect of the velocity profile on the discharge coefficient as indicated in Figure 12. The isentropic exponent is a thermodynamically derived quantity used in an expansion factor equation to predict properties at the downstream pressure tap.

Although densitometers have been available for many years, the densities of gases (natural gas, air, etc.) are almost always calculated from pressure and temperature measurements knowing gas composition (specific gravity or mole fractions). This requires that an equation of state be solved for the compressibility factor, Z, in order to compute the density, ρ. As indicated by Figure 13, generalized equations of state or specific state equations are written. The generalized two parameter (P,T) form shown is in terms of a reduced pressure, p_r, and reduced temperature, T_r. The generalized three parameter form noted includes an additional accentric factor, ω. The most widely used specific state equations are the ASME 1967 water (steam) equations and the AGA NX-19 equations for natural gas. The accuracy of these equations in predicting the density is part of the overall uncertainty calculation.

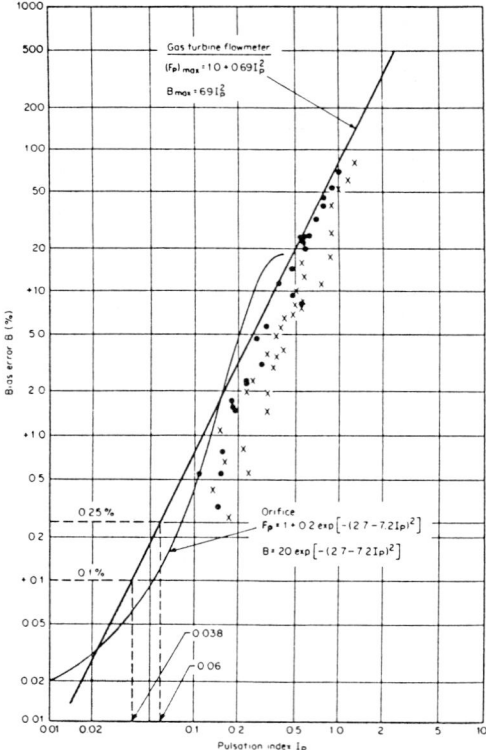

Figure 11—Bias error effects due to pulsating flow.

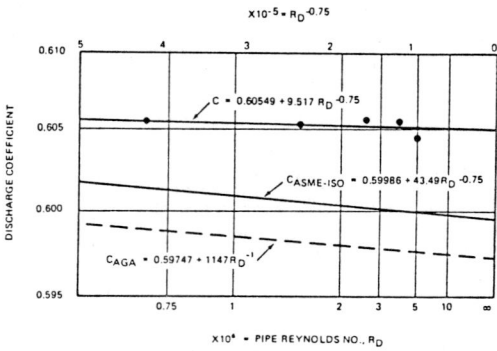

Figure 12—Examples of discharge coefficient variations with the Reynold's number.

EQUATIONS OF STATE

GENERAL
TWO PARAMETER (P, T)

$Z = 1 + A - \dfrac{AB}{A+Z} + \dfrac{A^2B}{AZ+Z^2}$

$A = \dfrac{0.0867 p_r}{T_r}, \quad B = \dfrac{4.934}{T_r^{1.5}}$

Redlich/Kwong ±0.1 to 5%

Three Parameter (P, T, ω)

Pitzer ±0.25 to 2%

Specific

Pure Substance (P, T)
IFC steam equation <0.25%

Mixtures (P, T)

USA	Natural Gas (NX-19)	0.1 to 2%
EUROPE	Redlich/Kwong (Modified)	0.1 to 1%

Figure 13—Indications of state equation forms.

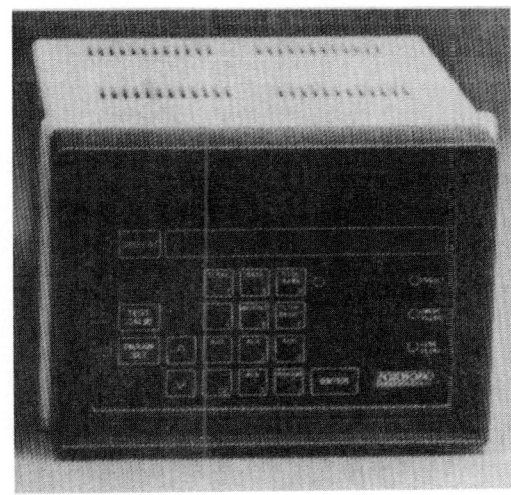

Figure 14—Presently available flow computer unit.

THE FUTURE

Flow measurement began with the Romans and had its modern development between the 1900's and 1950's. In the mid 1970's, a major change in thinking occurred within the four major user groups. Although each has differing problems, ranging from environmental to economic concerns, each now recognizes that improved flow measurements must be made in order to compete, maintain the environment, improve plant balances, and to assure buyer and seller that the bill is correct.

Today there is a major resurgence in flow measurement related activity. Research at the flow measurement companies has expanded, and national as well as international laboratories are now running tests on all types of flowmeters in order to better establish the in-situ accuracy values.

Flow computers, as shown in Figure 14, are increasingly being used to calculate flow rates using equations of state and correcting for Reynolds number, gas expansion, etc. Future products will be self-diagnostic be sold as systems, and include calibration correction algorithms, with some transmitters having in-situ calibration capability.

In conclusion, vortex, magnetic, and mass flowmeters will experience major growth as newer technology and products are introduced by instrument suppliers. One can only wonder what new flowmeters will be introduced, but it is certainly an exciting time to be involved in a field as broad as that of flow measurement.

Gas Flow Measurements:
Calibrations and Traceabilities
G. E. Mattingly
Senior Scientist for Fluid Measurement
and
Leader, Fluid Flow Group
Chemical Process Metrology Division
Center for Chemical Engineering
National Bureau of Standards
Gaithersburg, MD 20899
U.S.A

ABSTRACT

Increased concerns for improved gas flowrate measurement are driving the gas metering community-meter manufacturers and users alike-to search for better verification and documentation fluid measurements. These concerns affect both our domestic and international market places; they permeate our technologies - aerospace, chemical processes, automotive, bioengineering, etc. They involve public health and safety and they impact our national defense. These concerns are based upon the rising value of gas resources and products. These values directly impact the accuracy needs of gas buyers and sellers in custody transfers. These concerns impact the designers and operators of chemical process systems where control and productivity optimization depend critically upon measurement precision. The performance testing of engines - both automotive and aircraft are critically based upon accurate fuel measurements - both liquid and oxidizer streams.

Gas flowrate measurements are established differently from counterparts in length and mass measurement systems because these have the benefits of "identity" standards. For rate measurement systems, the metrology is based upon "derived standards". These use facilities and transfer standards which are designed, built, characterized, and used to constitute basic measurement capabilities and quantify performance - accuracy and precision. Because "identity standards" do not exist for flow measurements, facsimiles or equivalents must be concocted and used to quantify the systematic errors that might exist between or among measurement facilities for gas flowrate. This is the purpose of this paper - to describe the ways that flow measurement facilities can be characterized and how traceability of these facilities can be established.

NOMENCLATURE

In mass, length, time units:
ρ Fluid density, M/L^3
V Fluid volume, L^3
n Unit vector normal to surface, S
$\vec{v}$ Fluid velocity vector, L/t
S Surface of control volume, L^2
M_c Collected mass of fluid, M
$\dot{M}$ Mass flowrate, M/t
t Time, t
M_N Net mass of fluid collected, M

Re   Reynolds number
μ Dynamic viscosity, M/Lt
ν Kinematic viscosity, L^2/t
f   Meter frequency, N/t
$\dot{V}$ Volumetric flowrate, L^3/t
σ_r Random standard deviation, $f/\dot{V}$
σ_s Systematic standard deviation, $f/\dot{V}$
N_i Normal projection, $f/\dot{V}$
P_i Parallel projection, $f/\dot{V}$
e^i Ellipticity

INTRODUCTION

<u>Standards</u>. Fluid flowrate standards could be significantly simplified if the fundamental bases of these measurements were as simple as those for mass, length, etc. These systems of measurement are based upon discrete standards* or artifacts. For example, the platinum kilogram known as "K-20" is the ultimate artifact to provide the fundamental basis for mass measurement in the U.S. and the platinum meter bar (or its modern-day wavelength equivalent) is the ultimate artifact to provide the fundamental basis for length measurement. These artifacts can be considered "identity standards."

<u>Identity Standards</u>. These mass and length artifacts can be considered "identity" standards because under the appropriate conditions of use they define the basic quantity in their respective measurement systems. However, for flow rate measurements of fluids - i.e., gases or liquids - there does not exist an identity standard such as a gallon per minute, a liter per second, or a kilogram per hour. To supply the fundamental basis upon which to establish a flow measurement system, a "derived" standard is needed.

<u>Derived Standards for Flow</u>. For fluid flowrate measurements - as needed to form the basis of a national reference system - calibration facilities spanning a range of fluid and flow conditions are maintained by NBS for use by industry and others, (1-6). These facilities consist usually of:
(1) a source of flow - generally a compressor or a pump and a supply of the fluid with appropriate auxiliary equipment such as a regulated, pressurized tank of gas,
(2) a test section into which the meter and its adjacent piping can be installed so that the flow and fluid conditions into it duplicate those expected where the meter will actually be used,
(3) a flow determination system having a specified level of performance and appropriate proof of this to specify and assure the desired metering performance of the devices in question. Calibration systems are generally categorized according to the type of flow determination scheme used. Several of these schemes will be described below.

---
*The term standard has many meanings. It is used to refer to "paper" standards which are documents; it is also used to refer to reference facilities and equipment; it is also used to refer to the specific materials needed to transfer measurement quality from or between facilities. These specific materials are referred to in what follows as "artifacts".

Flow Determination Systems. The heart of the fluid flowmeter calibration facility is the flow determination system, (1-6). This generally uses a timed collection of the fluid which flows through the meter being calibrated. The amount of fluid collected is determined by gravimetric or volumetric techniques. This collected fluid is converted to flowrate using the collection time; the volumetric flowrate through the meter can be determined using the pertinent thermodynamic properties measured at the meter. This system can be made to perform at a high level of performance to determine the bulk flowrate of the fluid.

Levels of Performance. Measurement systems can be characterized via their accuracy and precision. These terms are briefly defined as follows:

Accuracy - the degree - generally expressed as a percent - to which a measured result approximates the true value of the quantity being measured.
Precision- The degree - generally expressed as a percent - to which successive determinations of the same quantity duplicate each other. "Precision" is sometimes further subdivided into:
"reproducibility" - which involves "how closely will successive determinations duplicate each other" or
"repeatability" - which involves "how closely can successive determinations be made to duplicate each other" - i.e., when conditions are the same and there is only a short time between measurements.

These characteristics apply to measurements made by flowmeters and to measurements made using calibration facilities, (7,8).

Facility Performance. For fluid flow calibration facilities, the precision can be theoretically evaluated from the appropriate error budget and from the precision of the component measurements that constitute the system. This evaluation technique is often referred to as the propagation of error approach, (9-11). It should be stressed that this approach can lead to serious under-estimates of the actual conditions. This is because the physical model for the actual process may not conform to that used for the propagation of errors. Furthermore, difficulty is encountered when facility accuracy is to be quantified because the true value of the fluid flowrate is not easily obtained. To estimate possible systematic offsets from true value, approximations - generally very conservative, are frequently used. Alternatively, and more preferably, a realistic and highly defensible traceability scheme either should be used or can be generated and then appropriately used to quantify the systematic offset of a calibration facility. This quantification should be done on a continuing basis to insure traceability to national standards.

Traceability. The concept of measurement traceability is based upon the need to check measurement results. As such, traceability has come to mean many things to many persons. There are a number of definitions for traceability, (12). For example, a prevalently used definition for traceability is to calibrate into a hierarchical scheme of measurements that leads, ultimately, to the national references for the respective measurements. For flowrate measurement systems that are based upon timed gravimetric or volumetric collection schemes, this definition could be implemented by checking, individually, the weighing or volumetric technique in addition to checking the timing device. However, limitations to this type of traceability for fluid flowrate measurement can be that errors can occur in the other components that contribute to end result. Examples would be the associated temperature, pressure, humidity measurements that may be influential. Equivalently, the mechanism that starts and stops the timing device can be in error so that even if the device itself is accurate and traceable, the timing can be wrong due to faulty activation.

Conventional Calibration Procedures. With conventional calibration procedures, a testing laboratory or a meter manufacturer might own and routinely use a master meter technique to assess the flowrate measurement performance of the laboratory. To do this, the master meter might be sent yearly to NBS for calibration. This done, the meter would be returned to the laboratory with a report on its performance in the NBS facility. The meter would be placed into the respective facility in the laboratory and then calibrated. The relative performance of these calibrations would hopefully compare very favorably and thereby document the closeness of agreement between the laboratory's facility and NBS. This procedure - while widely used at the present time - can leave a considerable number of factors affecting measurement completely unassessed. Traceability might also be established for a flowmeter calibration laboratory in the following manner. If calibrated weights (for example from a state office of weights and measures) were used to check a scale system and if a timing standard were used to check the lab's timing system, then traceability could be asserted for the weigh-time system. However, the overall ability of the lab to calibrate a flowmeter can be quite incomplete. For such reasons, it is widely believed that more complete assessment of the measurement capabilities of a flow measurement laboratory is preferred. This type of traceability can be established and maintained via flow measurement assurance programs - i.e., flow MAPs.

Flow MAPs. In the case of flow MAPs, a procedure is used that is different from conventional calibrations, (13,14). This involves NBS (or an initiating laboratory) sending a very reliable and well characterized artiface package (i.e., tandem meter arrangements consisting of two meters in series) to the laboratory in question with the request for a calibration of the device(s) according to tightly specified and prearranged conditions, (15,16). The results - which contain the effects of all the lab's routine calibration procedures - its facilities, its operating conditions, its personnel, and its techniques for calculating final results from raw data - are then sent to NBS. These can be objectively (and informedly) compared to NBS results or, more preferably, to similar results from a number of other comparable labs which have performed the same tests in a "round-robin" set of these calibrations. In these comparisons, NBS results are also incorporated as one of the participants. The results show quantitatively, the agreement (or disagreement) among the participants" results. Algorithms have been developed to handle these results, (17,18). Fig. 1 shows a comparison of conventional calibration procedures and those that can occur with MAPs. The comparison shows that the crucial advantages of the MAP program are that: (1) all aspects of the laboratory's measurement processes are checked, and (2) there is a "feedback" and, if necessary, a "follow-up" activity that can make improvements, etc. These follow-up activities can be directed either at the lab's procedures or at its calibration procedures and facilities, depending upon the results obtained from previous rounds of testing.

ANALYSIS AND RESULTS

Conservation of Mass Equation. Flow calibrations are usually performed using a system that includes a source of flow, the instrument being calibrated, connecting conduits, and a scheme for determining the fluid flowrate. When the calibration is based upon the bulk flowrate, i.e., either volumetric or gravimetric, the scheme for determining the fluid flow is based on conservation of mass considerations, (1-4). For each of these schemes, the ideal error budget should be known and maintained so that overall performance levels are as quoted, (1-3).

In Fig. 2, the meter and its downstream piping are considered as a part of the meter and volume a. Depending on the type of calibrator, control surface 4 of volume c may be a moving piston, the stationary end of a tank, etc. Conservation of mass principles applied to an arbitrary, stationary control volume, V which is surrounded by the control surface S can be written:

$$0 = \frac{\partial}{\partial t}\int_V \rho dV - \int_S \rho \vec{n} \cdot \vec{v} dS \qquad (1)$$

where ρ is the fluid density, $\partial/\partial t$ is the partial derivative with time, V is the control volume, which is comprised of all the sub-volumes in Fig. 2. The quantity $\vec{v}$ is the vector velocity of the fluid and $\vec{n}dS$ is the vectorial control surface element of area with direction taken inward and normal to the surface. Application of Eq. (1) to the control volume and surfaces shown in Fig. 2 gives

$$\dot{M} = \int_{S_1} \rho_1 v_{1n} dS_1 = \frac{\partial M_c}{\partial t} + \int_{S_4} \rho_4 v_{4n} dS_4 + \int_{V_a} \frac{\partial \rho}{\partial t} dV_a + \int_{V_b} \frac{\partial \rho_b}{\partial t} dV_b \qquad (2)$$

where $\dot{M}$ is the mass flow rate through the 1 surface and $\partial M_c/\partial t$ is the rate of fluid mass collected in volume c. Subscripts n refer to vector components normal to the numbered surfaces; integer subscripts refer to surfaces; lettered subscripts refer to volumes.

Performance levels for bulk flowrate calibrations facilities can be assessed using the above principles. These principles have been used to produce the quantifications of the uncertainties of the NBS flow facilities, (1-4).

Uncertainty Assessment. The performance of a calibration facility can be assessed in several ways. Before the facility is designed and built, performance can be assessed on the basis of the operational equation for the facility and the specifications of the component measurements. For example, a static gravimetric facility for measuring fluid volumetric flowrate can operate with the equation:

$$\dot{V} = \frac{M_N}{\rho t} \qquad (3)$$

where, in compatible units, $\dot{V}$ is the volumetric flowrate, M_N is the net mass of fluid collected i.e., the difference between the gross mass collected, M_G and the tare mass of the collection tank, M_T, ρ is the appropriate fluid density, and t is the collection time. Based upon this model the uncertainty in the determination of $\dot{V}$ can be specified in terms of the uncertainties in the values of M_N, ρ, and t. Assessment of the magnitudes of these results can be estimated via several techniques for combining component uncertainties. Two such examples are:

$$\frac{\Delta \dot{V}}{\dot{V}} \leq \left[\left(\frac{\Delta M_N}{M_N} \right)^2 + \left(\frac{\Delta \rho}{\rho} \right)^2 + \left(\frac{\Delta t}{t} \right)^2 \right]^{1/2} \qquad (4)$$

or,

$$\frac{\Delta \dot{V}}{\dot{V}} \leq \left| \frac{\Delta M_N}{M_N} \right| + \left| \frac{\Delta \rho}{\rho} \right| + \left| \frac{\Delta t}{t} \right| \qquad (5)$$

By inserting values for the precision of the respective components in the right hand sides of equations (4) and (5) one can obtain an initial estimate for the precision that can be expected in the determination of the volumetric flowrate, $\dot{V}$. These determinations are based upon a number of important assumptions - such as: (a) equation (3) is the proper model of the process, (b) an adequate data base is used to form the component uncertainties in eqns. (4) and (5), and (c) no other factors are involved. To varying degrees, a number of other factors can be involved and for these reasons, further assessments are needed.

After the facility is built, improved assessment of performance is possible, and this should be done in several stages. In the first stage, the components should be checked individually against the respective standards for each respective measurement. These can be considered "static" checks. They could consist of checking weigh systems with mass standards, checking timing and density measuring systems against appropriate standards, etc.

For gas flowrate measurement using piston-volumetric displacement techniques at NBS-Gaithersburg, the uncertainties (3 standard deviations) for the component measurements have nominal values as follows:

Item	Uncertainty (%)
Net mass determination	
1. Volume	0.04
2. Density	
a. Pressure effects	0.13
b. Temperature effects	0.05
Collection time	
1. Device	0.01
2. Switching	0.02

These can be combined using equations (4) or (5) to produce gas flowrate precision levels of ± 0.15% or ± 0.25%, respectively. It should be noted that these performance levels are those obtained after the respective instruments have been calibrated.

Specific examples of different types of gas flowrate facilities can be given using those currently in operations at NBS-Gaithersburg, (2):

AIR FLOWRATE CALIBRATION CAPABILTIES AT NBS-GAITHERSBURG, MD

Nominal Flow Rate Range	Capabilities (max flow) (SCMM)	Flow Determination System
Low	0.15 m^3/min	Piston Provers
Medium	3.0 m^3/min	Bell Provers
High	83 m^3/min	Pressure, volume, temperature and time (P,V,T,t) techniques with sonic nozzles

Summaries of the uncertainties for these facilties is tabulated as follows where uncertainties are three standard deviations. PISTON PROVERS; see Fig. 3.

Source of Uncertainty	Uncertainty, %
1. Collection Volume	
a) Cylinder area	0.023
b) Piston stroke length	0.001
c) Piston rocking	0.012
d) Thermal expansion	0.003
2. "Standard" Air Density	0.020
3. Pressure	
a) Barometric	0.100
b) "Gage" readings (on density)	0.002
c) Changes in piping	0.001
4. Temperature Effect on Density	0.017
5. Timing	
a) Device	0.007
b) Actuation	0.014

BELL PROVERS, see Fig. 4.

Source of Uncertainty	Uncertainty, %
1. Bell Volume	

		Source	Uncertainty, %

	a) Bell strapping	0.026
	b) Bell wall thickness	0.007
	c) Bell stroke Length	0.001
	d) Thermal expansion	0.005
	e) Oil film adherence	0.013
2.	"Standard" Air Density	0.020
3.	Pressure	
	a) Barometric	0.100
	b) "Gage" readings	0.002
	c) Changes in piping	0.002
	d) Effect on "constant" density	0.010
	e) Effect on density change	0.010
	f) Rise effect on oil level	0.066
4.	Temperature Effect on Density	0.017
5.	Timing	
	a) Switching	0.006
	b) Bell motion	0.040

P,V,T,t TANKAGE, see Fig. 5.

Source of Uncertainty	Uncertainty, %
1. Collection Volume	
a) Tank	0.008
b) Inventory (Associated piping)	0.001
2. "Standard" Air Density	0.020
3. Pressure Effect on Density	0.025
4. Temperature Effect on Density	0.017
5. Timing	
a) Device	0.001
b) Switching	0.029

When these static checks of instrument performance continue to give satisfactory results, one should proceed to the next phase of checking. The facility should be operated over its pertinent parameter ranges and data should be obtained for all the measurable quantities under realistic - i.e., "dynamic" conditions. This data quantifies the precision of the volumetric flowrate determined "dynamically". These values quantify the left hand side of equations (4) or (5). Additionally, these data should be compared to that obtained statically for the right hand sides of equations (4) and (5). Satisfactory agreement should be achieved for these precision assessments before the third stage of assessment is started.

The third stage of assessment should be directed at the systematic errors that may be present in the facility's measurement processes. This is properly done by conducting appropriate interlaboratory or "round-robin" tests. In this way the performance of the laboratory is quantified using its normal, routine - materials, procedures, personnel, and in its environmental conditions. Such quantifications are based upon the test results produced using transfer standards or "artifacts". These artifacts are comprised of flow meters. These artifacts are tested - i.e., calibrated according to strictly controlled algorithms. These algorithms are arranged to precisely stipulate all the details of the artifact testing procedures - complete with "go" - "no-go" check points to insure the validity of the meters and the techniques for analysing and presenting the data. Done properly and on a continuing basis, the third stage of quantifying flow measurement facility performance provides realistic traceability for the facility - and in turn for the measurement products - i.e., calibration data produced by the facility. When this data is properly processed and analysed to demonstrate that the facility's performance is satisfactory, considerable assurance can be placed in this facility. For this reason, these round robin activities have been named flow MAP's - i.e., measurement assurance programs. When these programs include or closely connect to the national reference systems - i.e., NBS, strong traceability links are produced.

NBS has initiated a number of round robin flow meter testing programs as described below. Based upon these tests, NBS uses and estimated systematic uncertainty of $\pm 0.1\%$ for both its liquid and gas measurement facilities. This produces the total accuracy quotes for liquid flow measurement of $\pm 0.13\%$ and for gas flow measurement of $\pm 0.25\%$, where in-house precisions, as tabulated above, are combined according to equation (4).

Flow Measurement Traceability. To establish the realistic traceability described above, a test program must be devised so that:

(1) high confidence can be placed in the artifact package - the meters assembled and the specifics of the procedures, check-points, responses to anticipated anomalies, etc.,
(2) the data base produced is adequate to the task of clearly evaluating the significant components of the systems that participate, and
(3) the algorithm for processing the data and producing the results is an unbiased and clear procedure that is adequate to this task.

Artifact confidence is established via calibration testing over an extended period of time for the kind of conditions that will be used in the round robin. This testing should occur in the initiating laboratory and it should establish a credible background data base for the units being tested. Specifically, high competence can be attained by calibrating two (2) meters in series according to tightly specified conditions. This type of configuration is shown in Fig. 6. Pre-testing of these configurations gives expected values for the respective meter factors as well as for the relative performance of the meters - i.e., the ratio of their outputs.

Adequacy of the data base is established by specifying the number of repeat calibrations done for each flowrate and meter configuration. These results should produce sufficient data so that statistical significance can be generated to exhibit the quality of measurement performance - (1) how this varies for successive calibrations done for the same conditions over short periods of time - i.e., repeatability, and (2) how this varies from day to day for conditions that may vary slightly - i.e., reproducibilty. It is recommended here that the data base be generated efficiently and for the expressed purpose of testing laboratory performance. To do this, a minimum number of flowrates are used and sufficient tests at each are done. An alternative approach might be to use numerous flowrates and minimal replications at each. However, this alternative approach tends to place emphasis on meter characteristics - as opposed to test laboratory characteristics.

The algorithm for data processing should be well established. This attribute is achieved when it is (has been) used for a number of MAPs for other measurement systems - i.e., the procedures produced by W.J. Youden and co-workers, (18).

By testing in both configurations shown in Fig. 6 the upstream data (and the downstream data), individually, have the statistical independence requirement that is needed to apply the Youden procedure, etc. The "SFC" unit shown in Fig. 6 is a "super flow conditioner" placed between the tandem meters, (15-17). It is intended to isolate the downstream meter from flow profile (or other anomalies) that might exist in the laboratory pipeline that connects to the upstream meter. Thus, the tandem meter configuration affords one the opportunity of generating data both without and with pipeflow profile effects because downstream meter and upstream meter performances can be treated separately. Comparisons can give unique global insights into laboratory pipeflow phenomena without having to measure these distributions.

The types of flowmeters for this type of laboratory testing should be selected according to the experiences of the participating laboratories. This consensus selection should produce the type of meter, the size, manufacture, associated instrumentation, etc. This selection process should be extended to include the fluid conditions, the flowrates, etc. as well as the tolerances to be used in arranging these.

The data generated via the round robin testing program is analyzed for each of the flowrates selected and for each of the meter positions. For each of these conditions, plots are produced of the respective meter performance characteristics - i.e., meter factor, discharge coefficient, (15-18). Individual results, or averages thereof can be plotted. Each point represents the combined results for both meters for each laboratory.

The data processing procedures consist of determining median values for the respective sets of data for the meters. By drawing horizontal and vertical lines through these median points, the plot is divided into four Cartesian quadrants. The origin of this Cartesian system is, according to the available data, the best estimate of the true values of the meter factors for the two meters tested according to the specified conditions, see Fig. 7. In the northeast Cartesian quadrant, the data can be considered systematically inaccurate in that points are each higher than those of the origin. Similarly in the southwest quadrant, points are lower. Thus, the degree to which data is distributed in these quadrants is a measure of the systematic off-sets prevailing in the laboratory data.

In the northwest and southeast quadrants the data can be considered inconsistent or random in that one value is low while the other is high. Therefore, the degree to which the data is distributed in a northwest to southeast manner about the median intersection is a measure of the random variation in the data.

The preferred result indicating good control would be to find that the measurement of systematic distribution (northeast to southwest) is equal to the random distribution (northwest to southeast) and that these measures are acceptably small. The respective levels of uncertainty can be quantified.

Where, as is usually the case, the two meters are identical, a procedure for quantifying the respective random and systematic levels of the data can be used as follows, (15-17). A line of slope +1 is drawn through the intersection of medians on Fig. 7. The data is then projected perpendicular to and parallel along this diagonal line. The respective projections are then used to produce standard deviations:

$$\sigma_r = \left[\frac{1}{N-1}\right] \sum_{i=1}^{N} N_i^2\right]^{1/2} \qquad (7)$$

$$\sigma_s = \left[\frac{1}{N-1}\right] \sum_{i=1}^{N} P_i^2\right]^{1/2} \qquad (8)$$

where N_i and P_i are the normal and parallel components of the data projected to the diagonal line. The ratio of these quantities produces the degree of ellipticity of the data:

$$e = \sigma_s/\sigma_r \qquad (9)$$

When this ratio is larger than unity, the interpretation is that systematic variations prevail among the labs; this is quantified by the magnitude of e. Analogous conclusions can be drawn for e < 1.

Depending upon the results obtained for ellipticity, a number of reactions can occur. If e is large and this is produced by one or more laboratories, then the reaction should be to examine the components of their flow measurement processes to find systematic causes, etc. If e is small and this is produced by one or more laboratories, the reaction should be to examine the components of their processes with respect to their precision. If e is near unity but the levels of uncertainty are considered too large, then the appropriate response would be for the labs responsible to search and repair the pertinent components.

When such search and repair efforts are completed, the round of tests should be repeated for the same conditions so that improvements can be quantified. Even when such search and repair efforts are not needed, repeat testing is needed to produce the continuous data record desired to substantiate realistic traceability.

CONCLUSION

The standards philosophies for flowrate measurements have been presented, briefly. Uncertainty analyses are given for successive stages of flowrate measurement laboratory assessment. Levels of performance have been given for typical facilities at NBS-Gaithersburg, MD.

The NBS flowrate measurement accuracy quotes of $\pm$ 0.25% for air are described, where precisions are produced via the root-sum-square method. The systematic portion of these quotes are estimated to be $\pm$ 0.1% on the basis of past round robin tests.

Techniques for establishing and maintaining flowrate measurement traceability have been presented. A specific scheme has been described in some detail so that realistic data, produced on a continuing basis, can be generated so that a laboratory's entire flowrate measurement process can be assessed.

It is concluded that once these types of traceability chains are produced so as to link flow measurement laboratories within and across national borders and boundaries, satisfactory fluid measurements can be achieved at specified levels. In this manner, the increasingly critical and costly measurements of valuable gas resources and products can occur satisfactorily for the widely varying conditions and reasons for making flowrate measurements.

REFERENCES

1. Ruegg, F.W. and Shafer, M.R., Flow Measurement: Procedures and Facilities at NBS; Procs Semi-Annual ASHRAE Meeting, San Fran, CA, 1970.
2. Benson, K.R., et al., NBS Primary Calibration Facilities for Air Flowrate, Air Speed, and Slurry Flow, Procs Amer. Gas. Assoc. Symposium on Fluid Measurement, Crystal City, VA, Nov 1986.
3. Mattingly, G.E., Gas Flow Measurement: Calibration Facilities and Fluid Metering Traceability at the National Bureau of Standards, Procs Inst. for Gas Technology Conference on Natural Gas Energy Measurement Chicago, 1986, 24 pages.
4. Uriano, G.A. (editor), NBS Calibration Services-Users Guide, NBS Special Publication 250, July 1986.
5. Mattingly, G.E., Primary Calibrations, Reference and Transfer Standards, in Developments in Flow Measurement-I, edited by R.W.W. Scott published by Applied Science Publishers, Englewood N.J. pp 31-73, 1981.
6. Shafer, M.R., and Ruegg, F.W., Liquid-Flowmeter Calibration Techniques, Trans. ASME $\underline{80}$, 1369, 1958.
7. ANSI/ASME Standard - Glossary of Terms Used in the Measurement of Fluid Flow in Pipes, ANSI/ASME-MFC-1M-1979, Published by ASME, United Engr. Ctr, New York, NY, 17 pages.
8. ISO International Vocabulary of Basic and General Terms in Metrology, Int'l Ingam. For Standardization; Geneva, Switz. 1984, 40 pages.
9. ANSI/ASME Standard - Uncertainties in Flow Measurement, ANSI/ASME-MFC-2M, United Engr. Ctr., New York, N.Y.
10. ISO Standard 5168 - Measurement of Fluid Flow - Estimation of Uncertainty of a Flowrate Measurement, Int'l Organ. for Standardization, Geneva, Switz. 1982.
11. Abernethy, R.B. and Thompson, J.W., Measurement Uncertainty Handbook (Revised 1980), Aerospace Industries Div. of the Instrument Society of America (ISA), 172 pages.
12. Belanger, B.C., Traceability - An Evolving Concept, ASTM Standardization News, Feb. 1979.
13. Cameron, J.M., Measurement Assurance, NBSIR No. 77-1240, Apr. 1977.
14. Croarkin, M.C., Measurement Assurance Programs, NBS Special Publications 676-I and II, 1984.

15. Mattingly, G.E. and Spencer, E.A., Steps Toward and Ideal Flow Transfer Standard, FLOMEKO Symposium, Groningen, The Netherlands, 1978, published by North Holland Publ. Co., Amsterdam, NL.
16. Mattingly, G.E., Dynamic Traceability of Flow Measurements, Invited Lecture, IMEKO Tokyo Flow Symposium, 1979, Society of Instrument and Control Engineers, Tokyo, Japan.
17. Mattingly, G.E., An Interlaboratory Round Robin Flowmeter Test Using Turbine Meters Flowing Water, in preparation as a NBSIR.
18. Youden, W.J., Graphical Diagrams of Interlaboratory Test Results, Journ. of Industrial Quality Control, Vol 15, No. 11, pp 133-137, May 1959.

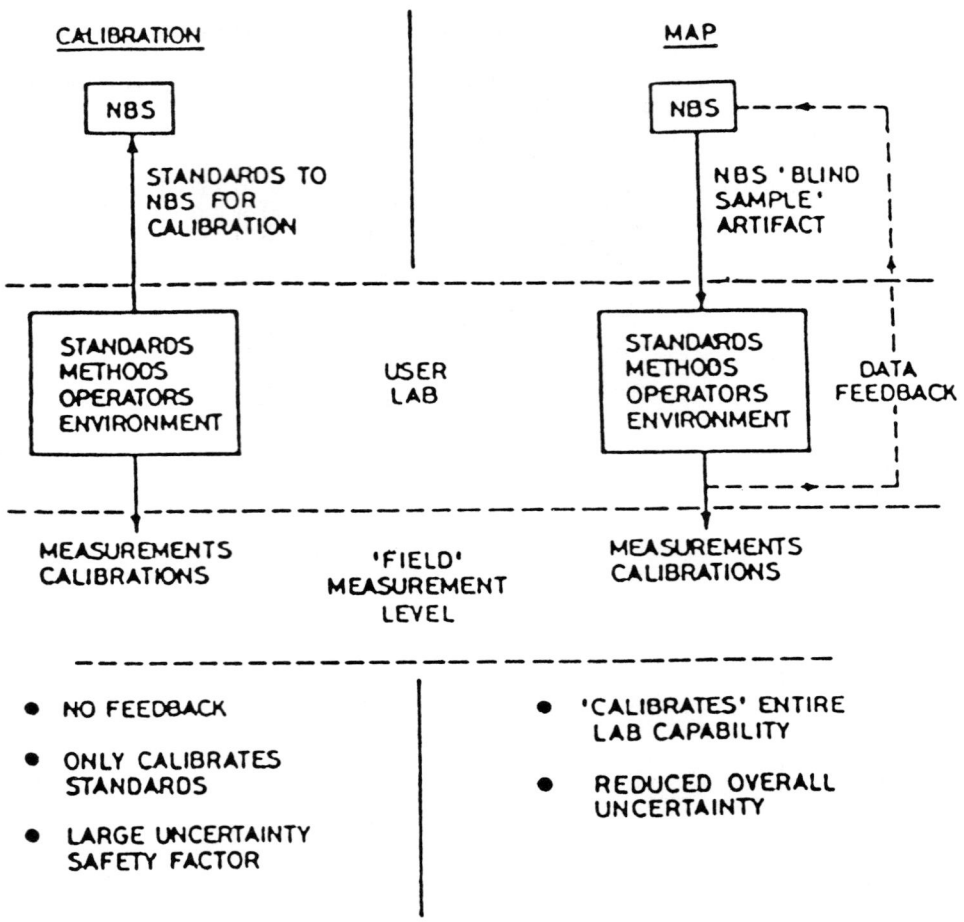

CONVENTIONAL CALIBRATION VS. MAP COMPARISON.

FIGURE 1

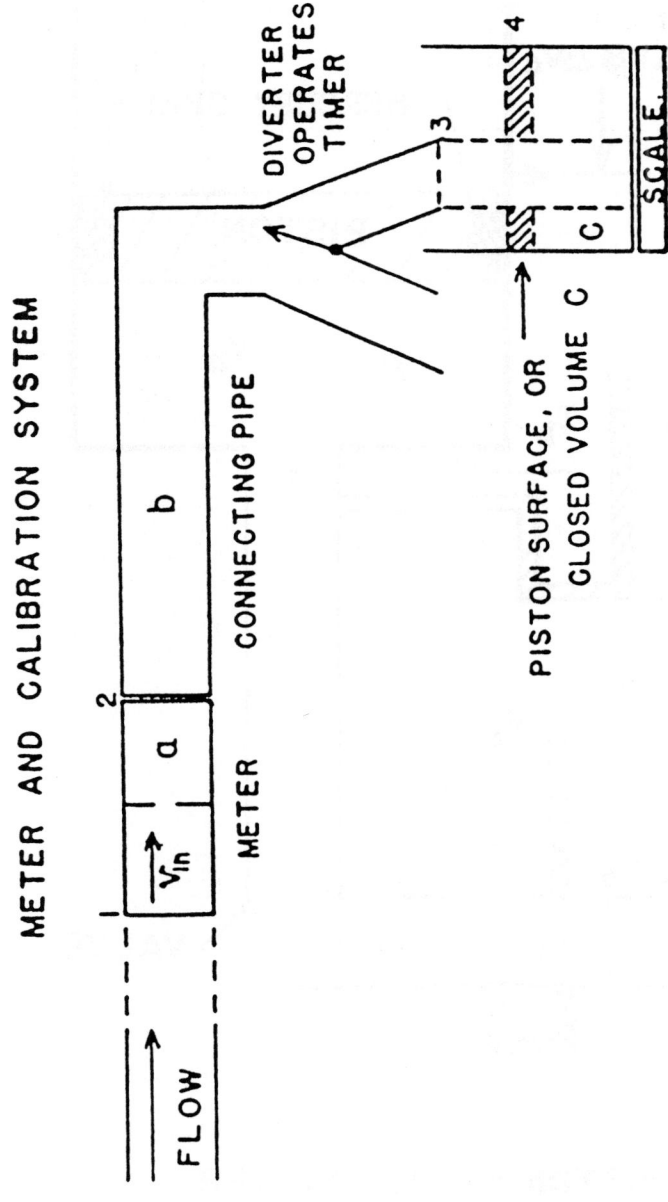

FIGURE 2

TYPICAL FLOWRATE CALIBRATION FACILITY

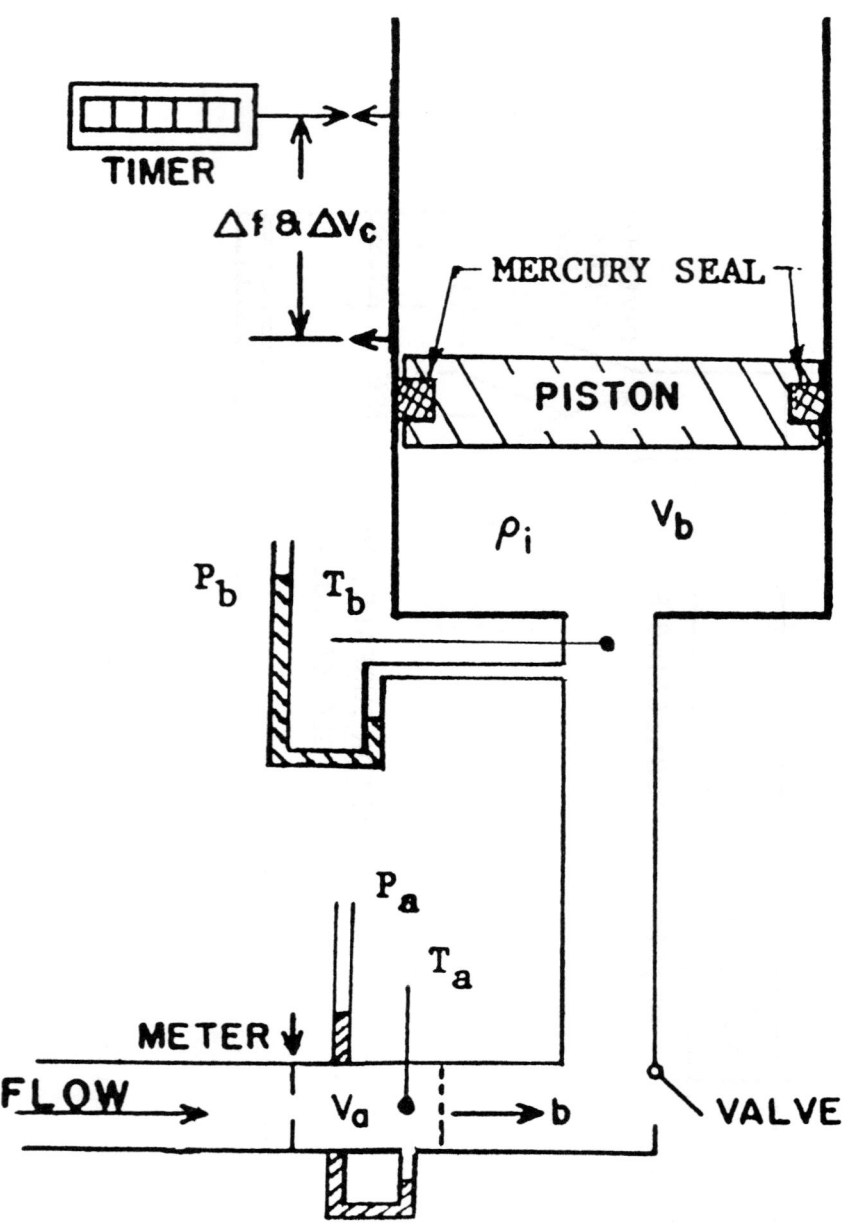

PISTON-TYPE PROVER

FIGURE 3

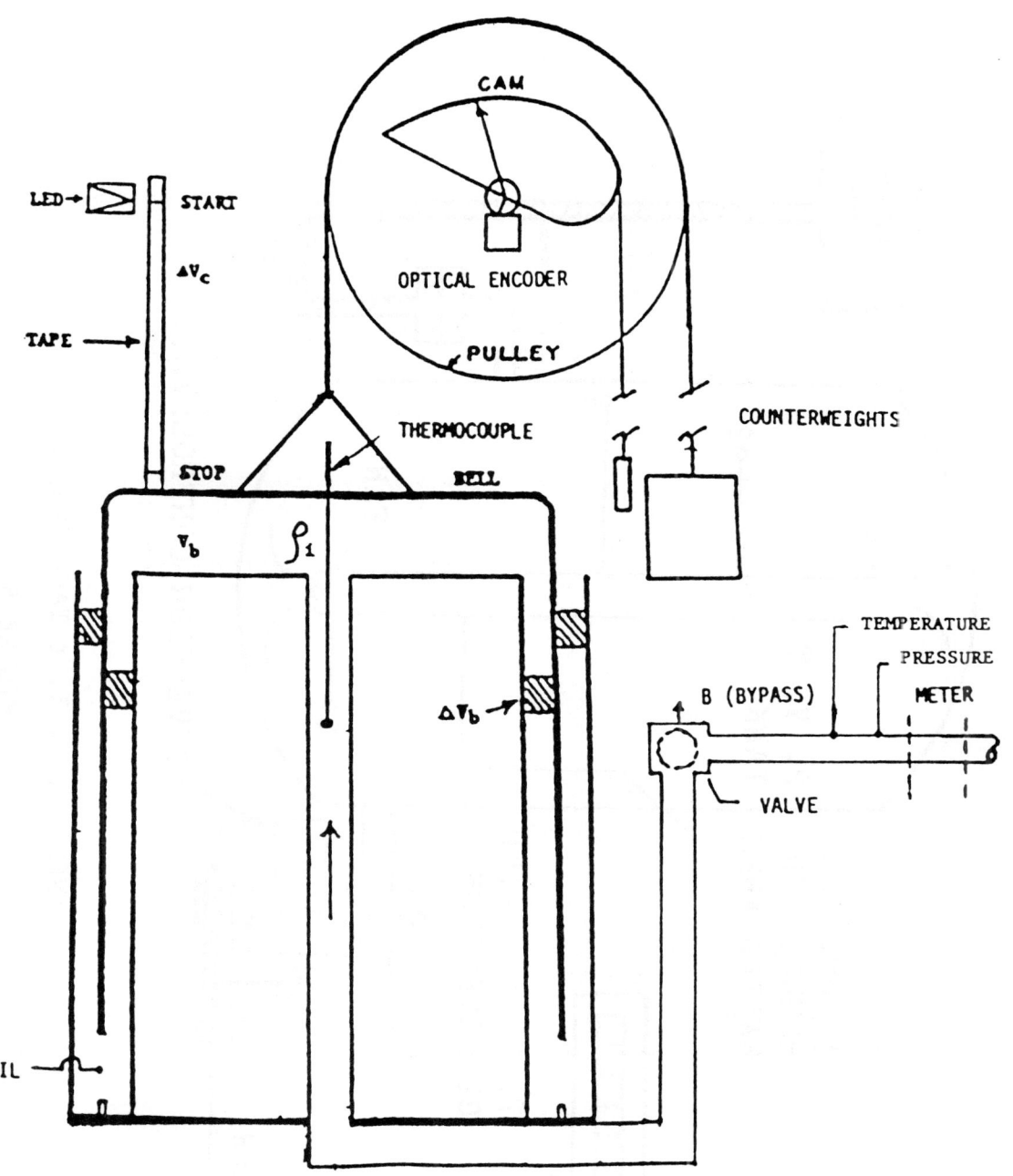

TYPICAL BELL PROVER ARRANGEMENT

FIGURE 4

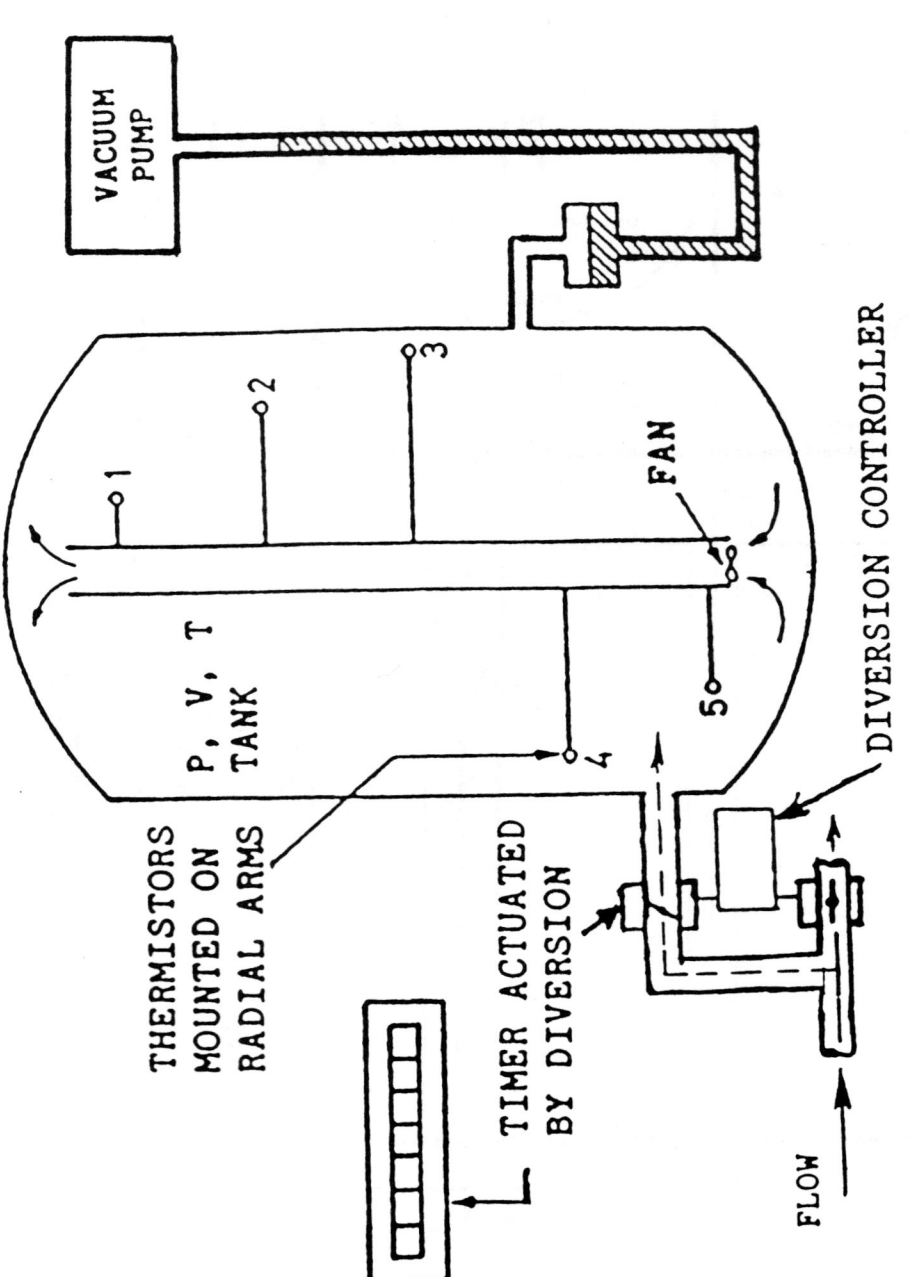

NBS' P, V, T, t TANK SYSTEM

FIGURE 5

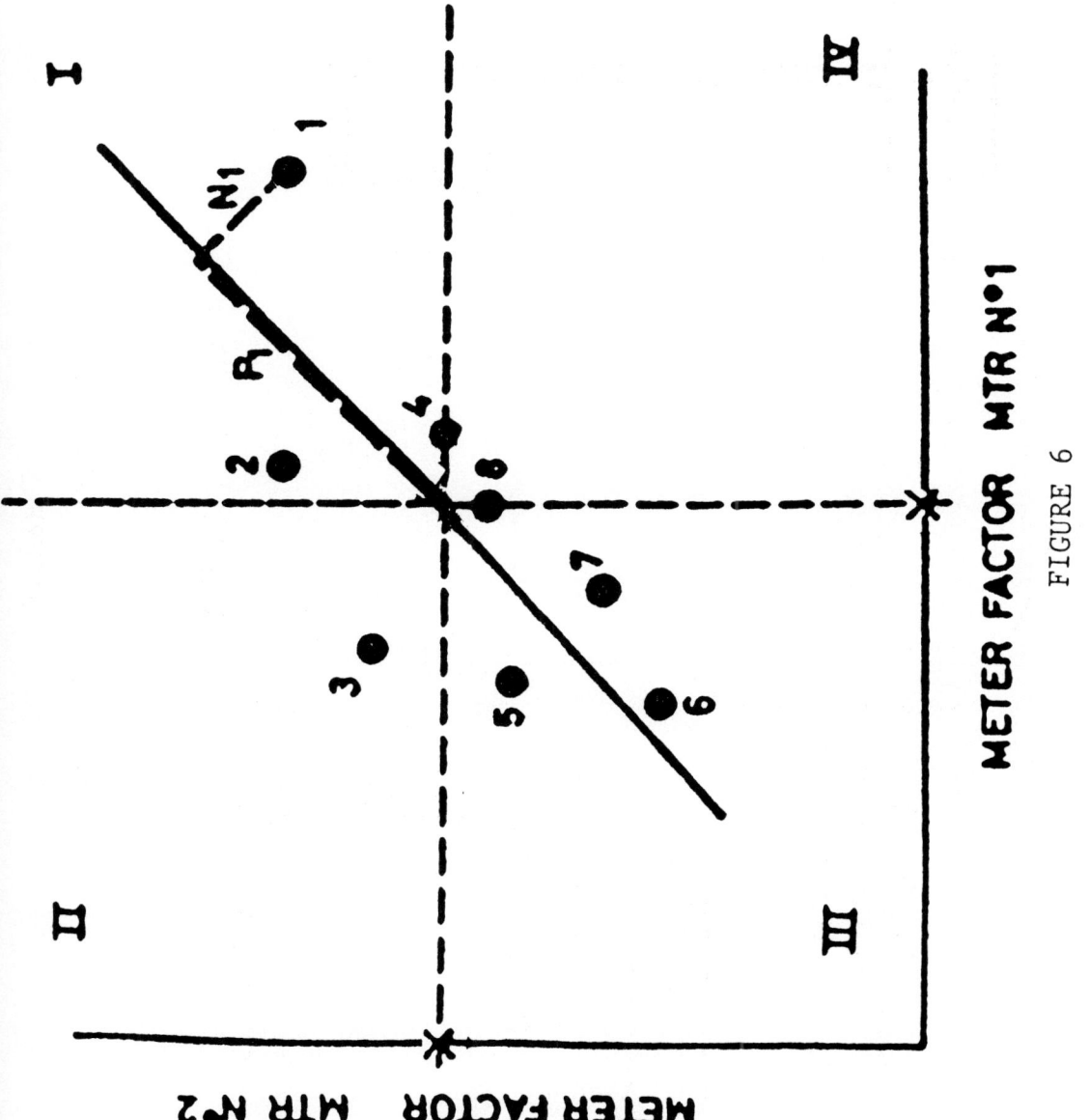

FIGURE 6

USE OF TURBINE METERS FOR HIGH ACCURACY GAS FLOWRATE MEASUREMENTS

DR. RICHARD A. FURNESS
Director
Centre for Flow Measurement
Department of Fluid Engineering and Instrumentation
Cranfield Institute of Technology
Cranfield, Bedford, MK43 0AL
United Kingdom

SUMMARY

The paper looks at the growing use of turbine meters for gas metering. This type of flowmeter is one of the most precise flowmeters currently available, but does have some drawbacks when used to measure gases. The paper opens with a discussion of the theory of turbine meters and a mathematical model is used to highlight the considerable deficiencies that exist in the design of turbine meters. Recent work in both experimental research and computational modelling are briefly covered.

Operating problems, particularly gas properties are listed, together with equations to estimate performance. Installation effects are then covered and reference is made to recent data and the current installation practices for gas metering stations.

Finally developments in new technology, the application of new materials and general perception of turbine meters in relation to other types of flowmeter are briefly dicussed and predictions for the continued use of this type of flowmeter are made. The paper is only a brief resume of the applications of gas turbine meter technology.

INTRODUCTION

The axial turbine meter offers the highest performance of flowmeters currently available. It is made in a wide variety of sizes and is widely applicable to the custody transfer of fluids, both liquid and gas. The turbine meter, as the name implies, is a rotor driven by the fluid being metered at a speed proportional to flowrate. The speed of the rotor is sensed by a pickoff on the outside of the meter body and the general characteristics make the turbine meter one of most common frequency output flowmeters.

Most meters are of the axial type but over the past thirty years, impulse, bearingless, twin rotor and insertion designs have all appeared, the design being developed for a particular application or fluid. The general basic characteristics, high accuracy, good rangeability and rapid response are the result of some forty years of continuous development. Their need arose in the late 1930's in the USA where engineers required accurate flow measurement and greater versatility. However, the early meters gained a reputation for dirt sensitivity and limited life as a result of poor bearing designs. Recent developments have made their performance so good that the use as international reference standards is growing, particularly in gas metering.

BASIC CHARACTERISTICS AND DESIGN

The basic construction of the modern turbine meter is fairly simple. All types of axial flow turbines have a rotor with blades running on a bearing and supported by a central shaft. The shape and design of the blades and bearings varies between manufacturers. The whole assembly is held centrally within the meter body by upstream and downstream spiders which are also claimed to act as flow straighteners. The motion of the rotor is sensed by a remote pickoff mounted in the wall but isolated from the line fluid. These features are shown in Figure 1 for one particular design of meter, the straight blade type. The speed of rotation is proportional to the throughput, but as we will see in the following section, this proportionality is not constant over the usable range of the meter. Each time the blade passes beneath the pickoff a pulse is generated. The output frequency therefore gives the flowrate the counting the number of pulses gives the volume passed.

When the turbine meter is running at a constant flowrate, the driving torque generated by the fluid impacting the blades exactly balances the resisting forces from bearing friction, viscous drag and magnetic drag. The actual behaviour is a complex function of many variables. The most important of these are:-

   (a) Temperature, pressure, density and viscosity of fluid
   (b) Lubricating qualities of the fluid
   (c) Mechanical wear on the bearings
   (d) Conditioning and dimensional changes of the blades
   (e) Changes in inlet profile and swirl
   (f) Pressure drop through the meter

Not all are important for gas metering but it is important to distinguish between actual flowing volume and standard volumes when sizing meters. The effect of temperature, pressure and gas density is covered later in the paper. Because the output is dependant on all these factors, the lowest uncertainty of measurement is obtained by proving or calibrating under the actual operating conditions. All turbine meters require calibration to establish the meter factor since our knowledge of their behaviour precludes a purely theoretical calibration as used for example for the orifice plate. This then brings into question the test stand performance. It should be remembered that the quoted meter performance must include the inherent random and systematic errors of the calibration stand. These must be very low since the turbine is a highly repeatable device, (< ±0.1% of reading). Any peculiarities of the test stand will affect the ability to determine the performance with any degree of certainty. Typical characteristics for a meter are shown in Figure 2.

This plots the change in meter coefficient (the pulse output per unit of throughput) the pressure drop, the output frequency and the output voltage as a function of the flowrate through the meter. The meter coefficient relationship with flowrate can be split into two main section. The "linear" portion, generally the upper three quarters of the operating range is to a large extent influenced by the fluid viscosity or the gas density, meter size and design. The meter should always be designed or sized to operate in this region where a mean meter factor can be used with little source of error. In the non-linear region, the flow profile, bearing and other retarding effects become more pronounced. The slope of the curve becomes steeper and meter factor linearity all but disappears. The repeatability of the meter is unaffected in this region.

At very low flowrates, the repeatability becomes poor as retarding forces begin to overcome hydrodynamic driving forces. Eventually the meter ceases to respond below a certain minimum flow and output stops. This is strongly influenced by gas density when considering gas flow measurements. At the other end of the performance curve, provided there is sufficient static pressure in the meter to supress cavitation then the meter can be run considerably over the rated throughput for short periods without affecting the bearings greatly. Obviously for gas measurement only compressibility effects need to be considered when pressure drop is high. Prolonged high speed usage is not recommended as both bearing life and meter accuracy will be affected. For many years manufacturers have been striving to design meters with wide linear ranges.

The frequency and voltage output depend on both meter and pickoff design. Two basic types of pickoff are available, magnetic and radio frequency modulated carrier. In the magnetic designs and coil may be mounted in the pickoff (reluctance type) of magnetic materials (or magnets) are used in the blades (inductive type). The magnetic properties of a circuit are changed by the presence of the blade and an AC output results. The magnitude of the signal varies between manufacturers but is usually in the range 10 mV to 1 V RMS. The frequency decreases with increasing meter size and decreasing flowrate, generally ranging from 10 Hz to 4 kHz. The higher the frequency the greater the resolution. The modulated carrier pickoff operates on the principle of the presence of a blade modifying a base carrier frequency. Because the energy transfer between sensor and rotor is negligible, this technique gives almost drag free sensing. Consequently the retarding torque is reduced and this method can improve low velocity (or low density) performance. The magnetic methods are the more common for the sole reason that they are much cheaper to implement. The pressure drop is proportional to the square of the flow rate, usually being in the range 0.2 to 0.7 bar (3 to 10 psi).

A typical pressure profile, shown in figure 3, has special significance for gases, since the point of minimum area (where the volumetric measurement is mad)e is also the point of maximum density sensitivity. This means that the design of the internals is critical to the performance of the meter in compressible fluids. Comments on the design of gas meters is made later in the paper.

The ability of the turbine to respond rapidly to transient flow conditions is another valuable characteristic. It is usual to express transient behaviour in the form of a time constant, i.e. the time required for the meter output to reach 63% of the final value of a step change in flowrate. Typical values vary with the size of the meter, the blade angle employed and the inertia of the rotor. The small turbine meter can respond to a step change in flow within 5-10 milliseconds whilst the larger meters (those with diameters in excess of 100 mm or so) have time constants of 20 milliseconds or longer. Generally speaking the low inertia straight blade designs achieve the more rapid response and this can be sustained on larger designs through the fabrication of hollow rotors.

It is the inherent high performance and wide rangeability however that are the important characteristics. Along with positive displacement meters, the turbine offers the highest performance currently available. The basic accuracy is comparable with the test stand or calibration method used to determine performance and for this reason the meter finds widespread use as secondary reference standard. A well designed, fully balanced meter can have a measurement uncertainty of 0.1% of reading but the usual industrial meter possesses an quoted accuracy of between 0.25 and 0.5 per cent of reading over flowranges up to 20:1. The overall quoted performance varies greatly between manufacturers and with over 40 suppliers of this type of meter worldwide, the user has much scope in matching desired performance with his particular application. The smaller meters (6-18 mm diameter) have quoted performances ranging from ± 0.25 to ± 1% over 10:1 flowrange.

TURBINE METER THEORY

On examination of the literature, several methods have been proposed to predict the behaviour of the turbine meter. All these models are based on two general principles, the momentum and the aerofoil approaches. In the momentum approach, the driving torque is expressed as a function of the change in angular momentum of the fluid. A rigorous analysis has yet to be performed and simplifying assumptions for the method means that all fluid particles crossing the plane of the blade leading edge are given the same change in momentum as those fluid particles adjacent to the blade. This is true for meters with many blades but is not the case for many commercial designs.

In the aerofoil approach the forces exerted on an element of blade are integrated over the entire blade to obtain the driving torque. This infers that increasing the number of blades gives a corresponding increase in rotor speed. This does not occur in practice since the influence of adjacent blades increases drag more than lift, the so called interference or cascade effect. Therefore, if blade number increases beyond the optimum, blade lift efficiency falls. The following model originally derived by Tan and Hutton (1971) is based on aerofoil theory but requires the velocity profile to be known or at least approximated by an empirical relation. These aspects are discussed later.

The driving torque is derived for an element of blade area with a thickness dr at a radius r. In order to perform the analysis the lift and drag forces must be resolved into components both parallel and perpendicular to the rotor axis. The diagram in Figure 4 shows the forces acting on an element of blade of angle Θ. As indicated the drag acts parallel to the mean relative velocity U_1 whilst the lift acts perpendicular to U_1. We can therefore write for the lift force:

$$dL = \frac{1}{2} \cdot \rho \cdot V_m^2 \, C_L \cdot c \cdot dr$$

This can be transposed to:

$$dL = \frac{1}{2} \frac{\rho \cdot W_b C_L \cdot U^2 dr}{\cos^2 \phi \cdot \cos \beta} \qquad \ldots (1)$$

Similarly for the drag force and by the same reasoning

$$dD = \frac{1}{2} \frac{\rho \cdot W_b \cdot C_D \cdot U^2 dr}{\cos^2 \phi \cdot \cos \beta} \qquad \ldots (2)$$

The element torque acting on the blade is then simply a force balance:

$$dT = N (dL \cos \phi - dD \sin \phi) \, dr \qquad \ldots (3)$$

Now Joukowski's theorem indicates that the lift coefficient for an airfoil in an ideal fluid when the blade thickness approaches zero with no camber (i.e. a thin flat plate) can be written:

$$C_L = 2\pi \sin \alpha$$

This only applies when the angle of attack is small and this would be the case for a turbine meter since consideration of the velocity profiles gives a variation in attack angle of around $15°$ at the blade root, falling to a negative attack angle (i.e. a drag force) of -5° at the tip. These values, of course, vary with the blade design. However, this assumes a wing in an infinite stream and clearly does not allow for interference effects. To take account of the finite aspect ratio and blade efficiency, the lift coefficient can be written as:

$$C_L = 2\pi \cdot E \cdot K \cdot \sin \alpha \qquad \ldots (4)$$

where E is an airfoil blade efficiency and K is a geometric constant for the blade cascade. Therefore, substituting (1), (2) and (4) into (3) yields:

$$dT = \frac{1}{2} \rho.N.W_b u^2 \, rdr \, \frac{2\pi.E.K.\sin\alpha}{\cos\phi.\cos\beta} - \frac{C_D \tan\phi}{\cos\phi.\cos\beta} \qquad \ldots (5)$$

Now $\dfrac{\sin\alpha}{\cos\phi.\cos\beta} = \dfrac{\sin(\beta-\phi)}{\cos\phi.\cos\beta} = \tan\beta - \tan\phi$

Also $\tan(\beta - \phi) = \dfrac{V_e + 2\pi rn}{u}$

and $\tan\phi = \dfrac{2\pi rn + \dfrac{V_e - V}{V_e}}{V}$

$$= 2\pi rn + \dfrac{u \, \mathrm{Tan}\,\dfrac{(\beta-\phi)}{2} - 2\pi rn - V}{u}$$

$$= \dfrac{\pi rn}{u} + \dfrac{\mathrm{Tan}\,(\beta-\phi)}{2} - \dfrac{V}{2u}$$

Therefore, finally:

$$\frac{\sin\alpha}{\cos\phi.\cos\beta} = \tan\beta - \tan\phi = \tan\beta - \frac{\pi rn}{u} - \frac{\tan(\beta-\phi)}{2} + \frac{V}{2u} \qquad \ldots (6)$$

Then substituting equation (6) into equation (5) gives:

$$\frac{2dt}{\rho.N.W_b} = u^2 rdr \left[2\pi \, EK. \left(\tan\beta - \tan\frac{(\beta-\phi)}{2} - \frac{\pi rn}{u} + \frac{V}{2u} - C_D \frac{\tan\phi}{\cos\beta \cos\phi} \right) \right] \qquad \ldots (7)$$

Integrating from blade hub to blade tip, we obtain:

$$\frac{2t}{\rho.N.W_b} = \int_{r_n}^{r_t} 2\pi EK \left[\tan\beta - \tan\frac{(\beta-\phi)}{2} \right] u^2 r\,dr - \int_{r_h}^{r_t} 2\pi^2 EKn\, u^2\, r^2\, dr$$

$$+ \int_{r_h}^{r_t} 2\pi E.K. \left[\frac{V}{2} \right] u\, r\, dr - \int_{r_h}^{r_t} \frac{C_D \tan\phi}{\cos\beta . \cos\phi} . u^2 r\, dr \quad \ldots (8)$$

It is normal to introduce a reference for both the velocity vector u and radius r. If we therefore replace u by u/U and r by r/r_0 (where U is the reference axial velocity and r_0 is the meter diameter) we have:

$$\frac{2T}{\rho.N.W.} = \frac{U^2 r_0^2}{2} . \pi.E.K. \int_{r_h}^{r_t} (2\tan\beta - \tan(\beta-\delta)) \left[\frac{u}{U}\right]^2 \frac{r\,dr}{r_0^2}$$

$$- 2\pi.n\, U^2 r_0^3 E.K \int_{r_h}^{r_t} \left[\frac{u}{U}\right]^2 \frac{r^2 dr}{r_0^3} + U^2 r_0^2 . 2.\pi E K \int_{r_h}^{r_t} \left[\frac{V}{u}\right]\left[\frac{u}{U}\right]^2 \frac{r\,dr}{r_0^2}$$

$$- U^2 r_0^2 \int_{r_h}^{r_t} \frac{C_D \tan\phi}{\cos\beta.\cos\phi} . \left[\frac{u}{U}\right]^2 \frac{r.dr}{r_0^2} \quad \ldots (9)$$

The equation means we have referenced the actual axial velocity is in terms of the velocity profile (u/U). For the purpose of further analysis we will replace the integrals by the terms A,B,C, and D. Therefore:

$$\frac{2T}{\rho.N.W} = \left[\frac{U^2 r_0^2}{2} . \pi E.K. A\right] - \left[2\pi r_0^3 n. U^2. EK . B\right] +$$

$$\left[U^2 r_0^2. 2\pi.E.K. C\right] - \left[U^2 r_0^2 . D\right] \quad \ldots (10)$$

or transposing the above equation, we have:

$$n = \frac{1}{2\, r_0 B}\left[\frac{A}{2} + C - \frac{2D}{EK}\right] - \frac{2T}{N.W.\rho.\pi\, r_0^3. U^2\, EK.B} \quad \ldots (11)$$

The total volume flow going through the rotor Q_r is simply the total flow area minus the area occupied by the rotor times the velocity:

$$Q_r = \int_{r_h}^{r_t} (2\pi r u - Ntu) \, dr$$

$$= \pi r_o^2 \cdot U \cdot \int_{r_h}^{r_t} \left[2r - \frac{Nt}{\pi} \right] \left\{ \frac{u}{U} \right\} \frac{dr}{r_o^2} = \pi r_o^2 \cdot U.E \qquad \ldots (12)$$

The total volume flow going through the tip clearance is:

$$Q_t = \int_{r_t}^{r_o} 2\pi r u \, dr = \pi r_o^2 U \int_{r_t}^{r_o} 2 \left\{ \frac{u}{U} \right\} \frac{rdr}{r_o^2} = \pi r_o^2 U F. \qquad \ldots (13)$$

The total flow going through the meter is then the flow through the rotor plus the flow path the rotor in the clearance gap.

$$Q = Q_t + Q_r = \pi r_o^2 U \left[E + F \right]$$

The performance of a turbine meter is usually expressed in the form of a meter coefficient versus flowrate. The meter coefficient is defined as the number of pulses per unit volume

$$K' = \frac{M}{Q_r} \frac{A}{4\pi r_o^3 \, UB.E} + \frac{C}{2\pi r_o^3 \, UBE} - \frac{D}{\pi r_o^3 \, U \, B.E}$$

$$- \frac{2T}{N.\rho.W.\pi^2.r_o^5 \, U^3 \, E.K.B.E.} \qquad \ldots (14)$$

However, this is the meter coefficient of the rotor alone and the meter coefficient actually measured is n/Q since boundary layer and the tip clearnce effect modify the performance of the rotor particularly around the tip area.

$$\therefore \quad \frac{n}{Q} = \frac{n}{Q_r} \cdot \frac{Q_r}{Q} \qquad \ldots (15)$$

Therefore finally for the meter coefficient we have:

$$\frac{n}{Q} = \frac{A}{r_o^3 \, U.B. \, (E + F)} + \frac{C}{2\pi.r_o^3 \, . \, U.B. \, (E + F)} - \frac{D}{\pi \, r_o^3 \, . \, U.B. \, (E + F)}$$

$$-\frac{2T}{N.W. \rho \pi^2 . r_o 5.U^3 . K. B. (E + F)} \qquad \ldots (16)$$

Thus, the characteristic equation can be expressed in the form:

$$\frac{n}{Q} = W + X - Y - Z \qquad \ldots (17)$$

where:

$$W = \frac{A}{4 \pi r_o^3 U.B. (E + F)}$$

$$X = \frac{C}{2 \pi r_o^3 U.B (E + F)}$$

$$Y = \frac{D}{\pi r_o^3 U. B. (E + F)}$$

$$Z = \frac{2T (E + F)}{N.\rho.W. r_o U E.K. Q^2 B.}$$

The constants A to F, all integrals, are summarized in Appendix A.

DISCUSSION OF THEORY WITH RELEVANCE TO METER DESIGN

Having derived the general expression for a turbine meter we can look at each term and also at the physical meaning of the expression. The most important feature of the equation is clearly the influence of the velocity profile (u/U). This appears in all of the integrals and this serves to emphasize how important it is to have a controlled profile at the meter inlet, whether the meter is measuring liquid or gas. The design of the meter itself is also very critical since a sudden change in section will greatly affect the change the velocity profile and hence the meter factor. The ideal meter would appear to be one of very small hub diameter with a small tip clearance. This means that the blades are sweeping almost the entire pipe area and only a fraction of the flow bypasses the blades. The small hub diameter would not induce asymmetry into the profile and if the flow volume is known approximately, an empirical expression could be substituted into equation 16 and a theoretical meter coefficient could be calculated. The model shows that unless the profile is known it is not possible to calculate a meter factor with any degree of certainty.

However with gas meters the hub is very large so that the maximum torque is extracted at the maximum radius to overcome the various retarding torques. The theory derived herein tends to suggest that most gas meters are well away from an optimum design.

Now we can look at the four different terms in the general equation. The first term on the RHS of equation 17 is the driving torque, the second term is the inlet swirl term since the integral includes the ratio (V/U). This is the ratio of the tangential velocity component to the axial velocity component, which is the fundamental definition of swirl. If the meter is installed in an ideal location with the correct pipe lengths upstream and downstream this term is essentially zero since little or no swirl will exist in the flow. The third term is a fluid drag term since the drag coefficient C_D appears in the integral. The value of the velocity profile is squared and hence fluid viscosity becomes a dominant parameter in this term. The higher the viscosity the larger the negative effect this term has on the meter factor. This is true in practice because the meter factor versus flowrate curve falls as the fluid viscosity increases or as gas density reduces. The fourth term is the retarding torque and includes such factors as bearing drag, pick-off magnetic drag and the drag at the blade tips. Each of these varies with respect to the others so that value of the resisting torque T is assumed to be constant throughout the range. This may or may not be a valid assumption.

If the relative magnitudes of each of the terms is examined the following picture emerges. At high flowrates term 1 dominates the value of the meter coefficient is close to the value of term 1. The presence of swirl increases the meter coefficient by a constant amount depending on the absolute value of (V/U). However, as flowrate decreases terms 3 and 4 begin to dominate and at very low flowrates the fourth term (with the $1/Q^2$ present) becomes the influential term. The relative values of each of these terms determines the shape of the flow calibration curve. The big unknown in all of the equations is the velocity profile. The classical assumption for turbulent pipe flow is that the profile varies with the Reynolds number according to the relationship:

$$\frac{u}{U} = \left[\frac{r_o - r}{\delta^*} \right]^{1/m} \qquad \ldots (18)$$

where δ^* is the boundary layer thickness and m is an exponent depending on the value of the Reynolds number. The normal value for turbulent pipe flow is 7 (the so-called one-seventh power law) but the range can vary between 6 and 10. However the design of most commercial meters and virtually all gas turbine meters gives rise to velocity profile changes within the meter body, a feature not desirable for the lowest uncertainty of measurement. The shape and size of the centre body is critical to the conditioning of the flow profile upstream of the rotor blade. Indeed in some designs of gas meter the hub to tip ratio is as high as 0.85 which entirely negates the reason for having long lengths of upstream pipe. The hydrodynamic design of turbines is one area where almost no attention has been paid, and very few meters are anything like the optimum.

If the fluid undergoes rapid acceleration due to a large centre body in the middle of the meter, this is merely increasing terms 3 and 4 in the meter equation relative to term 1. Although the meter factor will increase so will the bearing drag, fluid drag and pressure drop. For most commercial turbine meters a better approximation of profile would be (Tan and Hutton 1971):

$$\frac{u}{U} = \left[\frac{(r_o - r)}{\delta^*} \right] \cdot \left[\frac{(r_o)}{r_o - r_h} \right]^{\frac{1}{m}} \qquad \ldots (19)$$

This allows the contraction effect of the centre body

$$\left[\frac{r_o}{r_o - r_h} \right]^{\frac{1}{m}}$$

to be evaluated as a function of the flowrate. At this stage however some further research needs to be done to evaluate the velocity profiles encountered within contracting sections. Until this is performed the actual use of the equations is restricted. The theory however has been particularly useful in determining the important features of design.

OPERATING PROBLEMS WITH GAS TURBINE METERS

Pressure drop design considerations

The pressure drop developed in a turbine meter is due to two main factors. These are:-

(i) Energy required to overcome bearing and blade friction
(ii) Losses due to changes in flow area within the meter body

The pressure drop is usually measured at the inlet and outlet of the meter where the flow areas are the same as the nominal pipe bore. However as discussed earlier the lowest pressure occurs in the region of the rotor. Normally the nominal pressure drop ΔP_r is specified by the manufacturer and follows the turbulent flow loss relationship, i.e. $\Delta P \propto Q^2$. For gas meters however, operating pressure affects the pressure drop across the meter. The operating pressure drop ΔP_o can be calculated from the pressure drop at rated conditions and the ideal gas equation as follows:-

$$\Delta P_o = \Delta P_r \left[\frac{\rho_o}{\rho_r}\right]\left[\frac{Q_o}{Q_r}\right]^2$$

$$= \Delta P_r \left[\frac{G_o}{G_r}\right]\left[\frac{P_o}{P_r}\right]\left[\frac{T_r}{T_o}\right]\left[\frac{Z_r}{Z_o}\right]\left[\frac{Q_o}{Q_r}\right]^2 \quad \ldots (20)$$

This equation states that gas pressure, temperature, flowing gravity and compressibility all influence the pressure drop across the meter. It is essential that compressibility effects are minimized by ensuring that the pressure drop within the meter does not exceed that specified by the meter supplier. Should this limit be exceeded then the actual performance data is a function of flowing gas conditions, and becomes hard to estimate.

Maximum and minimum flowrates for gas meters

It was shown above that gas properties were very important in determining pressure drop across the meter. These same properties also determine the maximum and minimum flows through the meter. Most misapplications of gas turbine meter arises from failure to size the meter correctly, since actual and standard volume flows are often used synonymously. Most manufacturers size the meters not to exceed a certain rotor speed. This maximum rated flow Q_{rmax} remains the same for all operating pressure within the stated pressure limits (unless stated otherwise). Thus the maximum rotor speed remains constant regardless of pressure; i.e. :—

$$Q_{omax} = Q_{rmax}$$

Usually rated maximum flow is related to base conditions Q_{bmax}. This maximum base flowrate can be expressed as a function of Q_{rmax} by the equation:-

$$Q_{bmax} = Q_{rmax} \left[\frac{P_o}{P_b}\right]\left[\frac{T_b}{T_o}\right]\left[\frac{Z_b}{Z_o}\right]$$

where subscript o refers to operating conditions and subscript b to base conditions.

The minimum flowrate depends on more variables, but primarily the density of the gas and the magnitude of pickoff and bearing drag. The minimum base flowrate is approximately given by the equation:-

$$Q_{bmin} \cong Q_{rmin} \left[\left[\frac{G_r}{G_o}\right]\left[\frac{P_o}{P_b}\right]\left[\frac{P_r}{P_b}\right]\left[\frac{T_b}{T_o}\right]\left[\frac{T_r}{T_r}\right]\left[\frac{Z_b}{Z_o}\right]\left[\frac{Z_b}{Z_r}\right]\right]^{\frac{1}{2}} \quad \ldots (21)$$

Generally the rated temperatures and pressures are close to the base temperatures and pressures, (unless the supplier states otherwise) and this expression can be simplified to give:-

$$Q_{bmin} \cong Q_{rmin}\left[\left[\frac{G_r}{G_o}\right]\left[\frac{P_o}{P_b}\right]\left[\frac{T_b}{T_o}\right]\left[\frac{Z_b}{Z_o}\right]\right]^{\frac{1}{2}} \quad \ldots (22)$$

and the minimum operating line flow is given by:-

$$Q_{omin} \cong Q_{rmin}\left[\left[\frac{G_r}{G_o}\right]\left[\frac{P_r}{P_o}\right]\left[\frac{T_o}{T_r}\right]\left[\frac{Z_o}{Z_r}\right]\right]^{\frac{1}{2}} \quad \ldots (23)$$

In well designed and correctly operated meters the compressibility and the temperature ratios are close to unity and can be neglected for initial sizing purposes. The gas density however is important in determining the operating range over which the meter will perform within stated limits. In general these expressions indicate that rangeability varies with the square root of the gas density. As density increases, the linearity improves at the bottom end of the curve while the upper limit remains fixed as discussed. Thus we can derive a simple expression for rangeability as:—

$$\text{Rangeability} = \frac{Q_{omax}}{Q_{omin}} = \frac{Q_{bmax}}{Q_{bmin}} = \frac{Q_{rmax}}{Q_{rmin}} \left\{ \left[\frac{G_o}{G_r}\right]\left[\frac{P_o}{P_r}\right]\left[\frac{T_r}{T_o}\right]\left[\frac{Z_r}{Z_o}\right] \right\}^{\frac{1}{2}} \quad \ldots (24)$$

This states that the range of operating flows for more linear measurement increases approximately as the square root of the pressure ratio $\sqrt{(P_o/P_r)}$. The lowest rangeability is obtained at atmospheric conditions and this increases as system pressure increases. Such a trend is shown in figure 5 for data taken on low pressure air and natural gas.

CURRENT GAS TURBINE METERING PRACTICE IN THE UK

Gas meters, particularly in the past decade have relied heavily on orifice plates. Turbine meters have been installed in quantities recently and operational experience is growing. The new British Gas facility at Bishop Auckland now permits the calibration of meters at full line conditions with the consequent reduction in overall uncertinty. In the UK turbine meters for gas transmission are used in the size range 76 to 400mm (3 to 16 inch) in diameter, with maximum capacities from 249 to 6514 m^3/hr (8800 to 230000ft^3/hr). Recent field trials on 100 meters have shown that turbine meters can operate reliably, over extended periods, at pressures below 7 bar (100 psi). Their main disadvantages have been shown to be:-

1. relatively poor rangeability (on low pressure gas this rarely exceeds 15:1)
2. inability to measure reliably when the flow is pulsating
3. susceptability to increased measurement errors in distorted pipe installations.

However they do have advantages, namely:-

1. good basic performance characteristics including high repeatability
2. low weight for throughput capability
3. do not stop the gas stream in the event of failure

It has generally been found that they under-register if used for long periods near the specified minimum flowrate. This problem however can be overcome if the more modern designs discussed in the following section are used. There is also the problem of educating the user to install meters properly and even the suppliers information is suspect in some cases. There is no doubt that turbine meter systems do offer significant advantages over other gas meters but it will however be some years before they fully replace the orifice based systems in the UK and are used with confidence.

MODERN GAS METER DESIGNS

The present trend in gas turbine meters is toward self checking, low friction instruments. One of the latest design uses two sets of ball race bearings within a single meter. This meter, shown in Figure 6 has two rotating elements, an upstream indicating turbine and a downstream 'slave' turbine. The slave and central shaft run on one set of bearings whilst the indicating turbine rides on a second separate set of bearings attached to the shaft. This means that the relative motion between the indicating turbine and its bearings remain near zero. It is claimed that this large reduction in bearing friction gives more precise and repeatable performance over much wider flowranges than conventional designs. Personal experience with this meter in a gas pipeline application in the USA confirms this. It was shown in the theoretical section earlier how important bearing design and friction is to the overall meter performance particularly in the low flow portion (10 per cent of maximum rated flow and below) of the curve. Examination of the geometry shows that the centre body is much smaller than a conventional gas turbine meter shown in figure 7.

This twin rotor design also has a "no-drag" pick-off, whereas certain commercial design use magnetic sensors to measure rotational speed. The combination of no bearing or magnetic drag plus more efficient blade and centre body design contributes significantly to the performance now obtainable. This twin rotor design with electronic linearisation results in a flowrange of up to 600:1 in liquids and 1000:1 in gases with claimed accuracies of 0.1 per cent. These figures are orders of magnitude better than the first designs some 45 years ago.

Up to now the Quantum meter has had limited use on gas pipelines, due primarily to the high cost, but they find widespread use in aerospace applications where they are unrivalled in performance. Personal experience on a toxic gas pipeline in the Eastern United States showed the meter performance to be outstanding and they did operate satisfactorily for a number of years on this duty until line operation was suspended. In this application (a pipeline monitoring system) four of these meters were spaced at regular intervals on a 22 mile line and agreed to within 0.1% over medium to long periods of time (in excess of 6 hours).

A different twin rotor approach was adopted by Rockwell International a few years ago. This design is made self checking and self adjusting. Unlike the Quantum Dynamics meter where the two rotors are some distance apart, the Rockwell meter rotors are next to each other, with the measuring element behind the main rotor as shown in figure 8. The constancy of performance is attained because the sense rotor detects deviations in the exit angle of fluid leaving the main rotor. The sensing rotor has a blade angle considerably smaller than that of the main rotor but larger than the exit angle. It therefore rotates in the same direction as the main rotor but at a lower speed. When the speed of the sensor rotor is subtracted from the speed of the main rotor electronically, the difference depends only on the rotor blade angles. The performance is then the difference of the two speeds rather than from a single rotor speed as shown in figure 9. Any change in the main rotor retarding torque will give a corresponding change in rotor speed and hence exit angle. The sensor rotor adjust its speed by an equal amount, thereby cancelling out the change in bearing friction.

General experience in North America with these meters on gas transmission lines is favourable and Companies with this type installed include Florida Gas, Lone Star Gas, El Paso Natural Gas, Southern California Gas, Tennessee Gas Pipeline, Texas Eastern Gas and TransContinental Gas Pipeline.

They have been used offshore in the Gulf of Mexico and in various test sites throughout Canada and the USA. Both wet gas and dry gas with contaminant applications have been reported at pressure in excess of 1200 psig.

If there are weaknesses in both these twin rotor designs, they are as follows. The Quantum meter has been primarily designed and applied in aerospace applications and a more robust form of bearing with a lower quality of manufacture may be required for industrial usage. The quality of manufacture of this meter is superb, with attention paid to tip clearance, dynamic balancing and in the machining of key components. The Rockwell meter design has a mechanical drive system up into the readout head with components that could fail. These are both however personal judgements and there is no doubt that twin rotors do offer significant advantages if self diagnostic, high performance and wide rangeability are required.

INSTALLATION EFFECTS

Turbine meters are very sensitive to both swirl and velocity profile distortion, as was clearly shown in the theoretical section of this paper. Many are therefore fitted with internal straighteners which also act as supports for the shaft/rotor assembly. However additional flow conditioning upstream of the meter is also required. Figure 10 shows some data taken by Jepson and Bean (1969) of the effect of swirl on a 50 mm liquid turbine meter with and without flow straighteners. The resulting error was ±1.6% per degree of swirl, the sign depending on the direction of the swirl relative to the turbine rotation. This was reduced to ±0.3% per degree by a simple cruciform straightener fitted in the upstream pipe. Similar data on a 254mm gas meter is shown in figure 11. It is seen that with no straighteners the swirl error was 0.2% per degree, significantly less than for liquid meters. Generally gas turbine meters are less prone to installation effects than liquid meters. This is presumably due to the high contraction that is usually present in gas turbine meters. When integral flow straighteners and additional upstream conditioning is used the errors become around 0.05% and 0.02% per degree of swirl respectively.

Valves can affect the performance in a different way. Figure 12 shows data for a 50mm liquid meter. If the valve was more than 30 pipe diameters upstream of the turbine its influence is small. However as the valve is progressively closed the influence persists for greater lengths. When the valve is almost closed, the magnitude of the error changed sign, a possible indication of swirl being generated.

The interesting conclusion from this figure is that if meters are installed 10 to 20 pipe diameters downstream of valves (which is a common industrial practice), systematic shifts of around 1% can be expected if the valve is partially open. If valves are to be fitted upstream of meters, it is strongly recommended that they be full bore ball valves and that they be fully open during operation with flow control valves on the downstream side only.

We saw earlier that the basic equation for turbine meters is of the form:-

$$\frac{n}{Q} = W + X - Y - Z$$

The left hand side is the meter factor (pulses/unit volume) and the four terms on the right hand side are complicated integrals involving the velocity distribution and many other variables (Tan and Hutton 1971). The second term X is the swirl term, the magnitude and sign affecting the meter factor directly. Thus the way the meter is installed will affect the meter performance as a first order effect. When looking at the complete equation (Tan and Hutton 1971) it is not difficult to see why turbine meters are so influenced by velocity profile and swirl, and extreme care must be exercised if installation effects are to be reduced to acceptable levels.

The small amount of data presented in this paper has shown that profile distortion and swirl can have a profound influence on meter performance. It also shows that long lengths of pipe upstream of the meter are required before the performance is unaffected by the actual installation. These relatively unpalatable facts are not often appreciated and as a result most installed meters generally do not have the same performance compared to that when they were first made and calibrated. This is particularly true for turbine meters, where the accepted industry standard is to install the meter 10 diameters downstream of a flow straightener. Indeed some American standards suggest upstream pipe lengths of this magnitude. This is rather too short and although it is the Standard recommendation, recent data does show that 1 or 2 degrees of swirl can pass through some types of flow conditioner and this would have the result of systematically altering the meter factor by 1%.

For minimum effects however there are tables for orifice and venturi meters which tend to be quoted for turbine and other meters in Western Europe. In all cases it is the upstream pipe length which is important. Table 2, taken from ISO 5167, shows the <u>minimum</u> length for various pipe configurations upstream of orifice plates, venturis and nozzles. In this table the values outside the brackets denote no additional uncertainty and the values in brackets show minimum lengths if an additional uncertainty of 0.5% is added. Despite the fact that tests have been performed over the past fifty years, the specification of pipework is causing international disagreement. Current ASME/AGA standards recommend upstream lengths almost half that listed in the ISO 5167 document. Even the data in the widely accepted ISO standard is open to question. Work at several centres in the UK, including Cranfield, tends to suggest that even longer overall lengths may be needed, especially for the case of two bends in different planes.

Table 2 (ISO 5167) does not give recommendations for the cases of multiple upstream fittings. What, for example, should be the recommended lengths for a reducer downstream of a bend or a valve fitted after a single bend ?. Data on which to draft acceptable standards is very scarce for such cases. Thus for a fully open globe valve downstream of a single bend, it is very much open to question whether the recommended lengths would satisfy all installations.

Furthermore the user tends to fit the minimum of pipe lengths, assuming that because he complies with the standards there is no installation affect. This is a dangerous assumption, especially as recent investigations are showing that installation effects are much more common than has been previously realised. The prediction of the effect of pipe fittings is one area where the application of computer models would have a significant benefit. In the short term however, the position will continue to be unsatisfactory until adequate data is gathered on which to draft usable working standards.

DEVELOPMENTS IN TURBINE METER DESIGN

Theoretical work on the flow through turbine meters has led to a better understanding of the implications of the design of certain components on the performance of meters. Figure 13 (a and b) shows that the pressure distribution changes positive to negative as one moves from hub to tip. This work by Ferriera et al (1986) is the first to predict that blade shape and centre body shape is critical to turbine meter performance. The computational model has also showed that the velocity profile will govern pressure drop and the sensitivity to density and viscosity of the meter.

Figure 13 shows the velocity distribution along the passage of a meter for a stream surface near the hub and tip respectively. The torque can be calculated by integrating the lift distribution along the blades. Figure 14 shows, for one flowrate how the net pressure is distributed along the blade. In this figure the co-ordinates are given in mm for the radius and chord and in N/mm² for the Z axis and contour height. This example shows that the front of the blade is responsible for generating the lift with the tip and trailing edge region producing areas of drag. The work tends to suggest that blade shapes should not be as in conventional gas meters but rather more like the Quantum design with axially short and radially long blades to minimise pressure drop and reduce velocity profile changes in the region of the volume measurement.

Signal analysis will also permit more data to be gathered from these meters. Work in the UK using microprocessor techniques have led to the examination of turbine meter signals in a new way (Higham et al 1986). The work is based on the use of Sparse Fourier Transforms. In classical spectral analysis the complex magnitude $r(\omega,T)$ of the component of a time signal $r(t)$ is given by:-

$$R(\omega,T) = \frac{1}{T} \int_0^T r(t).e^{-j\omega t} dt$$

where T is the duration of the signal record. For pulse signals which are zero except at time intevals $t_1, t_2, t_3, \ldots t_N$, then

$$R(\omega,T) = \frac{1}{N} \sum_{i=1}^{N} e^{-j\omega t_i}$$

and thus
$$R(\omega,T) = \frac{1}{N} \sum_{i=1}^{N} (\cos(\omega t_i) - j \sin(\omega t_i))$$

A timer counter in the secondary electronics is configured so that its contents at a time instant t yields the principle value of the angle ωt. The pulse signal from the flowmeter is connected to an interrupt line and the microprocessor responds to each pulse by reading angle ωt from the counter, using the value as an index into a look-up table to obtain the sine and cosine values, and adding these to RAM locations designated as real and imaginary accumulators. The power spectrum estimate is the sum of the squares of the accumulated totals. Spectral estimates for a number of linearly related frequencies are obtained by repeated use of the look-up tables. Automatic monitoring of the signature, an example of which is shown in figure 15 for a turbine meter under steady flow, is simple to arrange. Every turbine meter has an individual signature and a change in this implies a change in rotor of bearing characteristics and hence a possible change in calibration. Methods to detect, identify and correct for pulsating flows and to detect and warn of asymmetric flow profiles are being developed, so that the turbine meter can be made "intelligent" and will perform it's own diagnostics.

New materials such as ceramics are being applied to bearings and bearing designs with self lubricating characteristics should lead to improvements in this area of weakness. Turbine meters have not yet reached the full peak of development and the use of powerful computer models will allow the full implications of blade shape and other parameters to be better understood.

PERCEPTION OF TURBINE METERS IN INDUSTRIAL USAGE

A recent market survey was performed by Halsey (1986) in the UK to examine the use of flowmeters in industry. The data collected included the fluid being metered, what types of flowmeters are used, the parameters each user looks for in meters and the existing and future use of flowmeters. Some 17,000+ installations were included in the survey and just two tables are presented from this work. Table 3 shows a summary of users opinions about the various types of flowmeters. Turbine meters (number 3 on the table) come out reasonably well on performance, but do not fair so well on reliability, installation requirements and maintenance aspects. Table 4 on expected future usage confirms that orifice plate will continue to be the meter most often installed in industrial applications, with the turbine meter being towards the centre of figure. In both tables ultrasonic meters seem to be poorly thought of, even though they are being developed in the UK for gas transmission lines. The developments taking place with computer modelling, microprocessors and new materials will certainly change the face of industrial flow measurement in the next decade and with its compact design, relatively low pressure drop, high throughput and potential for self diagnostics and possibly self in situ calibration, the turbine meter is well placed to respond.

CLOSURE

There is no doubt that turbine meters offer the highest performance of all meters used to measure gas flows. In the past they have been designed and developed on largely experimental grounds, but the use of turbine meter theory has led to the development of the Auto-adjust Turbo-meter® and in the future will led to further advances in meter design. The majority of gas turbine meters have large centre bodies with numerous small blades located at the maximum radius, and these are sensitive to gas properties. There is no theoretical reason why this should be the case and experience with twin rotor meters with more aerodynamic blades does lead to better performance and rangeability. The use of microelectronic techniques will permit "intelligent" flowmeters to be developed in the near future.

The paper cannot do justice in the limited space permitted to cover all aspects of this type of gas meter, but it is hoped that the author has given a different slant of gas turbine meter technology to that normally found in flow measurement books and conference papers.

ACKNOWLEDGEMENT

The Author would thank Professor Tapan Bose of the University of Quebec at Trois Rivieres for the invitation to speak, and Conference Sponsors, Gaz Metropolitain, Province of Quebec and Trans Quebec & Maritimes for making the trip possible. Support was also received from members of the Fluid Engineering and Instrumentation Department at Cranfield during the preparation of the paper. The latest computer modelling work is part of a PhD program being carried out by my student Vilson Ferreira.

REFERENCES

Ferriera, V.C.D., Furness, R.A. and Goulas, A., "The design of turbine meters - theory and practice", Paper 7.1, Proc of NEL Conference on Flow in the mid 80's, National Engineering Laboratory Conference, June, 1986.

Furness, R.A. "Turbine meters", Chapter 6 in Developments in Flow Measurement, R.W.W.Scott (Ed), Applied Science Publishers, Barking, Essex, UK, 1982.

Halsey, D.M., "A survey of industrial usage of flowmeters", Measurement and Control, Vol.19, No.5, 52-55, June 1986.

Higham, E.H. et al, "Signal analysis and intelligent flowmeters", Measurement and Control, Vol.19, No.5, 47-50, June 1986.

Jepson, P. and Bean, P.G., "Effect of upstream velocity profiles on turbine meter registration", J.Mech.Eng.Sci., vol.11, no.5, 503-510, 1969

Tan, P.A.K and Hutton, S.P, "Experimental, analytical and tip clearance loss studies in turbine type flowmeters", Paper 6.2, Conf. on Developments in Flow Measurements, C.G.Clayton (Ed), held at Harwell, 21-23 Sept. 1971.

LIST OF FIGURES

1. Elements of a turbine flowmeter
2. Typical turbine meter characteristics
3. Typical axial pressure profile
4. Turbine flowmeter force diagrams
5. Effects of gas density on gas turbine meter performance
6. Quantum dynamics twin rotor gas meter
7. Conventional gas turbine meter
8. Rockwell International gas turbo-meter®
9. Turbo-meter® theory
10. Effect of swirl on turbine meter coefficients
11. Influence of swirl in gas turbine meters
12. Influence of valves on the performance of turbine meters
13. Computed velocity distributions inside turbine blade passages
14. Computed pressure distribution on turbine meter blade.
15. Turbine meter signature curve under steady flow

APPENDIX A

Summary of the integrals appearing in general characteristic equation of the inferential type meter (equation 8):

$$A = \int_{r_h}^{r_t} \left[\tan \beta - \tan(\beta - \delta)\right] \left[\frac{u}{U}\right]^2 \frac{rdr}{r_o^2}$$

$$B = \int_{r_h}^{r_t} \left[\frac{u}{U}\right]^2 \frac{rdr}{r_o^3}$$

$$C = \int_{r_h}^{r_t} \left[\frac{V}{u}\right] \left[\frac{u}{U}\right]^2 \frac{rdr}{r_o^2}$$

$$D = \int_{r_h}^{r_t} \frac{C_D \tan \phi}{\cos \beta \cdot \cos \phi} \cdot \left[\frac{u}{U}\right]^2 \frac{rdr}{r_o}$$

$$E = \int_{r_h}^{r_t} \left[2r - \frac{Nt}{\pi}\right] \left[\frac{u}{U}\right] \cdot \frac{dr}{r_o^2}$$

$$F = \int_{r_t}^{r_o} 2\left[\frac{u}{U}\right] \cdot \frac{rdr}{r_o^2}$$

NOMENCLATURE

A	Constant in the turbine equation (defined in Appendix A)
B	Constant in the turbine equation (defined in Appendix A)
C	Constant in the turbine equation (defined in Appendix A)
C_D	Drag coefficient
C_L	Left coefficient
c	Blade chord length
D	Constant in the turbine equation (defined in Appendix A)
E	Constant in the turbine equation (defined in Appendix A)
F	Constant in the turbine equation (defined in Appendix A)
K	Blade constant
L	Lift
m	Exponent in pipe power law equation
N	Number of blades
n	Speed of rotation
Q	Volume flow through the meter
Q_r	Volume flow through the rotor
Q_t	Volume leaking past rotor
r	Radius
r_h	Hub radius
r_o	Inside meter radius
r_t	Rotor tip radius
T	Retarding torque
t	Blade thickness
U	Reference axial velocity
u	Axial velocity
U_e	Absolute exit velocity
U_i	Absolute inlet velocity
V_e	Outlet velocity relative to the blade
V_m	Mean fluid velocity relative to the blade
v	Tangential component of inlet swirl velocity
v_e	Tangential component of outlet swirl velocity
v_i	Inlet velocity relative to the blade
W	Constant in general equation
W_b	Blade width in axial direction
X	Constant in general equation
Y	Constant in general equation
Z	Constant in general equation
α	Angle of attack
β	Blade angle
δ	Outlet deviation angle relative to the blade
δ^*	Boundary layer thickness
ϵ	Blade efficiency
ρ	Fluid density
ϕ	Mean velocity angle relative to meter axis
θ_e	Outlet velocity angle relative to meter axis
ϕ_i	Inlet velocity angle relative to meter axis.

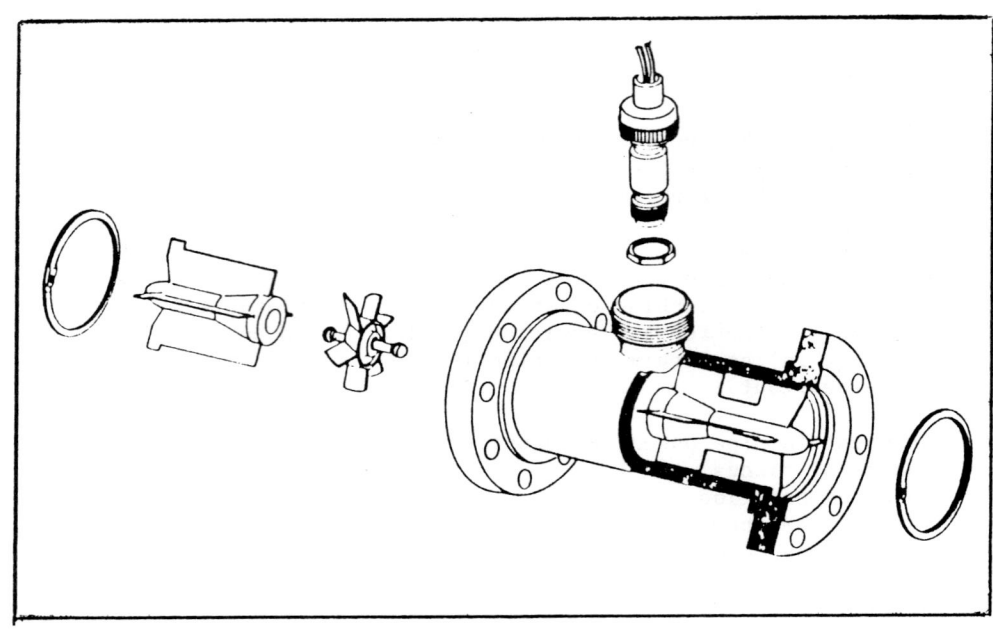

FIGURE 1   ELEMENTS OF A TURBINE METER

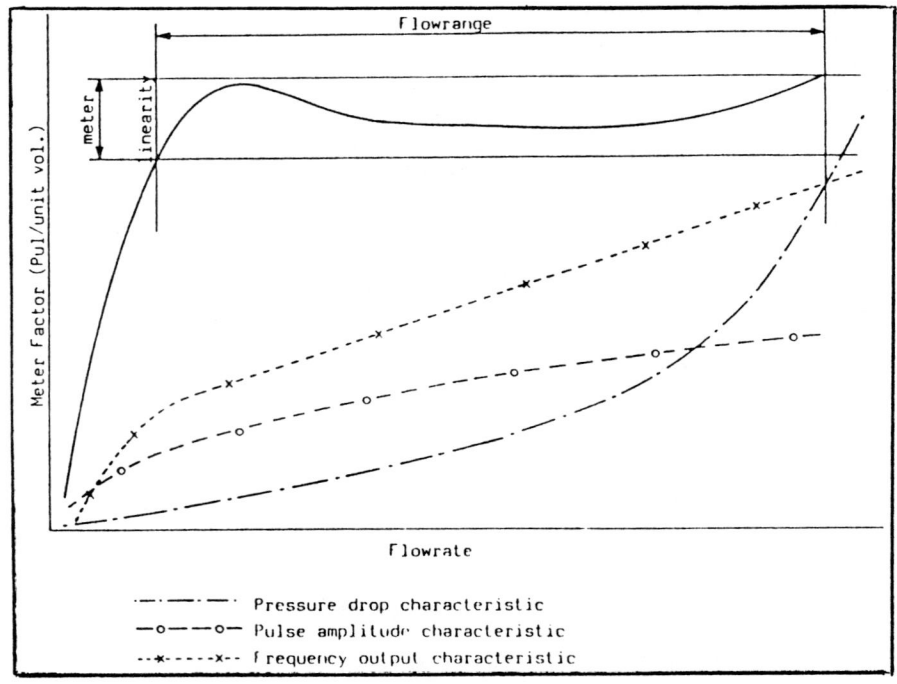

FIGURE 2   TYPICAL TURBINE METER CHARACTERISTICS

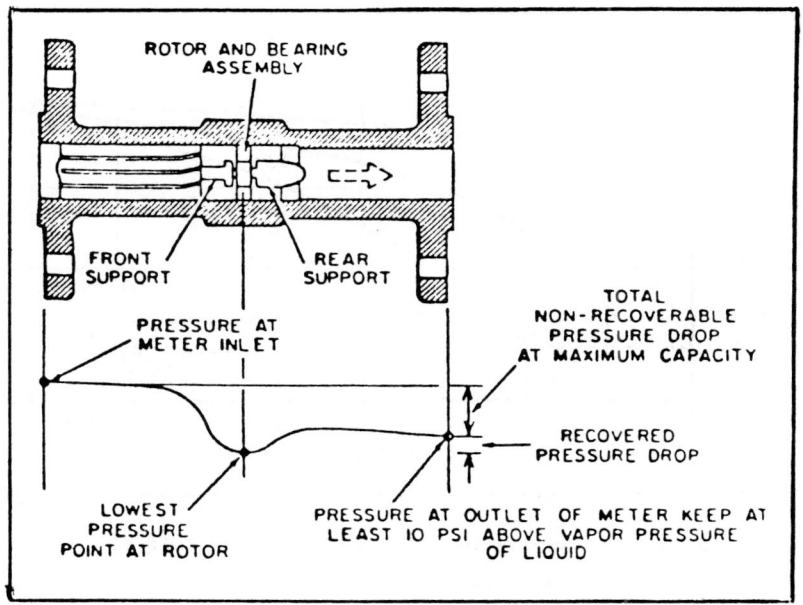

FIGURE 3   TYPICAL AXIAL PRESSURE PROFILE

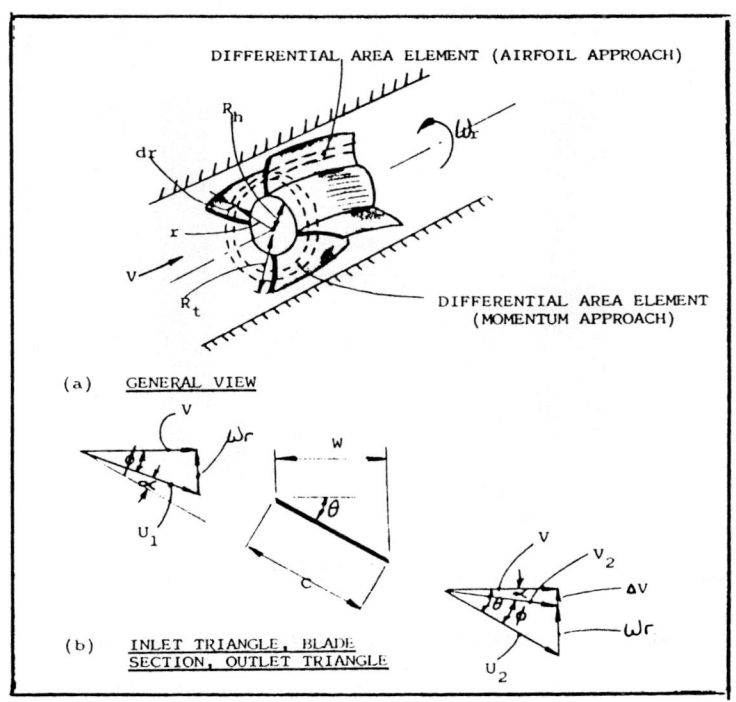

FIGURE 4   TURBINE FLOWMETER FORCE DIAGRAMS

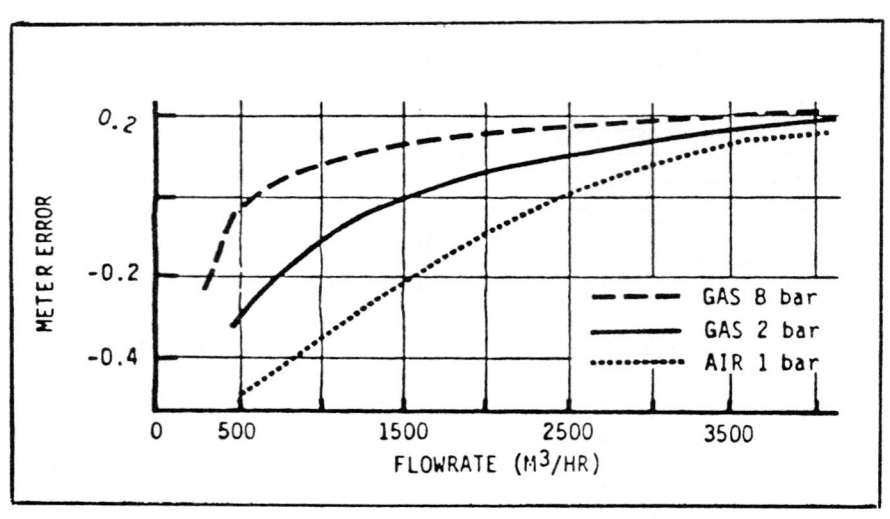

FIGURE 5   EFFECTS OF GAS DENSITY ON GAS TURBINE METER PERFORMANCE

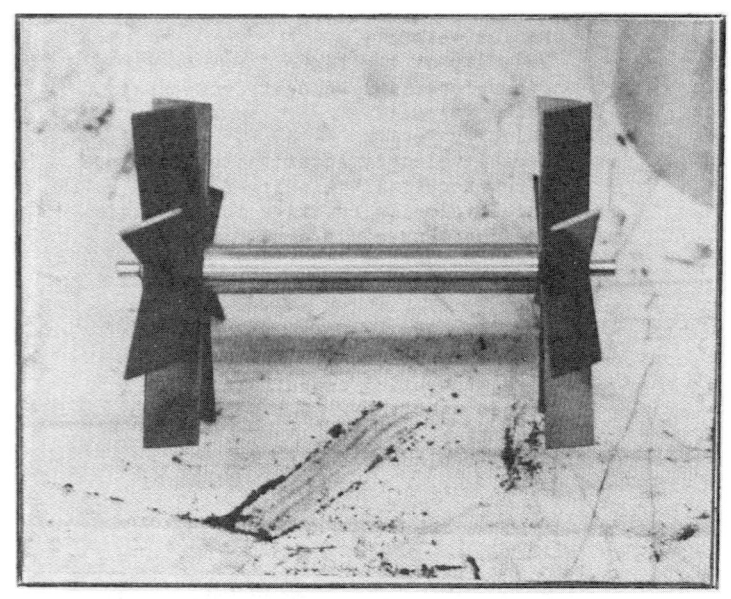

FIGURE 6   QUANTUM DYNAMICS TWIN ROTOR GAS METER

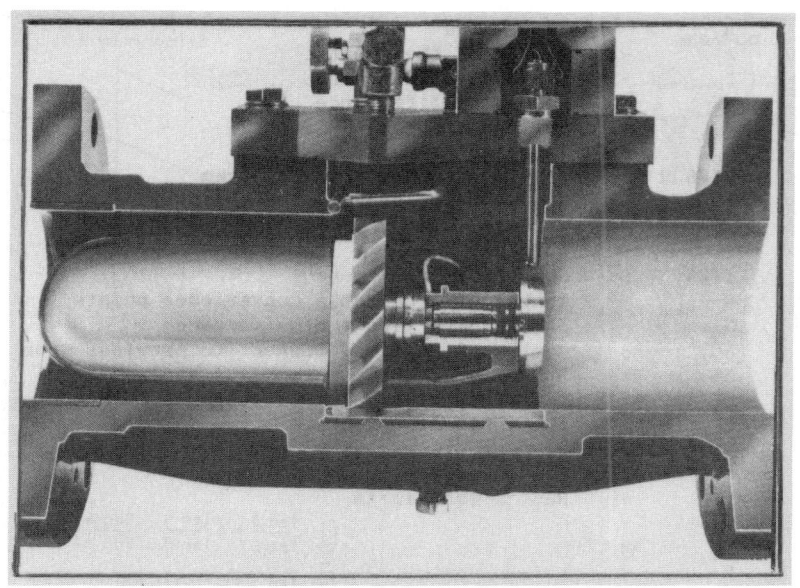

FIGURE 7   CONVENTIONAL GAS TURBINE METER

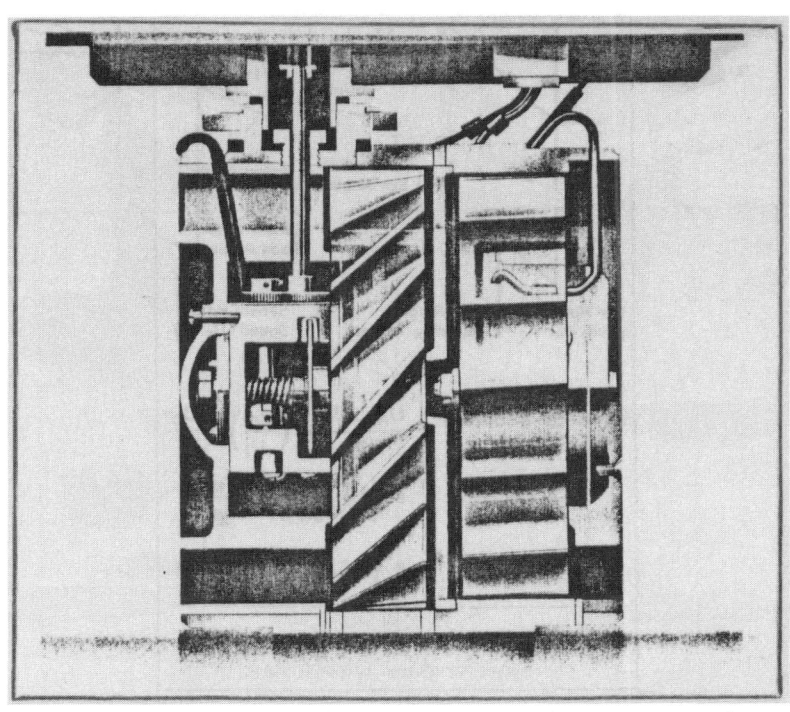

FIGURE 8   ROCKWELL INTERNATIONAL GAS TURBO-METER®

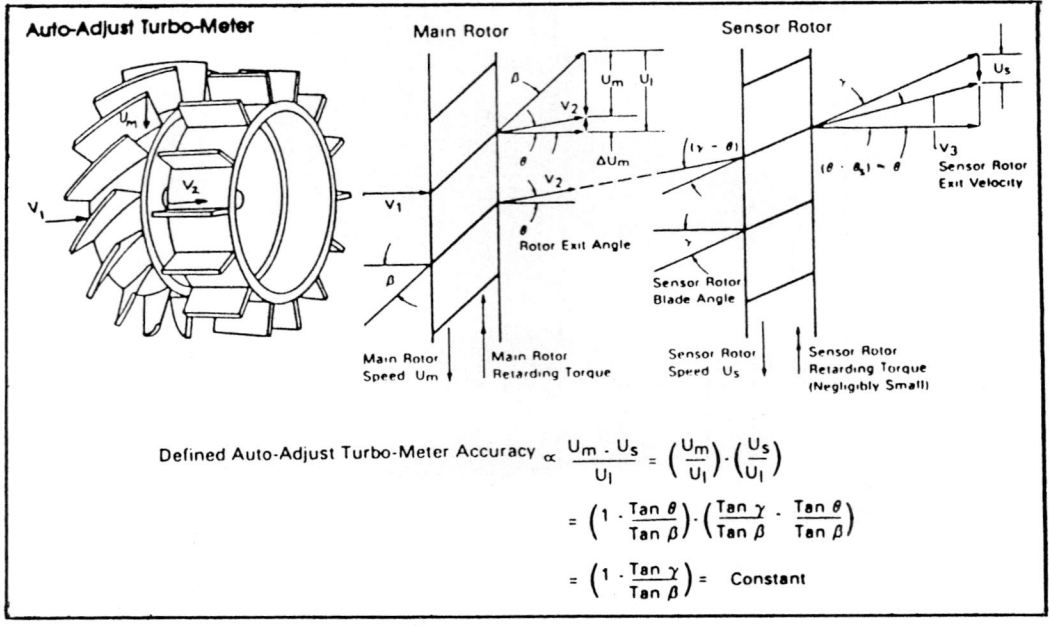

FIGURE 9   TURBO-METER® THEORY

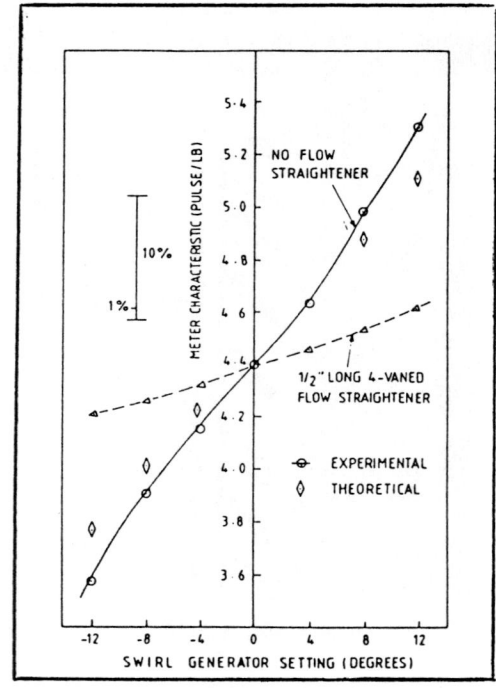

FIGURE 10   EFFECT OF SWIRL ON TURBINE METER COEFFICIENTS

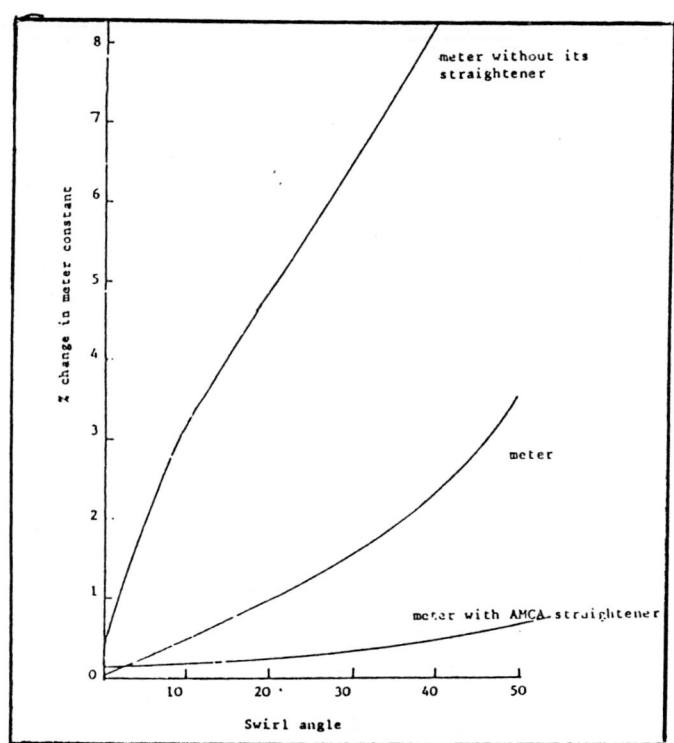

FIGURE 11   INFLUENCE OF SWIRL ON GAS TURBINE METERS

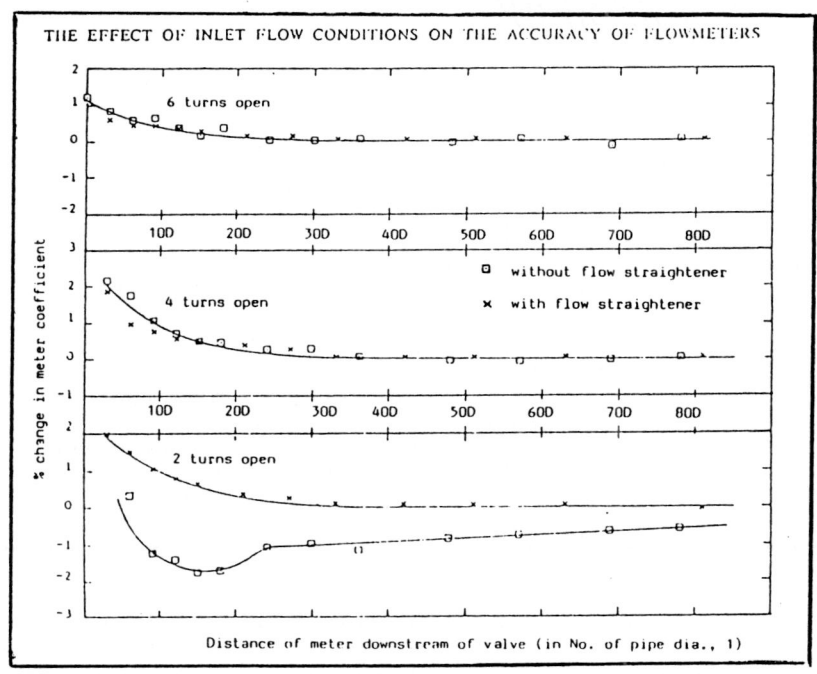

FIGURE 12   EFFECT OF VALVES ON TURBINE METER PERFORMANCE

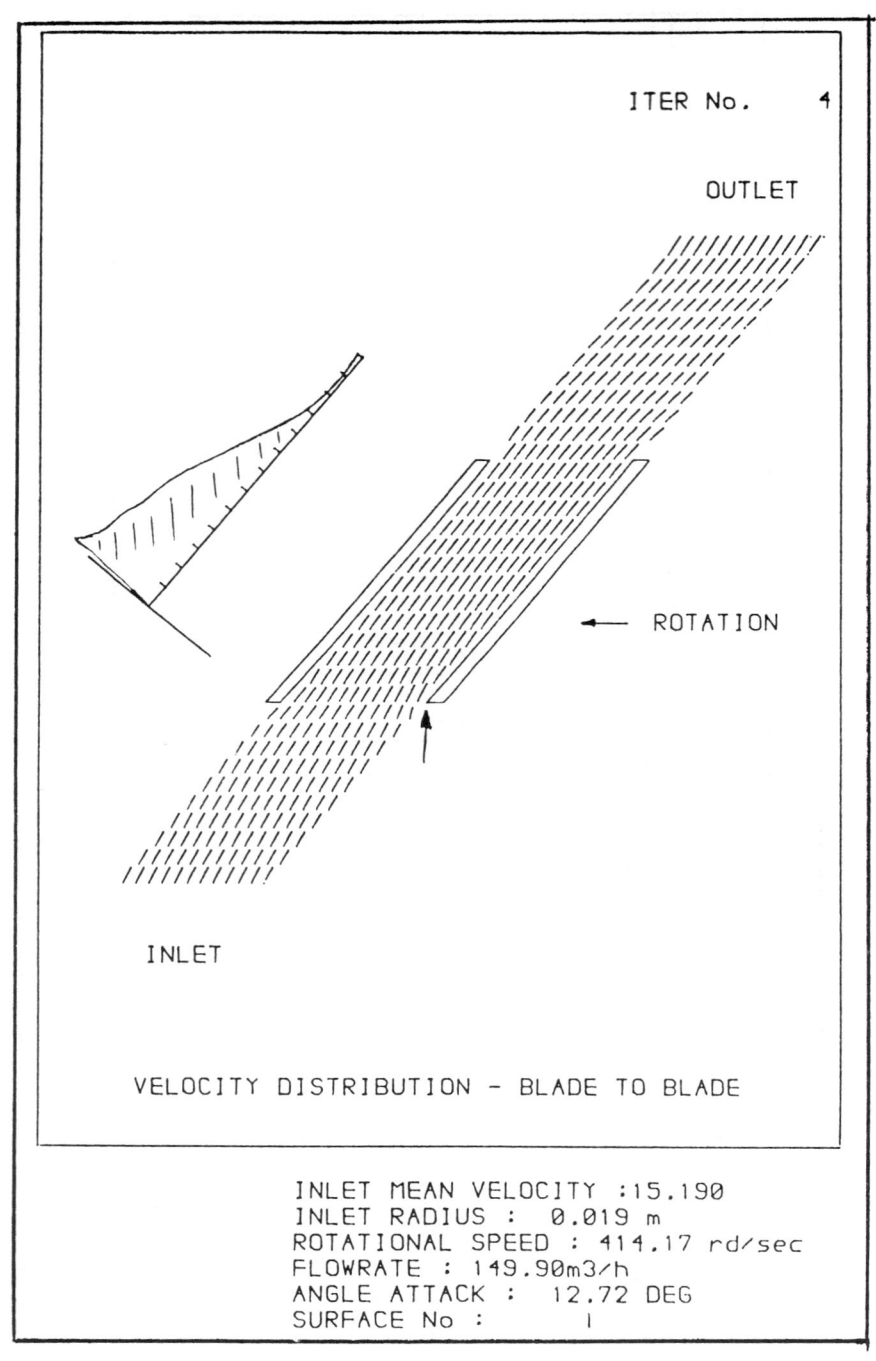

(a) near hub section of the rotor

FIGURE 13 COMPUTED VELOCITY DISTRIBUTION INSIDE TURBINE BLADE PASSAGES

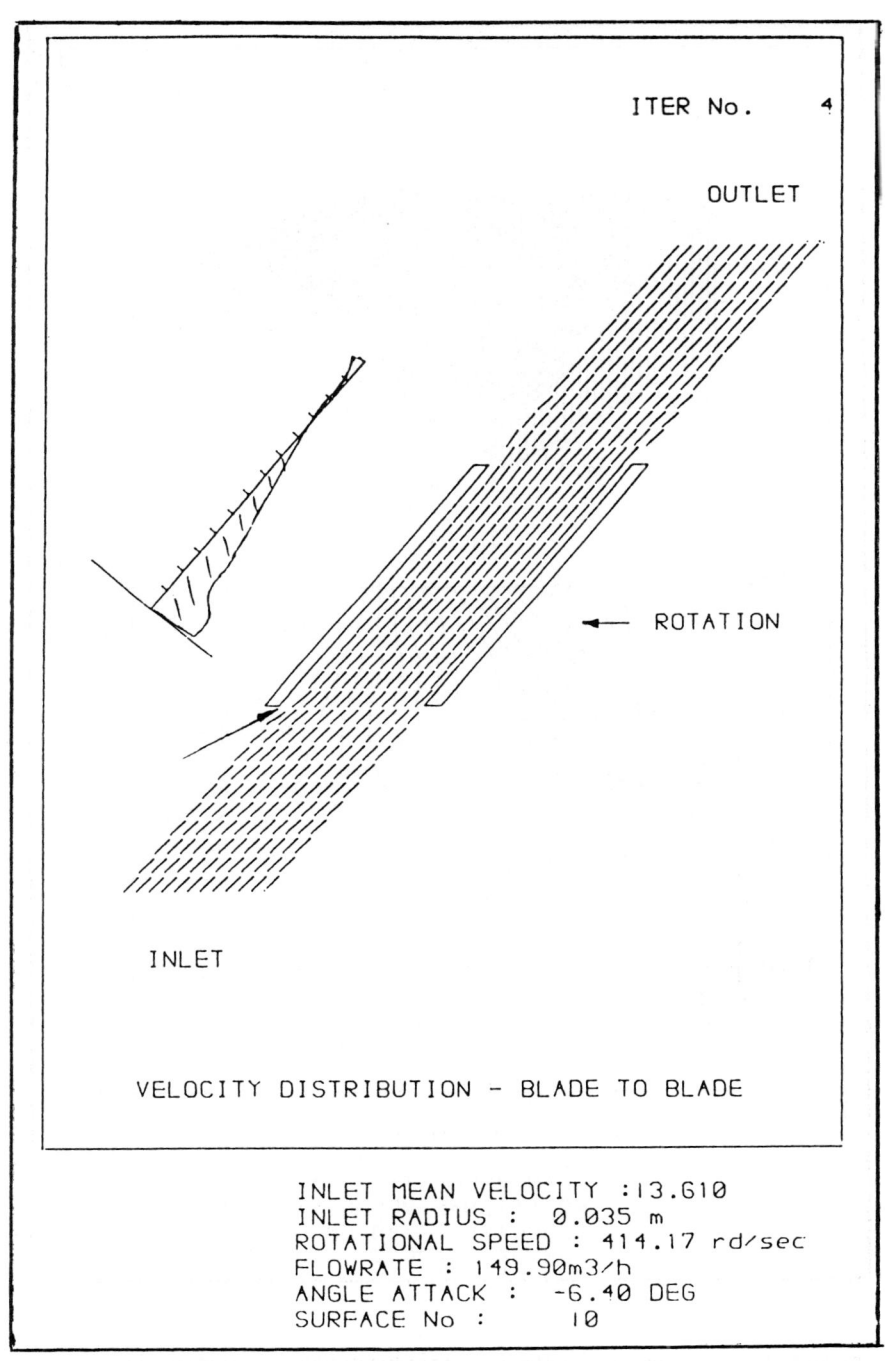

(b) near tip section of the rotor

FIGURE 13   COMPUTED VELOCITY DISTRIBUTION INSIDE TURBINE BLADE PASSAGES

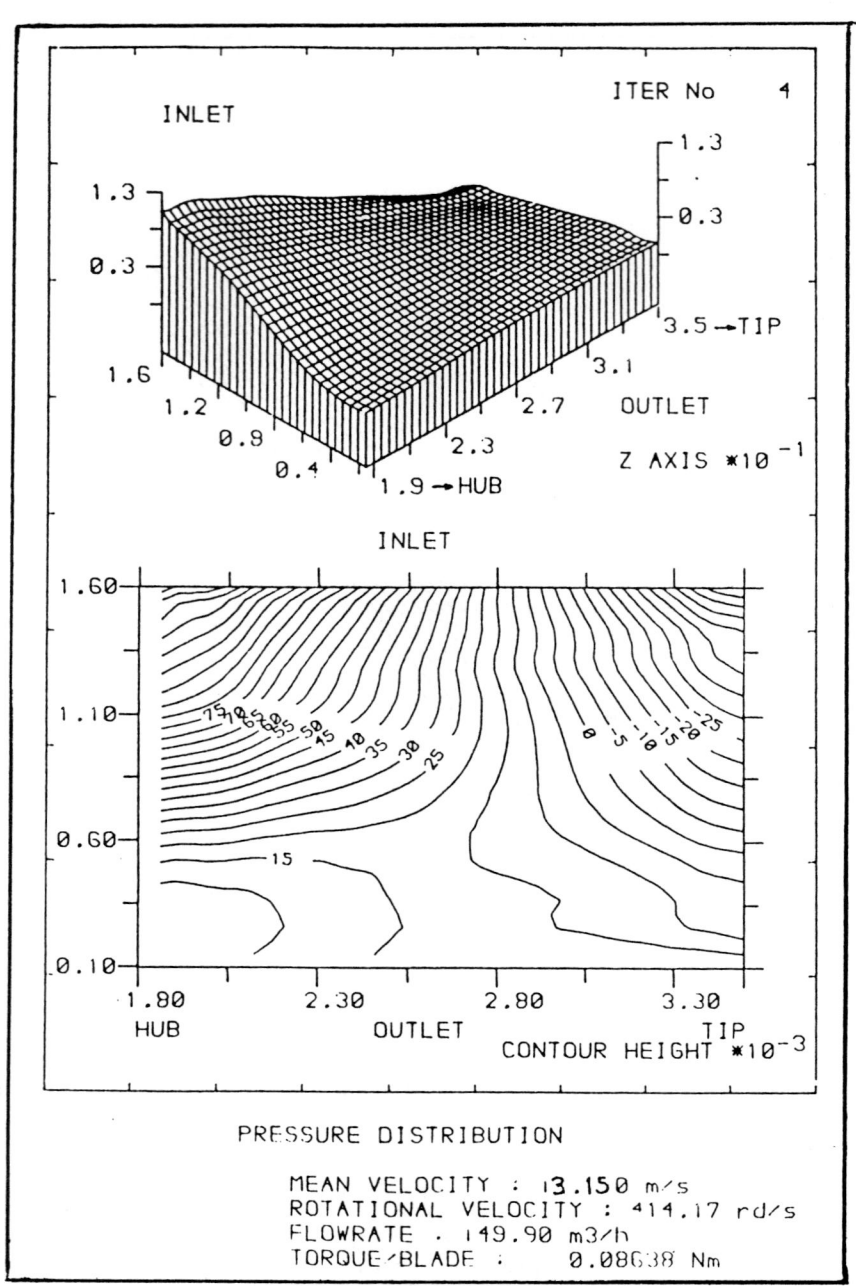

FIGURE 14   COMPUTED PRESSURE DISTRIBUTION ON TURBINE BLADE

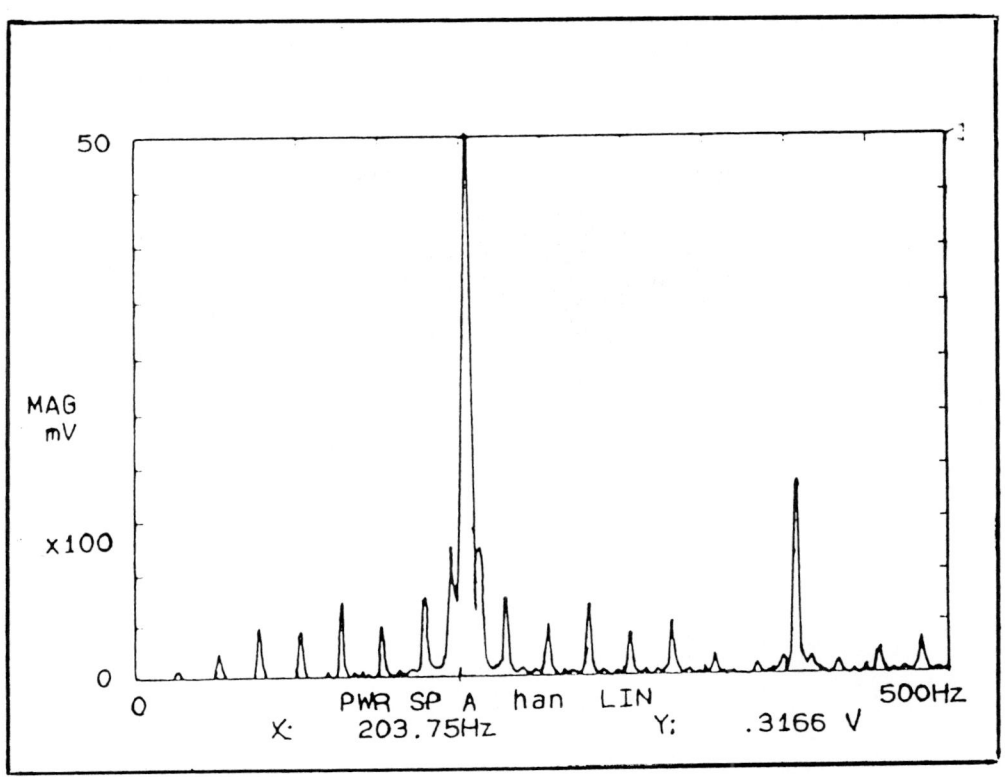

FIGURE 15   TURBINE METER SIGNATURE UNDER STEADY FLOW

NEW DIRECTIONS IN GAS FLOW METER RESEARCH AT THE GAS RESEARCH INSTITUTE

by

Carl H. Griffis
Project Manager
Gas Operations Technology
Gas Research Institute
8600 West Bryn Mawr Avenue
Chicago, Illinois 60631

International Symposium on Measurements, Properties
and Utilization of Natural Gas
Montreal, Quebec, Canada

November 25-27, 1987

ABSTRACT

The Gas Research Institute (GRI) has been supporting research in gas flow measurement since 1979. Several new concepts in flow meter designs ranging from energy flow meters to compact gas meters are summarized. Major activities in orifice meter research have been conducted at the U.S. National Bureau of Standards in Boulder, Colorado. This paper reviews some of the significant findings in swirl persistence, upstream pipe roughness, and positioning of flow conditioners. The initiation of a new Metering Research Facility at the Southwest Research Institute in San Antonio is also reviewed.

INTRODUCTION

The efficient transport and distribution of natural gas involves accurate measurement of large quantities of natural gas. As gas prices rise increased economic importance is attached to accurate gas measurement. Research into new methods of measuring natural gas volume and energy flow and improving existing measurement methods is a critical component of the GRI research and development program. This paper is an update of the current projects that address both new measurement technologies and improvements of existing measurement techniques in both distribution and transmission areas.

DISTRIBUTION MEASUREMENT

Compact Gas Meter

A metering issue relevant to multifamily dwellings and gas utilities is the difficulty and space requirements of metering gas in multiple-site, low-volume usage with individual meters. Existing gas meters consume valuable space.

The alternative of using a single meter for the multifamily dwelling fails to distribute energy costs equitable among the residents. There is, thus, the need to develop a low-cost, compact gas meter capable of being remotely read for multifamily buildings. This need is especially important as advanced interior piping technology permits gas service in both high-rise buildings and other multifamily units where individual metering is presently not available. GRI has initiated three projects to develop a compact gas meter utilizing three different technologies: mechanical, electronic and fluidic.[1]

Rockwell International has developed a mechanical compact gas meter that utilizes a gate and vane principle for measuring residential gas flow. The prototype meters with mechanical indexes have been fabricated for testing at several sites for long term accuracy and reliability. Additional meters will be fabricated with electronic indexes and will be subsequently tested at various field sites. GRI expects that the tests with the mechanical index meters will begin in early 1988 and with the electronic index meter in late 1988. After completion of this initial test period, GRI and Rockwell will evaluate the meter modifications needs, if any, from the present configuration.

Honeywell Inc. has developed a microstructure flow sensor which is applicable for an electronic compact gas meter.[2] This flow sensor measures gas flow utilizing a hot wire anemometer principle. Gas flowing across heated elements causes a temperature difference in the elements from which gas velocity can be inferred. Initial laboratory results indicate that the flow sensor gives very good response over the entire flow range of a typical residential meter. Additional questions on the sensor long term stability in a natural gas environment and the life of the battery required to power the meter are being addressed. Honeywell is also testing the laboratory prototype meter to evaluate the effects of gas composition, contamination, and various installation piping configurations on meter performance.

Illinois Institute of Technology (IIT) is developing a compact gas meter based on the fluidic principle. Fluid flowing through a specific geometry in the meter body oscillates between two predetermined flow paths. This oscillation, called the Coanda effect, can be correlated to the flow rate through the meter. Technical concern on pressure differential through the meter, improved rangeability and accuracy of the meter over the desired residential gas load range are being addressed. Initial studies have shown that the meter will operate in both laminar and turbulent flow regimes. It is, thus, feasible to design a meter to operate over the required flow rate range of 0.25 to 200 CFH.

Compressed Natural Gas Quick Fill Meter

An attractive market for natural gas use is in compressed natural gas (CNG) powered vehicles. There are several reasons for the slow growth of this market: the absence of factory produced CNG vehicles, the lack of public awareness of the safety of natural gas as a fuel option, and the scarcity of nationwide conveniently located public CNG filling stations. In order to increase the number of public CNG filling stations, the economics must be made more attractive. This means that the components of a CNG filling station must be examined for cost reduction, including the meter and fueling system. Fuel systems for CNG are currently available but the systems have not been optimized for quick fill natural gas fueling. Columbia Gas System Service Corporation is presently evaluating several CNG quick fill metering techniques under GRI contract. These metering techniques include: corriolis, coanda effect, sonic nozzle, ultrasonic, thermal effects, vortex shedding, turbine, positive displacement and differential head. Several concepts will be selected for testing in a test stand under conditions identical to those expected in actual fueling situations. These tests began in mid-1987 and should be completed by late 1988. Development of the most promising concepts will involve additional laboratory and field testing at Columbia Gas's six CNG fueling sites.

TRANSMISSION MEASUREMENT

Energy Flowmeters

Two projects are currently funded by GRI to improve the measurement of energy flow rate in transmission pipelines. Current measurement techniques involve the use of a volumetric flow measurement device, such as an orifice meter or turbine meter, and an energy content measurement device, such as a calorimeter or a gas chromatograph, to measure total energy flow.

Precision Measurement Inc. (PMI) under GRI sponsorship has been developing an instrument to measure energy flowrate.[3,4] By combining a standard Therm-Titrator calorimetric instrument with a unique flow splitting device, this concept has been demonstrated in laboratory and in a large scale field test. The key to accurate measurement in the PMI device is to accurately maintain a constant ratio of pipeline flow to bypass flow (the split ratio) over the range of transmission pipeline flow. The PMI device can only measure total energy flow (Btu/hr) and the individual measurements of volumetric flow rate or energy content cannot be determined. A field test of this device is being carried out at a Lone Star Gas Company meter run at Bryan, Texas. Natural gas flows at the site range from 500,000 to 1,000,000 SCFH in an eight inch line. The calorific value of the gas varies between 1000 and 1180 Btu/SCF due to fluctuations in a processing plant upstream of the test site. Initial results of this field test indicate a measurement precision of better than $\pm 0.3\%$. Additional field tests at Pacific Gas and Electric Company, Southern California Gas Company and Wisconsin Gas Company will evaluate the meter performance under wide range of operating conditions. In addition, work will also focus on determining the accuracy of the device.

Another energy flowmeter project at GRI with a longer term objective of accurately measuring energy flow with a wide rangeability involves the use of nonintrusive technologies – a laser technique and infrared spectroscopy to measure total energy flow in a nonintrusive installation. A laser transient anemometry technique measures volumetric flow by measuring the time of flight of particles in the gas stream. Spectron Development Laboratories (SDL) is the contractor developing the laser based volumetric flow measurement technique.[5] The activities are focused on characterizing the particles in typical natural gas pipelines, designing a traversing system to measure point velocities across the gas pipeline, and developing a correlation to calculate the flow rate by integrating the point velocity flow measurements made across the pipeline. Computer Genetics Corporation (CGC) under GRI contract is developing the infrared spectroscopy system for measuring the gas energy content. The absorption/correlation technique involves measuring the absorption characteristics of C-H bonds in natural gas and computing the energy content with an algorithm developed from a large data base of previously measured gases. The difficulty of measuring the natural gas energy content at typical transmission pipeline pressures is that the infrared absorption characteristics become less distinguishable. The research at CGC is focused on characterizing various gas mixture absorption wavelengths at high pressure. Very accurately known gas mixtures are measured at various infrared wavelengths to determine the optimum wavelengths at various pipeline pressures. The long term goal is to combine the SDL and CGC concepts into one instrument that nonintrusively measures energy flow in the gas pipeline. At the present time, both concepts are at the laboratory proof-of-concept stage. Upon successful completion of this phase in early 1988, both the SDL and CGC devices will be developed for field experimentation and testing.

Orifice Meter Research

In addition to developing new measurement techniques, GRI has sponsored research to improve existing measurement methods utilized by the gas industry. Most noteable of the existing methods is the flow measurement using the orifice meter.

In a recently completed project at the University of Oklahoma, a new correlation for the calculation of the supercompressibility factor of natural gas has been developed. The correlation, developed under GRI sponsorship, forms the basis of a new supercompressibility document (A.G.A. Transmission Measurement Committee Report No. 8, 1986).[6,7] This correlation is presently available in software products for micro, mini, and mainframe computers. The new correlation is applicable to essentially dry, sweet natural gases.

Work sponsored by GRI at the National Bureau of Standards/Boulder (NBS-B) has identified the need to evaluate flow conditioners as an alternative to long upstream pipe lengths. The effect of swirl on an orifice meter can be significant if there are insufficient straight pipe lengths upstream of an orifice meter.[8] NBS has evaluated several types of flow conditioners for their effectiveness at removing swirl and the associated pressure drop. This study has confirmed that flow conditioners can significantly reduce the required upstream pipe lengths to maintain orifice meter accuracy. Figure 1 shows several flow conditioners that were tested at NBS-B. In addition, NBS-B is currently investigating the relationship between flow conditioner placement and orifice meter discharge coefficients with a four-inch orifice meter. Initial results indicate that the flow conditioners eliminate swirl effects but distort mean and turbulent velocity profiles so that some recovery distance is needed. Additional research will be conducted with different meter tube sizes and lower flow rates to evaluate flow conditioner effects.

NBS-B has also identified that the pipe roughness can have an affect on orifice meter performance. Current work performed by NBS-B to evaluate surface roughness involves meter tubes fabricated from stainless steel.[9,10] Figure 2 is a schematic of the meter tube arrangement. Three upstream sections with different roughness are tested for each meter tube size. Results from a 4-inch meter tube indicate that as the beta ratio increases, the effect of surface roughness becomes more pronounced. Work with various sized meters is presently underway and should be completed in 1988.

Evaluation of a large number of parameters on orifice meter performance requires a large and expensive testing program. One way to reduce this large expense is to develop a numerical model that can simulate orifice meter flow and enable the evaluation of a large number of parameters at a fraction of the cost of an experimental program. Creare Inc. has developed the numerical model FLUENT which can simulate flow through an orifice plate utilizing both a $k-\varepsilon$ model and an Algebraic Stress Model. Numerical simulation results indicate that the model can predict discharge coefficients within 1 to 2 percent of the experimental data.[11] Simulations will also be performed to evaluate the model's capability to predict the effect of swirl and pipe roughness. Creare will also be involved in modeling the flow through the fluidic meter presently under development at IIT. Creare will also simulate various nozzle geometries that will provide a uniform or 'top hat' velocity profile for the SDL flowmeter project funded by GRI. A uniform velocity profile region is desireable for the optical flow meter under development by SDL.

Speed of Sound

The sonic nozzle is a method of accurately measuring the flow of natural gas, providing the gas stream composition is well characterized. Sonic nozzle calibration, however, will require speed of sound data for natural gas. Due to the limited amount of accurate data on the speed of sound in natural gas, however, it is difficult to evaluate the accuracy of existing speed of sound correlations. GRI has sponsored research at the National Institute for Petroleum and Energy Research (NIPER) and at NBS-B to develop accurate speed of sound measurements and verify the correlation developed by the University of Oklahoma.[12] Several natural gas compositions at various temperatures and pressures will be evaluated for agreement between the correlation and the experimental data.

Meter Research Facility

The gas industry has identified the need for a metering research facility to conduct research and testing for both distribution and transmission applications. The facility would provide the means for evaluating the performance of existing meters over a wide range of operating conditions, determine the feasibility of new metering concepts and provide input for other research programs. Southwest Research Institute (SwRI) has been selected as the GRI contractor to design and construct the Metering Research Facility (MRF) for future research needs. SwRI was selected from a group of six qualified organizations by GRI and a Industry Review Panel in late 1986. Figure 3 shows the proposed MRF to be built in San Antonio, Texas.[13] The facility will be constructed as two independent recirculating closed loops: the Support Facility and the Primary Facility. The Support Facility will be capable of conducting tests at pressures up to 200 psi, line sizes from 1/2 to 6 inch, and pipe Reynolds number to 2×10^6. The Primary Facility will be constructed to achieve higher pressure and flow rates required for custody transfer stations applications. The Primary Facility design requirements include 100 to 1440 psig pressures, 2 to 16 inch line sizes, and flow Reynolds number to 2×10^7 (based on 16 inch line size) with flow rates to 165 MMCFD.

Research is scheduled to begin in the Support Facility in early 1988 and in the Primary Facility in 1989. Activities for the MRF is divided into five research areas:

1. Orifice meter research
2. Other meter research
3. Instrument development and testing
4. Pipeline research
5. Information dissemination and technology transfer

The success of such a research facility will depend on its usefulness and acceptance to the gas industry. This can best be achieved by obtaining inputs from industry and continued critique of results obtained. GRI will continue to solicit input during the design, construction and operation of the MRF.

CONCLUSIONS

GRI has been sponsoring research and development on measurement technolcgies for both transmission and distribution applications for several years. The ultimate goal of all of this research is to provide more accurate, less expensive measurement devices and provide the gas industry with better correlations, data bases, etc., with which to use existing measurement techniques.

REFERENCES

1. Griffis, C.H., "New Metering Options for Residential Application" Proceedings of A.G.A. Operating Section, Paper 1986 86-DT-104.

2. "Development of an Electronic Compact Gas Meter," Phase I Topical Report, July-December 1986, Honeywell, Inc., GRI Report No. 87/0103

3. "Development of an Energy Flowmeter-Phase III," Final Report, June 1984-December 1985, Precision Machine Products, Inc., GRI Report No. 86/0223

4. Clingman, W.H., Griffis, C.H., Keneedy, L.R., Hall, K.R. and Holste, J.C., "Direct Measurement of Energy Flow-Recent Field Experience," Proceedings of 1986 IGT Natural Gas Energy Measurement Symposium, Chicago, Illinois

5. Azzazy, M. and Modarress, D., "Optical Volumetric Flowmeter," Proceedings of 1986 International Symposium on Fluid Flow Measurement, Washington, DC

6. "Development of Improved Capabilities for Computation of Gas Supercompressibility Factors and Other Properties," Final Report, July 1981 – September 1984, University of Oklahoma, GRI Report No. 84/0224

7. "Compressibility and Supercompressibility for Natural Gas and Other Hydrocarbon Gases," A.G.A. Transmission Measurement Committee Report No. 8, Catalog No. XQ 1285

8. Batemann, B.R., Brennan, J.A., McManus, S.E., Mann, D and Pantoja, I.V., "The Decay of Swirling Gas Flow in Long Pipes, "Proceedings of 1985 A.G.A. Operating Section, Paper 85-DT-54

9. Brennan, J.A., McFadden, S.E. and Sindt, C.F., "NBS Research on the Effects of Pipe Roughness and Flow Conditioners on the Orifice Discharge Coefficient," Proceedings of 1987 A.G.A. operating section, Paper 87-DT-6

10. "The Effect of Meter Tube Roughness on Gas Flow Measurements," Gas Research Institute Bulletin, August 1987

11. Kothari, K., Patel, B.R. and Sheikholeslami, Z., "Numerical Modeling of Turbulent Flow Through Orifice Meters, Proceedings of 1986 International Symposium on Fluid Flow Measurement, Washington, DC

12. "Speed-of-Sound Measurements in Natural Gas Fluids," Final Report, October 1984-January 1986, National Institute for Petroleum and Energy Research, GRI Report No. 86/0043

13. Kothari, K.M. and Norman, R.S., "GRI Plans for a Meter Research Facility," Proceedings of 1987 A.G.A. Operating Section, Paper 87-DT-86

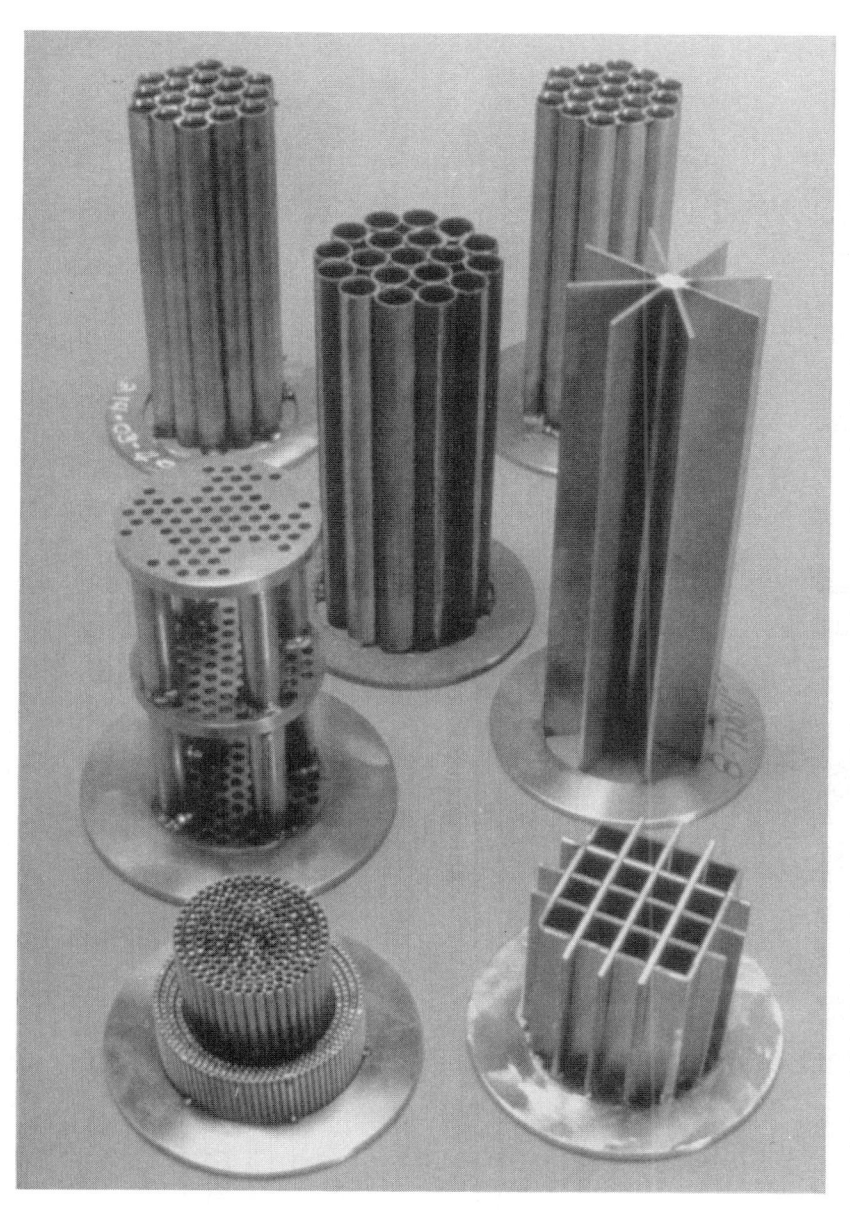

FIGURE 1   FLOW CONDITIONERS TESTED AT NBS-B

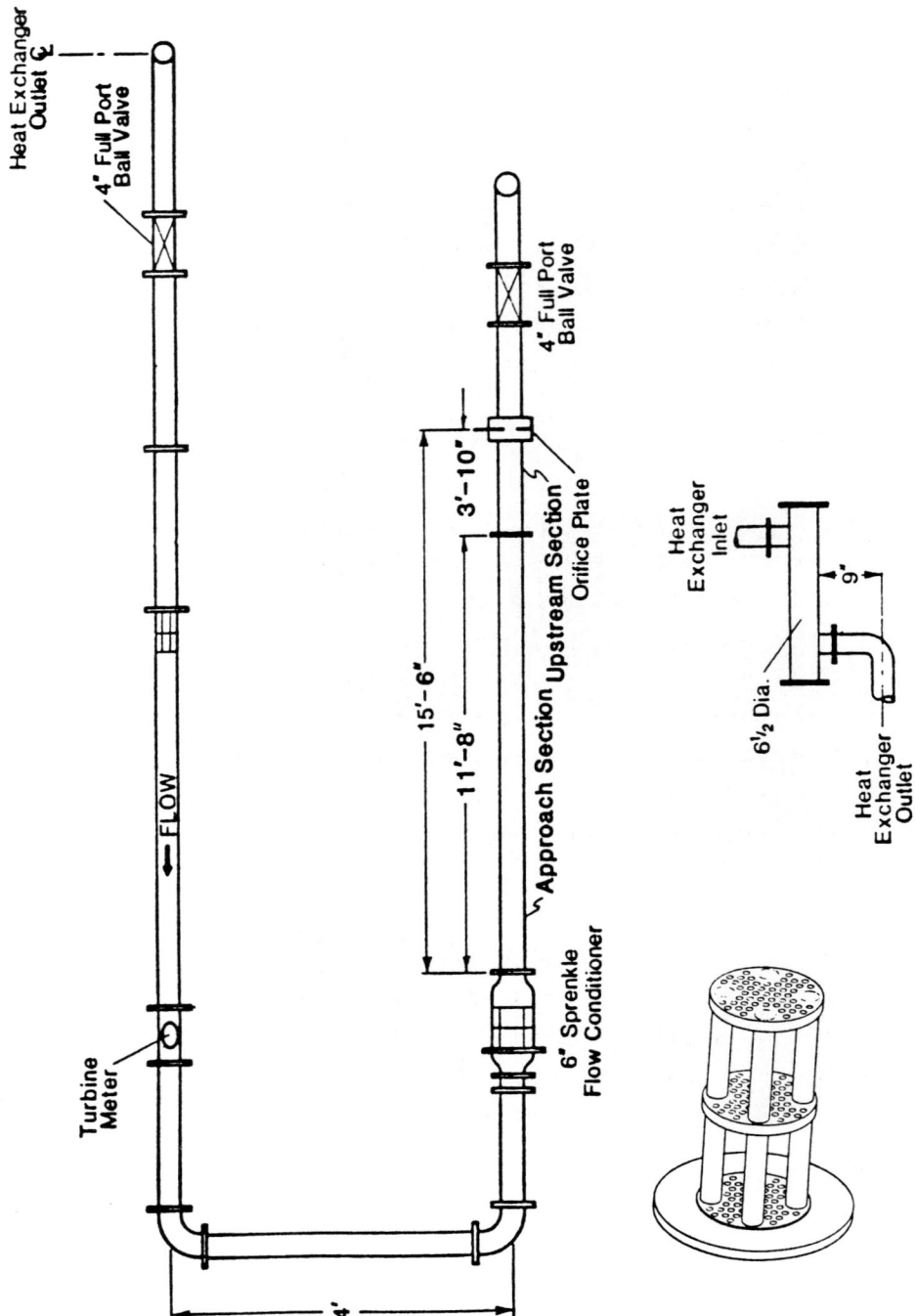

FIGURE 2 SCHEMATIC OF NBS-B METER TUBE ARRANGEMENT

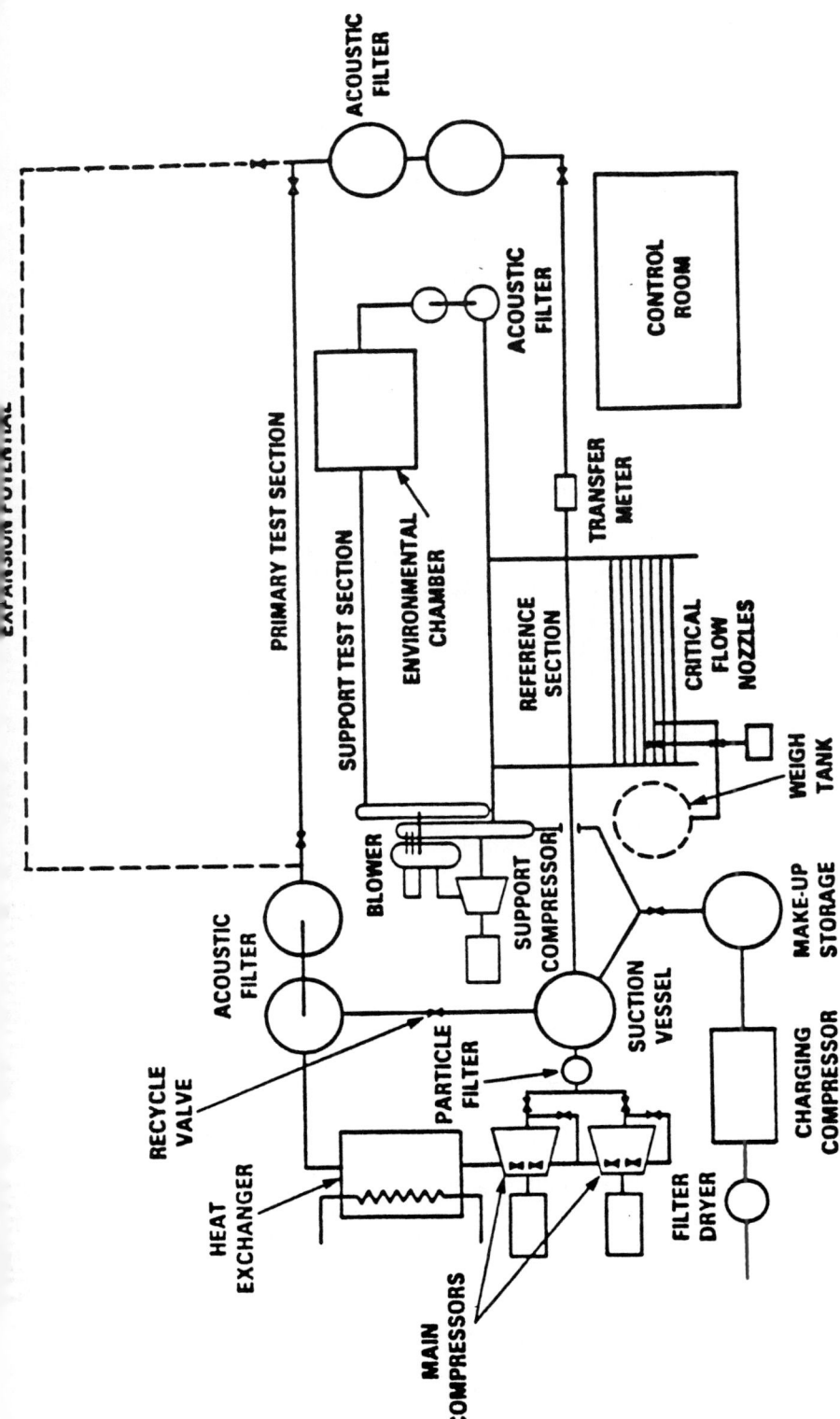

FIGURE 3   PROPOSED MRF AT SOUTHWEST RESEARCH INSTITUTE

Importance of Accurate Thermodynamic Correlations
for Gas Flow Measurement

Kenneth R. Hall*
Kenneth N. Marsh**
James C. Holste***

Texas A&M University
College Station, TX 77843
USA

Abstract

Accurate metering of natural gas flows requires knowledge of the density as a function of temperature, pressure and composition. It is not feasible to provide this information experimentally, so correlations based upon critically evaluated, existing data are necessary. This paper examines the source equations for flow measurement and some thermodynamic considerations which are applicable.

* Associate Dean, Engineering; Assistant Director, Texas Engineering Experiment Station; Professor, Chemical Engineering
** Director, Thermodynamics Research Center
*** Professor, Chemical Engineering

Importance of Accurate Thermodynamic Correlations for Gas Flow Measurement

Introduction

Custody transfer of natural gas is a major a commercial enterprize throughout the world. In the USA alone, nearly a trillion (million million) standard cubic meters pass between buyer and seller yearly at a cost approaching $50 billion (thousand million). Given the magnitude of these transactions, seemingly small uncertainties translate into huge sums of money. Assume, for example, a 0.1% uncertainty in measuring the volumetric flow rate of the gas; the consequence is a $50 million uncertainty in commercial exchange.

The underlying theory for most flow measurement devices in the First Law of Thermodynamics. Because of this, thermodynamic properties are essential information for flowrate determination and for energy flow calculations. The principal properties required are: the density (often expressed in terms of the real gas factor) and the heating value.

Thermodynamic properties are measurable quantities and have experimental error associated with them. In addition, the density or real gas factor is a function of temperature, pressure and composition and requires a correlation to establish the value at specific conditions. Under these circumstances, standards become necessary. Because accuracy is imposed by experimental constraints, it is important to be consistent in using correlations. Consistency in this case promotes (but does not guarantee) cancelation of uncertainties in multiple transactions.

Theoretical Development

Orifices are the most commonly used flow measurement devices and serve well as a general model for all differential pressure devices, therefore we use them to discuss the topic of performance equations. Derivation of the performance equations begins with the First Law of Thermodynamics:

$$\Delta[u + ke + pe]_{sys} = \Sigma q + \Sigma w + \Sigma[h + ke + pe]_{mt} \qquad (1)$$

where u is internal energy, ke is kinetic energy, pe is potential energy, q is energy transferred as heat, w is work and h is enthalpy; all are per mass units. Subscript sys refers to the system while mt refers to mass transfer. The Δ denotes change from beginning to end of a process. For flow of a compressible fluid through an orifice, we assume:

- steady state flow
- no work
- circular cross section
- horizontal flow
- turbulent flow

Under these assumptions, Equation 1 becomes

$$h_2 - h_1 + \frac{[\dot{z}_2^2 - \dot{z}_1^2]}{2g_c} - {_1}q_2 = 0 \qquad (2)$$

where $\dot{z}$ is velocity, g_c is the force/mass conversion, and subscripts 1 and 2 refer to upstream and downstream respectively. The mass flowrate, $\dot{m}$, is (at steady state)

$$\dot{m} = \dot{z} A d \tag{3}$$

where A is the cross section area of the conduit and d is the mass density. The real gas factor, Z, is

$$Z = \frac{MP}{RTd} \tag{4}$$

where M is molar mass, P is pressure, R is the universal gas constant and T is temperature.

The enthalpy difference in Equation 2 can have various forms, but for present purposes we select

$$h_2 - h_1 = \int_{s_1}^{s_2} T ds + \int_{P_1}^{P_2} v dP \tag{5}$$

where s is entropy per mass and v is volume per mass. The first integral on the rhs has a relationship to dissipative forces

$$_1f_2 \equiv \int_{s_1}^{s_2} T ds -_1 q_2 = \dot{z}_1^2 \varphi_1 / 2 g_c \tag{6}$$

where $_1f_2$ is the energy dissipation in process 1→2 and φ_1 is a complex function of geometry, flow characteristics, fluid properties and possibly other variables. The second integral on the rhs of Equation 5 is not tractable because of the physical path passing through the orifice which necessitates a definition

$$\int_{P_1}^{P_2} v dP = F_1^2 Y_1^2 v_1 [P_2 - P_1] \qquad (7)$$

F and Y are empirical factors accounting for irreversibility and for gas expansion in flow through the orifice.

Substituting Equations 3, 4, 5, 6, and 7 into Equation 2 and rearranging yields

$$\dot{m} = \left[\frac{\pi^2}{8R}\right]^{1/2} \Phi_1 Y_1 \beta^2 \left[\frac{MP_1}{Z_1 T_1}(P_2 - P_1)\right]^{1/2} \qquad (8)$$

where β is the ratio of orifice diameter to pipe diameter and

$$\Phi_1 = F_1 D_1^2 \bigg/ \left\{\beta^2 \left[\left(\frac{Z_2 T_2 P_1}{Z_1 T_1 P_2}\right)^2 \left(\frac{D_1}{D_2}\right)^4 - 1 - \varphi_1\right]^{1/2}\right\} \qquad (9)$$

where D is the pipe diameter.

Equation 8 is a valid expression of mass flowrate given adequate correlations for Φ, Y_1 and Z_1. However, the industry is reluctant to buy or sell gas on a mass basis. This is an historical prejudice and is unfortunate because conversion to volumetric flowrate introduces additional error and some arbitrary definitions.

Practical Considerations

The natural gas industry deals in volumetric flowrates. This requires multiplication of the mass flowrate by a specific volume (per mass). What is the appropriate specific volume? The answer is, unfortunately, ambiguous. The choices include: ideal gas volume at actual conditions, ideal gas volume at base conditions, real gas volume at actual conditions, real gas volume at base conditions. Of these choices, either ideal gas value introduces the least additional error, but the industry feels strongly that it should work with real gas volumes at base conditions. What are base conditions? Literally any condition - although most governing agencies select a pressure near atmospheric and a temperature between 0° and 25°C.

Combining Equations 4 and 8 produces the volumetric flowrate (real gas) at base conditions

$$\dot{V}_b = \dot{m}/d_b = \left[\frac{\pi^2 R}{8M_a}\right]^{1/2} [\Phi_1 \beta^2][Y_1][\frac{1}{P_b}][T_b][\frac{1}{T_1}]^{1/2}[\frac{1}{G}]^{1/2}[\frac{Z_b}{Z_1}]^{1/2}[P_1(P_2 - P_1)]^{1/2} \quad (10)$$

in which M_a is the molar mass of air, subscript b denotes base conditions and

$$G = \frac{d_b}{d_a} = \left(\frac{M}{M_a}\right)\left(\frac{1}{Z_b}\right) \quad (11)$$

assuming that base conditions and ambient conditions are identical in measuring G. Equation 10 is within a few constants of being the classical orifice performance equation which appears in ANSI 2530:

$$\dot{V}_b = F_b F_r Y F_{pb} F_{tb} F_{tf} F_{gr} F_{pv} [P_{f1} h_w]^{1/2} \qquad (12)$$

$$\begin{aligned}
F_b F_r &= \text{constant} \left[\frac{\pi^2 R}{8 M_a}\right]^{1/2} \Phi_1 \beta^2 \\
Y &= Y_1 \\
F_{pb} &= \text{constant} \left[\frac{1}{P_b}\right] \\
F_{tb} &= \text{constant}[T_b] \\
F_{tf} &= \text{constant} \left[\frac{1}{T_1}\right]^{1/2} \\
F_{gr} &= \left[\frac{1}{G}\right]^{1/2} \\
F_{pv} &= \left[\frac{Z_b}{Z_1}\right]^{1/2} \\
h_w &= \text{constant}(P_2 - P_1)
\end{aligned}$$

The thermodynamic property correlations appear in the F_{pv} term.

Custody transfer usually requires energy content for pricing in which the energy content is defined as the product of flowrate and heating value. The heating value is the enthalpy of combustion in an ideal reaction. The cost, C, is then

$$C = \dot{n} H n^* \Delta t = \dot{m} H m^* \Delta t = \dot{V}_b^* H v^* \Delta t = (\dot{V}_b / Z_b) H v^* \Delta t \qquad (13)$$

where $\dot{n}$ is the molar flowrate, Hn^* is the heating value per mole, Hm^* is the heating value per mass Hv^* is the heating value per volume superscript * denotes as ideal gas value and Δt is the time period for accounting. The last equation in Equations 13 requires some explanation. Because the heating value is an ideal gas property, it is necessary to multiply by an ideal gas flowrate. However, industry has chosen to utilize the real gas flowrate so a conversion is necessary:

$$\dot{V}_b^* = (\dot{V}_b^* / \dot{V}_b) \dot{V}_b = \left(\frac{\dot{m} R T_b M P_b}{M P_b \dot{m} Z_b R T_b}\right) \dot{V}_b = \dot{V}_b / Z_b \qquad (14)$$

It is a common misconception that division of Hv^* by Z_b converts the heating value to a real gas property. This is not true; the fact is that division of $\dot{V}_b$ by Z_b converts the real gas flowrate to an ideal gas flowrate as in Equation 14.

Effect of Thermodynamic Correlation

Assuming that the cost equation represents the most important practical calculation, we examine it for the effect of thermodynamic correlations. Combining Equations 10, 12 and 13 produces

$$C = \Delta t \left[F_b F_r Y F_{pb} F_{tb} F_{tf} F_{gr} (P_{f1} h_w)^{1/2} \right] \left[\frac{1}{Z_1 Z_b} \right]^{1/2} Hv^* \quad (15)$$

The final two terms represent the thermodynamic properties. Define C_1 as

$$C' = \left[\frac{1}{Z_1 Z_b} \right]^{1/2} Hv^* \quad (16)$$

Then the relative error in C_1 arising from thermodynamic properties is

$$\frac{\delta C'}{C'} = \left[\left(\frac{\delta Z_1}{2 Z_1} \right)^2 + \left(\frac{\delta Z_b}{2 Z_b} \right)^2 + \left(\frac{\delta Hv^*}{Hv^*} \right)^2 \right]^{1/2} \quad (17)$$

If we now assume that we can obtain Z from correlation and Hv^* by measurement each within 0.1%, then the error introduced into C by thermodynamic properties is 0.12%.

It is interesting to note that the industrial goal is 0.1% measurement. Many suppliers assure customers that their instruments are within 0.1%. However, the fact is that 0.1% is essentially state-of-the-art laboratory capability, and is unreachable in gas flow measurement. The thermodynamic properties alone exceed this value in laboratory conditions. Of course, the 0.12% number assumes independent measurements of Z_1, Z_b and Hv^* at the 0.1% level. It is more likely that a correlation would produce Z with P, T and composition as input; it is also possible to calculate Hv^* given T and composition.

To illustrate the effect of composition upon the thermodynamic properties, assume a relatively low pressure such that

$$Z = 1 + BP/RT \tag{18}$$

$$B = \sum_i \sum_j x_i x_j B_{ij} \quad \left(B_{ij} \approx [B_{ii} B_{jj}]^{1/2}\right) \tag{19}$$

and use the rigorous relation

$$Hv^* = \sum_i x_i Hv_i^* \tag{20}$$

Assume a binary mixture of methane and "other stuff" with 90 mol % methane. Assume the temperature is such that B(methane) is - 50 cm^3/mol and B(other stuff) is - 100 cm^3/mol; further assume that Hv^*

(methane) is 1 MJ and H_v^* (other stuff) is 2 MJ. Finally, assume that the errors associated with the various determinations required are: composition, 0.2% (this is achievable in the laboratory, but field values probably exceed 0.5% cm³/mol); B(methane), 1 cm³/mol; B(other stuff), 1 cm³/mol; B(methane, other stuff), 1.5 cm³/mol; $H_{v_i}^*$, negligible. Under these conditions, the error in Z is 0.16% from P, T and composition, and the error in H_v^* is 0.15% from composition. Thus, the error induced in gas cost by thermodynamic properties calculated from composition (assuming very low errors in composition measurement) is 0.19%

Conclusions

The thermodynamic properties contribute on-the-order of 0.2% uncertainty in calculation of gas cost in custody transfer. This figure is somewhat less with direct measurement of the properties, and higher if the properties are calculated from composition. These statements assume that the correlation is exact. Any significant error in the correlation adds to the overall effect. A 0.1% correlation, which is difficult to achieve, contributes 10% of the total error, while a 0.2% correlation can account for 40% of the total error. The AGA-8 correlation and the GERG correlations for natural gas both achieve 0.1% in the custody transfer range (assuming the composition is correct). NX-19, on the other hand, can exhibit significantly higher errors for some compositions.

Given that industry seeks an overall measurement accuracy of

0.1%, this analysis indicates that it is not achievable. However, the importance of accurate thermodynamic data and correlations is also obvious. Inaccurate values for these properties can inflate the overall error significantly and even overcome the discharge coefficient errors at the 0.5% level.

The obvious conclusion is that the most accurate possible data and correlations are essential. It is also apparent that direct measurement of the properties is preferable to calculation using composition.

ACCURATE MEASUREMENTS OF FLUID DENSITIES

J. C. HOLSTE, K. R. HALL and K. N. MARSH

Chemical Engineering Department
and
Thermodynamics Research Center
Texas A&M University
College Station TX 77843 USA

January 1988

ABSTRACT

In the past decade, a number of new experimental techniques for measuring the densities of fluids at high pressures have been developed or improved. These techniques are reviewed, and their relative merits discussed. Several techniques that have been developed or improved upon at Texas A&M are discussed in greater detail.

INTRODUCTION

Accurate knowledge of the densities of fluids at pressures well above atmospheric pressure is required for several practical applications. One application that is of extreme economic importance relates to the custody transfer of fluids, and, as a result, considerable effort has been devoted over the past five years to investigations of the densities of natural gas mixtures. High pressures also occur naturally in petroleum and natural gas reservoirs, and the efficient and profitable exploitation of these resources depends upon an accurate knowledge of the various thermophysical properties of the fluids at reservoir conditions. Accurate experimental densities are required for the development and testing of equations of state that describe the fluid behavior, and reliable equations of state can, in turn, be used to calculate phase equilibrium properties as well as densities.

In this paper, we review several experimental methods that recently have been developed or improved significantly. The relative strengths and weaknesses of each method are discussed. We also present details of several apparatus that have been developed or improved upon at Texas A&M and discuss the philosophy of our experimental approach to PVT studies.

METHODS CURRENTLY EMPLOYED BY OTHER WORKERS

The discussion of methods employed by other workers will exclude measurements which were made using conventional equipment and methods. Instead, we devote our attention to those methods that have been improved significantly or which represent significant developments in measurement capabilities.

Isochoric/Burnett apparatus

This method has been used for some time by Kobayashi and co-workers to study the PVT properties of mixtures containing methane or hydrogen at cryogenic temperatures. This method also provides information about phase equilibrium properties because the phase boundary can be detected by observing the discontinuous temperature derivative of the isochore that occurs at the phase boundary. Magee and Kobayashi (1984) recently reported measurements on mixtures of hydrogen and methane that provide information about the locus of isochoric inflections as well as PVT and phase behavior. Straty and Palavra (1984) report the development of a new Burnett/isochoric apparatus which operates to high temperatures and which is capable of measurements on corrosive fluids.

Z-meter

Although their measurements have not been reported in the open literature to date, workers at several laboratories in Europe and the United States have used a commercial device for studies of the densities of natural gas mixtures near room temperature and at pressures to approximately 10 MPa. These devices, when operated by competent personnel in a laboratory environment, appear to be capable of accuracies in the range 0.02 to 0.05 %. However, the temperature range is quite limited (0 to 35 °C), and regions near the liquid-vapor two-phase region must be avoided, otherwise condensation may occur during the expansion process. In spite of their limitations, these devices provide an excellent opportunity to obtain rapidly large amounts of useful data on multicomponent natural gas mixtures because of the rapid rate at which the measurements can be made.

Buoyancy force (Archimedes' principle) devices

Devices utilizing magnetic suspension of a buoy in a fluid first were applied extensively to measurements of interest to the chemical and process industries by Haynes and co-workers (1976, 1977, 1983), who measured the densities of a large number of liquefied natural gases at or below ambient temperature (Haynes, et al., 1983). Wagner and Kleinrahm (1986) recently have developed a buoyancy force apparatus which is designed for highly accurate measurements. Adsorption effects on the surface of the suspended quartz sphere impose the ultimate limit upon the accuracy of their device.

Direct weighing methods

For many years, direct weighing of the fluid in a container of known volume has been used as a method of measuring densities. For densities at ambient pressures in particular, pycnometers provide accurate data through a simple measurement procedure. However, these direct weighing methods have required that the filling lines for high pressure measurements be disconnected during the measurement, resulting in a measurement procedure that is tedious, time-consuming, and prone to operator errors. Recent advances in the design of electronic force balances have reduced the vertical motion of the weighing pan nearly to zero, thereby making possible the accurate weighing of a cell with a pressure line attached. Machado and Streett (1983) report densities for pure liquid methanol which were obtained over a wide range of temperatures and pressures using a direct weighing device.

Vibrating tube densimeters

Densimeters based upon the resonant frequency of vibrating U-shaped tubes have been used for some time, and they are available from commercial suppliers. These devices can provide densities precise to a few parts per million, but, for the highest accuracy, they must be calibrated using reference fluids of approximately the same density as the unknown fluid. Vibrating tube densimeters are suited extremely well for the investigation of excess volumes, where the mixture densities are compared to the densities of the respective pure fluids. Recently, the useful range of the commercial devices has been extended to include pressures to 35 MPa and temperatures to 425 K. Albert and Wood (1984) have investigated the density behavior of salt solutions at temperatures to 700 K and pressures to 40 MPa using a vibrating tube densimeter of their own design.

Isochoric substitution method

Distortions of the sample cell volume with pressure represent a significant source of uncertainty in PVT measurements at pressures above 10 MPa. Morris and coworkers (1980, 1983, 1984) have measured the densities of argon, methane and nitrogen at pressures to 700 MPa using an isochoric substitution method. With this technique, an isochoric cell is filled with the fluid of interest, the cell is weighed to determine the mass of fluid present, and the internal pressure is measured at several temperatures along the isochore. A piece of metal of well-defined volume (often spherical in shape to simplify the distortion calculations) is placed in the cell, which then is filled with fluid and the entire sequence repeated. At the filling temperature, the difference between the fluid masses in each case represents the amount of fluid which occupied the volume now occupied by the reference metal, and the density of the fluid can be calculated from this series of measurements. The densities at the other temperatures also can be calculated by a slightly more involved procedure. The pressure distortions which directly enter the calculations are those of the inserted metal only, thereby the accuracy of corrections for these distortions is improved.

Refractive index techniques

Dielectric effects, including refractive index, also depend directly on the number of molecules present, therefore they can be used to investigate densities. Bose and co-workers (1986) have developed an optical technique that provides information about both the density and dielectric properties of a fluid, which can in turn be related to polarizabilities. This device makes possible rapid measurements in the range where Burnett measurements become extremely slow and tedious, and the accuracy of the two methods is comparable. The dielectric device also utilizes much smaller samples and shorter residence times in the apparatus. These attributes are advantageous for the investigation of toxic, reactive or corrosive fluids.

Other methods of interest

Many other methods for PVT measurements exist, particularly for special situations. In particular, Burnett apparatus still are employed by many workers to provide highly accurate measurements at low to moderate pressures, and the variable volume cells often used for phase equilibrium measurements provide accurate fluid densities as well. These methods have been described often, and they generally are widely known; therefore we have chosen not to discuss them here because of space limitations.

HIGH PRESSURE PVT MEASUREMENTS AT TEXAS A&M

Because of various limitations inherent in the basic nature of each apparatus, no single density measurement technique is the best for all temperatures, densities and pressures. We therefore have concluded that the optimal approach to PVT measurements is to develop a variety of experimental apparatus, and to apply each of them to the particular conditions for which that apparatus represents the best available technique. We also have devoted considerable effort to the development of techniques that increase the rate of measurements without significantly reducing the accuracy of the experiment. For density measurements, we currently use the following techniques: Burnett expansions, isochoric measurements and direct weighing (pycnometer).

Burnett expansions provide the best measurements of densities which are less than one half the critical density. This method also provides by far the best determinations of the virial coefficients. The isochoric technique can be used to extend the densities determined by Burnett expansions to other temperatures more conveniently than by making additional Burnett expansions. At higher densities, the pycnometer, or direct-weighing device, provides measurements more rapidly and with accuracy equivalent to the Burnett apparatus. Again, isochoric measurements are used to extend the densities measured along the isotherms to other temperatures. Each method is discussed in more detail below.

Burnett and Burnett-isochoric

We have used this technique to measure densities for several fluids, including both pure components and binary and multicomponent mixtures. We present here only a few representative results to indicate the quality of the measurements.

Figure 1 shows a comparison of our experimental values for the second virial coefficient of carbon dioxide to those considered to be the best determinations by other workers. Our values were accumulated over a period of eight years by four workers using three different apparatus. The internal consistency of these values is noteworthy. The experimental values are compared to an equation, derived from the BACK equation of state (Chen and Kreglewski, 1977), which was fit to the experimental data of Waxman, et al., (1973), and ourselves. The correlation of Levelt-Sengers, et al.
several sets of data, considered to be reliable at the time of the correlation, which lie outside the range of the plot. Figure 2 shows our data for the third virial coefficient of carbon dioxide, along with the values reported by selected other workers. The solid line comes from a correlation due to Orbey and Vera (1983) and the dashed line from a correlation proposed by de Santis and Grande (1979).

Figure 3 shows Burnett-isochoric data for a carbon dioxide + nitrogen mixture. These data also provide information about the saturation boundary through observations of the changes in slope of the isochores upon entering the two-phase region. The phase boundaries are shown as a solid line. An expanded view of the saturation boundary is shown in Figure 4, where phase equilibrium points obtained by Al-Sahhof, *et al.*, (1983) using conventional techniques also are shown for comparison. Figure 5 shows the pressure-composition diagram generated by conventional techniques, with our points shown for comparison. The only noticeable divergence occurs very near the critical point for this mixture. We also have derived interaction second virial coefficients for this mixture from the PVT data. The interaction viral coefficent results are shown in Figure 6 and compared with the results of other workers. Again, the agreement with other workers is quite good.

High pressure pycnometer

We recently have completed the development of a direct weighing apparatus capable of operation over a wide range of temperature and pressure. In some respects, our new apparatus is similar to that of Machado and Streett (1983), but we have reduced the sample volume by nearly one order of magnitude, without reducing the precision and accuracy of the measurement technique. As a result, equilibrium can be achieved much more rapidly after compression or expansion operations.

The high pressure pycnometer design is shown schematically in Figure 7. The beryllium-copper sample chamber, which has an internal volume of approximately 10 cm^3, is suspended from an electronic balance using piano wire. The pressure connection to the cell is made through a stainless steel capillary which is anchored by a tee at the opposite end. This connection is made as a long straight length to minimize loading of the balance due to bending of the capillary caused by vertical displacements of the cell or changes in internal pressure. Such loading effects are estimated to be smaller than the 0.1 mg resolution of the electronic balance.

Details of the cell closure are shown in Figure 8. The actual pressure seal is made by a metallic C-ring (gold-plated stainless steel) which is compressed into the proper position by the end plug and thrust nut. The end plug is keyed to prevent rotation when the thrust nut is tightened, thereby providing a nonrotating seal. This design has been pressure tested successfully to 300 MPa at room temperature.

The sample chamber and connecting lines are surrounded by an isothermal shield fabricated of copper which is controlled at the experimental temperature. The space inside the isothermal shield is filled with helium exchange gas. Helium provides the best heat transfer characteristics as well as minimizing the buoyancy effects on the cell. The buoyancy corrections are reduced below the resolution of the balance (and thereby effectively eliminated) if the helium pressure is maintained constant to approximately 10 kPa. The copper isothermal shield is surrounded in turn by an aluminum radiation shield that also is maintained at the experimental temperature. The spaces surrounding the copper isothermal shield and the aluminum radiation shield are evacuated to provide barriers to heat transfer.

The sample chamber initially is evacuated and the balance is tared. The sample then is introduced into the cell through the feed line and the mass of material in the cell is measured directly by the electronic balance as a function of the pressure. The effective volume of the cell is determined using a calibration fluid for which the density is known over the temperature and pressure range of interest. Above 273 K, water provides excellent calibrations.

Comparisons of densities measured with this apparatus to results reported by other workers are given for carbon dioxide, methane and propane near 300 K in Figures 9, 10, and 11 respectively. Figure 9 compares our pycnometer results and the Burnett apparatus results from our own laboratory (which lead to the data shown in Figures 1 and 2) to the correlation of Angus, et al., (1973). Note that the agreement between the experimental results is much better than 0.1%. The systematic deviations near 10 MPa represent shortcomings of the equation of state for conditions near the critical point. Figure 10 shows results of several workers for propane at 300 K. Note the excellent agreement between our results and those of Ely and Kobayashi (1978) and Thomas and Harrison (1982). The stability of our apparatus is shown by the agreement between our two sets of results; a complete isotherm was measured at 344 K between runs #1 and #2. Finally, Figure 11 compares our results for methane at 303.14 K and the results of Douslin, et al., (1964) with the equation published by Trappeniers, et al., (1979), which represents their experimental data quite precisely. The agreement between the three sets is well within 0.1%, even though the mass density for our lowest point is less than 0.05 gm/cm^3. In general, the internal precision of our pycnometer is 0.02% or less within a single isotherm and 0.04% for repeated isotherms. The agreement with other published results is better than 0.1% for liquids, supercritical gases and dense vapors. Measurements for each point along the isotherm require from approximately 10 minutes for relatively incompressible fluids to about 30 minutes for fluids where the compression heating is more significant.

Isochoric apparatus

We have designed and constructed a new isochoric apparatus intended to provide rapid measurements along isochores. The new apparatus is shown schematically in Figure 12. The apparatus is extremely simple, requiring only the cell and a radiation shield. The density of the fluid in the cell is calculated from the measured pressure at one temperature (the base isotherm), based upon experimental data from the pycnometer and the Burnett apparatus at the base isotherm. Because we are not required to remove the cell from the apparatus for direct weighing, the measurement procedure is simplified greatly, thereby minimizing mechanical operations and the possibility of introducing leaks and other apparatus difficulties.

The volume of the sample cell is small (approximately 25 cm^3), and it contains provision for internal mixing so that equilibrium can be achieved more rapidly at each measurement temperature. The cell is constructed of beryllium-copper to exploit the high strength and the high thermal conductivity of this material. The differential pressure indicator is of our own design, and it is incorporated directly into the body of the cell.

The experimental procedure consists of filling the apparatus to the maximum density of interest, completing the pressure measurement at each temperature along the isochore, exhausting a small amount (5 to 10%) of sample, and repeating isochores until the lowest density of interest is completed. The simplicity of this procedure facilitates complete automation of the measurement.

SUMMARY

The capability for accurate density measurements at high pressures has advanced considerably over the last decade, both in our laboratories and elsewhere. These new techniques provide potential for gathering significant amounts of data accurate to 0.1% or better for use in the development of equations of state required for custody transfer applications, phase equilibrium calculations and various other design requirements.

ACKNOWLEDGEMENTS

Financial Support for this work was provided by the Gas Research Institute, the National Science Foundation, the Gas Processors Association, AMOCO Production Company, Shell Oil Company, Sundstrand Aviation Corporation, the Texas Engineering Experiment Station and the donors of the Petroleum Research Fund, administered by the American Chemical Society.

REFERENCES

Albert, H.J., and R.H. Wood, "High-precision flow densimeter for fluids at temperatures to 700 K and pressures to 40 MPa," Rev. Sci. Instrum., 55, 589 (1984).

Al-Sahhaf, T.A., A.J. Kidnay and E.D. Sloan, "Liquid + vapor equilibria in the N_2 + CO_2 + CH_4 system," I&EC Fundamentals, 22, 372 (1983).

Angus, S., B. Armstrong, and K.M. de Reuck, International Thermodynamic Tables of the Fluid State: Carbon Dioxide, Pergammon Press: Oxford, UK, 1973.

Bose, T.K., J.M. St-Arnaud, H.J. Achtermann and R. Scharf, "Improved method for the precise determination of the compressibility factor from refractive index measurements", Rev. Sci. Instrum., 57, 26 (1986).

Chen, S. S., and A. Kreglewski, "Application of the augmented van der Waals theory of fluids. I. Pure fluids", Berichte der Bunsen Gesellschaft fur Physikalische Chemie, 81, 1048 (1977).

Cottrell, T.L., R.A. Hamilton and R.P. Taubinger, Trans. Farad. Soc., 52, 1310 (1956).

de Santis, R., and B. Grande, "An equation for predicting third virial coefficients of non-polar gases", AIChE J., 25, 937 (1979).

Dittmar, P., F. Schulz and G. Strase, "Druck/Dichte/Temperatur-Werte fur Propan and Propylen", Chemie-Ing.-Techn., 34, 437 (1962).

Douslin, D.R., R.H. Harrison, R.T. Moore and F.P. McCullough, "P-V-T relations for methane", J. Chem. Eng. Data, 9, 358 (1964).

Edwards, A.E., and W.E. Roseveare, "The second virial coefficient of gaseous mixtures", J. Am. Chem. Soc., 64, 2816 (1942).

Ely, J.F., and R. Kobayashi, "Isochoric pressure-volume-temperature measurements for compressed liquid propane", J. Chem. Eng. Data, 23, 221 (1978).

Gunn, R.D., "Volumetric properties of non-polar gas mixtures", M.S. Thesis, University of California (Berkeley), 1958. Values are calculated from experimental data given by W.K. Tang, Tech. Rep. WIS-OOR-13 (1956), University of Wisconsin.

Haynes, W. M., "Simplified magnetic suspension densimeter for absolute density measurements", Rev. Sci. Instrum., 48, 39 (1977).

Haynes, W.M., "Measurement of densities and dielectric constants of liquid propane from 90 to 300 K at pressures to 35 MPa", J. Chem. Thermo., 15, 419 (1983).

Haynes, W. M., and N. V. Frederick, "Apparatus for density and dielectric constant measurements to 35 MPa on fluids of cryogenic interest", J. Res. Nat. Bur. Stand. (U.S.), 88, 241 (1983).

Haynes, W. M., M. J. Hiza and N. V. Frederick, "Magnetic suspension densimeter for measurements on fluids of cryogenic interest", Rev. Sci. Instrum., 47, 1237 (1976).

Haynes, W. M., R. D. McCarty and M. J. Hiza, "Liquefied natural gas densities: Summary of research programs at the National Bureau of Standards", Nat. Bur. Stand. (U.S.) Monograph 172, 1983, 240 pages.

Kratzke, H., and S. Muller, "Thermodynamic quantities for propane. 3. The thermodynamic behavior of saturated and compressed liquid propane", J. Chem. Thermo., 16, 1157 (1984).

Kvalnes, H.M., and V.L. Gaddy, "The compressibility isotherms of methane at pressures to 1000 atmospheres and at temperatures from -70 to 200°, J. Am. Chem. Soc., 53, 394 (1931).

Levelt-Sengers, J.M.H., M. Klein and J.S. Gallagher, "Pressure-volume-temperature relationships of gases", AIP Handbook, 3rd ed., McGraw-Hill: New York, 1972.

MacCormack, K.E., and W.G. Schneider, "Compressibilities of gases at high temperatures, IV. Carbon dioxide in the temperature range 0° - 600° and up to 50 atmospheres", J. Chem. Phys., 18, 1269 (1950).

Machado, J.R.S., and W.B. Streett, "Equation of state and thermodynamic properties of liquid methanol from 298 to 489 K and pressures to 1040 bar", J. Chem. Eng. Data, 28, 218 (1983).

Magee, J.W., and R. Kobayashi, "Measurement and correlation of isochoric P-V-T behavior of a binary H_2 - CH_4 mixture from near ambient to cryogenic temperatures and pressures to 700 atm", Adv. Cryo. Eng., 29, 943 (1984).

Mason, D.M., and B.E. Eakin, "Compressibility factor of fuel gases at 60°F and 1 atm", J. Chem. Eng. Data, 6, 499 (1961).

Michels, A., and C. Michels, "Isotherms of CO_2 between 0° and 150 °C and pressures from 16 to 250 atm", Proc. Roy. Soc., A153, 201 (1935).

Miller, J. G., W. C. Pfefferle and J. A. Goff, "Compressibility of gases. I. The Burnett method. An improved method of treatment of the data. Extension of the method to gas mixtures", J. Chem. Phys., 23, 509 (1955).

Morris, E.C., "Accurate measurements of the PVT properties of methane from -20 to 150 °C and to 690 MPa", Int. J. Thermophys., 5, 281 (1984).

Morris, E.C., and R.G. Wylie, "Accurate method for high pressure PVT measurements and results for argon for T = -20 to +35 °C and P in the range 200 - 400 MPa", J. Chem. Phys., 73, 1359 (1980).

Morris, E.C., and R.G. Wylie, "The PVT properties of nitrogen from -20 to +35 °C and 200 to 570 MPa, and some comparisons with argon and the Lennard-Jones fluid", J. Chem. Phys., 79, 2983 (1983).

Orbey, H., and J.H. Vera, "Correlation for the third virial coefficent using T_c, P_c and as parameters", AIChE J., 29, 107 (1983).

Perez Masia, A., and M. Diaz Pena, An. R. Soc. Esp. Fis. Quim., 54B, 661 (1958).

Straty, G.C., and A.M.F. Palavra, "Automated high-temperature PVT apparatus with data for propane", J. Res. NBS, 89, 375 (1984).

Thomas, R.H.P., and R.H. Harrison, "Pressure, volume, temperature relations of propane", J. Chem. Eng. Data, 27, 1 (1982).

Tomlinson, J.R., "Liquid densities of ethane, propane and ethane-propane mixtures", Technical Publication TP-1, Natural Gas Processors Association, Tulsa, OK, 1971.

Trappeniers, N.J., T. Wassenaar and J.C. Abels, "Isotherms and thermodynamic properties of methane at temperatures between 0 ° and 150 °C and at densities up to 570 Amagat", Physica, 98A, 289 (1979).

Vukalovitch, M.P., and Ya.F. Masalov, Teploenergetika, 13, 58 (1966).

Wagner, W., and R. Kleinrahm, "Apparatus for determining the densities of saturated liquid and vapour of pure fluids along the whole coexistence curve", presented at the Ninth Int. Symp. on Thermophys. Prop., Boulder, Colorado, June, 1985. (To be published in Int. J. Thermophys.).

Waxman, M., H.A. Davis and J.R. Hastings, "A new determination of the second virial coefficient of carbon dioxide at temperatures between 0° and 150 °C and an evaluation of its reliability", Proc. of 6th Symp. Thermophys. Prop., Atlanta, GA, 1973.

FIGURE CAPTIONS

Figure 1. Comparison of selected experimental values of the second virial coefficient of carbon dioxide. The present values (●) and those of (▲) Waxman, et al., (1973) were used to provide the baseline. The results of other workers shown are as follows: (□) Michels and Michels (1935), (△) Perez Masia and Diaz Pena (1958), (▽) MacCormack and Schneider (1950), (○) Pfefferle, et al., (1955), and (▷) Vukalovich and Masalov (1966). The solid line represents smoothed values derived from an equation of state by Angus, et al., (1973), and the dashed line a correlation presented by Levelt-Sengers, et al., (1972).

Figure 2. Comparison of selected experimental values of the third virial coefficient of carbon dioxide. The symbols denote the same work as in Figure 1. The solid and dashed lines are calculated from correlations due to Orbey and Vera (1983) and de Santis and Grande (1979) respectively.

Figure 3. PVT data for a nitrogen + carbon dioxide mixture. The data at 300 and 400 K are Burnett isotherms, the remaining data are isochoric.

Figure 4. Saturation curve for a nitrogen + carbon dioxide mixture determined from the behavior of the isochores.

Figure 5. Pressure-conmposition diagram for nitrogen + carbon dioxide comparing saturation values derived from PVT measurements with values obtained using conventional techniques.

Figure 6. Comparison of experimental values for the interaction second virial coefficients for nitrogen + carbon dioxide.

Figure 7. Schematic diagram of high pressure pycnometer.

Figure 8. Details of sample cell closure design.

Figure 9. Comparison of carbon dioxide densities measured at 320 K using the high pressure pycnometer with densities measured at the same temperature using a Burnett apparatus. The closed circles denote the pycnometer results and the closed squares the Burnett results.

Figure 10. Comparison of liquid propane densities measured at 300 K with the results of selected other workers. The deviations of the experimental data are from the equation given by Kratzke and Muller (1984).

Figure 11. Comparison of methane densities measured at 303.14 K using the pycnometer with densities reported by other workers. The deviations are from the equation published by Trappeniers, et al., (1979), which represents their experiment data with a scatter of less than 0.01%.

Figure 12. Schematic diagram of isochoric apparatus.

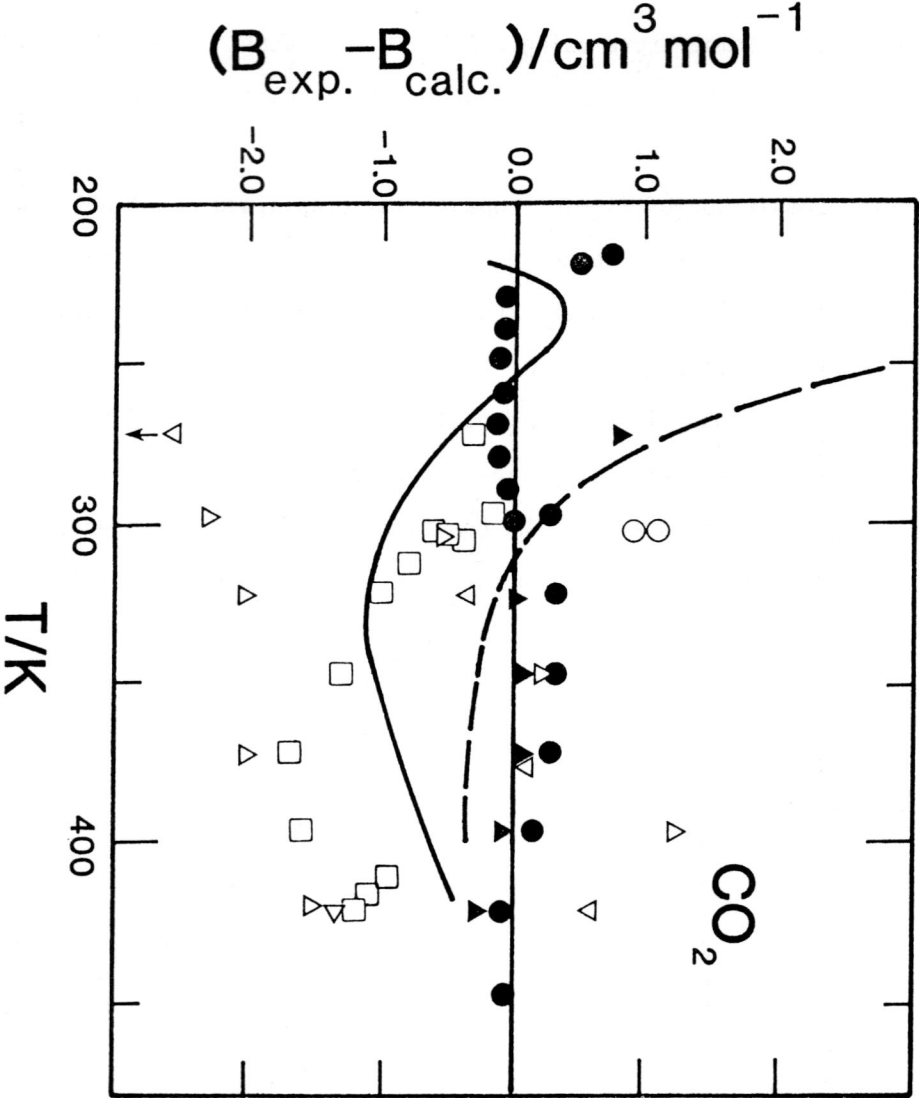

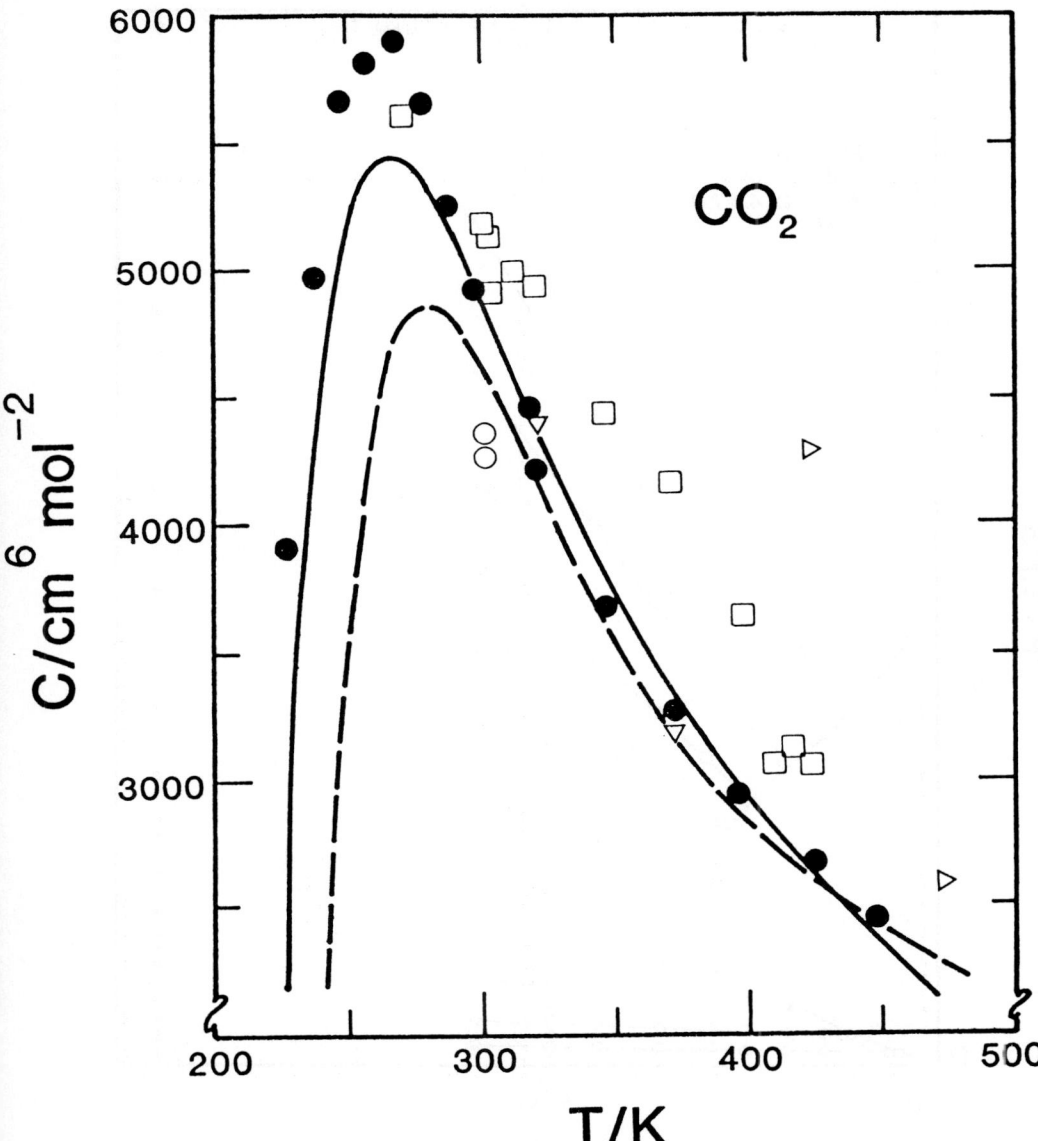

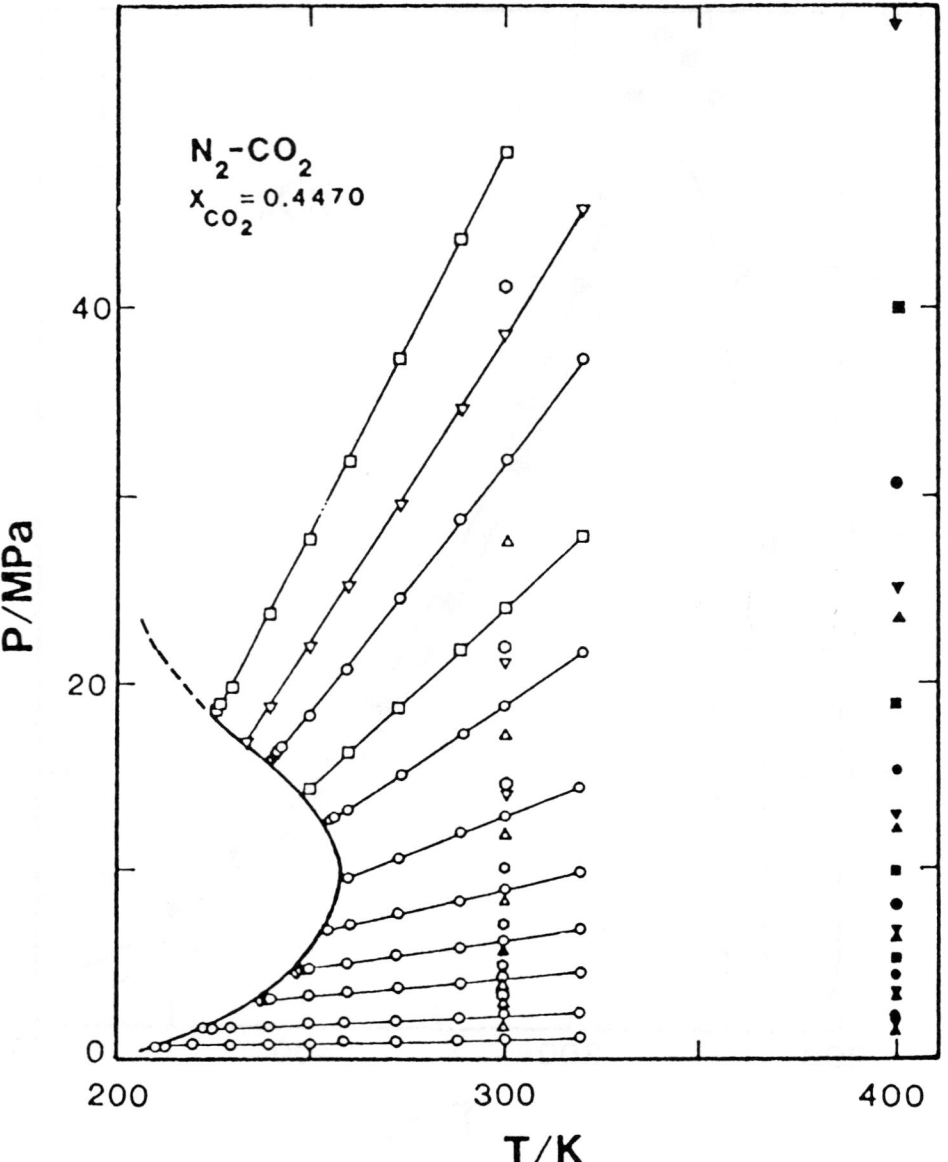

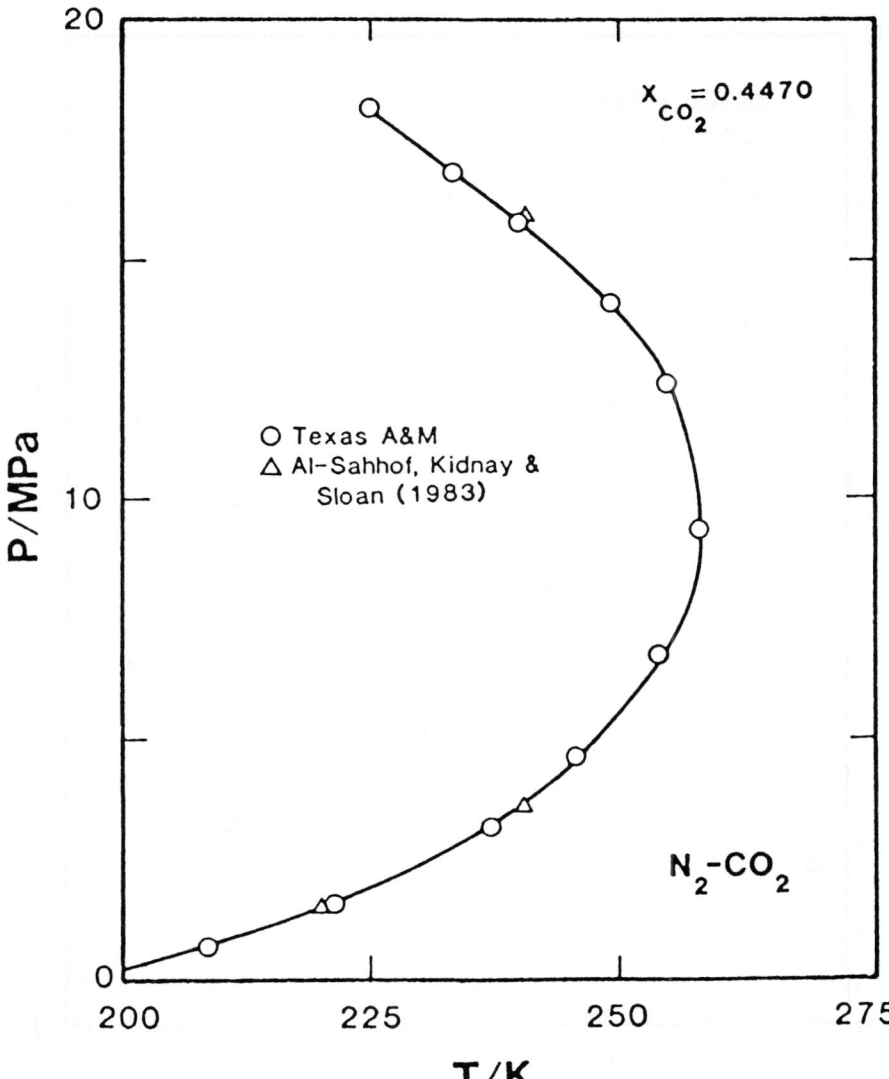

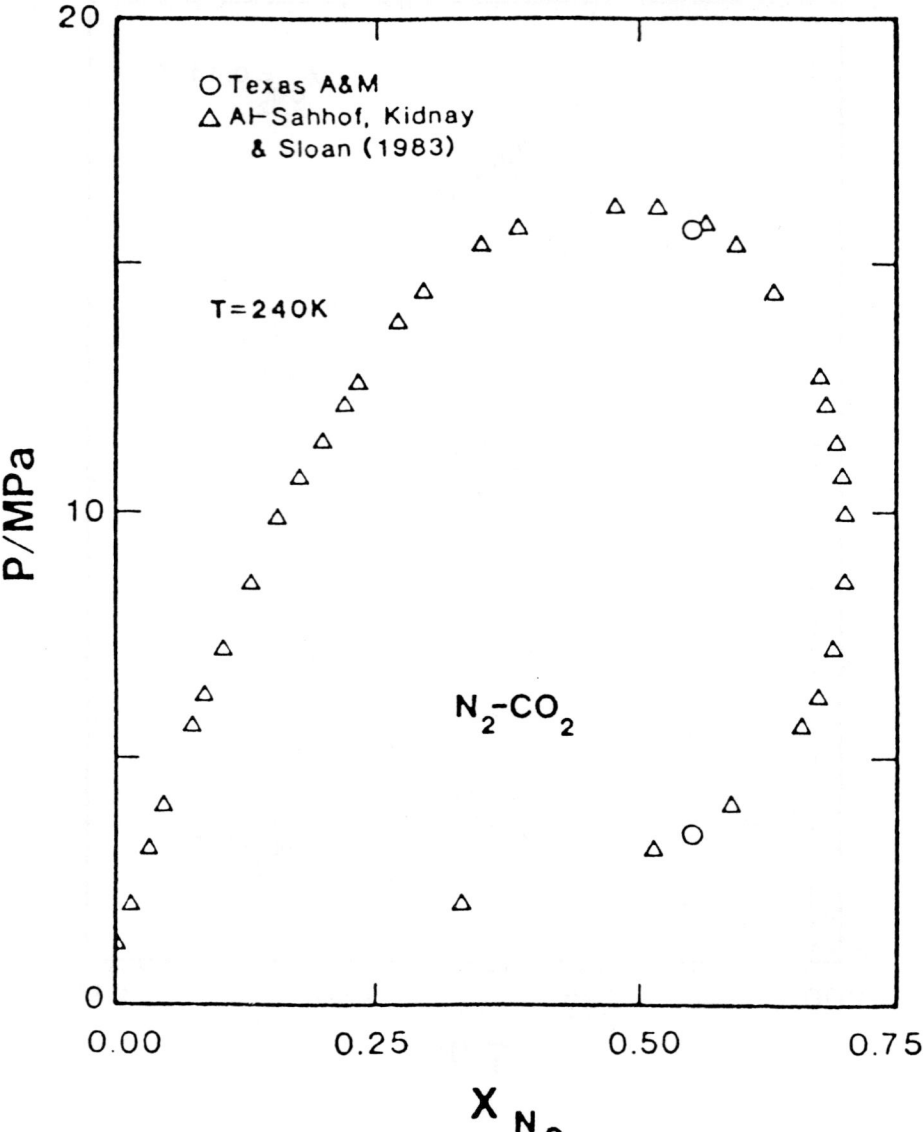

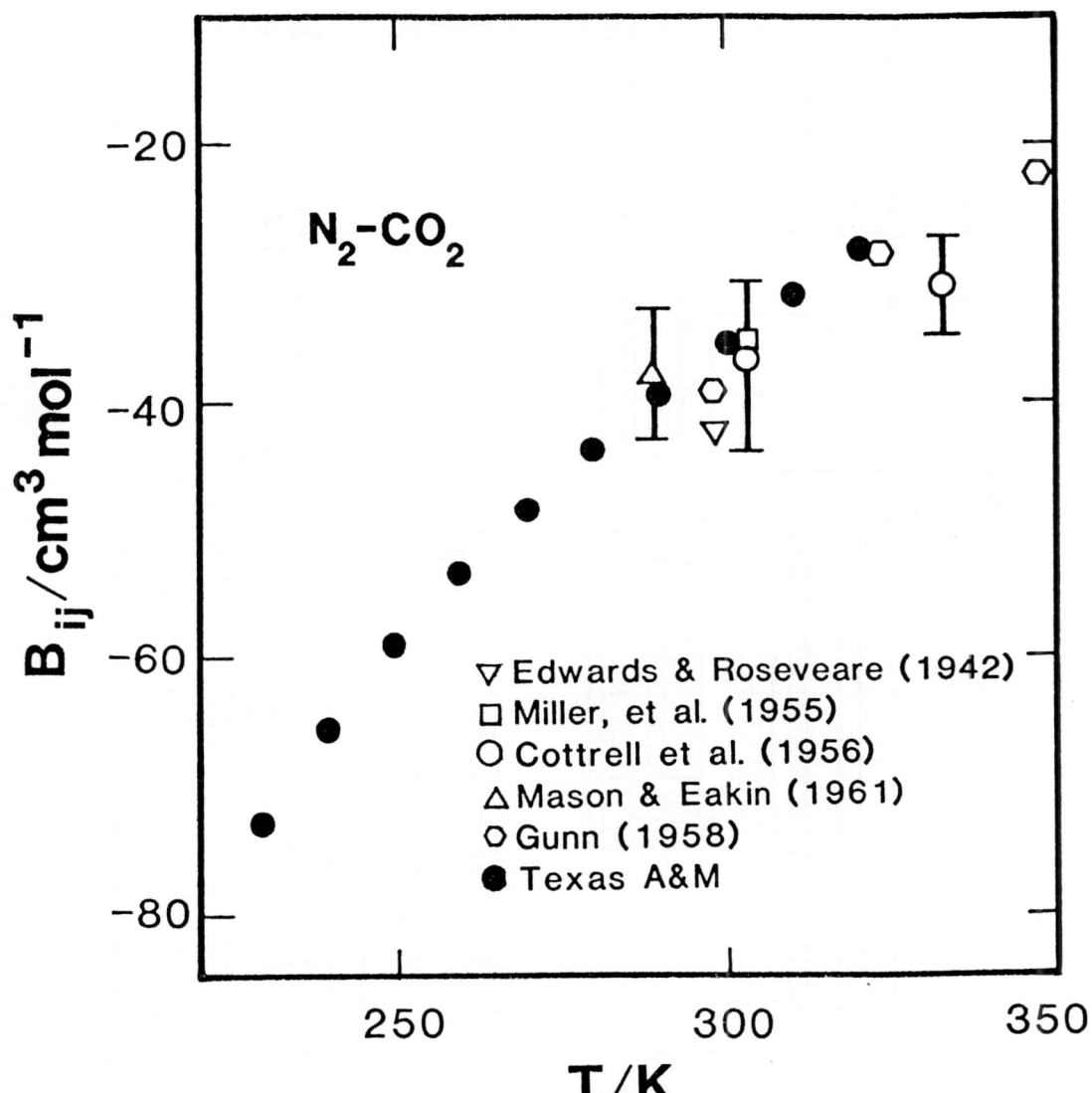

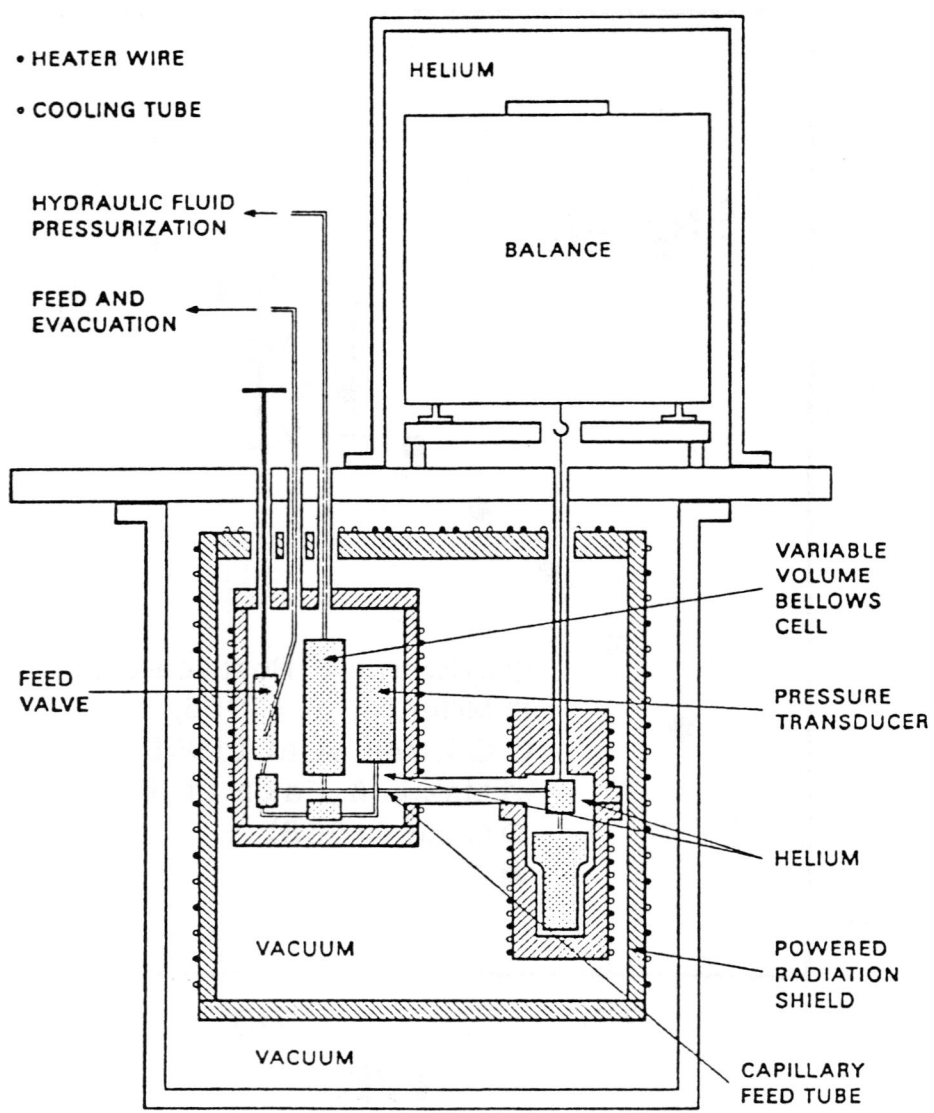

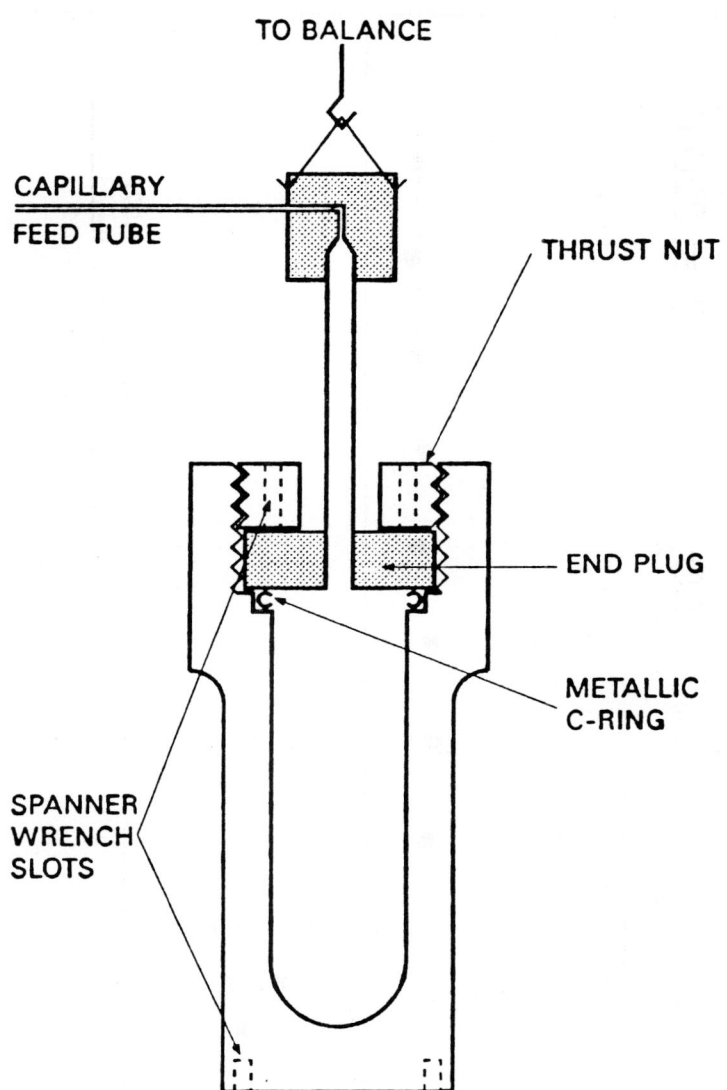

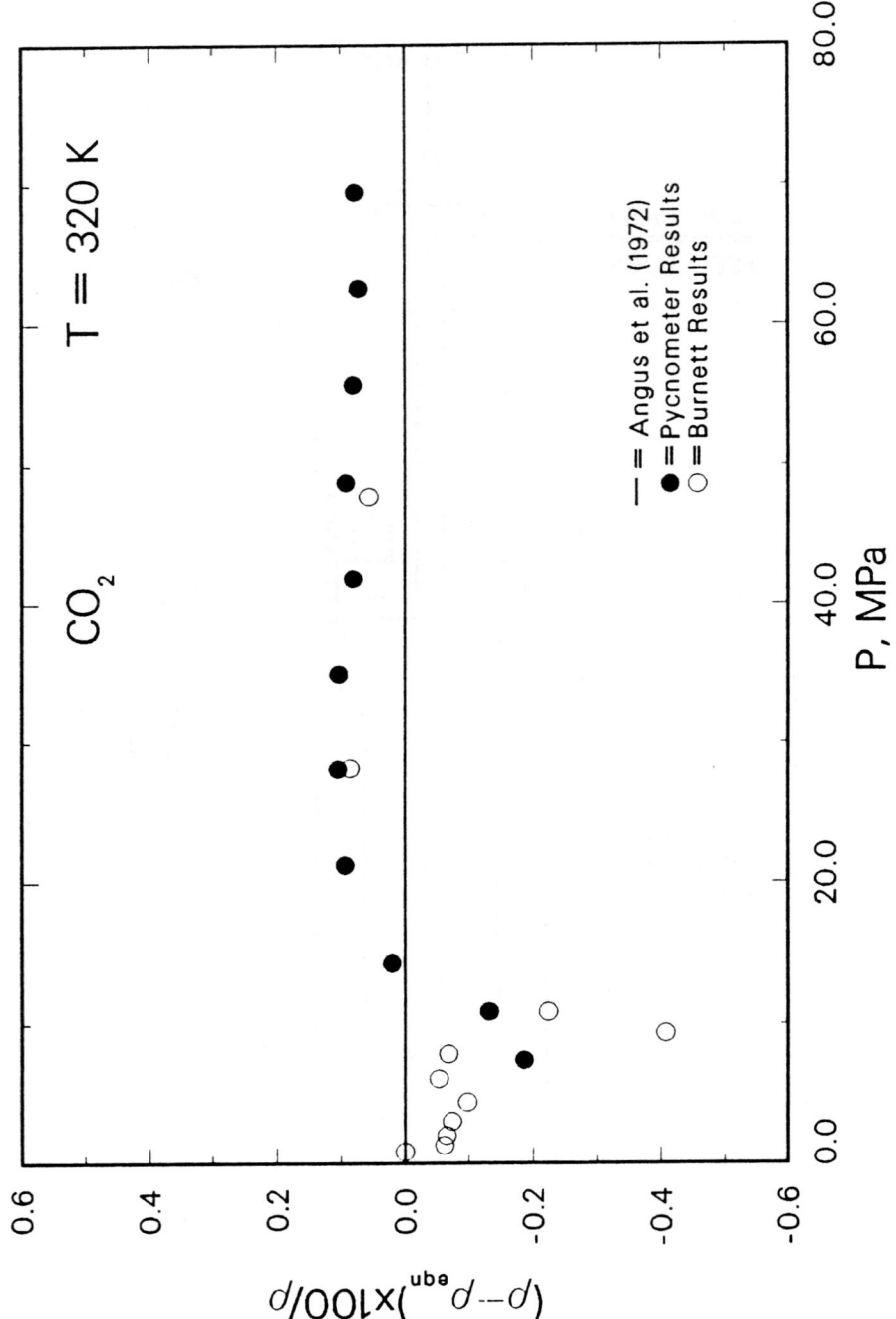

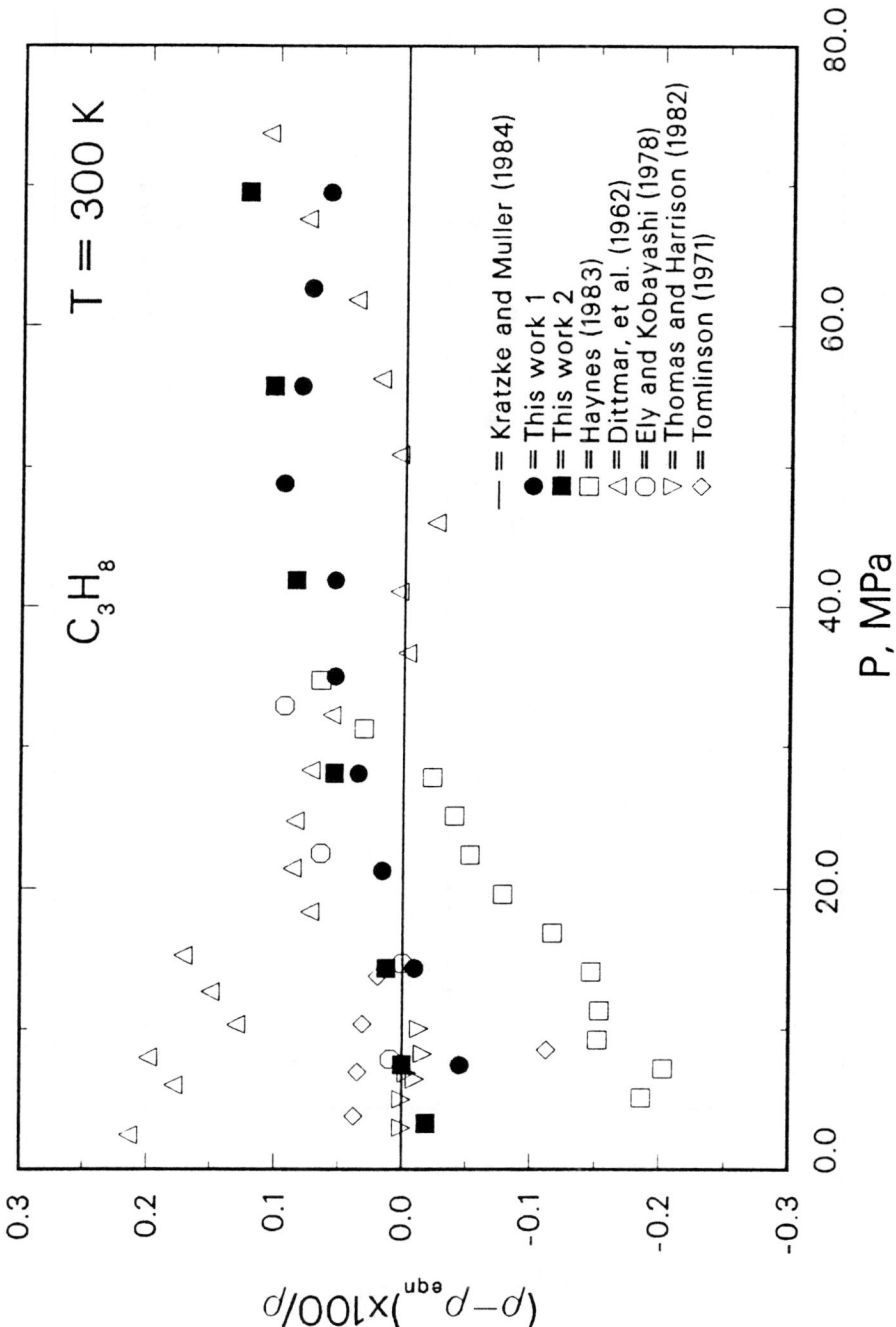

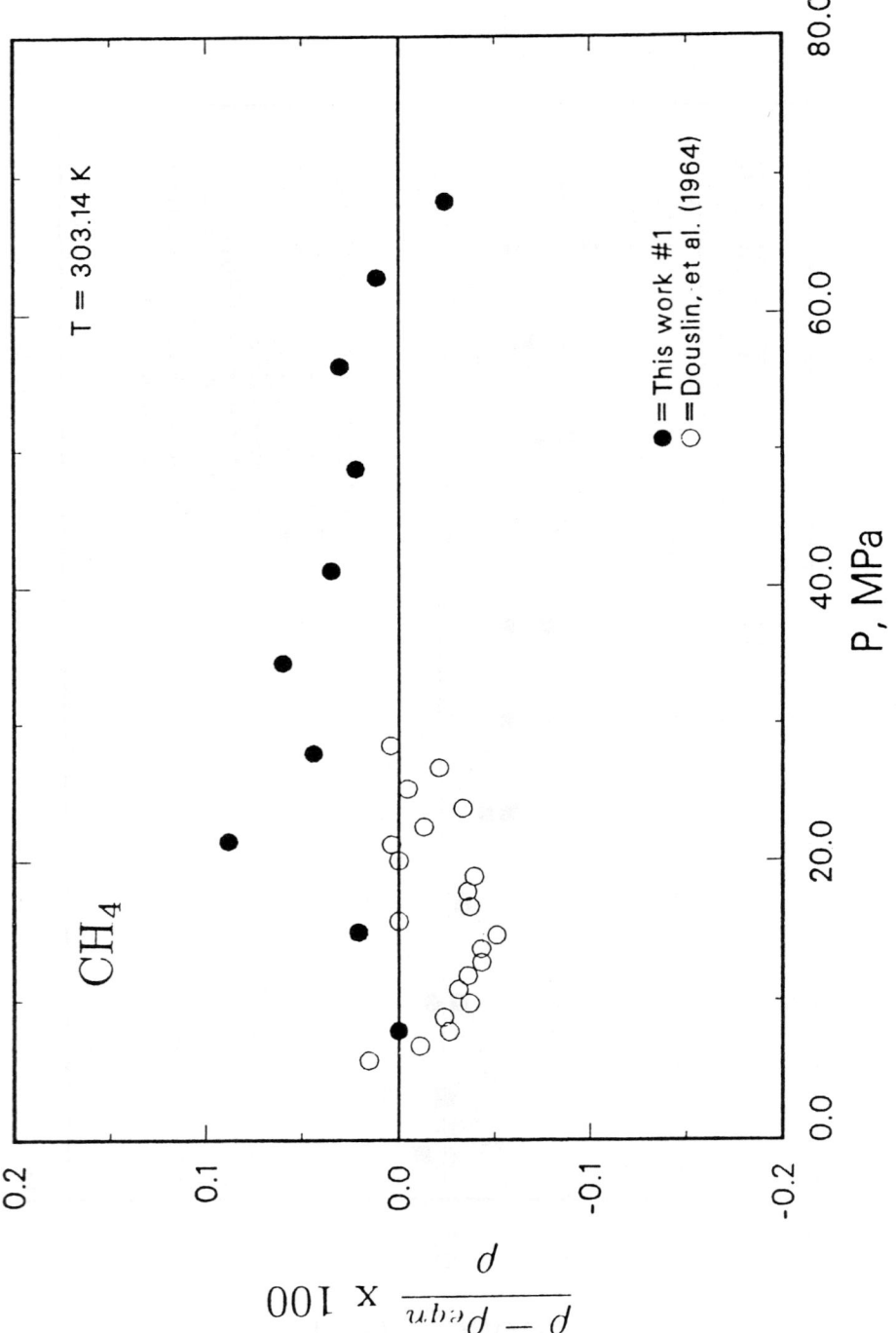

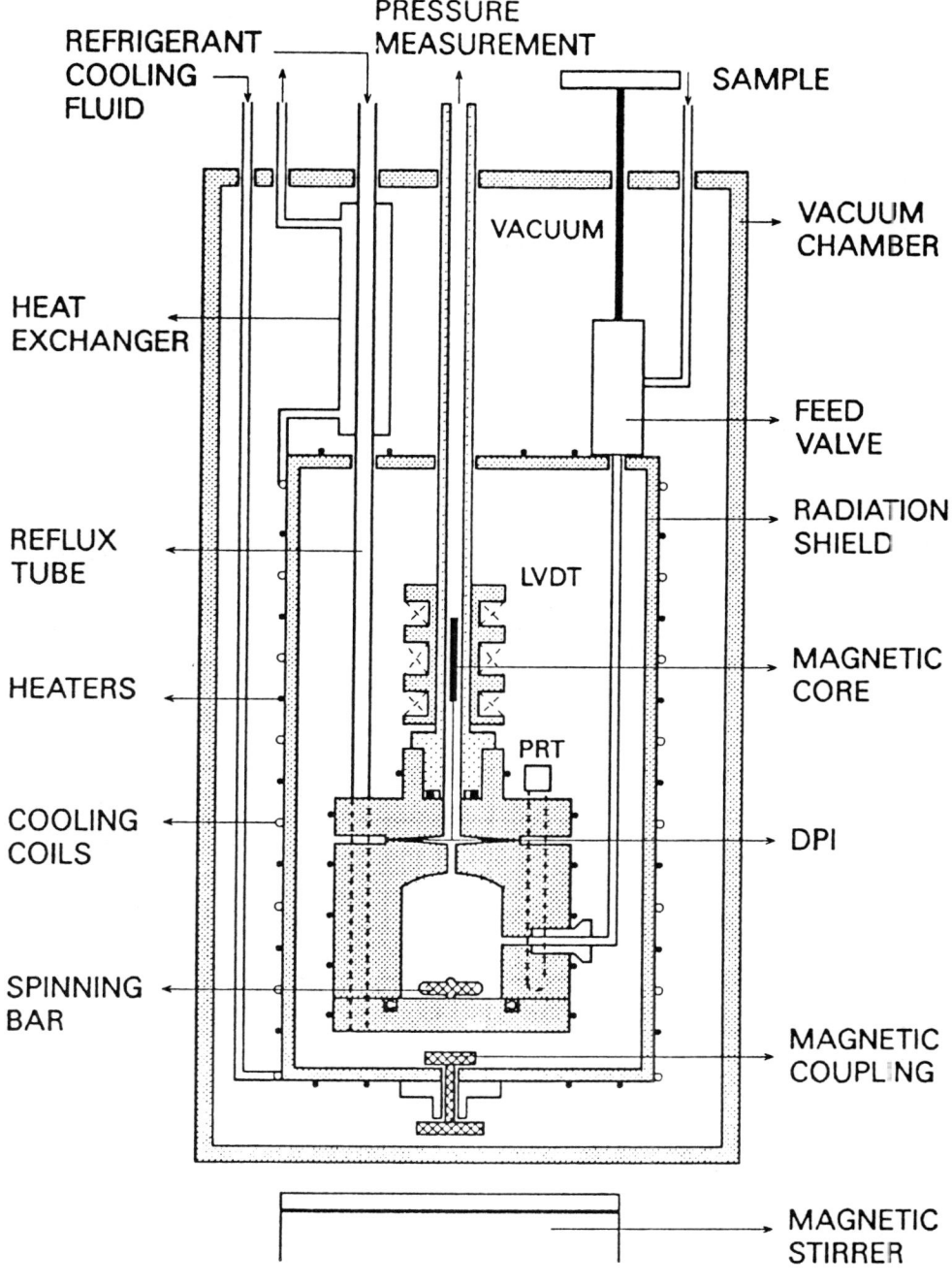

ISOCHORIC APPARATUS

TURBINE METER BASED DISPENSER FOR NATURAL GAS MOTOR VEHICLES

Presented by: Edward J. Farkas, Sc.D., P.Eng.
Canadian Gas Research Institute

International Symposium on Measurements,
Properties and Utilization of Natural Gas

Montréal, Québec

November 25-27, 1987

ABSTRACT

Canadian Gas Research Institute (CGRI) has been involved in development of a dispenser for natural gas as a fuel for motor vehicles since 1982. The objects of the work were to:

- Determine whether a meter type other than the Micro-Motion meter can be used as a basis for a dispenser for natural gas for motor vehicles.

- Develop a dispenser which operates automatically to the maximum extent possible, in order to facilitate self serve operation.

It is desirable to have an alternate metering principle to encourage price competition and for use in fuelling of heavy vehicles where the Micro-Motion meter may not be suitable.

CGRI considered a variety of meter types and selected the turbine meter for the project. A dispensing system based on the turbine meter was assembled and has been taken through various stages of field testing. The test results indicate that the turbine meter is completely suitable for metering natural gas for motor vehicle use.

The CGRI dispenser incorporates various automatic features. One of these features is automatic filling pressure control. The dispenser stops fills automatically at the correct final vehicle tank pressure, without the use of dome load valves or other similar mechanical components.

1. INTRODUCTION

Canadian Gas Research Institute has been involved in development of technology for the natural gas for vehicles industry since 1982. Specific project areas are:

- Development of a dispenser for use at public filling stations.
- Development of an improved method of vehicle tank filling pressure control.
- Development of an improved probe/receptacle system for fuelling of natural gas vehicles.

The first two projects are discussed in the present paper.

2. BACKGROUND

In 1982, Canadian Gas Research Institute (CGRI) received a request from its member companies to investigate alternatives to the Micro-Motion meter.

The Micro-Motion meter, and similar meters manufactured by other firms, utilize principles of physics to sense mass flow directly. The measurement is claimed to be independent of fluid density and viscosity. By 1982, the Micro-Motion meter had already established a dominant position in dispensing of natural gas for motor vehicle use in Canada.

In requesting CGRI to look at alternatives, the member companies were primarily concerned with the cost of the Micro-Motion meter. During the project, additional factors were identified so that the basis for the project can now be summarized as follows:

1. The existence of a proven alternative metering principle would place a limit on the price that the natural gas

industry is prepared to pay for the Micro-Motion metering principle.

2. The total cost of the dispenser, including installation, rather than the cost of the meter, is the real concern. A dispenser offering various desirable automatic features may be less expensive if based on an alternate metering principle.

3. An alternate metering principle may be more suitable for fuelling of heavy vehicles at high flow rates.

The fundamental objective is a means of dispensing accurately known amounts of natural gas at high pressure. CGRI considered, for example, a system in which a known amount of gas is held in a tank in the dispensing system, and then this gas is moved by displacement to the vehicle tank. All variants of this type of approach appeared to involve equipment that was much larger and much more expensive than a system based on a flow meter.

CGRI considered a variety of principles on which a flow meter could be based. Various types of commercially available flow meters were considered, including the vortex meter, the Coanda meter, the target flow meter, flow meters based on thermal principles and the turbine meter.

Various organizations have considered these metering principles, as well as others, for the natural gas for vehicles application. In 1982, dispensers or at least metering systems based on the turbine meter were already offered by firms in the United Kingdom and in New Zealand. The use of the Coanda effect has been studied in New Zealand. CGRI selected the turbine meter as most appropriate for further study. This selection does not necessarily mean that CGRI regards all other metering principles as inappropriate or not capable of development into practical metering systems.

3. LABORATORY METERING SYSTEM

CGRI assembled a metering system from commercially available components. The system consisted of a turbine meter, pressure and temperature sensors and transmitters, and a flow computer. This system was initially tested in the laboratory with nitrogen.

The laboratory system was then assembled into a container for ease of transportation to locations where compressed natural gas was available (Figure 1). The laboratory system was utilized in two types of tests at several field locations:

A. The laboratory system was used in vehicle fills. The CGRI laboratory metering system was placed in series with the existing dispenser at the field location. The amount of fuel dispensed, as displayed by the flow computer in the CGRI system, could be compared with the reading produced by the existing dispenser.

B. The laboratory system was used in test fills of a tank not installed in a vehicle. Subsequent to the filling of the tank, the tank was disconnected from the metering system. The amount of gas in the tank was then determined by a totally independent means. The reading produced by the CGRI laboratory system could then be compared with the independent measurement of the amount of fuel in the tank.

Throughout the test program, attention was also given to reliability of the components in the metering system.

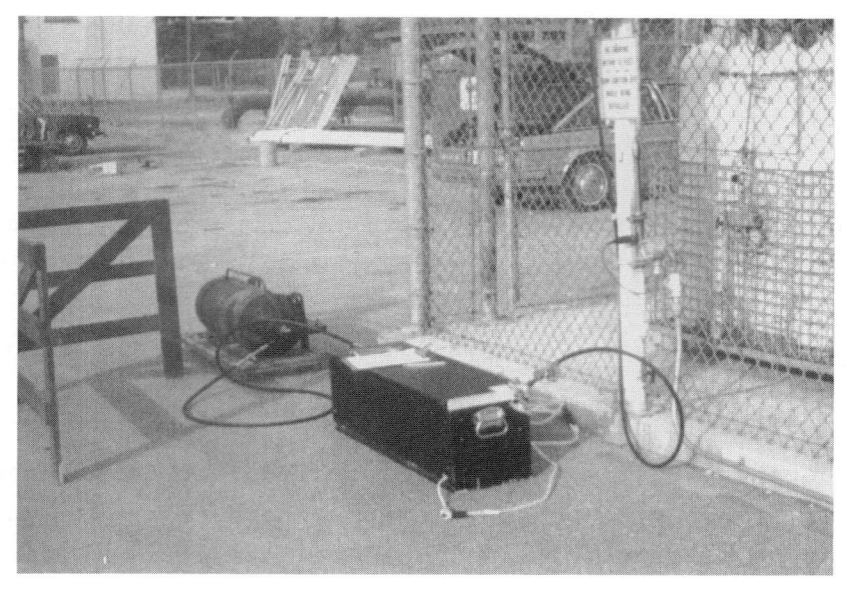

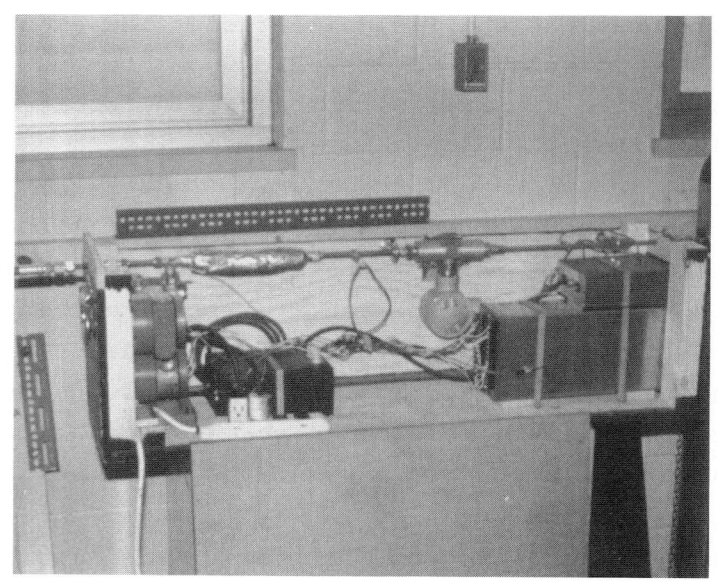

FIGURE 1 - LABORATORY METERING SYSTEM

4. THEORETICAL ASPECTS OF ACCURACY TESTING

In the present paper, only the results of type B tests are discussed.

The ratio R was defined as follows:

$$R = R_{CGRI}/R_{IM} \qquad (1)$$

where R_{CGRI} = reading produced by the CGRI turbine based metering system

R_{IM} = reading produced by the independent means of determination of the amount of fuel in the test tank

In analyzing values of R obtained in the test program, it is important to consider both precision and accuracy. It is also important to keep in mind that precision and accuracy of R are additive functions of the precision and accuracy of both the metering system and the independent means of measurement of the amount of fuel in the tank.

Most types of flow meters utilize a calibration constant. Other components in a metering system or a dispenser may also have calibration adjustments. The calibration factor for each component in the metering system can be considered as combined into one calibration factor for the system as a whole. If the system is not producing accurate readings, but is working correctly in all other respects, the calibration factor can be adjusted so that the system will then produce accurate readings.

Therefore the first consideration is the precision of the metering system. If the precision is not satisfactory, major modifications of the design may be needed to produce satisfactory precision and accuracy.

Precise and accurate gas measurements in general require sophisticated equipment and careful technique. In particular, it is likely that the independent means of measurement will be no better in terms of accuracy and precision than the natural gas metering system being tested.

Any measurement contains random error. If the random error is small in a series of measurements, the precision of the measurements will be good. Random error in R_{IM} and random error in R_{CGRI} contribute additively to random error in R. In particular, according to the principles of statistics and the laws of probability, if values of R in a series of measurements exhibit good precision, then it must be that both the metering system and the independent means of measurement are exhibiting good precision. It is absolutely impossible to produce values of R which exhibit good precision if the precision of either the metering system or the independent means of measurement is poor.

5. TEST PROCEDURE

The obvious method of independent determination of the amount of fuel in the test tank is to weigh the tank before and after the test. The problem with this method is that the tank may weigh 50 kg when empty and 5 kg of fuel may be involved in the test. One has then an example of the classic problem of a determination by difference when the difference is relatively small. The result is that extremely precise weighing equipment is needed and it is difficult to secure satisfactory performance of this equipment at field locations.

To avoid a determination by difference, CGRI used the following method. The gas in the test tank was allowed to flow out of the tank, through a pressure reduction train and then at a gauge pressure of 5 inches of water through a temperature compensated diaphragm meter. Whereas a test fill may require 1 to 2 minutes, the process of "draining" the tank out through the diaphragm meter required typically 30 minutes. The diaphragm meter has an apparent resolution of 0.01 SCF, although it is not known if the internal mechanical components really work this well. The amount of fuel in a test fill is typically 250 to 400 SCF.

6. TEST RESULTS

The CGRI laboratory metering system was involved in 93 tests, including both type A and type B tests, at 3 different locations, from January through November 1984. All components performed reliably and no drift in performance of any of the components could be detected over that period of time.

When the Legal Metrology Branch of Consumer and Corporate Affairs Canada tests a natural gas dispenser, consideration is given to a series of tests made on a given day. A more severe test is to consider a series of tests made on different occasions.

As an example of the performance of both the CGRI laboratory metering system, and the CGRI independent means of measurement of tank contents, a particular series of type B tests can be considered. There were 8 tests in all:
 4 tests on July 3, 1984
 1 test on July 12, 1984
 3 tests on September 24, 1984
A crude measure of the precision is obtained by considering the difference between the highest and lowest values of R obtained in any series of tests. The difference in this series of tests was found to be
 $1.023 - 1.009 = 0.014$
Again, in an intuitive format rather than in a strictly

correct mathematical format, it can be then be stated that the precision was ± 0.7%.

It must be noted again that this value includes the performance of both the CGRI turbine based metering system and the diaphragm meter used as an independent means of determining the amount of fuel in the test tank.

In the opinion of CGRI, this excellent result provides a great deal of support for the turbine meter in the natural gas for vehicles application.

7. THE CGRI DISPENSER

CGRI then undertook to design and build a dispenser with the following characteristics:
- Based on the same metering principle as used in the laboratory metering system.
- Dispenser to be able to receive Ontario Pressure Vessels Safety Branch approval and Ontario Hydro electrical approval for Class I, division 1, group D operation.
- Dispenser to include various automatic features to make it suitable for self serve operation by members of the general public.

The design was based on principles already developed in connection with the laboratory system. These principles are brought into sharper focus in connection with the dispenser and so are discussed in this section.

In any system based on a turbine meter, there is a need to incorporate provisions which will prevent overspeeding of the meter. The turbine meter responds to actual volumes of gas and to prevent overspeeding it is necessary to ensure that a certain actual volumetric flow rate is never exceeded.

It can be shown that the maximum possible actual volumetric flow rate of a given gas through a given restriction, such as a partially open needle valve, is approximately

$$V = \text{constant} \times T^{1/2}/F_{pv} \qquad (2)$$

where V = actual volumetric flow rate, ACFM or actual cubic meters per minute or similar units
T = absolute temperature upstream of the restriction
F_{pv} = supercompressibility factor (Reference 1)

F_{pv} is evaluated at the temperature and pressure upstream of the restriction.

According to equation 2, V is rather insensitive to both upstream pressure and temperature. The effect of pressure is felt only through its effect on F_{pv}. The effect of temperature is modest because it is expressed as the square root of the absolute temperature and also only indirectly through F_{pv}. Therefore, if an appropriately sized restriction is placed downstream of a turbine meter, then the turbine meter can never be subjected to overspeeding, regardless of pressure.

The CGRI dispenser design includes an electrically operated on-off valve within the dispenser cabinet, downstream from the turbine meter and near the exit from the cabinet. This valve has a safety function. If there is an electric power failure during a fill, the valve closes instantly and automatically, stopping the flow of gas. The valve also functions in various automatic features of the dispenser. If power is removed from the valve for any reason, it closes immediately.

The highest normal flow rate for any dispenser installation and vehicle fleet is observed at the beginning of a fill, in the case of a vehicle which has a relatively non-restrictive fuel line and other fittings, and in a case where the vehicle fuel tank is nearly empty at the start of the fill. In the CGRI dispenser design philosophy, the turbine meter is selected so that the maximum allowable flow rate for the meter is approximately double the highest normal flow rate defined above. In consequence of equation 2, both of these flow rates are in terms of actual volumes of gas.

The on-off valve is either fully open or fully closed. When open, it offers a certain restriction. The on-off valve is sized so that the maximum allowable flow rate for the meter is not exceeded even if the on-off valve is the only component downstream of the turbine meter (i.e. in the event of a hose break or other damage). With these criteria, the pressure drop across the on-off valve during normal operation is not excessive.

The CGRI dispenser design contemplates drawing gas from three separate storage banks. When the actual volumetric flow rate drops to a certain fraction of the flow rate observed at the start of the fill, the object is to switch to the next higher bank. Results of calculations for a hypothetical dispenser operated according to this scheme are presented in Table 1. It can be seen that the range of actual volumetric flow rates experienced during the fill is surprisingly narrow. This phenomenon is favourable for the turbine meter since the meter factor (calibration factor) for the turbine meter can readily be assumed constant over a narrow range of flow rates.

If the storage pressure is not substantially larger than the final vehicle tank pressure, then flow rate would drop off to low levels toward the end of the fill. Reduced accuracy is not likely to result for the following reasons:

TABLE 1 - CALCULATED DISPENSER OPERATING CONDITIONS

PHASE OF FILL	DRAWING FROM BANK (psig)	ASSUMED PRESSURE IN METER (psia)	PRESSURE DOWNSTREAM OF ON-OFF VALVE (psia)	PRESSURE IN FUEL TANK (psia)	FLOW RATE SCFM	FLOW RATE ACFM
1*	1200	1215	940	0	767	7.2
1**	1200	1215	1085	1000	533	5.0
2*	2400	2415	1900	1000	1550	6.7
2**	2400	2415	2300	2200	800	3.5
3*	3600	3015	2650	2200	1492	5.6
3**	3600	3015	2880	2800	817	3.1

* - initial
** - final

NOTE: all values are approximate

- The flow rate down to which meter factor is approximately constant is much lower at high pressure, as compared to atmospheric pressure.

- A relatively small proportion of the total amount of fuel in the fill goes through the dispenser while flow rate is low.

It is important to note that this design philosophy can be applied to a dispenser for passenger cars and other light vehicles, or to a dispenser for heavy vehicles such as transit buses. The only difference between the two cases would be a somewhat larger turbine meter and on-off valve. The actual physical size of the units is very insensitive to flow capacity.

For example, one manufacturer offers the following turbine meters:

MAXIMUM FLOW RATE ACFM	LENGTH OF METER INCHES	NOMINAL BORE INCHES
15	5½	0.75
120	8	2.00

Thus the design of turbine based dispensers can be very similar for both light and heavy vehicles.

8. THE COMPUTER

In the laboratory metering system, the flow computer was a standard unit which is available commercially. This computer did not have all the features required for the next stage of the project. Therefore, CGRI commissioned Displayco Alles Corp. of Downsview, Ontario, to develop a computer specifically for the dispenser. This computer receives signals from the turbine meter, and from the pressure and temperature transmitters, and carries out the standard gas calculation corrected for F_{pv} (Reference 1). The computer produces signals in a dual channel format which then go to a standard Kraus Industries display head.

CGRI personnel further developed the computer and added programming for various automatic features. These features are described in following sections.

It is to be emphasized that the mathematical models and programming developed by CGRI to implement these automatic features are not tied solely to dispensers based on turbine meters. Using CGRI technology, these automatic features can be implemented in dispensers based on the Micro-Motion meter or on other metering principles.

CGRI has developed a version of the flow computer which incorporates the functions of the Kraus display head. The consolidation of the two units reduces the cost of the dispenser and makes additional space available within the dispenser cabinet. This version of the computer has been tested in the laboratory with excellent results but has not yet been field tested.

9. BANK SELECT

In any dispenser, gas flow may be started by the instantaneous operation of a quarter turn on-off valve or gas flow may start gradually as a valve is slowly opened by the motorist or attendant. In either case, the moment when the valve has reached the fully open position will be denoted by $t = 0$ sec.

Between $t = 0$ and $t = 1$ sec, the flow rate will be changing rapidly with time. Probably the transients die out by t = 0.5 sec, but t = 1 sec will be used for discussion purposes.

Beginning at t = 1 sec, and continuing for a period of seconds or tens of seconds, depending on the initial pressure in the vehicle tank, the flow rate will be reasonably constant. The CGRI bank select feature and other automatic features require the computer to determine when the transients have died out and to retain for later use the flow parameters observed at the beginning of the constant flow period. The flow rate during this pseudo steady state period is referred to as the initial flow rate.

Each of the three storage banks at a typical filling station may be at the same pressure or may be at different pressures. The bank which the compressor fills last is referred to as the low bank. Every fill starts on low bank. The CGRI computer utilizes a pre-programmed criterion. If the initial flow rate is below this pre-programmed criterion, the computer instantly switches the fill to the next higher bank (the medium bank). The computer then repeats the process of determining and storing the initial flow parameters. If the flow is then above the pre-programmed criterion, then this is taken as the official start of the fill.

If the flow is still below the pre-programmed criterion, then the computer immediately switches the fill to the high bank. Again, after transients have died out, the initial flow parameters are retained and the fill officially begins on high bank.

For example, the fill would be switched to the medium bank if the initial pressure in the vehicle tank is relatively high in comparison with the pressure in the low bank. The object is to provide reduced fill times, so the vehicle fill is successively switched to higher banks until a satisfactory flow rate can be achieved.

The switch, if necessary, at the beginning of the fill, from low bank to medium bank, and also if necessary, to high bank, is completed within approximately 2 seconds and it is hardly discernible to the motorist.

If the fill begins on the low bank or on the medium bank, the initial flow rate is retained for further use in the bank select feature. If the fill begins on the high bank, then of course the entire fill occurs on the high bank and the bank select feature does not further enter into the picture.

In the case of a fill starting on the low bank or the medium bank, when the flow rate later drops to 75% of the initial flow rate, the computer automatically switches the fill to the next higher bank. Once on the high bank, the fill continues until it is stopped by other action, even if flow rate drops below 75% of the initial flow rate.

The bank select feature is implemented through two motor-operated quarter turn valves and two check valves, on the three lines from the storage banks. The motor-operated valves are controlled by the computer. At the end of the fill, the computer closes both valves in preparation for the next fill.

10. EXCESS FLOW

If, during the fill, the flow rate increases to 2½ times the initial flow rate, the computer sees this increase as evidence of excess flow and stops the fill. Excess flow could be caused by a hose break, for example.

11. VEHICLE FILLING PRESSURE CONTROL

In order to provide reduced fill times, the storage pressure should always be higher than the final vehicle tank pressure. Therefore, some means are required to automatically stop the fill when the correct final vehicle tank pressure has been reached.

The correct final pressure is defined by a schedule of pressure as a function of temperature. Various pressure versus temperature schedules are possible:

A. Vehicles are filled to the same pressure, regardless of temperature
B. Vehicles are filled to a pressure which is a function of ambient temperature
C. Vehicles are filled to a pressure which is a function of flowing gas temperature.

Again, no matter which schedule is in use, some means are required to automatically stop the fill at the correct vehicle tank pressure.

In many dispensers currently in operation, the dome load valve/reference cylinder system is used to stop fills at the correct pressure according to B or C. The dome load valve has several disadvantages:
- The dome load valve/reference cylinder system can only readily implement one schedule of pressure as a function of temperature.
- Where a fill is controlled by the dome load valve/reference cylinder system, the flow rate drops off to low values as the correct tank pressure is approached. Thus fill times are longer.
- The dome load valve restricts flow at all points during the fill and requires frequent maintenance.

Because of these disadvantages, CGRI developed a computer based filling pressure control method. No variable restrictions such as the dome load valve are required. When the computer concludes that the correct vehicle tank pressure has been reached, it cuts off the flow of gas by removing power from the electrically operated on-off valve located downstream of the turbine meter. As already indicated, this valve is either fully open or fully closed and offers little resistance to flow when open, under normal operating conditions.

As is well known, when a vehicle tank is filled in a time on the order of several minutes, i.e. fast fill, there is a temperature increase in the tank. The CGRI computer based filling pressure control method offers the advantage that special schedules which at least in part take this temperature increase into account can be utilized. The motorist can then receive more nearly a full fill, regardless of temperature.

The temperature increase in the tank is a function of initial pressure in the tank, size of tank, number of tanks on the vehicle, and temperature and pressure of the flowing gas in the dispenser. To avoid overfilling, it is necessary to assume conditions leading to the smallest expected increase. The calculated tank temperatures expected, and the resulting revised pressure versus temperature schedules, are presented in Figure 2 and Table 2, respectively. Some experimental data obtained by Consumers' Gas Co. are also presented in Figure 2.

The calculation of mass of fuel flowing through the dispenser is carried out frequently during the fill. In two different versions of the CGRI computer, calculations are carried out every 1/4 second and every 1/16 second, respectively. The

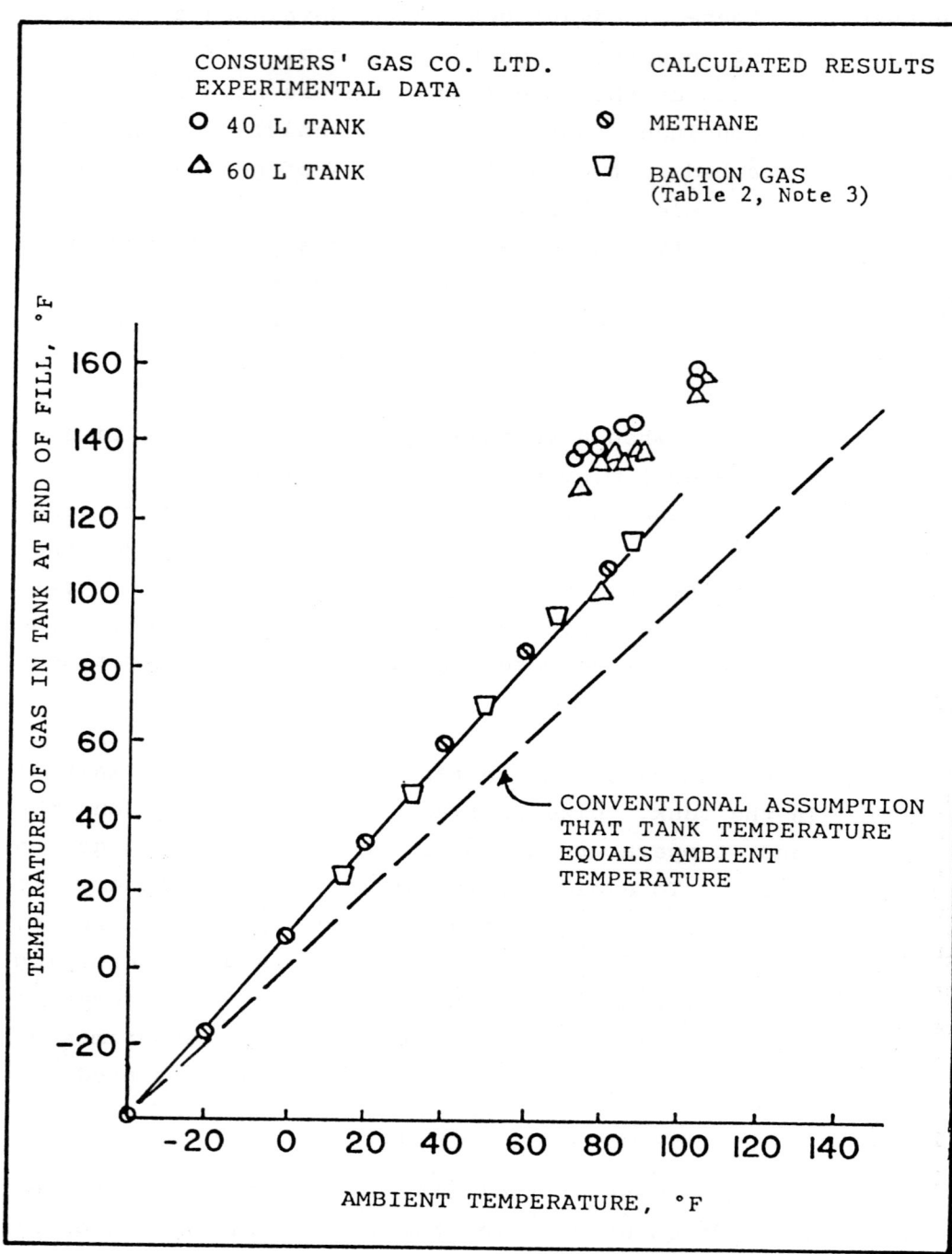

Figure 2

TABLE 2 - CONVENTIONAL AND CGRI REVISED PRESSURE-TEMPERATURE SCHEDULES

MAXIMUM ALLOWABLE VEHICLE TANK PRESSURE, psig

AMBIENT TEMPERATURE °F	CONVENTIONAL SCHEDULES			CGRI REVISED SCHEDULES	
	(1)	(2)	(3)	(1)	(3)
-40	1626	1610	1554	1626	
-20	1875	1861	1814	1915	
0	2127	2116	2077	2248	
20	2380	2372	2343	2543	2510
40	2630	2626	2608	2878	2840
60	2877	2876	2870	3174	3163
80	3124	3125	3128	3455	3478
100	3374	3377	3389	3600	3600

Notes:
Conventional schedules are based on the assumption that temperature of gas in tank is equal to ambient temperature. CGRI revised schedules are based on calculated temperature increase in the tank, making assumptions which minimize the calculated increases (see Figure 2). These calculations require enthalpy data.
(1) Methane; G = 0.554; enthalpy data from ASHRAE Handbook, 1977 Fundamentals, p. 16.47
(2) Typical pipeline-quality natural gas; G = 0.576
(3) Mean Bacton gas in the British Gas system; G = 0.5943; enthalpy data available for 14°F and above from British Gas Data Book, volume 1, 1974, section 5.

amounts of fuel obtained in each calculation cycle are summed to obtain the total amount of fuel dispensed during the fill.

The CGRI computer based filling pressure control method utilizes a proprietary mathematical model developed by CGRI. Each calculation cycle, the computer uses current flow information, as well as initial flow information, to estimate the pressure in the vehicle tank at that moment. The estimate of pressure is compared with the maximum allowable pressure, as per the schedule pre-programmed into the computer. When the estimated pressure reaches the maximum allowable pressure, the computer cuts off the fill by removing power from the electrically operated on-off valve downstream of the turbine meter.

12. FIELD TESTING OF THE CGRI DISPENSER

The computer, turbine meter, pressure and temperature sensors, Kraus display head, various valves and other fittings, and explosion proof housings and conduit system were assembled into a standard gasoline dispenser cabinet.

Through the cooperation of Consumers' Gas Co. Ltd. and its personnel, the CGRI dispenser was placed for field testing in March 1986 at the Mississauga, Ontario, facility of the company (Figure 3). From March 1986 to the time of writing, the dispenser has been used for fuelling of company vehicles.

The cabinet is intended to ultimately accommodate two hoses. Only the equipment for one hose has been installed for test purposes. Initially, a dome load valve was installed in the dispenser cabinet, downstream of the turbine meter.

The CGRI computer based filling pressure control method was developed to the point of readiness for field testing by February 1987. At that time the main program chip in the

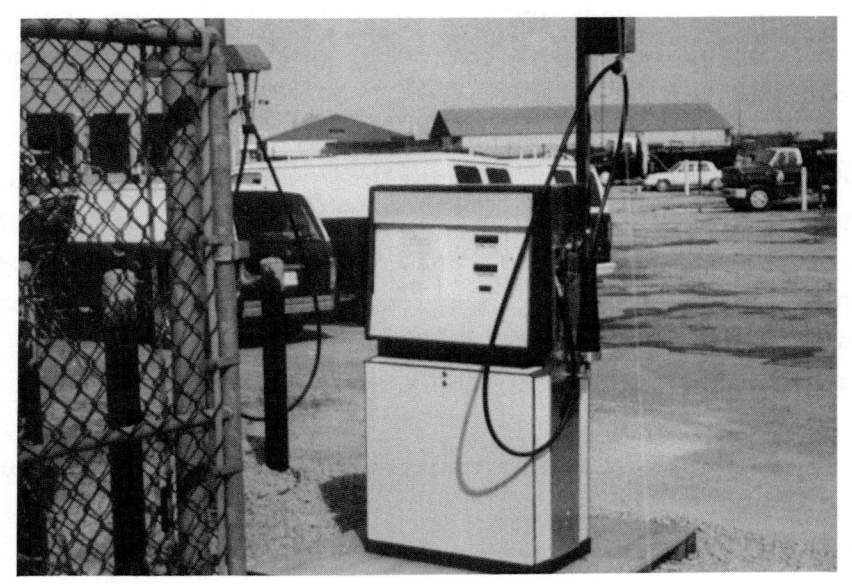

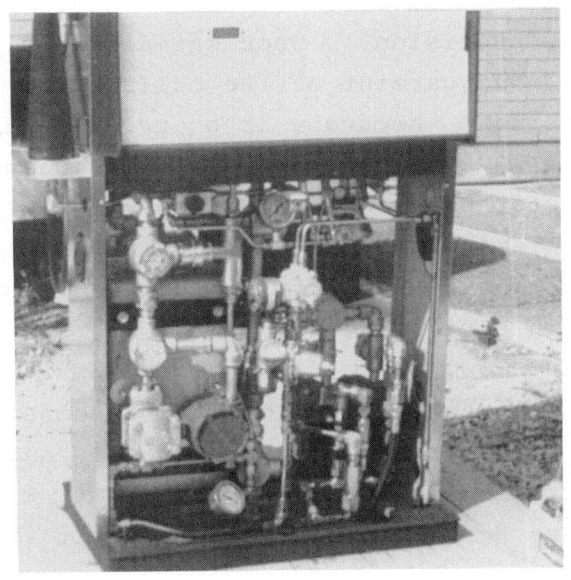

FIGURE 3 - CGRI DISPENSER AT FIELD TEST LOCATION

computer was replaced by a chip containing the required additional programming and the dome load valve was removed from the dispenser.

The CGRI dispenser is a stand-alone unit. All required components are located within the dispenser cabinet. There is no need to place electronic components or any other components in a separate location on the filling station premises. The connections required for operation of a two hose dispenser, according to the CGRI design, are:

- three gas supply lines, one from each of three storage banks
- 110 volt AC power.

13. PRECISION AND ACCURACY TESTING OF THE DISPENSER

As indicated in Section 4, the first concern in testing of the dispenser is precision. Once satisfactory precision can be demonstrated, adjustment of the calibration factor in the computer to achieve accuracy is a trivial exercise. In testing of the CGRI dispenser, minor changes in the calibration factor were not made on any regular basis. It was desired to make as few changes in the dispenser as possible, in order to simplify detection of any long term drift or trend in performance.

Precision and accuracy testing of the dispenser followed the same pattern as described in Sections 4 and 5 for the laboratory metering system. Values of R were again determined, where R is defined by equation 1.

On June 29, 1987, 14 tests were carried out. This series of tests is similar to series of tests carried out on many other occasions. The June 29 tests are of particular interest because the outdoor temperature and hence the flowing gas temperature varied substantially through the day. Also, because of varying patterns of use of the filling facility, the storage pressure varied through the day. The independent means of determination of the amount of fuel in the test tank was again the diaphragm meter as described in Section 5.

The gas in the fill hose at the end of a test fill has gone through the meter in the dispenser but does not go through the diaphragm meter. To reduce errors due to this effect, the hose pressure should be approximately the same before and after each test fill. The total amount of gas in each test on June 29 was under 5 kg in order to reduce the time required to "drain" the test tank out through the diaphragm meter. Part way through the series of tests, it was realized that differences in hose pressure could lead to significant errors under these conditions.

The June 29 tests are presented in Table 3. Run 5 is omitted from the discussion because it is definitely known that the hose pressures were greatly different before and after this test. For all other June 29 runs, the difference between the highest and lowest R values is 0.01767. Again in the informal terminology of Section 6, it can be said that the precision was ±0.8835%.

Starting with run 8, care was taken to ensure that hose pressures were the same before and after each test. For runs 8 through 14, the maximum range in R values is 0.00807 and the precision can be said to be ±0.4035% for these runs.

As a further check on dispenser performance, CGRI introduced a second independent means of determination of the amount of fuel in the test tank. In this procedure, a Sartorius Type 3807 MP8 electronic scale was used. This scale has a capacity of 60 000 grams and is claimed to be capable of a reproducibility of ±1 gram. This scale utilizes the force

TABLE 3 - DISPENSER TEST RESULTS

RUN	TEMPERATURE °F (1)	PRESSURE psig (1)	DISPENSER DISPLAY READING kg	R (2)
1	55	2500	4.716	0.99426
2	63	2700	4.752	0.99137
3	53	1900	4.845	0.98018
4	59	1900	4.310	0.98205
5	60	1700	3.836	0.97370
6	70	2000	3.918	0.97682
7	69	2200	3.889	0.97957
8	76	2500	3.967	0.99449
9	81	2800	4.327	0.99174
10	83	3000	4.157	0.99295
11	80	3100	4.069	0.98843
12	79	2900	3.930	0.98647
13	84	2900	4.321	0.99334
14	79	2800	4.336	0.98642

Notes:

(1) Typical flowing gas conditions during the test fill.

(2) The R values carry additional figures to avoid introducing a relatively large round-off error into the result of subtracting one R value from another.

coil principle, rather than load cells, as load cells are usually stated to be capable of no more than 1 part in 10 000 reproducibility.

An aluminum test tank weighing under 40 000 grams was used with the scale in order to reduce tare weight. The weight of the tank was distributed on the scale through use of two steel channel sections, as CGRI believes it is important to avoid pan distortion if the claimed reproducibility is to be achieved.

In the dispenser tests, the aluminum tank remained on the scale at all times. After each fill, the tank was disconnected from the dispenser. A short length of hose remained with the tank and was included in the weighing.

Tests with dead weights in the laboratory supported the manufacturer's claim of 1 gram reproducibility. In testing the dispenser at the field location, the scale reading was affected by gusts of wind. CGRI plans to utilize a temporary shelter in future tests, to eliminate this problem.

In four tests carried out on June 18, 1987, the difference between the highest and lowest R values was 0.0119. Therefore, the precision can be stated to be ±0.60%. In view of the wind effect, this result is regarded by CGRI as excellent and as a further confirmation of the satisfactory performance of the CGRI dispenser.

Application was made to the Legal Metrology Branch of Consumer and Corporate Affairs Canada for approval of type for the CGRI dispenser. On March 26, 1987, 13 tests were carried out by Consumer and Corporate Affairs personnel. The independent means of determination of the amount of fuel in the test tank in these tests was a scale based on load cells.

The test tank is weighed, removed from the scale, filled, and then replaced on the scale.

The range of R values in the government tests was 0.065 and so the precision was determined as ±3.25%. This result was of course not satisfactory to Consumer and Corporate Affairs or to CGRI. It must be remembered that random error in both the dispenser and the independent test equipment contribute additively to the random error seen in values of R. In CGRI tests, values of R showed a precision substantially better than ±1%. CGRI therefore puts forward the hypothesis that the independent equipment used in the Consumer and Corporate Affairs tests, namely the scale based on load cells, contributed substantially to the poor precision noted in values of R resulting from these tests.

As of this writing, a new application has been made to the Legal Metrology Branch.

14. TESTING OF THE CGRI FILLING PRESSURE CONTROL METHOD

The principle of the method can be tested equally well using either the ambient temperature or the flowing gas temperature. In utilizing the CGRI dispenser as a test bed for the filling pressure control method, it was convenient to utilize the flowing gas temperature, in order to avoid having to add a sensor and computer input port for ambient temperature. CGRI believes that in actual practice, for maximum safety, any filling pressure control method should be based on the ambient temperature.

Similarly, the principle can be tested equally well using any pressure versus temperature schedule. The conventional schedule (Table 2) was programmed into the computer for the test program.

Filling of Consumers' Gas vehicles from February 1987 to the time of writing was entirely under the control of the CGRI filling pressure control method. There was no dome load valve anywhere in the system. On the order of 5 to 10 vehicles use the dispenser daily. During this period of time, CGRI did not receive any complaints of over- or under-filling.

On occasion, CGRI personnel visited the test site to monitor fills. Measurements of flowing gas temperature and pressure were made during fills, using equipment totally independent of and separate from the temperature and pressure sensors utilized by the computer. The pressure gauge installed on each vehicle was read before each fill and immediately after gas flow stopped at the end of each fill.

From the flowing gas temperature as observed by CGRI personnel, the maximum allowed pressure was determined from Table 2 (conventional schedule (2)). This pressure was compared with the pressure reading on the vehicle gauge at the end of the fill, in order to check whether the CGRI filling pressure control method was performing in a satisfactory manner.

The vehicle gauges are known to be somewhat inaccurate, but were deemed acceptable since absolute accuracy is not required of the filling pressure control method either.

A typical set of monitoring results is presented in Table 4. These results indicate that the CGRI filling pressure control method is performing well.

At the time of writing, CGRI was nearing completion of an improved version of the program, which would allow more accurate determination of the initial flow conditions and

TABLE 4 - TEST RESULTS - FILLING PRESSURE CONTROL

DATE 1987	RUN NUMBER	OUTDOOR TEMP °F	VEHICLE PRESSURE BEFORE FILL, psig	LOW BANK (1)	LOW BANK (2)	MEDIUM BANK (3)	MEDIUM BANK (4)	HIGH BANK (5)	HIGH BANK (6)	ACTUAL FINAL VEHICLE PRESSURE	TARGET FINAL VEHICLE PRESSURE (7)
Apr 8	1	36	0	36	2800	36	2800	35	2700	2600	2560
	2	36	700		2300	32	2500	31	2550	2400	2510
Apr 14	1	42	1000	42	3300	42	3200			3000	2650 (8)
	2	44	600	38	3000	41	3100		3200	2700	2650(8)(9)
	3	44	300	40	2700	43	3200	43	3200	2650	2660
	4	45	1000	45	3000				3300	2700	2660 (10)
	5	46	0	40	2800	43	3200		3200	2650	2660 (10)
	6	46	100	28	2300	38	2900	40	2500	2500	2620 (11)
Jun 29	1	62	0	57	3000				3400	3200	2870 (12)
	2	64	600	50	2600	59	3200	59	2900	2700	2870

Notes:

All temperatures and pressures in this table (except column (7)) were manually recorded by CGRI personnel during vehicle fills. Missing data in the table are due to inadequate time to record all data during the rapidly progressing vehicle fills.

(1) Flowing gas temperature just before the switch to Medium bank.
(2) Flowing gas pressure just before the switch to Medium bank.
(3) Flowing gas temperature just before the switch to High bank.
(4) Flowing gas pressure just before the switch to High bank.
(5) Flowing gas temperature immediately after the switch to High bank. (Immediately upon switching to a next higher bank, the computer makes a new determination of the target vehicle pressure).
(6) Flowing gas pressure just before the end of the fill - the clearest demonstration of the CGRI filling pressure control method occurs when this pressure is substantially higher than actual final vehicle pressure.
(7) Determined manually by reference to Table 2 at the temperature in column (5) (conventional schedule (2)).
(8) Temperature assumed to be 42°F.
(9) Fill was stopped by computer virtually simultaneously with switch to High bank; therefore difficult to know what temperature the computer was using to determine the target vehicle pressure.
(10) Very clear-cut examples of computer control; temperature assumed to be 43°F.
(11) Flow rate was low at the end of the fill, but the fill was definitely stopped by computer control. Equivalence of pressures may be only apparent, as the gauges used are typically good only to ±100 psi.
(12) If vehicle gauge was correct, it must be concluded that this fill was allowed to go too far.

hence would enable the computer to control the filling process more accurately.

It must be emphasized that the CGRI filling pressure control method can be added to any dispenser, regardless of metering principle used. If the dispenser does not already have sensors for ambient temperature, and for flowing gas temperature and pressure, these would have to be added. The details of the mathematical manipulation of the signals from these sensors are slightly different for different metering principles. It is not necessary that fills be stopped at exactly the correct pressure. A deviation of 5 to 10% could readily be tolerated while still assuring complete safety. Therefore, inexpensive temperature and pressure sensors can be used to implement the method.

15. CONCLUSIONS

CGRI believes that the results of its development program demonstrate that the turbine meter is viable as a basis for a dispenser for natural gas for motor vehicle use. Turbine based dispensers can readily be offered in a stand-alone version and higher flow rates for fuelling of heavy vehicles can be accommodated.

The CGRI computer based filling pressure control method constitutes significant new technology for the natural gas for vehicles industry. It offers many advantages over the dome load valve, including reduced fill time, reduced plumbing complexity, reduced maintenance, and ability to accommodate an infinite variety of pressure versus temperature schedules.

16. REFERENCE

1. A.G.A. Manual for the Determination of Supercompressibility Factors for Natural Gas, PAR Research Project NX-19, 1980 edition.

Propriétés du gaz naturel
Natural gas properties

IMPORTANCE OF HYDRATES TO THE GAS INDUSTRY

D.B. Robinson
DB Robinson & Associates Ltd.
Edmonton, Alberta, Canada

INTRODUCTION

Clathrates are a class of solid compounds whose molecules are interlocked through hydrogen bonds to form a three dimensional lattice-like structure. The molecules forming the structure are thought of as "host" molecules and those occupying the cavities in the structure are called "guest" molecules. When the "host" molecules are water, the clathrate is called a hydrate.

The existence of gas hydrates has been known for over 175 years, ever since their discovery and study by scientists such as Sir Humphrey Davy (1) and Michael Faraday (3) in the early 1800's. However, until the rapid development of the automobile and consequently the petroleum industry in North America in the 1930's, hydrates were largely regarded as a scientific curiosity. At this time the problems hydrates could create in the production, transportation and processing of natural gas and oil were soon recognized.

The increased awareness of hydrates and their importance to industry has prompted many experimental and theoretical studies on incipient hydrate formation, hydrate decomposition, hydrate inhibition and all related matters. In addition, as part of the ever-increasing quest for supplementary sources of energy, a great deal of effort is being expended in identifying the reserves of gas presently locked in the earth's crust particularly in northern latitudes and beneath the floor of the deeper oceans of the world.

The purpose of this paper is to provide an overview of the importance of gas hydrates to the natural gas industry, both from the point of view of the problems they create and of the potential energy source they represent.

2.0 <u>HYDRATE STRUCTURE AND CHARACTERISTICS</u>

As indicated above, gas hydrates are inclusion compounds in which one component fits into a cavity formed by water. They are solid and resemble ice or snow in appearance but they form both above and below the freezing point of water, depending on the nature of the hydrating compounds.

It was not until relatively recently that the molecular architecture of hydrates became known in detail through the use of molecular models and X-ray diffraction techniques. In hydrates the water molecules are linked together into rings and the pentagonal planes thus formed join to form dodecahedra. Such a unit cell structure is shown schematically in Figure 1. The dodecahedra may be arranged in either of two cubic crystal systems, generally referred to as hydrate Structure I or hydrate Structure II.

The configuration of the Structure I crystal is also shown schematically in Figure 1. It may be seen that the dodecahedra cannot be arranged without leaving some interstitial space. This space gives rise in Structure I to tetrakaidecahedron (14 faces, 2 hexagonal and 12 pentagonal) cavities and in structure II to hexakaidecahedron (16 faces, 4 hexagonal and 12 pentagonal) cavities.

The significant fact about these crystal structures is that the cavity dimensions impose limits on the nature of gases that form hydrates. Small molecules like nitrogen, methane and hydrogen sulfide will fit into all the spaces, whereas other molecules like ethane and carbon dioxide will only fit into the tetra- and hexakaidecahedra and propane and isobutane will only fit into the hexakaidecahedra. Larger molecules like pentane and heavier hydrocarbons will not form hydrates because they are too large to fit into the lattice.

Whenever water and any hydrating molecules such as those indicated above are brought together within a range of specific temperatures and pressures, the solid hydrate will become stable and the crystals will grow indefinitely as long as water and hydrating molecules are simultaneously available. The specific range of temperatures and pressures where hydration can occur varies with the nature of the gas or the gas mixture containing the hydrate forming molecules.

The most convenient way to envisage the various regions of hydrate formation for the components of natural gas is by means of a pressure-temperature diagram such as that shown in Figure 2. This diagram is indicative of hydrate formation in the presence of materials like methane. The line ABC separates regions of stable hydrate formation to the left from regions where hydrates do not form to the right. Thus the line ABC represents a pressure-temperature locus of incipient hydrate crystal formation.

The line BD separates the region to the right where hydrates form in the presence of aqueous liquid from the region to the left where hydrates form in the presence of ice. The point represented by B is a unique condition where hydrate, ice, gas and aqueous liquid can co-exist.

An example of hydrate forming conditions in a methane-rich gas mixture is shown in Figure 3. This figure shows the pressures and temperatures where hydrates commence to form in methane and in gaseous mixtures of methane and propane in the presence of liquid water. It is interesting to note the way relatively small amounts of propane cause a dramatic decrease in the hydrate forming pressure at a specified temperature. For example at a temperature of 7°C, 1 percent propane reduces the initial hydrate forming pressure from 5.10 MPa to 3.08 MPa, a reduction of 40 percent.

Figure 4 shows schematically where hydrates may form in a natural gas mixture which can condense at temperatures where hydrates may form. As in Figure 2, the line ABCDE separates regions of hydrate formation from regions where hydrates do not form. The line FGDCH forms a boundary between the region where condensate liquids exist from the region where they do not. Aqueous liquid, condensate liquid and gas exist anywhere within the envelope FGDCH but along the locus CD and to the left of this line hydrates may also exist. Above point D and to the left of line DE, hydrates exist in the presence of aqueous liquid and the dense natural gas fluid. The line BJ separates the region of ice from aqueous liquid.

An example of initial hydrate forming conditions in an actual condensate-type fluid is shown in Figure 5. This gas contains over 70 percent methane together with substantial quantities of carbon dioxide, ethane and other heavier hydrocarbons. In this case the aqueous solution contains 35 percent methanol by weight and the initial hydrate forming locus traverses the phase envelope for the natural gas as it crosses the lower dew point locus at about 1.3 MPa and -18°C, and the retrograde dew point locus at about 7.0 MPa and -6°C. Within the phase envelope, hydrates form in the presence of aqueous liquid, hydrocarbon liquid and gas. Above the retrograde dew point locus, hydrates exist in the presence of aqueous liquid and the dense gas fluid phase.

3.0 SIGNIFICANCE OF HYDRATE FORMATION TO INDUSTRIAL GAS OPERATIONS

From the foregoing, it will be readily appreciated that the production, transportation and processing of natural gas and related systems frequently take place at conditions where hydrates can form. In practice these situations must be identified so that remedial measures can be taken before serious problems resulting from the obstruction or plugging of pipelines, heat exchangers or other process equipment develop.

Production Problems

It is well known that many of the world's larger gas reserves lie under water in offshore locations such as the North Sea, the Coast of Alaska, the Gulf of Mexico and elsewhere. The temperature at the ocean floor is normally in the 0° to 5°C range and the fluid pressures in the production tubing are well within the range of hydrate formation at these temperatures. During normal operation when the production facilities and the separator facilities are in the same location, the temperature of the produced fluids may be high enough to prevent hydrate formation. However, during upsets in the production program or during shutdowns, the production tubing can approach the ocean temperature, whereupon hydrate formation followed by plugging may occur.

A related problem in gas production arises when the effluent from several wells is sent by under water pipeline to a central location for separation and partial treating. Owing to the distances involved, the temperature of the pipeline contents will reach the hydrate forming temperature even during normal operation. In this case the pipeline may become inoperable due to plugging. In cases where remedial measures are taken, such as the addition of methanol to depress the hydrate forming temperature to safe levels, plugging could still result in the event of failure of the methanol injection facilities.

The resolution of the problem of a plugged pipeline in any of the above situations can be extremely time consuming and in some cases prohibitively expensive.

Hydrate problems similar to those described above are rarely encountered at normal onshore production facilities. This is largely because in most geographical locations, the reservoir fluid temperatures, even by the time the wellhead and separator facilities are reached, are well out of range of hydrate formation. This would not be the case however where light hydrocarbon mixtures or carbon dioxide are used in enhanced oil recovery operations*. Here, the prepared injection fluids would be delivered by pipeline and injected under ground. During this process, the relatively cool fluids contact normal ground temperatures which would be in the 3° to 8°C range. At the injection pressures required, hydrates could easily form in the injection piping unless dehydration or inhibition were practiced. Inhibition creates an additional problem here because the inhibitor would disappear into the formation and could rarely if ever be recovered.

In northern regions of the world where a layer of permafrost exists, problems of hydrate formation may be encountered both during drilling and production operations. Figure 6 illustrates schematically how the layer of permafrost may vary in depth as one moves from South to North along a line of longitude. The diagram shows how hydrates could exist in the rock formations where both the temperature and pressure are such that hydrates would be stable whenever water and light hydrocarbons co-exist.

---

* Although enhanced oil recovery would not be practiced in a true natural gas well, it would be practiced in other situations where the produced gas from the gas-oil mixture can be regarded as natural gas.

In drilling operations, if the drill bit encounters a region where hydrates exist, gas will be generated when the warmer drilling fluids come in contact with the hydrate zone causing decomposition. Special precautions must be taken to deal with these situations in such a way that the evolved gas does not cause a blowout. A further related problem may result when the drill enters the producing formation allowing the release of hydrocarbons into the drilling fluid. When the hydrocarbon-drilling fluid mixture reaches a hydrate forming zone, partial or total plugging of the circulation passages may result.

Transportation Problems

Hydrate problems may occur during the transportation and storage of natural gas and hydrocarbon liquids in much the same way as they do during production.

Figure 7 illustrates schematically a typical situation where gas and liquid streams leaving a separator battery may contribute to hydrate formation. Here the gas and liquid streams A and B respectively are dehydrated separately in conventional equipment and following dehydration are recombined before entering an underground pipeline. Owing to the dehydration process, no free water phase would exist at the pipeline temperature. However, the residual water content of the recombined stream C may be sufficient to cause hydrate formation in the gas-hydrate region. In a typical example the pipeline flow conditions were at a pressure of 9.65 MPa (1400 psia) and a buried pipeline temperature of approximately 5°C (41°F). Calculations showed that hydrates would form in the presence of the residual water content at a temperature of 15°C (59°F) although they would have formed at 29°C (84.2°F) if a liquid water phase had been present.

Another example illustrating the importance of hydrate formation in transportation process may be found by referring to Figure 8. Here, liquefied petroleum gases are stored underground, for example in washed out salt caverns. The temperature reached in these storage facilities is typically in the 55° to 60°C (131° to 140°F). The stored products will ultimately become saturated with water at these temperatures. This temperature is too high for hydrate formation. However, as the fluids are produced to the surface, probably by injection of surface water through an annular piping system, a heat exchanger is created such that the hydrocarbon stream may reach a temperature and pressure where hydrates could form.

In addition to this problem, if the hydrocarbon product is transported by underground pipeline at typical ground temperatures (say 5°C (41°F)) after recovery from the storage cavern, hydrate formation could occur at the prevailing pipeline pressure. This represents hydrate formation in the liquid-liquid-hydrate region as illustrated previously in Figure 4. Partial or complete plugging of the pipeline could result.

Processing Problems

The possibility of hydrate formation always exists in natural gas processing plants. Typical processing conditions involve temperatures from well above ambient to as low as -100°C (-180°F). Clearly, the possibility of hydrate formation in the liquid-gas-hydrate, liquid-liquid-hydrate and ice-gas-hydrate region exists.

Figure 9 illustrates schematically an arrangement whereby the possibility of hydrate formation necessitates removal of water and/or the addition of an inhibitor such as ethylene glycol. This is a typical situation where gas is chilled in a propane cooler prior to separation and subsequent fractionation of the resulting liquid.

Another common example where extensive front-end treating for water removal is practised is in a typical turbo-expander low temperature processing plant. Here the possibility of hydrate formation, ice formation or solid carbon dioxide formation exists.

Hydrate Prevention

It will perhaps be obvious from the wide range and variety of situations described above where hydrate problems arise in natural gas handling that a great deal of effort and expense goes into minimizing the potential difficulties. Two major remedial measures are taken, namely water removal by separation and dehydration, and suppression of hydrate formation through the use of inhibitors such as methanol or ethylene glycol.

Normally, water removal is practised at production and other surface facilities where glycol contacting and/or dry desicants can be used. Water removal by molecular sieves is invariably used ahead of very low temperature processing facilities.

When natural gas is being transported by pipeline where underground temperatures are below 0°C, an additional problem arises because of the possible presence of hydrates. When the temperature of water is below 0°C, the stable phase is normally ice over which an equilibrium partial pressure of pure water is established. However, in the presence of natural gas at temperatures below 0°C, the thermodynamically stable phase is hydrate and the equilibrium partial pressure of water vapor over hydrate is less than it is for ice at the same conditions. This means that dehydration must be carried out to lower water vapor values if the gas transmission line is expected to encounter sub-freezing temperatures.

These characteristics are shown in a semi-quantitative way in Figure 10. Here, the maximum amount of water allowable in the gas without condensation, hydrate formation or ice formation is indicated by the constant pressure lines. For example, if one imagines following the 1000 psia isobar from a temperature where liquid water might condense to lower temperatures, it will be seen that the hydrate-liquid-gas locus will be crossed. At that temperature, it is possible for hydrate, liquid and ice to co-exist. However, if the temperature is lowered further, only hydrate and gas can co-exist.

In situations where water removal is impractical, such as in sub-sea gathering systems or in certain medium-temperature process applications, the use of methanol or ethylene glycol as hydrate inhibitors is practised. The extent to which methanol can reduce the temperature where hydrates will form in the presence of methane is illustrated in Figure 11. Each line shown on the graph represents the locus of incipient hydrate formation temperatures and pressures in the presence of various concentrations of methanol in the aqueous liquid phase. It will be seen that at a pressure of 6.89 MPa (1000 psia), the initial hydrate forming temperature is reduced from about 10°C (50°F) in pure water to -10°C (14°F) in a 50 wt. percent methanol solution. Figure 12 shows the reduction in hydrate forming temperature in a gas condensate-type system using ethylene glycol. Here, at 6.89 MPa (1000 psia), the temperature is reduced from 17.8°C (64°F) in pure water to -2.8°C (27°F) in the presence of 50 wt. percent ethylene glycol.

Hydrates as a Source of Energy

The foregoing has caste the importance of hydrates to the gas industry in an unfavorable light because the emphasis has been on the problems they can create through all aspects of the industry. However, there is another side to the story, namely that hydrates represent possibly the largest storage reservoir of gas known to exist in the earth's crust. These reserves have arisen in two ways. The first through the growth of hydrates in perma-frost regions and the second under the deep oceans of the world.

Hydrates in Perma-Frost Regions

Perma-frost regions occur where the mean temperature of the atmosphere is below 0°C (32°F). In these regions, thick layers of frozen ground can develop as shown schematically in Figure 6. The thickness of this layer will tend to decrease as one moves away from the polar region, finally disappearing at warmer latitudes. As the crust of the earth is penetrated, the temperature will gradually increase according to the geothermal gradient, ultimately exceeding 0°C and reaching higher temperatures at greater depths.

In addition to the variation in temperature with depth, the pressure will also increase, generally in accordance with the hydraulic gradient at a rate of about 0.3 MPa (43 psia) per 31 m (100 ft). Thus depth can be related to pressure such that, for example, 500 m (1600 ft) would correspond to about 4.8 MPa (700 psia). At this pressure, in a gas containing methane with small amounts of propane or other hydrocarbons, hydrates would form at approximately 13° to 15°C (55° to 59°F).

It is clear from these temperature-pressure considerations that a zone could exist within which formation water and hydrate forming components in gas or oil could form a band or layer of hydrates. These solid hydrates would represent large volumes of trapped natural gas. Calculations show that each cubic meter of hydrate, upon decomposition, would release about 160 standard m^3 of natural gas.

Estimates of the total amount of natural gas that may exist in hydrates associated with perma-frost regions are based on very limited data. Suffice it to say, however, that even the more conservative estimates indicate enormous amounts. The average of estimates made by three different authorities (6) are [$3.5(10^{13})$ standard m^3] ($1.2(10^{15})$ standard ft^3).

Hydrates in Offshore Locations

Hydrates of natural gas may occur naturally in sediments beneath the world's oceans where temperatures are near 0°C and where water depths of over about 500 m (1600 ft) prevail, i.e. at pressures over about 4.8 MPa (700 psia). It is postulated that decaying organic matter falls to the ocean floor where over geologic time it releases methane and possibly some carbon dioxide. At the prevailing temperature and pressure these gases hydrate and ultimately occupy a significant portion of the sediment volume up to depths in the order of 300 m (1000 ft).

Naturally occurring hydrates of natural gas have been (1983) reported in 24 different locations, primarily along the Atlantic and Pacific-Continental shelf off North and South America and in the Black Sea. Their presence has been inferred offshore in Japan, Australia, New Zealand, Angola and Oman (6). Again, estimates of the total volume of gas existing in hydrated form in offshore locations vary widely but appear to be in the range of $3-9(10^{15})$ standard m^3 ($1-3(10^{17})$ standard ft^3).

Recovery of Natural Gas from Hydrate Deposits

An accurate assessment of the reserves of natural gas stored in the form of hydrate requires considerably more knowledge than presently exists on the potential reservoir properties. This knowledge is not readily obtained because the deposits tend to be in remote and inaccessible places. Because of the lack of data, estimates of the total reserves vary widely. However, when it is realized that these estimated reserves, however uncertain, are several orders of magnitude greater than the U.S. Geological Survey's estimate of the world's proven reserves of natural gas (6), it becomes obvious that they must at least be given serious consideration and that they must be included in the long-term estimates of total energy resources.

The difficulties faced in producing natural gas from hydrates are similar in many respects to those encountered in producing heavy oil from tar sand deposits. The fundamental problem in both cases is the inability to deliver the required energy to release the gas or oil to the location where it is needed. It has only been in recent years that energy reserves such as these have been considered sufficiently important to justify serious study and expenditure. Much work has been done and is being done on calculating the net energy balance that would result if the hydrates could be decomposed either by depressurization or by the application of heat. The results of the calculations depend largely on the assumptions that are made but generally indicate a net recoverable energy of about 1.4 to 1.8 gigajoules/m^3 of reservoir (40,000 to 50,000 BTU/ft^3 of reservoir).

However remote the possiblity of achieving an energy release of this magnitude may be, it would appear to justify intensive efforts to achieve it.

REFERENCES

(1) Davy, H., "On Some of the Combinations of Oxymuriatic Gas and Oxygene, and on the Chemical Relations of These Principles, to Inflammable Bodies," Phil. Trans. Roy. Soc. London, 101, 1 (1811).

(2) Deaton, W.M. and Frost, E.M. Jr., "Hydrates of Natural Gas, Pure Gases and Synthetic Gas Mixtures," Proc. Nat. Gas Dept., American Gas Association, 122 (1940).

(3) Faraday, M., "On Fluid Chlorine," Phil. Trans. Roy. Soc. London, 113, 160 (1823).

(4) Frost, E.M. Jr. and Deaton, W.M., "Gas Hydrate Composition and Equilibrium Data," Proc. Nat. Gas Dept., American Gas Association, 49 (1946).

(5) Kobayashi, R. and Katz, D.L., "Methane Hydrate at High Pressure," Petroleum Transactions AIME, 186, 66 (1949).

(6) Lewin and Associates, Inc., "Handbook of Gas Hydrate Properties and Occurrence," United States Department of Energy, Office of Fossil Energy, Morgantown, West Virginia, DOE/MC/19239-1546, 233 pp., 1983.

(7) Ng, H.-J. and Robinson, D.B., "Equilibrium Phase Composition and Hydrating Conditions in Systems Containing Methanol, Light Hydrocarbons, Carbon Dioxide, and Hydrogen Sulfide," Gas Processors Association Research Report RR-66, April, 1983.

(8) Ng, H.-J., Chen, C.-J. and Robinson, D.B., "The Effect of Ethylene Glycol or Methanol on Hydrate Formation in Systems Containing Ethane, Propane, Carbon Dioxide, Hydrogen Sulfide or a Typical Gas Condensate," Gas Processors Association Research Report RR-92, September, 1985.

(9) Ng, H.-J. and Robinson, D.B., "The Influence of Methanol on Hydrate Formation at Low Temperatures," Gas Processors Association Research Report RR-74, March, 1984 and RR-74 (Revised), February, 1986.

(10) Ng, H.-J., Chen, C.-J. and Robinson, D.B., "Vapor Liquid Equilibrium and Condensing Curves for a Gas Condensate Containing Nitrogen," Gas Processors Association Research Report RR-105, 31 pp., April, 1987.

(11) Wu, B.J., Robinson, D.B. and Ng, H.-J., "Three- and Four-Phase Hydrate Forming Conditions in the Methane-Isobutane-Water System," J. Chem. Thermodynamics, $\underline{8}$, 461-469 (1976).

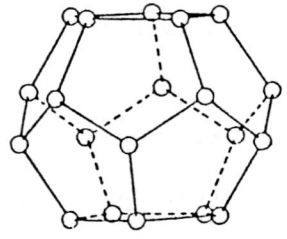

PENTAGONAL DODECAHEDRON

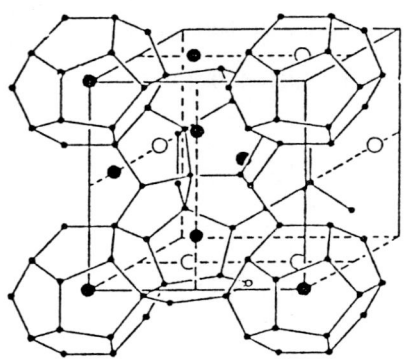

STRUCTURE I CRYSTAL

FIGURE 1   SCHEMATIC REPRESENTATION OF
           STRUCTURE I HYDRATE CRYSTAL

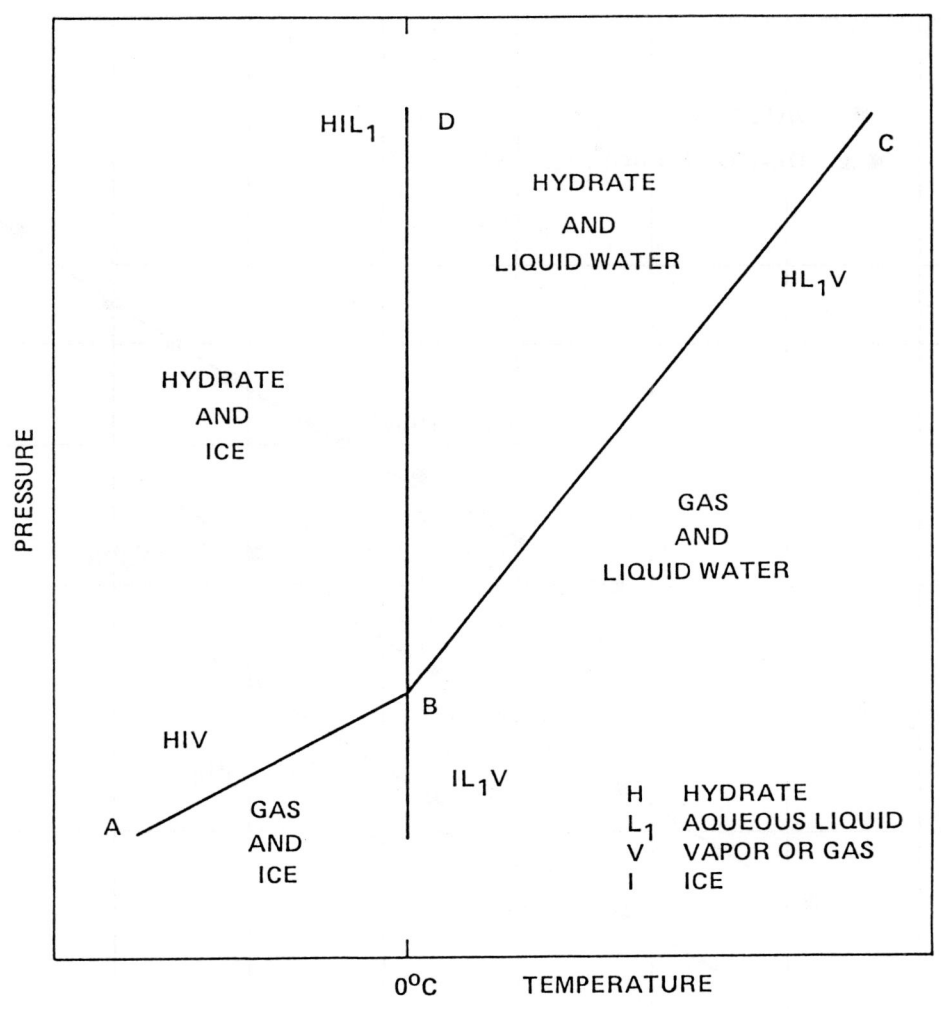

FIGURE 2 SCHEMATIC ILLUSTRATION OF HYDRATE FORMING CONDITIONS IN A SIMPLE SYSTEM

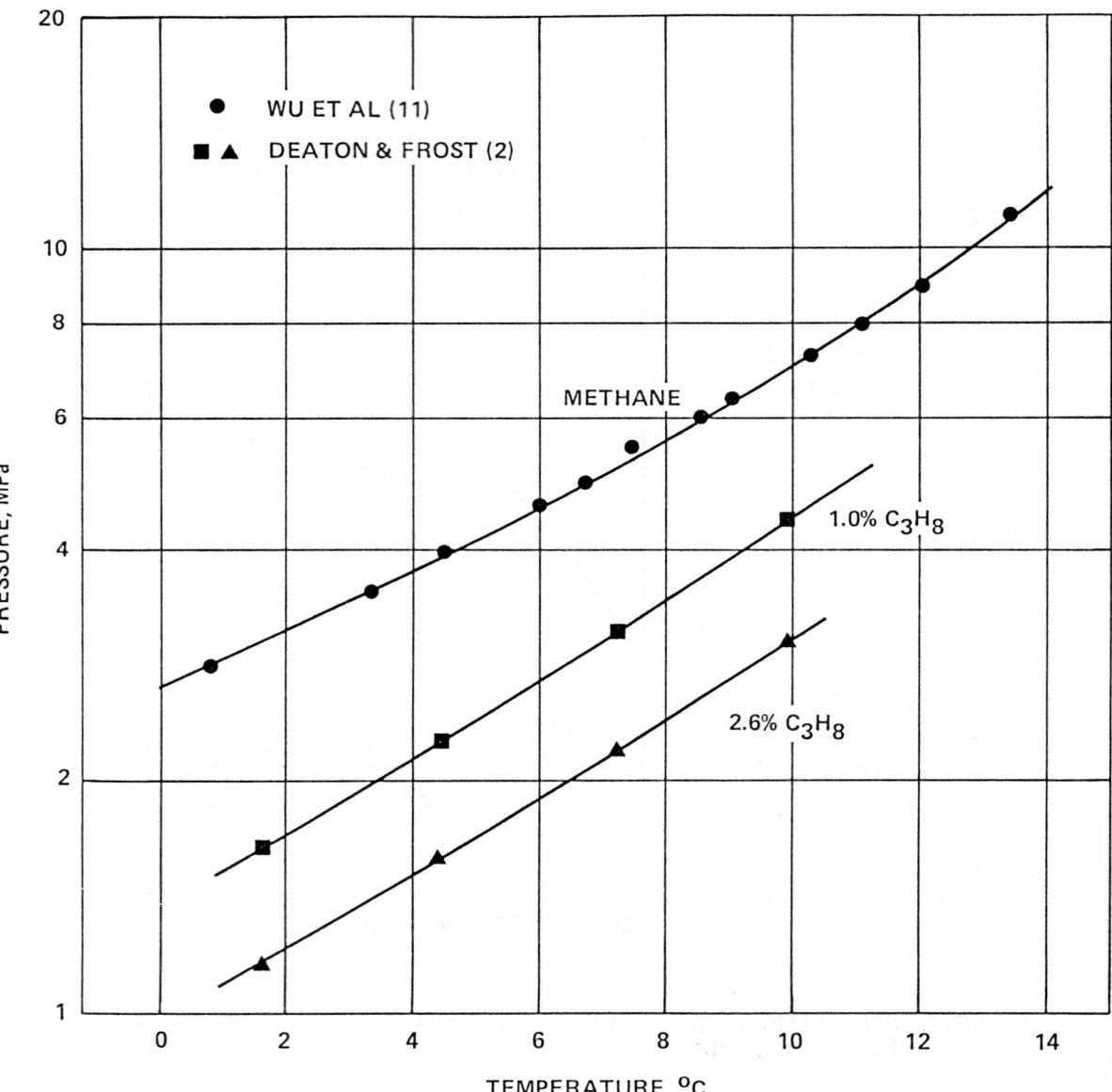

FIGURE 3 HYDRATE FORMATION IN MIXTURES OF METHANE AND PROPANE

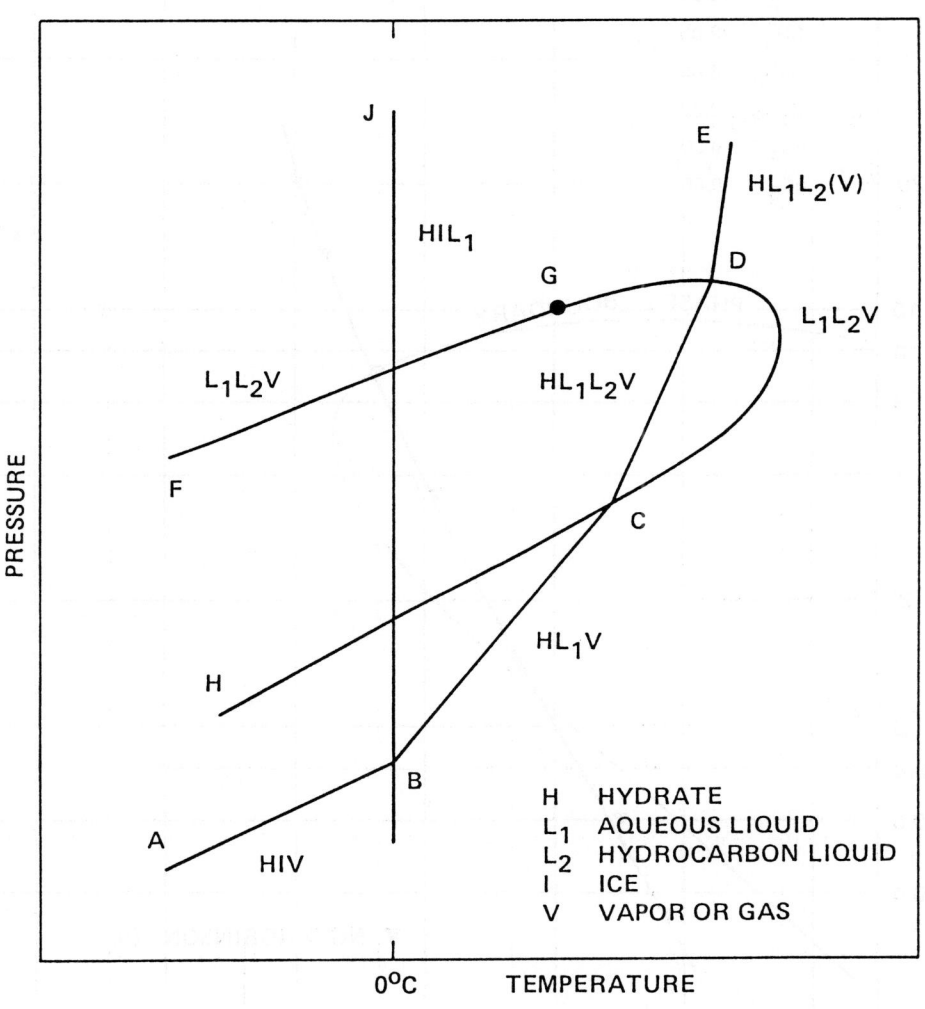

FIGURE 4 SCHEMATIC ILLUSTRATION OF HYDRATE FORMATION IN A TYPICAL GAS CONDENSATE SYSTEM

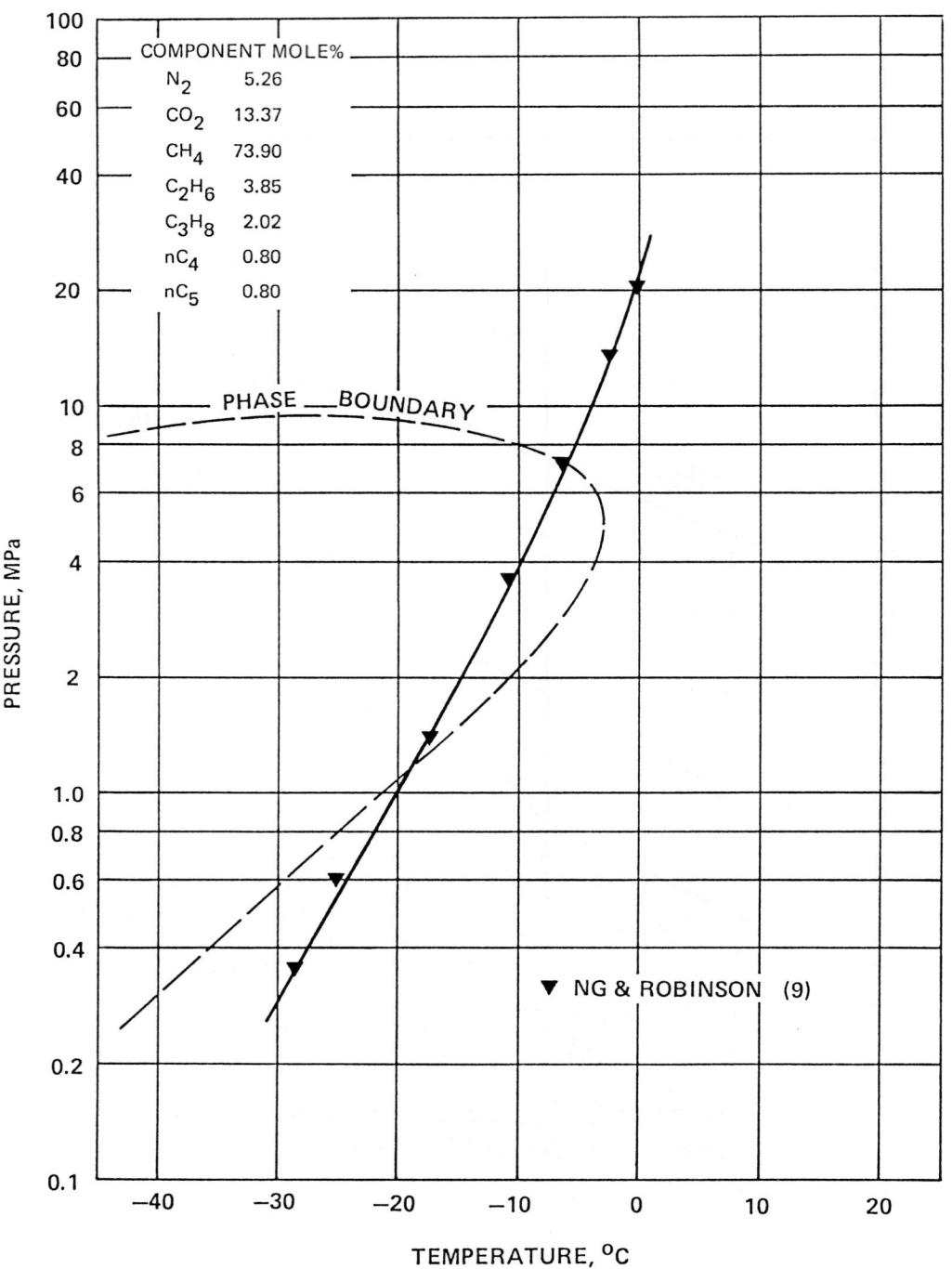

FIGURE 5   HYDRATE FORMATION IN A SIMULATED NATURAL GAS MIXTURE

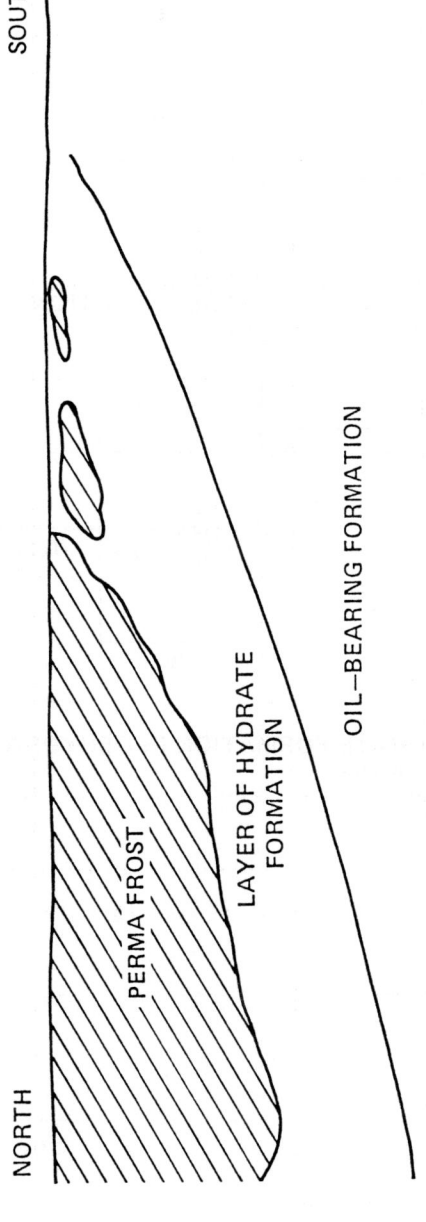

FIGURE 6 SCHEMATIC ILLUSTRATION OF HYDRATE FORMATION IN PERMA FROST REGIONS

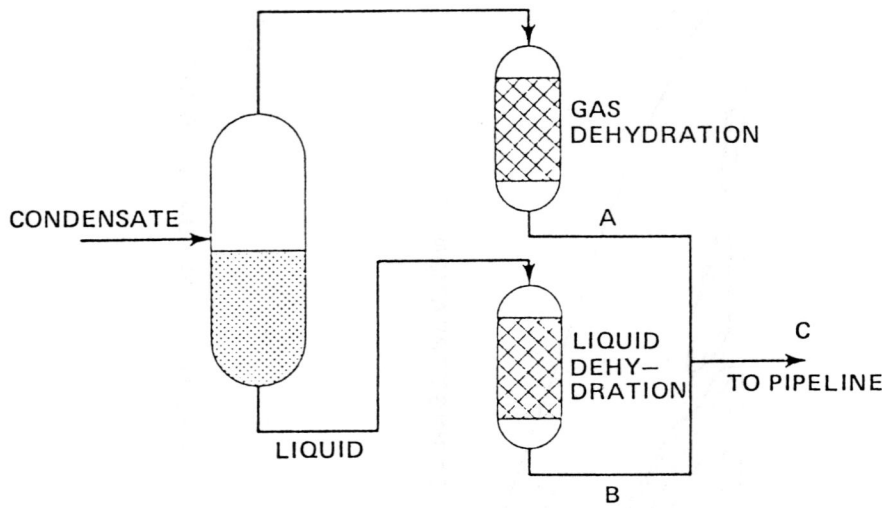

FIGURE 7 POTENTIAL HYDRATE FORMATION IN DEHYDRATED SEPARATOR STREAMS

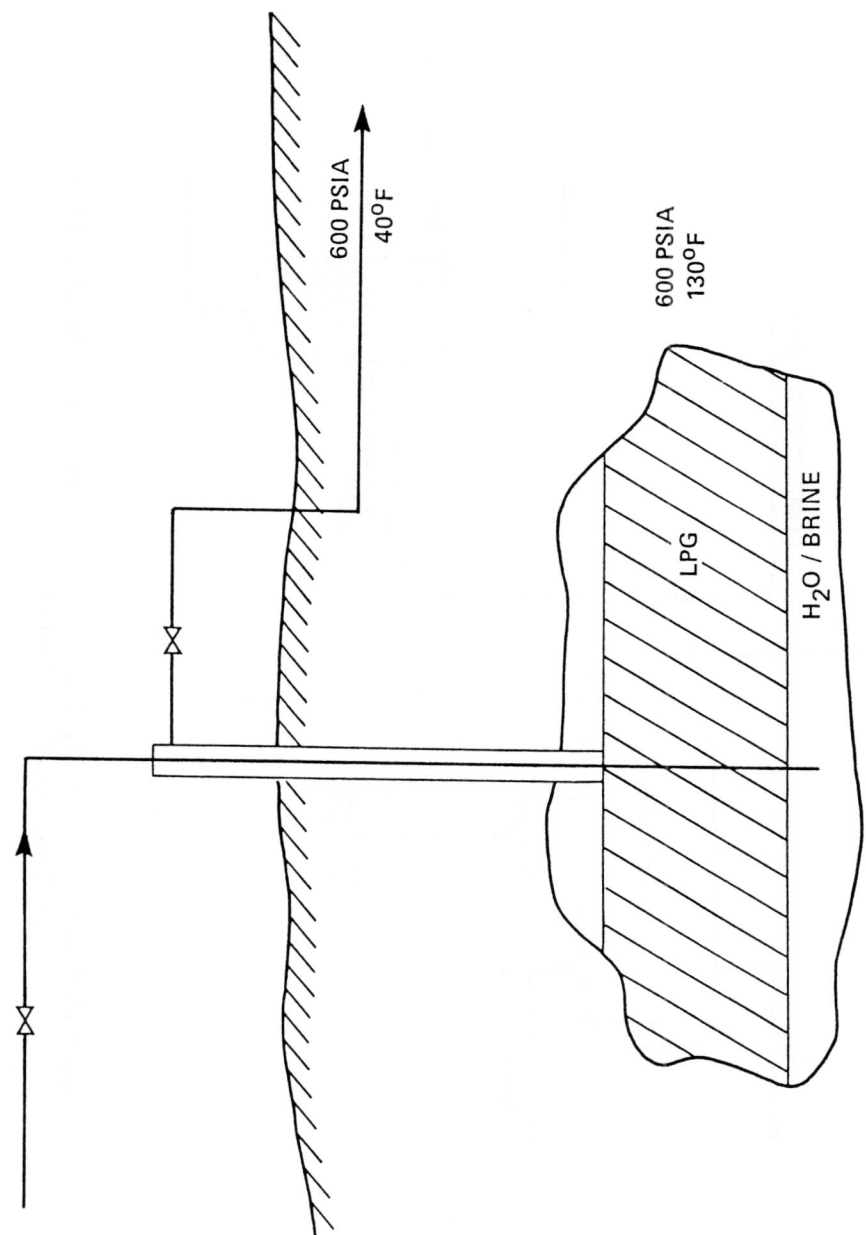

FIGURE 8 HYDRATE FORMING PROBLEMS IN LIQUIFIED PETROLEUM GAS STORAGE

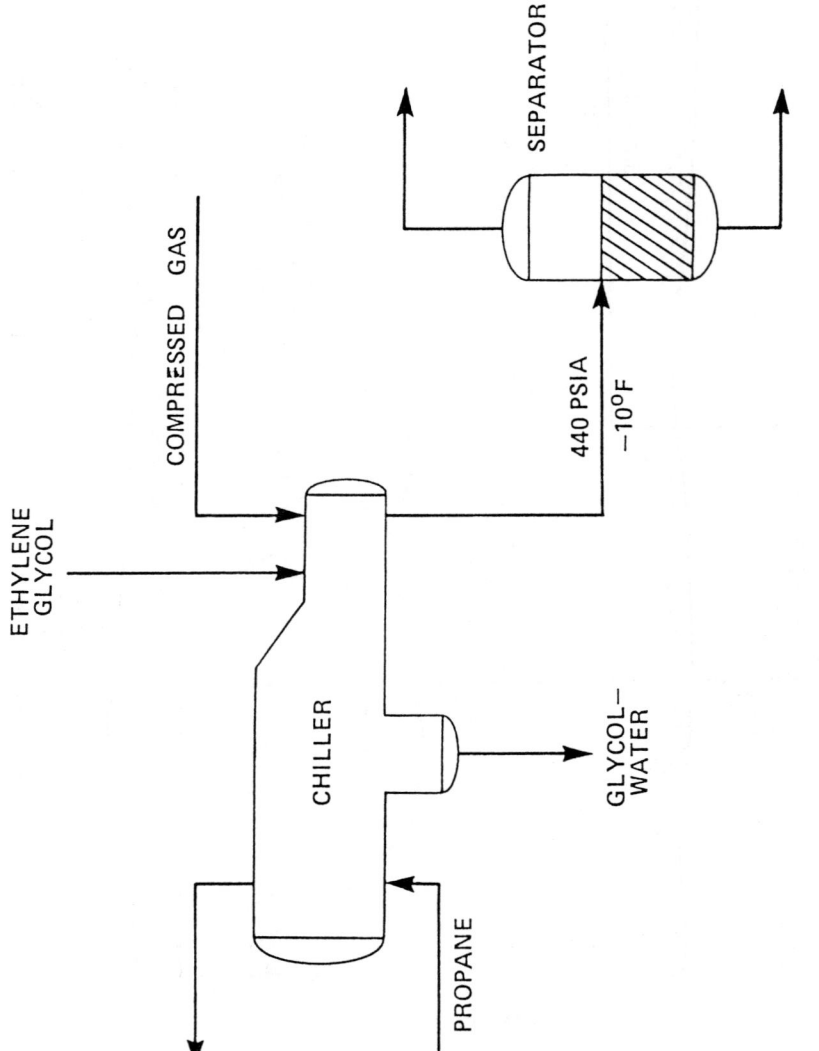

FIGURE 9 CONTROL OF HYDRATE FORMATION USING ETHYLENE GLYCOL IN A GAS PROCESSING PLANT

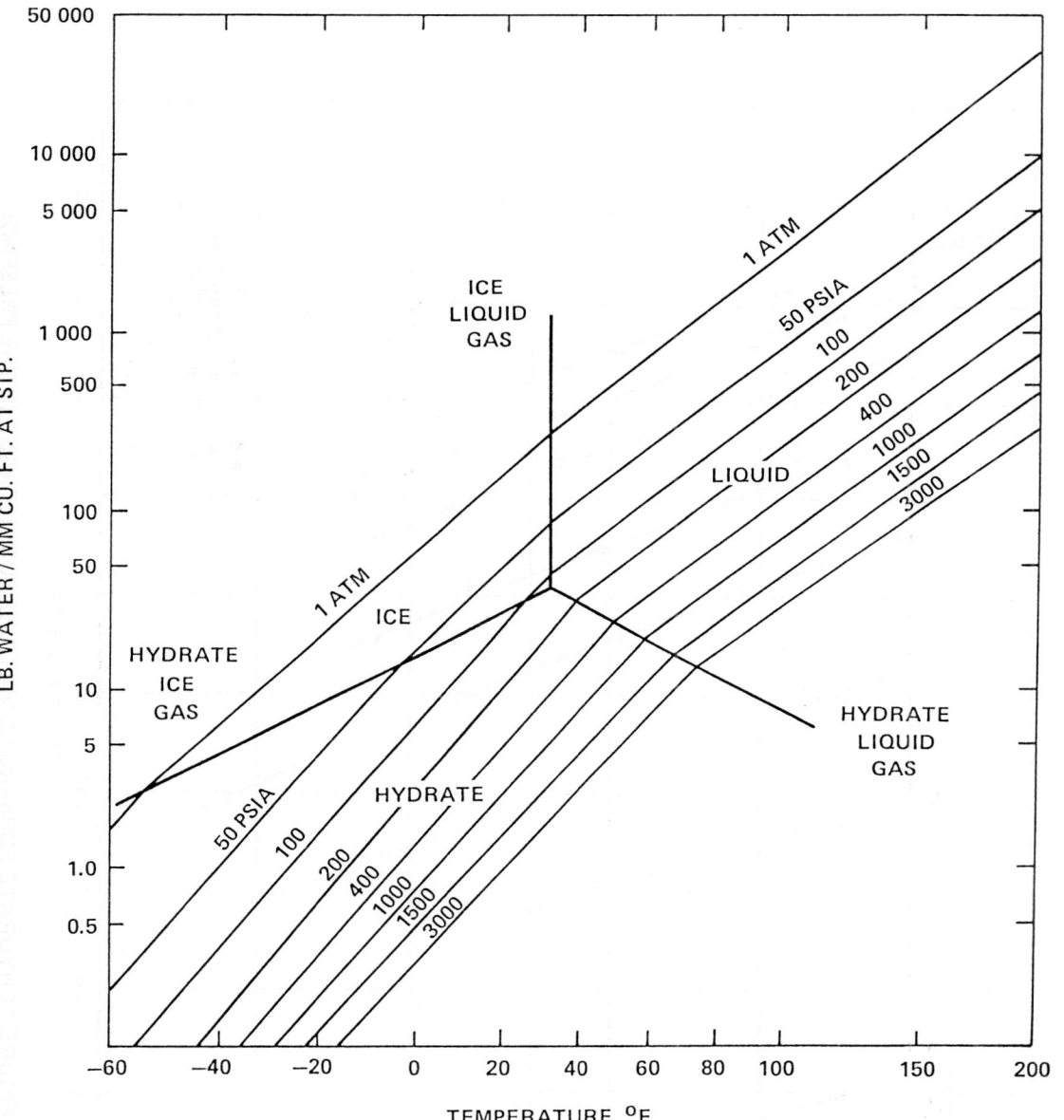

FIGURE 10 EFFECT OF HYDRATE ON ALLOWABLE WATER CONTENT OF NATURAL GAS

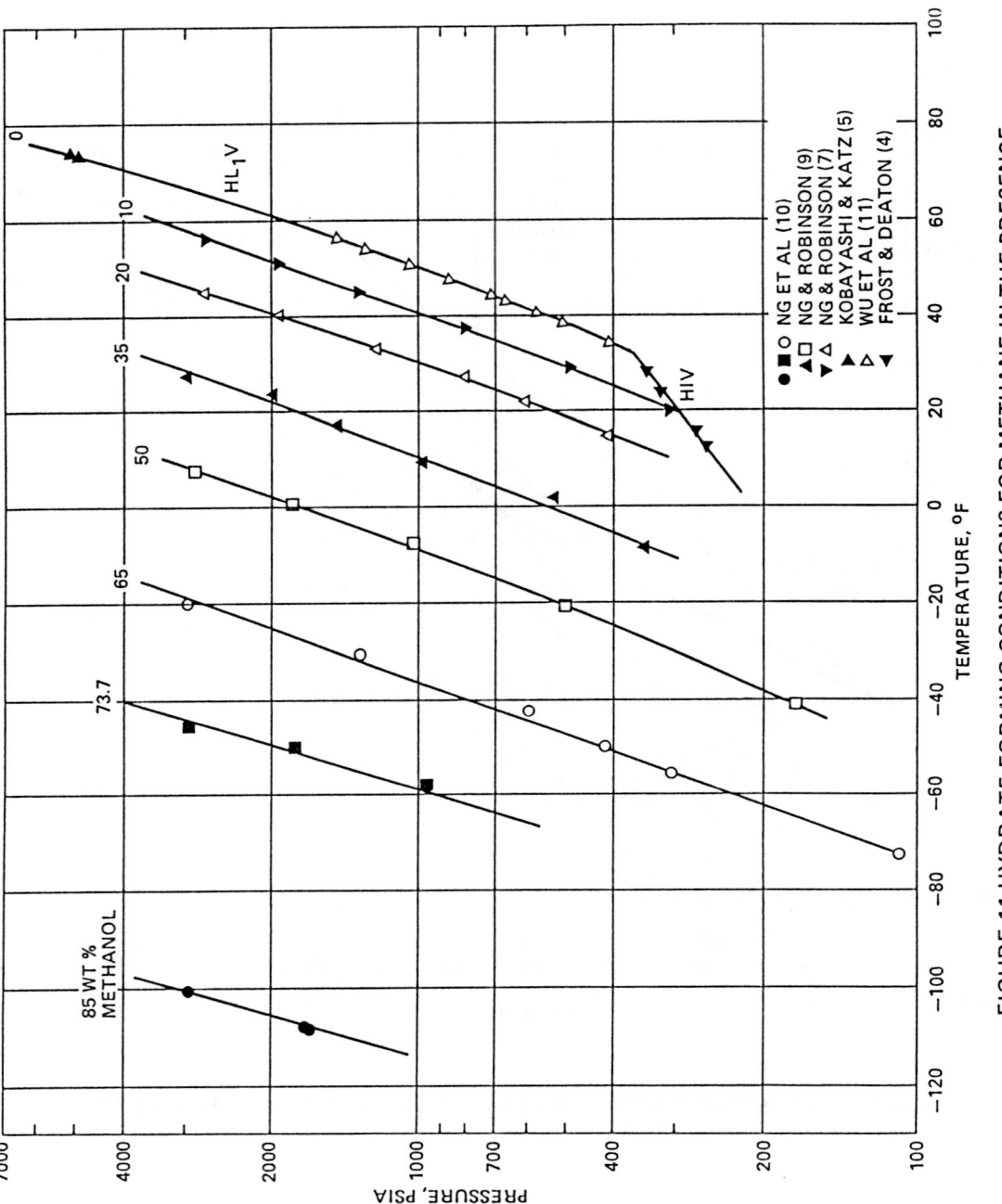

FIGURE 11 HYDRATE FORMING CONDITIONS FOR METHANE IN THE PRESENCE OF METHANOL SOLUTIONS

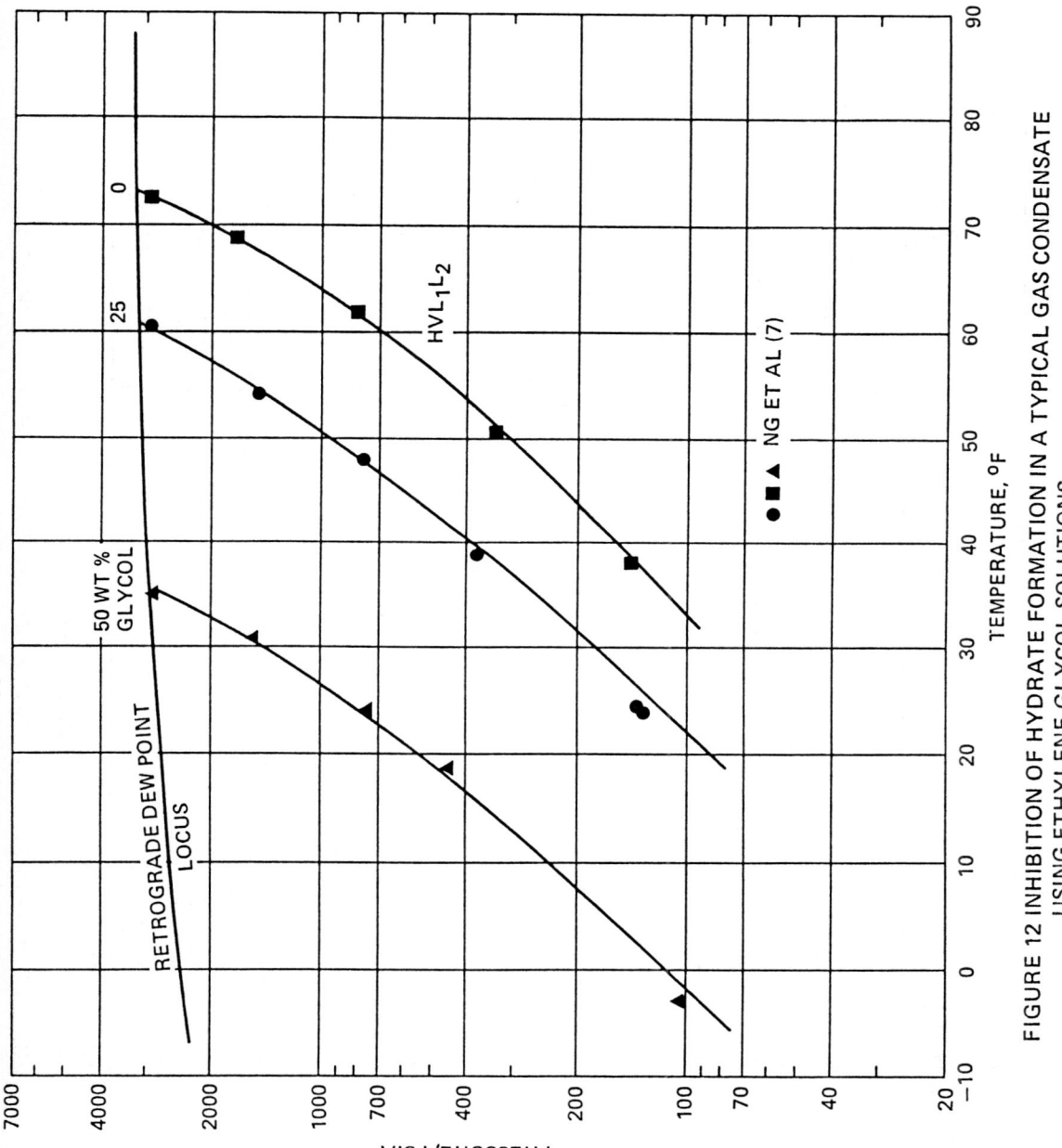

FIGURE 12 INHIBITION OF HYDRATE FORMATION IN A TYPICAL GAS CONDENSATE USING ETHYLENE GLYCOL SOLUTIONS

L'ODORISATION DANS L'INDUSTRIE GAZIERE AUJOURD'HUI

Jean-Paul COQUAND

Chef du Service de Physique Appliquée

du Centre d'Etudes et de Recherches
sur les Sciences et Techniques Appliquées

DIRECTION DES ETUDES ET TECHNIQUES NOUVELLES
DU GAZ DE FRANCE

1 - INTRODUCTION

Le gaz manufacturé, fabriqué par distillation de la houille, était du fait de la présence en grande quantité de composés sulfurés (en particulier d'H_2S) suffisamment odorant pour que le public soit alerté de sa présence et ce bien avant que la situation ne présente un danger quelconque. On peut noter au passage, qu'avec ce type de gaz le danger est double : on a en effet un risque à la fois d'intoxication par le monoxyde de carbone et d'inflammabilité du mélange air/gaz. Compte tenu de la toxicité du CO pour l'homme le premier risque se situe à un niveau de concentration de gaz dans l'air bien inférieur au second. Une épuration poussée dans certains procédés rendait le gaz manufacturé inodore et c'est de cette époque que datent les premières expériences d'odorisation, car le recours à l'odeur pour permettre de détecter une présence de gaz était passé dans les moeurs.

Distribuer un gaz odorant est devenu de nos jours une obligation à laquelle doivent se soumettre les Compagnies Gazières. La législation ou les règles de l'art fixent une valeur de concentration de gaz dans l'air au-dessus de laquelle il est indispensable que la présence de gaz soit détectée par l'odorat. Dans de nombreux pays la concentration de gaz naturel qui doit être repérée à coup sûr par toute personne douée d'un odorat normal est égale au cinquième de la limite inférieure d'inflammabilité soit 1 % de gaz dans l'air. Il existe certains pays comme le JAPON où la législation est plus sévère et mentionne une concentration inférieure.

Le gaz naturel, souvent dépourvu de composés odorants ou insuffisamment odorant, doit donc être odorisé. De ce fait l'odorisation est devenue une technique à part entière dans la panoplie de celles utilisées dans l'industrie gazière pour fournir au consommateur final un produit de qualité et sûr d'emploi.

L'odorisation est le point de rencontre d'un certain nombre de grands domaines en relation avec les sciences exactes mais également les sciences humaines. Si, comme nous le verrons par la suite, la plupart des problèmes purement techniques ont aujourd'hui reçu des solutions satisfaisantes, il n'en est pas de même quant à ceux relevant des sciences humaines.

2 - LES PROBLEMES TECHNIQUES RELATIFS A L'ACTION D'ODORISATION

2.1 - LES ODORISANTS

Pour odoriser un gaz il est nécessaire de disposer d'un odorisant pour lequel on peut dresser le cahier des charges suivant :

- ses caractéristiques odorantes en premier lieu. Son odeur doit être puissante puisque sa concentration dans le gaz reste faible, l'accoutumance à l'odeur doit être la plus réduite possible,

- il doit présenter une bonne stabilité chimique à l'état condensé ou à l'état gazeux vis à vis des matériaux ou composés avec lesquels il va se trouver en contact et ce afin de ne pas disparaître,

- ses caractéristiques physiques doivent être telles qu'on le retrouvera en phase gazeuse sans risque de disparition (condensation, adsorption, absorption ...),

- il est évident que ce produit doit être disponible sur le marché à un coût acceptable,

- enfin il doit être manipulable aisément donc non toxique.

Il n'existe pas d'odorisant ayant à la fois toutes ces qualités et les produits utilisés réalisent toujours un compromis entre les différentes caractéristiques.

Au départ les produits utilisés étaient des résidus malodorants récupérés lors de la distillation de pétroles chargés en soufre. Ces odorisants ont pratiquement laissé la place aujourd'hui à des produits de synthèse utilisés purs ou en mélange, issus de deux grandes familles de produits soufrés :

- les mercaptans de formule générale R-SH dont le représentant le plus caractéristiques est le tertiobutyl mercaptan (TBM),

- les sulfures organiques dont le tétrahydrothiophène (THT) et le diméthylsulfure sont deux exemples.

.../...

On peut dire globalement que les mercaptans ont à leur avantage leur odeur très puissante et leurs caractéristiques favorables en ce qui concerne l'adsorption par les conduites ou par les sols, mais que leur stabilité limitée vis à vis de l'oxydation peut parfois être à l'origine de perte "d'odeur" dans des réseaux particulièrement anciens et faiblement balayés par le gaz. En raison de sa plus grande résistance à l'oxydation le TBM est le mercaptan le plus employé, mais il ne peut être utilisé seul en raison d'une température de congélation de 1 °C. Les odorisants mercaptiques sont donc des mélanges ce qui présente un avantage supplémentaire, celui d'autoriser les anosmiques à l'un des composants du mélange à détecter la présence de gaz grâce aux autres constituants. A l'inverse certains travaux semblent montrer un certain "éblouissement" par les mercaptans de la muqueuse olfactive, qui perd rapidement toute sensibilité. Le phénomène n'est que lentement réversible, ce qui permettrait d'expliquer un certain nombre d'accidents où des gens après avoir nettement perçu l'odeur du gaz ont perdu cette sensation et n'ont pas de ce fait pris les mesures qui s'imposaient en présence d'une fuite de gaz.

Le THT est le seul sulfure qui s'emploie seul. Il ne semble pas présenter le phénomène d'éblouissement dont il vient d'être question ou s'il le présente c'est à un degré moindre. Sa stabilité chimique est sa qualité principale. Son comportement vis à vis des phénomènes d'adsorption en particulier dans le sol est moins bon que celui de mercaptans.

Les sociétés mettent sur le marché un nombre important de produits. On peut se demander aujourd'hui si un nombre aussi grand est réellement justifié par des observations objectives et si seule une dizaine de produits ou peut-être moins ne permettraient pas de traiter tous les cas auxquels sont confrontés les Compagnies Gazières.

2.2 - LES ODORISEURS

Disposant d'un odorisant il faut l'introduire dans le gaz en quantité adéquate : les odoriseurs, véritables installations de génie chimique, ont ce rôle. Citons pour mémoire une première famille d'appareils qui furent utilisés dans de petites exploitatons gazières, et qui assuraient par des moyens simples (goutte à goutte, léchage, mèche, barbottage) l'introduction d'un odorisant dans le gaz à une teneur dont la constance n'était que très approximative, et en tout cas dépendante de la température. Ce genre de matériel peu coûteux, de mise en oeuvre rapide et aisée est encore utilisé pour la réalisation de surodorisations temporaires dans des zones particulières.

Une deuxième famille d'installations vise à assurer une teneur en odorisant constante en asservissant le débit de l'odorisant à celui du gaz. Dans le cas où l'injection se fait sous pression ou dans celui où la température du gaz varie de façon importante, il importe de corriger en conséquence l'information débit de façon à avoir une teneur en odorisant aussi constante que possible en sortie de l'installation. L'injection est réalisée à l'aide d'une pompe dont le moteur peut être soit électrique, soit mû par le gaz (secours). Au débit on asservit suivant le type de pompes soit la vitesse de rotation du moteur soit la course du piston soit encore le temps de fonctionnement de la pompe. On trouve aujourd'hui sans difficulté des pompes d'injection bien adaptées aux besoins exprimés pour l'odorisation (plage de débit, résistance à la corrosion). Certains constructeurs proposent des installations complètes de ce type clés en main, qui conduisent à de bons résultats lorsqu'aucun composé odorant n'est présent dans le gaz en amont de l'installation. En effet l'asservissement en boucle ouverte (ou ce qui revient au même à une variable qui n'est pas celle qu'on cherche à réguler) ne permet pas de traiter commodément un gaz déjà odorisé et ce d'autant plus si le gaz est de ce point de vue variable.

La troisième famille d'odoriseurs la plus évoluée, se définit comme celle des appareils à asservissement en boucle fermée. Dans ce cas le débit d'odorisant ajouté dans le gaz est asservi à la teneur en composés odorants dans le gaz émis par la station d'odorisation elle-même. Ce sont des installations du type précédent auxquelles a été rajouté un capteur permettant de connaître les composés odorants en aval du point d'injection et un système comparant cette information à une valeur de consigne. Diverses réalisations ont vu le jour. Elles sont en général l'oeuvre des Compagnies Gazières elles-mêmes. A titre d'exemple nous allons décrire le système "MORGANA" développé par le GAZ DE FRANCE (figure 1).

FIGURE 1   SCHÉMA GÉNÉRAL DE L'INSTALLATION D'ODORISATION

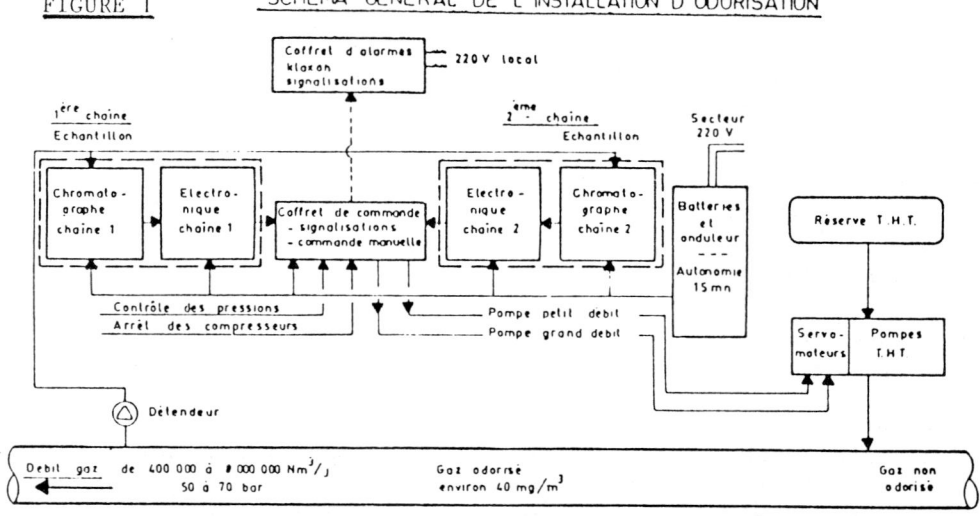

Ces appareils sont élaborés autour d'un capteur électrochimique qui permet de doser toutes les cinq minutes les composés soufrés présents dans les gaz ; on obtient ainsi la teneur en THT, la teneur globale en RSH, il est ensuite possible de calculer la quantité de THT devant être rajouté dans le gaz pour se conformer aux recommandations.

Ce principe est le seul qui permet de réaliser une odorisation complémentaire : il n'est pas nécessaire de connaître le débit du gaz à odoriser, l'installation peut donc être totalement indépendante du comptage, sous réserve d'un régime ne présentant pas de variations débits trop brutales. En effet l'analyse étant séquentielle et le résultat connu seulement 4 minutes après le prélèvement, seule l'acquisition complémen la température du gaz varie de façon importante, il importe de corriger en conséquence l'information débit de façon à avoir une teneur en odorisant aussi constante que possible en sortie de l'installation. L'injection est réalisée à l'aide d'une pompe dont le moteur peut être soit électrique, soit mû par le gaz (secours). Au débit on asservit suivant le type de pompes soit la vitesse de rotation du moteur soit la course du piston soit encore le temps de fonctionnement de la pompe. On trouve aujourd'hui sans difficulté des pompes d'injection bien adaptées aux besoins exprimés pour l'odorisation (plage de débit, résistance à la corrosion). Certains constructeurs proposent des installations complètes de ce type clés en main, qui conduisent à de bons résultats lorsqu'aucun composé odorant n'est présent dans le gaz en amont de l'installation. En effet l'asservissement en boucle ouverte (ou ce qui revient au même à une variable qui n'est pas celle qu'on cherche à réguler) ne permet pas de traiter commodément un gaz déjà odorisé et ce d'autant plus si le gaz est de ce point de vue variable.

La troisième famille d'odoriseurs la plus évoluée, se définit comme celle des appareils à asservissement en boucle fermée. Dans ce cas le débit d'odorisant ajouté dans le gaz est asservi à la teneur en composés odorants dans le gaz émis par la station d'odorisation elle-même. Ce sont des installations du type précédent auxquelles a été rajouté un capteur permettant de connaître les composés odorants en aval du point d'injection et un système comparant cette information à une valeur de consigne. Diverses réalisations ont vu le jour. Elles sont en général l'oeuvre des Compagnies Gazières elles-mêmes. A titre d'exemple nous allons décrire le système "MORGANA" développé par le GAZ DE FRANCE (figure 1).

FIGURE 1 — SCHÉMA GÉNÉRAL DE L'INSTALLATION D'ODORISATION

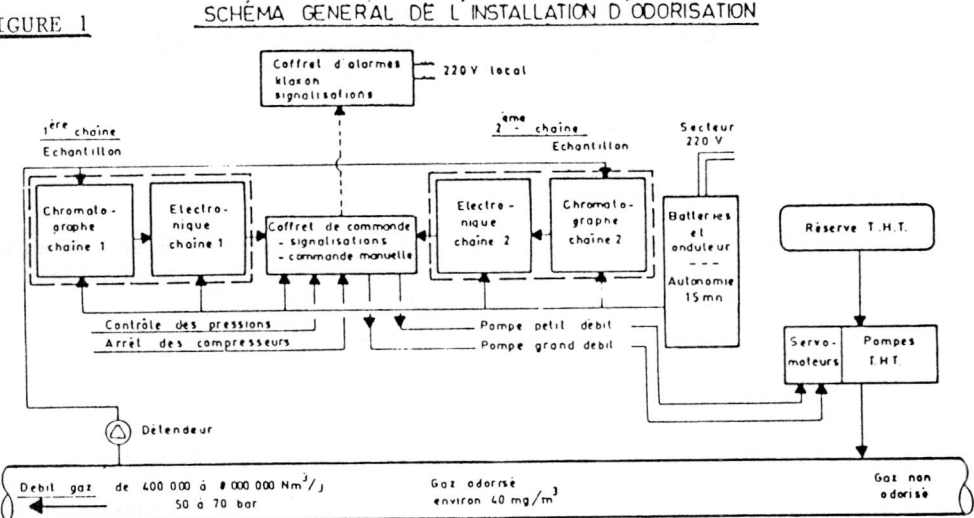

Ces appareils sont élaborés autour d'un capteur électrochimique qui permet de doser toutes les cinq minutes les composés soufrés présents dans les gaz ; on obtient ainsi la teneur en THT, la teneur globale en RSH, il est ensuite possible de calculer la quantité de THT devant être rajouté dans le gaz pour se conformer aux recommandations.

Ce principe est le seul qui permet de réaliser une odorisation complémentaire : il n'est pas nécessaire de connaître le débit du gaz à odoriser, l'installation peut donc être totalement indépendante du comptage, sous réserve d'un régime ne présentant pas de variations débits trop brutales. En effet l'analyse étant séquentielle et le résultat connu seulement 4 minutes après le prélèvement, seule l'acquisition complémen

2.3.1. - La chromatographie

La séparation par voie chromatographique des composés sulfurés ne pose en elle-même aucun problème particulier. Ce qui pose problème est dans une matrice hydrocarbonée la détection des composés sulfurés à une concentration de l'ordre de quelques parties par million. La solution passe par l'emploi d'une détection sélective. On trouve sur le marché des matériels de laboratoire fournis par des fabricants d'instrumentation générale équipés de détecteurs à photométrie de flamme. Un tel détecteur mesure le rayonnement spécifique des atomes de soufre dans une flamme riche en hydrogène selon un principe breveté par BRODY et CHANEY. Ces matériels ne sont en général pas de véritables matériels d'exploitation.

Il a été mis au point un chromatographe équipé d'un détecteur électrochimique fonctionnant comme une pile à combustible brûlant de façon spécifique les composés sulfurés d'un gaz naturel. Cet appareil développé par le GAZ DE FRANCE appelé appareil MEDOR est spécifique de cette application et a été largement diffusé en EUROPE (figure 2).

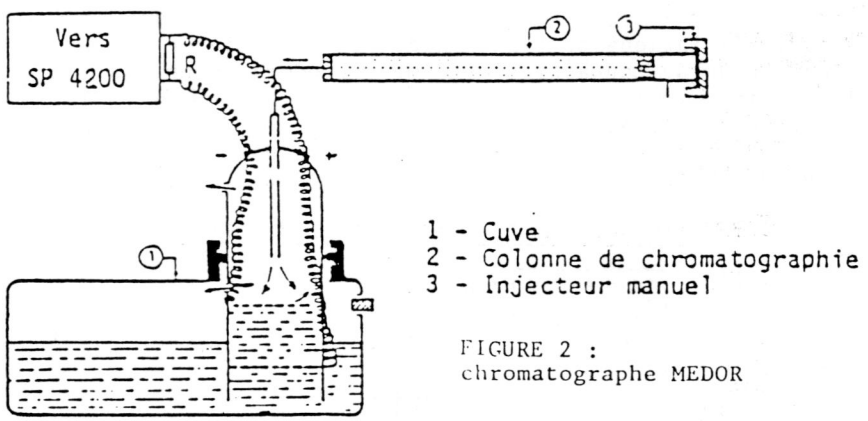

1 - Cuve
2 - Colonne de chromatographie
3 - Injecteur manuel

FIGURE 2 :
chromatographe MEDOR

Sa diffusion sur le continent Nord Américain en est à ses débuts. On donne ci-dessous à titre d'exemple un chromatogramme correspondant à l'analyse des composés sulfurés d'un gaz naturel (figure 3).

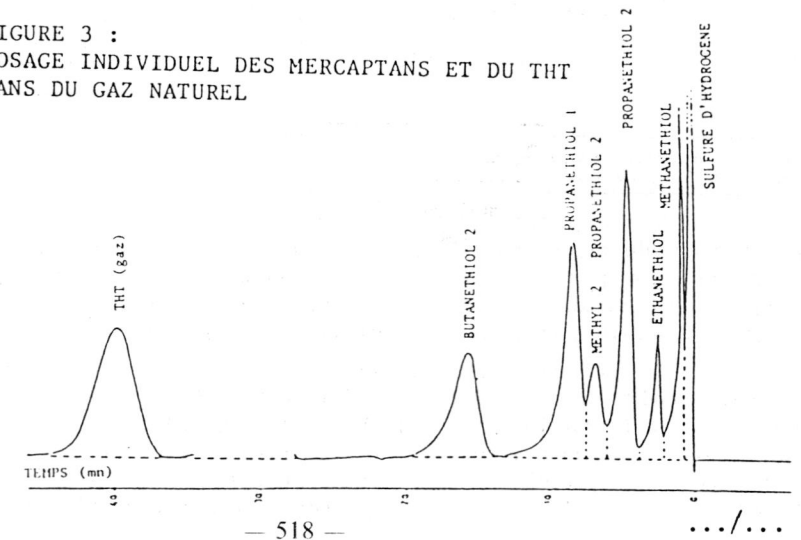

FIGURE 3 :
DOSAGE INDIVIDUEL DES MERCAPTANS ET DU THT DANS DU GAZ NATUREL

2.3.2. - La coulométrie

Cette méthode repose sur le fait qu'H_2S, les mercaptans peuvent être oxydés par le brome. On mesure la quantité de courant nécessaire pour générer par électrolyse d'une solution de bromure une quantité de équivalente à celle qui a été consommée par l'oxydation. On dose donc :

- soit le soufre total si l'on a pris soin de réduire à l'état d'H_2S la totalité du soufre présent dans le gaz. La mesure est alors continue,

- soit par différence chacune des familles chimiques si l'on a pris soin d'interposer dans le circuit d'échantillonnage un filtre chimique correspondant à chacune d'entre elles. La méthode est alors bien évidemment discontinue.

La coulométrie ne permet donc pas d'identifier chaque composé à l'inverse de la méthode précédente. Bien qu'industrielle, elle est considérée comme une mesure nécessitant une maintenance relativemet importante.

2.3.3. - Les méthodes optiques

La mesure du noircissement d'un papier imprégné avec de l'acétate de plomb indique la quantité d'hydrogène contenu dans un gaz. Ce système peut donc être utilisé pour le dosage du soufre total après réduction du soufre en H_2S ou en diminuant le temps de réponse, comme détecteur de chromatographie. Bien connue pour la première application la méthode a été développée pour permettre la seconde. Le développement a débouché récemment sur un matériel relativement sophistiqué qu'il importe de tester en exploitation.

Il existe également dans les méthodes optiques une méthode par absorption d'un rayonnement lumineux par un complexe organique du THT. Cette méthode n'est pas apparue sur le plan industriel en dehors de la compagnie qui l'a développée.

3 - PROBLEMES RELATIFS A L'ODEUR

Si dans les domaines des odorisants, des odoriseurs et du contrôle on possède aujourd'hui un ensemble de solutions satisfaisantes, pour tout ce qui concerne l'odeur on n'a pas en général de solutions correctes aux problèmes posés à savoir :

- équivalence des odeurs,
- niveau optimal de l'odorisant,
- addition des odeurs individuelles (synergie, masquage),

- contrôle sensoriel de l'odeur,
- impact de l'odorisation sur le public.

L'origine de cet état de fait doit être recherchée dans le fait que l'odorat est de nos sens celui qui est le plus mal connu. Très vite déclaré sens mineur, il est perçu par les naturalistes et les philosophes du passé comme le sens de l'animalité ou comme un résidu de l'évolution. Cependant ce sens est resté celui de la conservation, celui de la vigilance inquiète, ce qui en quelque sorte justifie tout à fait qu'on ait eu recours à lui pour la détection d'un danger.

On ne possède pas comme par exemple pour l'ouie de modèle pour l'odorat, sens chimique, qui présente de plus un pouvoir important sur le psychisme. Cette absence a la conséquence immédiate suivante :

on ne pourra se passer du nez humain pour "mesurer" une odeur,

Par ailleurs, l'importance du psychisme particulièrement difficile à maîtriser se traduira par une variabilité des résultats en fonction du protocole de mesure qui rendra délicate l'interprétation des valeurs obtenues et la comparaison de données d'origine différente. Le facteur humain étant essentiel, il importera de réaliser un traitement statistique des résultats de raisonner non seulement sur les moyennes mais également sur les dispersions pour tenir compte de tous les sujets.

Pour mesurer une odeur, il faudra tout d'abord la fabriquer puis la présenter à un sujet. L'appareil devra présenter deux caractéristiques imposées par la physiologie de l'odorat :

* un système de liaison nez du sujet/source de gaz odorant,

* un débit de gaz odorant en rapport avec le débit de gaz inspiré.

Un appareil de ce type sera appelé olfactomètre, il est essentiellement constitué par un système de dilution qui permet de faire varier la concentration d'un odorisant dans l'air, donc l'intensité du stimulus odorant soumis au juré. Le terme olfactomètre est en lui même un abus de langage puisque l'appareil n'effectue par lui-même aucune mesure, mais permet simplement d'élaborer des stimuli.

L'olfactomètre le plus simple est la carte-senteur. Il s'agit d'une carte informative sur laquelle ont été déposées des microcapsules (diamètre   ) contenant l'odorisant à étudier, suivant une technologie qui est directement dérivée de celle du papier autocopiant. Le passage d'un objet dur (ongle, pièce de monnaie, ...) brise l'enveloppe des microcapsules et libère l'odorisant. Le magazine américain National Geographic a utilisé cette technique pour une étude de l'odorat. Parmi les odeurs testées se trouvait celle associée au gaz. $1,5.10^6$ réponses ont été reçues. Un dépouillement sur plus de 100.000 réponses a montré que 1,2 % de la population était insensible aux odeurs, chiffre que l'industrie gazière devra prendre en compte pour définir sa politique vis à vis de la sécurité. Cette technique qui est d'une grande aide en raison de sa simplicité d'emploi mais qui ne répond pas aux critères imposés par la physiologie de l'odorat mentionnées ci-dessus, ne permet d'obtenir que des résultats qualitatifs.

L'olfactomètre le plus simple et le moins coûteux permettant de conduire des études quantitatives consiste à dissoudre dans un solvant inodore diverses concentrations d'un produit odorant dans des erlenmeyers. Cette expérimentation de laboratoire permet d'aborder une étude mais ne permet pas des conclusions précises.

Plusieurs types d'olfactomètres industriels ont été construits. Certains sont destinés à la mesure en exploitation (ODORATOR de Heath Consultants). Le protocole de mesure qui leur est associé ne permet pas de contrôler certains paramètres importants comme le bruit de fond odorant, la concentration en produit odorant et encore moins compte tenu de la méthode employée l'attitude psychologique du sujet en particulier l'attente où il se trouve de rencontrer une odeur. La mesure absolue d'une odeur semble aujourd'hui une gageure c'est pourquoi nous avons quant à nous construit un olfactomètre avec pour objectif non pas la détermination des valeurs absolues des odeurs mais bien plutôt la comparaison entre eux des odorisants.

L'olfactomètre réalisé est schématisé sur la figure 4. Il est composé de trois blocs élémentaires ; le coffret mélangeur, le coffret analyseur et le coffret de commande. Le premier permet d'obtenir les mélanges nécessaires à l'expérience, ces mélanges sont contrôlés directement et en temps réel par le coffret analyseur. Ces deux coffrets sont placés sous le contrôle du coffret de commande qui en assure le pilotage ainsi que l'acquisition des réponses fournies avec l'opérateur chargé de surveiller le bon déroulement d'une séquence d'essai. L'olfactomètre constitue donc un ensemble totalement interactif avec le sujet soumis à l'expérience et avec l'opérateur. La présence de ce dernier n'est à la limite pas nécessaire au bon déroulement d'une séance d'essai.

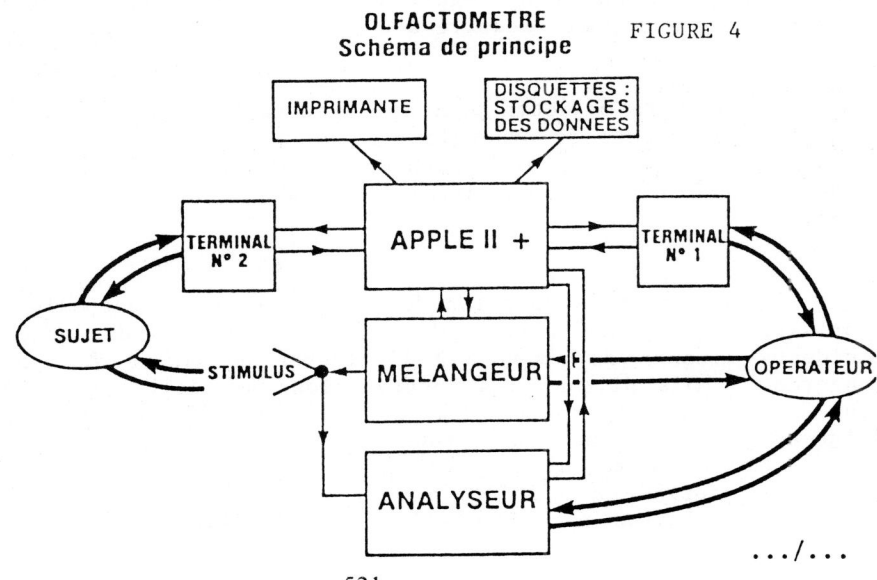

FIGURE 4

.../...

On a cherché à comparer les deux grandes familles d'odorisants gaziers à savoir : les mercaptans et les sulfures. La comparaison du THT et du tertiobutyl mercaptan a conduit à l'établissement d'une courbe d'équivalence décrite sur la figure 5.

FIGURE 5 : EQUIVALENCE THT / TBM SUR LE PLAN DE L'IMPRESSION OLFACTIVE

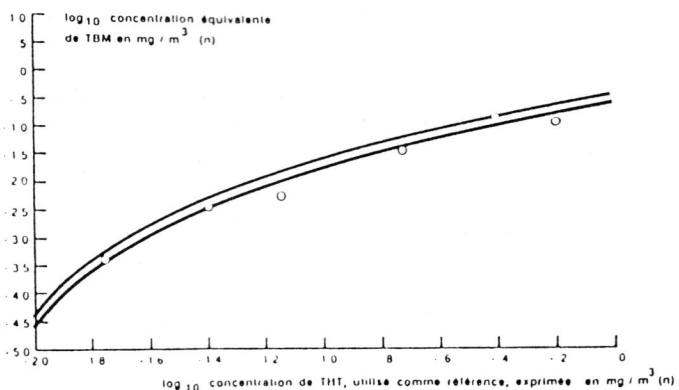

Contrairement à notre attente il ne semble pas que l'on puisse parler d'un seul coefficient d'équivalence rapport des concentrations des deux odorisants mais bien plutôt d'un coefficient qui varie selon la concentration du stimulus de référence. Si l'on considère le rapport TBM/THT ce coefficient est très important aux faibles concentrations de THT et décroît ensuite quand la concentration en THT augmente. Ce résultat remet en cause la loi de Stevens qui admet que l'intensité absolue d'une sensation est proportionnelle au logarithme de la concentration du stimulus et qui par conséquent doit conduire à un rapport constant entre TBM et THT.

Un autre objectif poursuvi avec cette expérimentation a été la recherche des effets de synergie souvent publiés entre sulfures et mercaptans. Pour des mélanges THT/TBM contenant plus de 70 % de THT il semble que le modèle d'addition linéaire des odeurs soit applicable sans restriction.

Cependant la question de la concentration optimale d'un gaz en odorisant reste posée : trop d'odorisant conduit à des appels pour des incidents mineurs ne pouvant à l'évidence déboucher sur une situation dangereuse, mais diluant les interventions auxquelles peut être réellement associé un danger débouchant donc sur une multiplication des équipes d'intervention ou à un nombre constant d'équipes à un risque d'intervention tardive. Une teneur trop faible est par principe un risque inacceptable. Ce problème a donc été à nouveau posé à des laboratoires de recherches américains par le Gas Research Institute. Nous avons quant à nous pour éclairer le sujet et obtenir des données complémentaires sur l'équivalence des odorisants, tenté une analyse statistique des appels pour intervention au niveau de plusieurs Centres de Distribution.

L'analyse des résultats enregistrés sur les jours ouvrés a montré que dans une distribution où alternaient THT et mercaptans le comportement de la population était équivalent selon que l'on avait dans le gaz 25 mg du THT par m^3 ou 4 mg de mercaptans par m^3, confirmant par une expérience en vraie grandeur des résultats obtenus par olfactométrie.

L'ensemble de ces travaux a permis d'établir une politique rationnelle pour l'odorisation. C'est ainsi que le GAZ DE FRANCE tente en ce moment une expérience de changement d'odorisant sur un nombre limité d'abonnés. Il a été décidé d'injecter à un mélange 70 THT - 30 TBM à une concentration de 10 mg/m^3 en remplacement du THT à 25 mg/m^3. Compte tenu d'un prix équivalent pour les deux odorisants l'intérêt économique est évident. Afin de conserver une sécurité équivalente dans les deux cas la concentration du mélange a été calculée en raisonnant non pas sur des valeurs moyennes mais sur les valeurs extrêmes des distributions supposées gaussiennes des concentrations équivalentes de l'ensemble du jury qui a participé aux expériences d'olfactométrie.

4 - CONCLUSION

Il ressort qu'aujourd'hui les problèmes technologiques dans le domaine de l'odorisation sont pour la plus grande part résolus. Par contre ceux liés à l'odorat et au comportement de la population restent encore relativement flous en l'absence de moyens de mesure de l'odeur fiable et précis. L'industrie gazière devra emboîter le pas des chercheurs, psychophycisiens et physiologistes, si elle veut affronter l'avenir dans ce domaine avec plus de confiance.

BIBLIOGRAPHIE

*****

Contrôle des composés sulfurés

    M. MAMAN, M. CHARRON - Un détecteur électrochimique pour le dosage des composés sulfurés du gaz naturels - 13° Symposium de chromatographie - CANNES 1980.

    Bulletin HEWLETT-PACKARD avril 1987.

    M.R. LEE - Continuous Automatic Gas Odorant Analyzers. Their evaluation. The MEDOR-IGT Symposium on odorization 1987.

    A. VINCENT - Continuous Analysis of Hydrogen Sulfide, Mercaptans and Residual Sulfur. A.G.A. Oper. Sect. Proc. 636-9 (1986).

Installation d'odorisation

    G.J. EVANINA - Automated Natural Gas Odorization and Monitoring - IGT Symposium on odorization Proceedings 1987.

    D.F. HENDERSON - Large Volume Odorization - Installation operation and maintenance - IGT symposium on odorization Proceedings 1987.

    Mesure d'odeur et sa régulation dans les réseaux de gaz naturel - documentation technique - Société SPIE BATIGNOLLES 1987.

Comportement du public - Olfactométrie

    J.P. COQUAND, C. FARRUGIA, B. CALINAUD - Congrès ATG 1983 - Nouvelles études sur l'odorisation.

    J.P. COQUAND - Congrès ATG 1987 - Vers une nouvelle règle d'odorisation.

Accurate Measurements and
Prediction of Compressibility Factors
in the Gas Industry

Paper

presented by

Dr. Manfred Jaeschke,
Applied Physics Section, Ruhrgas AG,
Essen, Federal Republic of Germany

at the International Symposium
on Measurements, Properties and
Utilization of Natural Gas
in Montreal, Canada,
on 26 November 1987

Accurate Measurements and Prediction of Compressibility Factors in the Gas Industry

Table of Contents

1. Introduction

2. Thermal Billing by Ruhrgas

3. Volume Correction
3.1 Volume Correction for Ideal Gases
3.2 Real Gas Volume Correction
3.2.1 Correction Using Compressibility Factors
3.2.2 Correction Using Densities

4. Density and Compressibility Factor Measurement
4.1 Laboratory Measurement
4.2 Field Measurement
4.2.1 Field Measurement of Compressibility Factor
4.2.2 Field Measurement of Density

5. Prediction of Density and Compressibility Factor
5.1 AGA NX 19
5.2 GERG Virial Equation
5.2.1 The Equation
5.2.2 Uncertainty of the GERG Virial Equation
5.3 Super-Z Equation

6. Uncertainty of Volume Correction

7. References

Accurate Measurements and
Prediction of Compressibility Factors
in the Gas Industry

by

Manfred Jaeschke, Ruhrgas AG

1. Introduction

Ruhrgas purchases natural gas from West German reservoirs and from fields in other West European countries and in the Soviet Union and sells the gas to local utilities, regional pipelines, power station and industrial users. The gas received from suppliers and the gas delivered to customers must be measured accurately.

At a large delivery station, the hourly flowrate may be as high as 1 million $m^3(n)$ and even an error in the per mille range implies that some 1,000 $m^3(n)/h$ will not be invoiced or will be paid for although the gas was not delivered. Under unfavourable conditions, these errors may, over one month, add up to as much as 0.5 million m^3.

For this reason, Ruhrgas sponsors gas measurement projects. Presently, large gas flows can be measured with an accuracy of $\pm$ 0.3 % under laboratory-type conditions.

Ruhrgas also promotes thermodynamic research and development to improve the accuracy of density and compressibility factor measurements and equations of state, as accurate density and PVT data are necessary for accurate custody transfer measurement.

This paper presents the method of thermal billing used by Ruhrgas and discusses the techniques employed by Ruhrgas for the measurement of the density of natural gas at flowing conditions and natural gas compressibility factors. It also examines the accuracy of equations of state used for the prediction of densities and compressibility factors and reports on recent work undertaken by the European Gas Research Group to develop a new equation of state.

2. Thermal Billing by Ruhrgas

If gas is billed on a thermal basis, errors can occur in the determination of the heating value and in the volume at flowing conditions as well as in the correction of the volume at flowing conditions to reference conditions, for instance, as the real gas behaviour or the density are not accurately known.

For thermal billing, a measuring station is equipped with a meter to measure gas flow, a system to correct flow at operating conditions to flow at reference conditions and a computer to multiply the flowrate at reference conditions and the heating value of the gas (see Fig. 1) measured at large Ruhrgas stations by calorimeters. Flowmeters, volume correctors and the computer necessary to determine energy flow may be integrated in one unit.

Ruhrgas measures for thermal billing the volume rate of flow at flowing conditions. The measured flowrate is corrected to a flowrate at normal conditions which is multiplied by the measured higher heating value to obtain the energy flow.

As Fig. 1 shows, certain base data are needed for the determination of energy flow. If a turbine flow meter is used for measuring the volume flowrate at operating conditions, the volume (v) and the time of measurement (Δt) must be known to determine the flowrate (q). If a pressure difference meter is employed, the differential pressure (Δp), the static pressure (p), the temperature (T) and the real gas behaviour of the metered gas must be known. For volume correction, the density at flowing conditions and the density at normal conditions are, for example, required for calculating flow at normal conditions.

As Fig. 1 shows clearly, the real gas behaviour is crucial both for flow measurement and for volume correction. Section 3 discusses how the real gas behaviour influences volume correction. The measurement or the prediction of the density or the compressibility factor of the measured gas will then be reviewed in detail in Sections 4 and 5, followed by a final section, presenting the present uncertainties of volume correction.

3. Volume Correction

A gas volume or a rate of flow are an insufficient description of a gas quantity. It is necessary to know at what temperature and at what pressure the volume or the rate of flow were measured.

For invoicing, the volume at flowing conditions must be corrected to reference conditions. In the Federal Republic of Germany, a normal temperature of 273.15 K (0 °C) and a normal pressure of 1.01325 bar are the standard reference conditions.

3.1 Volume Correction for Ideal Gases

For an ideal gas, the thermal equation of state

$$pV = n\,RT \tag{3.1}$$

Where:

p = pressure
V = gas volume
n = number of gas moles
R = universal gas constant
T = thermodynamic temperature

The volume corrected to normal conditions ($V_{n,\,id}$) is calculated from the volume at flowing conditions by the following formula:

$$V_{n,\,id} = V \times G_{id} \tag{3.2}$$

Where:

$$G_{id} = \frac{p}{p_n} \cdot \frac{T_n}{T}$$

Equation (3,2) is derived from equation (3,1) by applying equation (3,1) both to flowing conditions and to normal conditions. The factor G_{id} is only valid for ideal gases.

3.2 Real Gas Volume Correction

3.2.1 Correction Using Comressibility Factors

A similar approach as for a perfect gas may be used for the correction of a real gas volume to reference conditions. The thermal equation of state for a real gas reads as follows:

$$pV = n Z RT \qquad (3.3)$$

Where:

Z = compressibility factor

The compressibility factor is mainly a function of pressure and temperature. It reflects the deviation of the behaviour of a real gas from the ideal gas law and introduces a correction for real gas behaviour.

Similar to equation (3,2), the corrected volume of a real gas

$$V_n = V \cdot G_{id} \cdot K^{-1} \qquad (3.4)$$

Where:

$K = Z/Z_n$

The Z/Z_n quotient is sometimes referred to as the gas law deviation factor or the K value. Z_n is the compressibility factor of the real gas at normal pressure and temperature conditions.

As Fig. 1 shows, the volume of a gas can be corrected to normal conditions even if the real gas behaviour of the gas is unknown. For this purpose, the density of the gas must be measured.

3.2.2 Correction Using Densities

The density (ρ) is the quotient of the mass of the gas and the volume it occupies. This relationship may be expressed as follows:

$$\rho = \frac{m}{V} = \frac{nM}{V} \qquad (3.5)$$

Where:

m = gas mass
n = number of gas moles
M = molar mass

Equation (3.5) is also valid for the gas at normal conditions. Hence, the volume correction is made by

$$V_n = \frac{nM}{\rho_n} = \frac{\rho}{\rho_n} V \qquad (3.6)$$

The correction of a real gas volume to normal conditions can therefore be made by using measured densities only, although the compressibility factor of the gas is unknown. Equation (3.6) and equation (3.4) yield, for the correction factor:

$$\frac{\rho}{\rho_n} = \frac{G_{id}}{K} \qquad (3.7)$$

Ruhrgas mainly uses equation (3.6) at stations where large gas flows are measured. If the flow rate is small, Ruhrgas still usually applies equation (3.4) for the determination of flows at normal conditions.

4. Density and Compressibility Factor Measurement

4.1 Laboratory Measurement

Under laboratory conditions, the compressibility of a gas can be determined by a Burnett apparatus (1,2) or a Desgranges & Huot Z meter (2,3). Both units comprise two test chambers. The gas sample is expanded isothermally from one chamber into the second chamber. Under these conditions, the compressibility of the gas can be derived from the change in pressure.

Compressibility factors can also be measured by a grating interferometer, measuring the refractive index of the gas sample. The compressibility factor of the gas is computed from the refractive index by the Lorentz-Lorenz law which defines specific refraction as a function of the refractive index and molar density. A schematic of the grating interferometer is shown by Fig. 2. The grating interferometer and the method of computing compressibility factors from measured refractive indexes are described in detail in (4,5).

The gravity method (6) and the buoyancy method (7) are other high-precision techniques for determining the compressibility of a gas from measured densities. Density measured by the gravity method is a primary laboratory technique. A vessel of a known volume is filled with gas and the mass of the gas is determined by subtracting the weight of the empty vessel from the weight of the gas-filled vessel. The density of the gas is given directly by the quotient of the mass and the volume of the gas.

The buoyancy method described in (7) uses two sinkers of identical mass and surface area but considerably different volumes. The two sinker method compensates for all surface and suspension effects. The uncertainty of some of the laboratory methods of measuring the compressibility factor of a natural gas is less than 0.1 %. Table 1 reviews the accuracies of the laboratory techniques both for pure gases and natural gases. The uncertainties given for natural gas comprise the additional uncertainty introduced by the uncertainty of the natural gas composition.

Table 1

Uncertainties of Different Laboratory Techniques
Used for the Determination of Compressibility Factors
at Pressures Below 80 bar

	pure gases	natural gases
Burnett apparatus*	0.05 %	0.09 %
interferometer*	0.06 %	0.09 %
Z-meter	0.1 %	0.2 %
gravity method	0.1 %	0.15 %
buoyancy method	0.03 %	0.07 %

* The Burnett apparatus and the interferometer can be employed for pressures below 300 bar. The uncertainty of the two systems at high pressure is 0.1 % for pure gases and 0.16 % for natural gases.

4.2   Field Measurement

Densities and compressibility factors measured under laboratory conditions are used to check field densitometers and to correlate new equations of state. This Section 4.2 presents typical field equipment employed for compressibility factor and density measurement.

4.2.1   Field Measurement of Compressibility Factor

Distrigaz of Belgium uses measured compressibility factors for the correction of volumes at flowing conditions to reference conditions. A Z meter was developed to Distrigaz specifications and has been used for flow measurement since 1975. Fig. 3 is a schematic of the Z meter.

The meter consists of two chambers separated by an expansion valve and fitted with a gas inlet and a gas outlet valve respectively. The mode of operation is as follows:

1. Sample gas to be measured at pressure p_1 and temperature T_1 is filled into the small chamber (V_1), while the large chamber (V_2) contains the same gas at atmospheric pressure p_2.

2. The gas inlet and outlet valves are then closed and the expansion valve is opened. The gas then expands into the two chambers ($V_1 + V_2$) and the pressure equilibrates at pressure p_3.

The compressibility factor Z_1 (p_1, T_1) is calculated from the three measured pressures p_1, p_2 and p_3 using the following equation:

$$Z_1 = p_1 \left\{ p_3 (A + 1)/Z_3 - p_2 A/Z_2 \right\}^{-1} \qquad (4.1)$$

The volume ratio $A = V_2/V_1$ is determined by calibration using, for example, methane. The compressibility factors Z_2 and Z_3 are computed by iteration by

$$Z_i = 1 + B\, p_i, \quad i = 2.3 \qquad (4.2)$$

The second Virial coefficient B is approximated by

$$B = (Z_1 - 1)/p_1 \qquad (4.3)$$

Distrigaz claims a maximum uncertainty of 0.1 % for the measured compressibility factors (8). Energy flow is computed by Distrigaz using compressibility factors measured by the Z meter and measured higher heating values. Z meters are installed at all major measuring stations of Distrigaz (8).

At small metering stations, Ruhrgas determines energy flow by a similar method using predicted compressibility factors. At large custody transfer points Ruhrgas and other corporations such as British Gas (United Kingdom), Gasunie (Netherlands) and Phillips Petroleum (Norway) measure the density of the gas for volume correction.

4.2.2 Field Measurement of Density

Vibrating-element densitometers used for the field measurement of the density of a gas measure the change in the eigenfrequency of the vibrating element (vibrating cylinder or tuning fork) surrounded by the gas which is measured. This eigenfrequency decreases as the density increases.

Fig. 4 is the schematic of a tuning fork densitometer. The tuning fork is fitted between two coils in the densitometer housing. One coil excites tuning fork vibrations; these are picked up by the other coil which controls the feedback of energy into the vibration circuit. The vibration is unattenuated if the tuning fork is excited by appropriate forces at appropriate periods. The frequency of these vibrations is measured. The eigenfrequency depends on the tuning fork size and the gas density.

The eigenfrequency is a non-linear function of the density at flowing conditions. The density at flowing conditions $\rho_{fl,r}$ is related to the frequency f, by a second order polynomial as follows (see Fig. 5):

$$\rho_{fl,r} = A + B(1/f) + C(1/f^2) \tag{4.4}$$

where coefficients A, B and C are constants determined conventionally by calibration with a pure gas such as pure methane.

A verification of the density readouts of vibrating element densitometers using densities measured by the gravity method showed that the systematic error of natural gas density readout may be as high as 0.6 %, while the systematic error for pure gas was in some cases even 1.5 % (see Fig. 6).

This error cannot be accepted for sales gas metering. An analysis of the test data showed that the error of the density readout increased as the difference between the velocity of sound in the sample gas and the velocity of sound in the calibration gas (methane) increased.

A correction for the velocity of sound effect can be made by the application of the following formula (see Fig. 7):

$$\rho_{fl,c} = \rho_{fl,r} \times \frac{1 + \left[\dfrac{L}{C_c}\right]^2}{1 + \left[\dfrac{L}{C_s}\right]^2} \qquad (4.5)$$

Where:

$\rho_{fl,c}$ = density at flowing conditions, corrected
$\rho_{fl,r}$ = readout of density at flowing conditions
L = densitometer constant $L = 53.36$ m/sec
C_c = calibration gas velocity of sound at $\rho_{fl,r}$
C_s = sample gas velocity of sound at $\rho_{fl,r}$

To predict the calibration gas and the sample gas velocities of sound with sufficient accuracy, a polynomial expressed as $C = f(\rho_{fl,r}, t, d)$ was developed. The variables of this polynomial, such as the density at flowing conditions, ($\rho_{fl,r}$) and the relative density (d) are measured at each sales gas metering station. The temperature (t) may be assumed to be constant for an approximation or may be measured if a high quality correction for the velocity of sound effect is required.

At some stations, the velocity of sound is now even measured by meters based on the Coanda effect. Naturally, velocity of sound measurement must be preferred over a mathematical approximation, since the measurement accounts directly for changes in gas composition. Further details of the method employed for velocity of sound correction have been published in literature (9), (10).

The correction allows a reduction of the velocity of sound uncertainty of current vibrating element densitometers from 0.6 % to less than 0.1 % for all types of gases distributed in the Federal Republic of Germany (see Fig. 8). Physikalisch Technische Bundesanstalt, the West German gas measurement agency, has authorized the use of the correction formula for sales gas metering in the Federal Republic of Germany.

Densitometers are mainly employed at installations where large gas flows are measured at high pressures in excess of 16 bar and where the composition of the gas measured changes frequently. At small custody transfer metering stations, predicted compressibility factors are used for volume correction. Prediction techniques are also employed for checking densitometers. Section 5 discusses standard custody transfer prediction techniques and two new methods of calculation developed for the European Gas Research Group and the Gas Research Institute.

5. **Prediction of Density and Compressibility Factor**

5.1 AGA NX-19

Ruhrgas and other European gas utilities presently use modified versions of the AGA NX-19 (11) for the prediction of compressibility factors.

In the case of low-BTU natural gases with a higher heating value of 31.8 MJ/m^3(n) to 39.8 MJ/m^3(n), the compressibility factor is calculated by the AGA NX-19-mod technique (12), while the AGA NX-19-mod/3H method (13) limited to pressures between 0 bar and 90 bar and to temperatures between -10 °C and +30 °C is employed for high BTU natural gas with a higher heating value between 39.8 MJ/m^3(n) and 46.2 MJ/m^3(n).

The agreement between compressibility factors predicted by the AGA NX-19-mod method and measured compressibility factors of group L natural gas is sufficient for low pressures and high temperatures (see Fig. 9). Even in the case of these gases, the difference between predicted and measured compressibility factors increases as pressure rises and may be as large as 0.7 % for low temperatures.

The validity of the AGA NX-19-mod/3H method developed by a simple correction of the AGA NX-19-mod method using a best fit for group H natural gas data is only valid in a pressure range between 0 and 90 bar and in a temperature range between -10 °C and +30 °C. In this range it predicts, for instance, group H Ekofisk type natural gas compressibility factors correctly (see Fig. 10). The differences between Ekofisk type gas compressibility factors calculated by the AGA NX-19-mod/3H method and measured values are less than 0.2 %. For high pressures and high temperatures the difference may be as much as 1 %.

In view of this unsatisfactory precision of methods for the prediction of compressibility factors, the European Gas Research Group (GERG, Groupe européen de Recherches gazières) decided to develop an equation of state with a specified uncertainty of less than 0.1 % for predicted compressibility factors. Initial results of this work were discussed in a paper presented at the International Gas Research Conference in Toronto in 1986 (14). Final results and the impact on the uncertainty of flow measurment are reviewed below.

5.2 GERG Virial Equation

The objectives specified by the European Gas Research Group for the development of the Virial equation are summarized in Table 2.

Table 2
GERG Virial equation

specified maximum uncertainty	± 0.1 %
temperature conditions	-10 °C to +60 °C
pressure conditions	0 bar to 120 bar
gas composition	

CH_4	>	50 % (molar)			
N_2	<	50 %	CO_2	<	20 %
C_2H_6	<	20 %	H_2	<	10 %
C_3H_8	<	5 %	CO	<	3 %
C_4H_{10}	<	2 %	He	<	0.5 %
C_5H_{12}	<	0.5 %	C_6H_{14}	<	0.1 %
C_7H_{16}	<	0.1 %	C_8H_{18}	<	0.1 %

5.2.1 The Equation

As discussed above, real gas behaviour can be described by the following equation of state:

$$Z = \frac{p}{\rho_m RT} \qquad (5.1)$$

Where:

- Z = compressibility factor
- p = pressure
- ρ_m = molar density
- T = thermodynamic temperature
- R = universal gas constant

Figs. 11 and 12 plot the real gas behaviour of natural gases. The compressibility factor decreases nearly as a linear function of pressure. At absolute zero pressure, the compressibility factor is equal to unity, because every gas behaves like an ideal gas at this pressure. The compressibility factor also decreases as a function of temperature. Further, as the ethane content rises, the behaviour of natural gas deviates more from the ideal gas behaviour.

A virial equation of state is a particularly simple representation of this real gas behaviour. The equation truncated after the third term takes the general form of

$$Z = 1 + B(T)\rho_m + C(T)\rho_m^2 \qquad (5.2)$$

B(T) and C(T) are the second and the third virial coefficients which are functions of temperature and gas composition.

For gas mixtures, the second and the third virial coefficients are determined by the following mixing rules:

$$B_{mix}(T) = \sum_{i=1}^{n} \sum_{j=1}^{n} x_i x_j B_{ij}(T) \qquad (5.3)$$

$$C_{mix}(T) = \sum_{i=1}^{n} \sum_{j=1}^{n} \sum_{k=1}^{n} x_i x_j x_k C_{ijk}(T) \qquad (5.4)$$

x_i, x_j and x_k represent the molar fraction of the i-th, j-th and k-th component. The virial coefficients of a mixture are thus combined from the coefficients for the pure components and the interaction virial coefficients. For a binary system,

$$B_{mix}(T) = x_1^2 B_{11} + 2x_1 x_2 B_{12} + x_2^2 B_{22} \qquad (5.5)$$

$$C_{mix}(T) = x_1^3 C_{111} + 3x_1^2 x_2 C_{112} + 3x_1 x_2^2 C_{122} \qquad (5.6)$$
$$+ x_2^3 C_{222}$$

A second order polynomial is used to describe the influence of temperature:

$$B(T) = b_0 + b_1 T + b_2 T^2 \qquad (5.7)$$

$$C(T) = c_0 + c_1 T + c_2 T^2 \qquad (5.8)$$

The GERG virial equation of state was developed from the above relationships. The work necessary to correlate the measured compressibility factors for pure gases and binary mixtures stored in the GERG data bank to predict compressibility factors was carried out by Van der Waals Institute in Amsterdam, the Netherlands, under a contract awarded by the European Gas Research Group.

5.2.2 Uncertainty of the GERG Virial Equation

75 sets of experimental natural gas data were used for reviewing the GERG virial equation of states. The sources of these data sets and the number of experimental data (given in brackets) are as follows:

published data	14 (889)
N.V. Nederlandse Gasunie	23 (1249)
Gaz de France	5 (50)
Ruhrgas AG	33 (1966)
total	75 (4154)

N.V. Nederlandse Gasunie and Ruhrgas AG measured most natural gas compressibility factors stored in the GERG data bank. Ruhrgas AG is the only company which made measurement at very high pressures up to 120 bar. The average root mean square error for the differences between the compressibility factors predicted by the GERG virial equation and all measured natural gas compressibility factors is

RMS = $\pm$ 0.051 % for pressures between 0 and 120 bar.

Fig. 13 is a schematic plot of the correlation between the RMS error and pressure. The errors are as follows for the two pressure ranges:

RMS = $\pm$ 0.049 % for pressures between 0 and 80 bar
RMS = $\pm$ 0.061 % for pressures between 80 and 120 bar.

Fig. 14 plots the RMS errors for 6 specific natural gases for pressures between 0 and 80 bar and between 80 bar and 120 bar. As the graph shows, the error is less than 0.04 % for pressures not exceeding 80 bar and less than 0.06 % for the high-pressure range. The NAM gas, the natural gas/coke-oven gas mixture and the Ekofisk gas each contain some 10 % of nitrogen or hydrogen or ethane. The Drohne gas contains some 5 % of nitrogen and of carbon-dioxide and the TENP gas some 5 % of nitrogen and of ethane, while the Soviet gas is practically pure methane.

Fig. 15 shows the influence of pressure on the difference between compressibility factor predicted by the GERG virial equation and measured Z values for the 270 K and the 273.15 K isotherms. Even for pressures between 80 and 120 bar, the differences are less than 0.1 % for these six gases. This excellent agreement is particularly satisfactory as the differences between predicted and measured compressibility factors are highest for low temperatures and high pressures, while the differences are relatively small for high temperatures. The GERG virial equation is discussed in more detail in (15).

5.3 Super-Z Equation

The Super-Z equation was correlated by K.E. Starling et al. under the sponsorship of the Gas Research Institute in close liaison with the American Gas Association's Transmission Measuring Committee (16).

The resulting errors for six specific natural gases are given in Fig. 16. For four natural gases of group L or H, the resulting Z errors at a pressure of up to 120 bar are within $\pm$ 0.1 %. For the natural gas/coke-oven gas mixture, the Z errors are positive and may be as high as 0.4 %. For the Ekofisk-type natural gas from the North Sea, the Z error at 80 bar and 270 K is -0.2 %. The maximum negative Z error was 0.35 % at approx. 100 bar.

Thus, the Super-Z equation is less accurate than the GERG virial equation as pressure increases (see Fig. 15 for comparison). This view is supported by the RMS errors of the differences between the calculated Z values and the measured Z values for all natural gas data in the GERG data file, as tabulated below:

pressure range/bar	percentage RMS error GERG equation	percentage RMS error Super-Z equation
0 - 80	0.049	0.066
80 - 120	0.061	0.132
0 - 120	0.051	0.075

6. Uncertainties of Volume Correction

The compressibility behaviour of natural gas can be determined with an uncertainty of ± 0.1 % using a Z meter or a densitometer. The uncertainty of current predictive methods for field application is ± 3 %. The new GERG virial equation reduces this uncertainty to ± 0.1 %. The uncertainty of the density at flowing conditions measured in the field is ± 2 % if a correction for the velocity of sound effect is made.

For field volume correction using pressure, temperature and the compressibility factor, the overall uncertainty is therefore as follows:

		uncertainty
absolute pressure	p	0.1 %
thermodynamic temperature	T	0.1 %
density at normal conditions	ρ_n	0.2 %
compressibility factor (GERG Virial equation or Z meter)	Z	0.1 %
total volume correction error		0.3 %

If the density is used for volume correction, the overall uncertainty is as follows:

density at flowing conditions	ρ	0.2 %*
density at normal conditions	ρ_n	0.2 %
total volume correction error		0.3 %

Irrespective of the approach adopted, the uncertainty of volume correction under field conditions is less than ± 0.3 %.

---

* If no correction is made for the velocity of sound effect, the systematic error of the density at flowing conditions may be as high as 0.6 %.

7. References

(1) Burnett, S.: Compressibility Determinations without Volume Measurements, ASME Trans. J. appl. mech., $\underline{3}$, 136 - 140 (1936)

(2) GERG Information Committee on the Thermodynamic Properties of Natural Gas: Accurate Measurement and Prediction of the Compressibility Factor for Natural Gas Mixtures for Use in Transmission, Paper IGU/C4-82, presented at the 15th World Gas Conference, Lausanne (1982)

(3) Jaeschke, M.: Experimental Pressure, Volume and Temperature Data for Natural Gases. Paper TP-15C-2, 8th Symposium on Thermophysical Properties, Gaithersburg, Maryland (1981)

(4) Jaeschke, M.: PVT Data for Carbon Dioxide-Ethane Mixtures. Gas Quality, Elsevier Science Publishers B.V. Amsterdam (1986), pp. 247-261

(5) Achtermann, H.J., Bose, T.K., Jaeschke, M., St-Arnaud, J.M.: Direct Determination of the Second Refractivity Virial Coefficient of Methane, Nitrogen and Five of their Mixtures. Int. J. Thermophysics 7, 357-366 (1986)

(6) Hinze, H.M., Jaeschke, M.: Messung der Dichte von Erdgasen nach der Wägemethode und mit Betriebsdichteaufnehmern. Fortschritts-Berichte VDI, Reihe 6, Energietechnik/Wärmetechnik No. 162 (1985)

(7) Kleinrahm, R., Duschek, W., Wagner, W., Jaeschke, M.: Measurement and Correlation of the (Pressure, Density, Temperature) Relation of Methane in the Temperature Range from 273.15 K to 323.15 K and Pressures up to 8 MPa, The Journal of Chemical Thermodynamics (to be published)

(8) Ballez, G., Rombouts, P.: System for Natural Gas Metering in Energy Units. Distrigaz, Metering Department, Brussels, Belgium (June 1985)

(9) Jaeschke, M.: Messung und Berechnung der Dichte von Erdgases, gwf-gas/erdgas $\underline{126}$, 93-102 (1985)

(10) Jaeschke, M., Hinze, H.M.: Using densitometers in gas metering. Hydrocarbon Processing, (June 1987), pp. 37-41

(11) Manual for the Determination of Supercompressibility Factors for Natural Gas. AGA (1963)

(12)   Herning, F.u.E., Wolowski: Kompressibilitätszahlen und Realgasfaktoren von Erdgasen nach neuen amerikanischen Berechnungsmethoden. Ges. Ber. Ruhrgas 15 (1966), pp. 7-14

(13)   Jaeschke, M., Harbrink, B.: Korrektur des AGA NX-19-mod-Rechenverfahrens für Realgasfaktoren von Erdgas H. gwf-gas/erdgas 123, 20-27 (1982)

(14)   Melvin, A.: Predictive Methods for the Compressibility Factors of Natural Gases in Transmission. IGRC, Toronto, (1986), paper 93

(15)   Jaeschke, M.: Realgasverhalten - Einheitliche Berechnungsmöglichkeiten von Erdgas L und H. gwf-gas/erdgas 129 (1), (1988)

(16)   Starling, K.E.: Compressibility and Supercompressibility for Natural Gas and other Hydrocarbon Gases. A.G.A. Transmission Measurement Committee Report No. 8, December (1985)

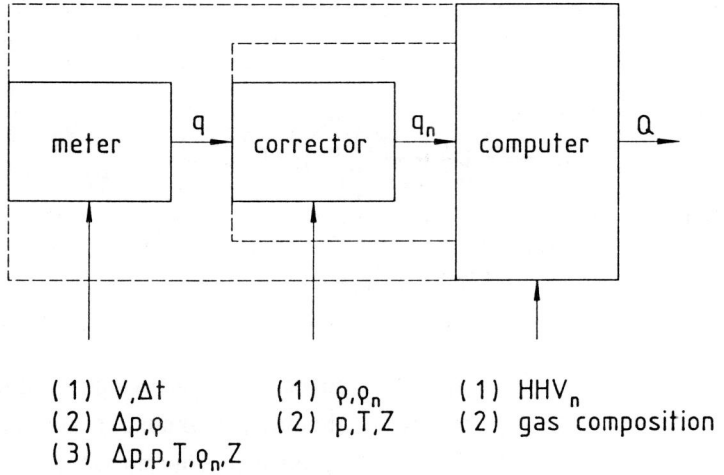

(1) V,Δt   (1) ρ,ρ$_n$ (1) HHV$_n$
(2) Δp,ρ   (2) p,T,Z   (2) gas composition
(3) Δp,p,T,ρ$_n$,Z

Fig. 1   Schematic of Energy Flow Measurement

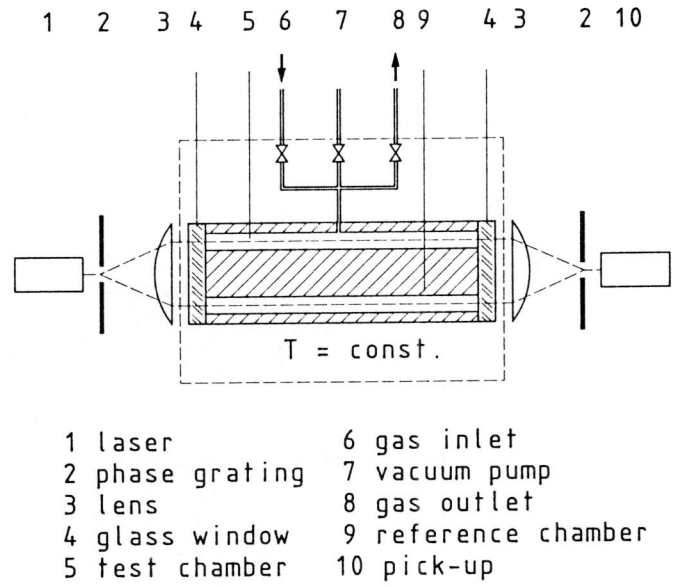

1 laser   6 gas inlet
2 phase grating   7 vacuum pump
3 lens   8 gas outlet
4 glass window   9 reference chamber
5 test chamber   10 pick-up

Fig. 2   Schematic Drawing of the Grating Interferometer

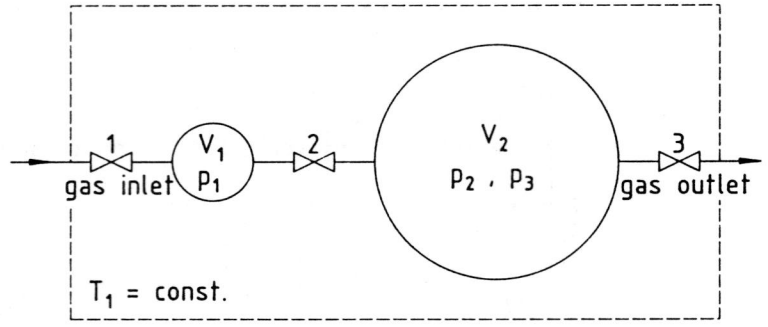

p_1 : automatic dead-weight balance
p_2, p_3 : absolute pressure transmitter
T_1 : resistance thermometer
$p_1 Z_n / Z_1$: calculated from pressures p_1, p_2 and p_3

Fig. 3   Field Method of Measuring Compressibility Factors by the Z Meter (DEH)

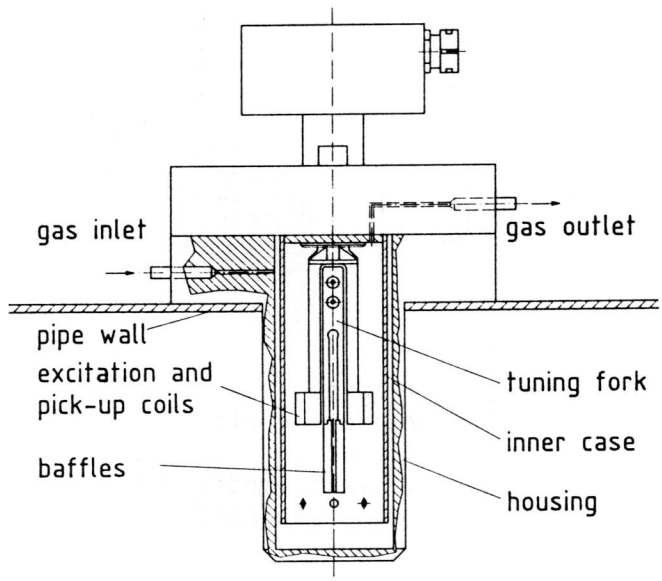

Fig. 4   Vitrating-Element Densitometer

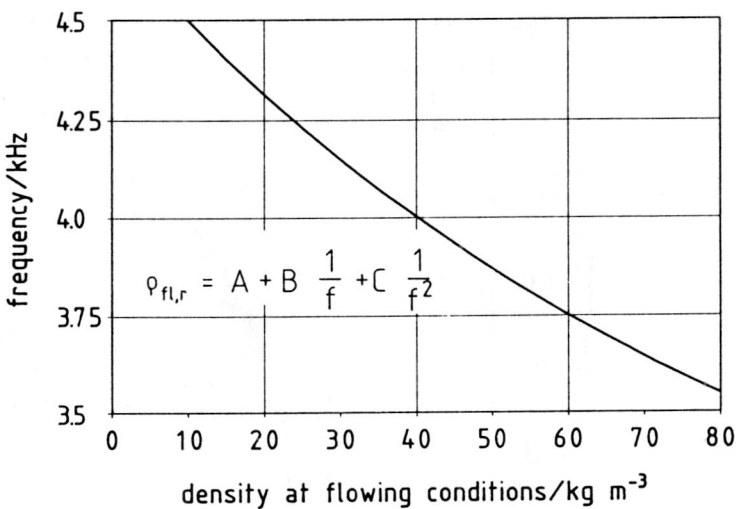

Fig. 5   Density at Flowing Conditions Versus Frequency

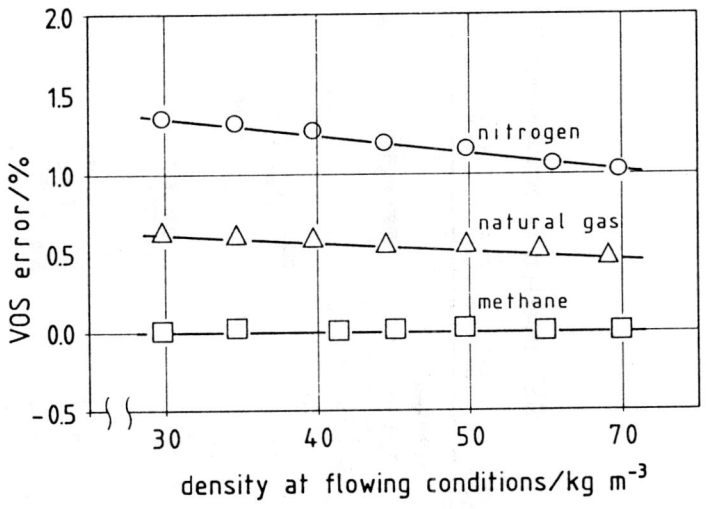

Fig. 6   Velocity of Sound (VOS) Effect on Densitometers

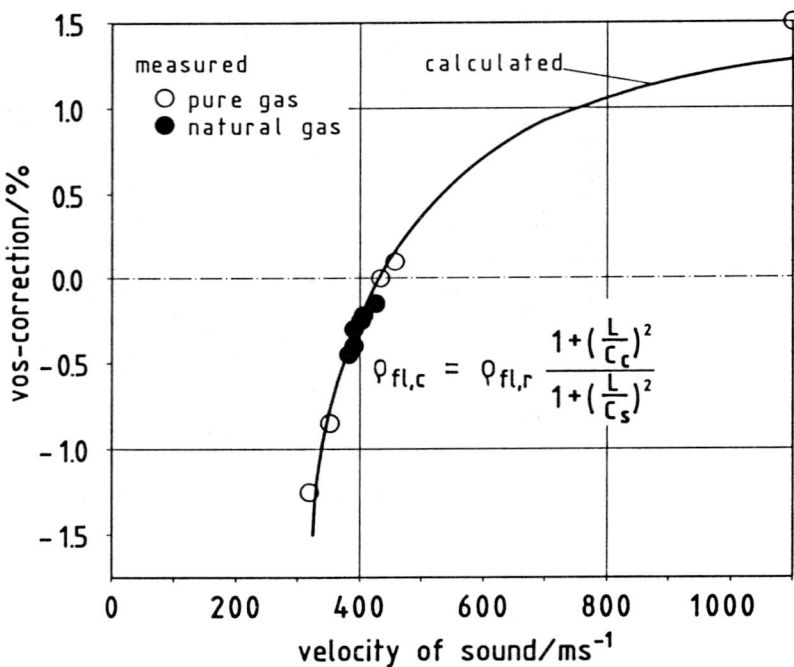

Fig. 7   Velocity of Sound (VOS) Correction of Density
(C_c = 433 ms^{-1}, L = 53.36 ms^{-1} and $\rho_{fl,r}$ = 30 kg m^{-3})

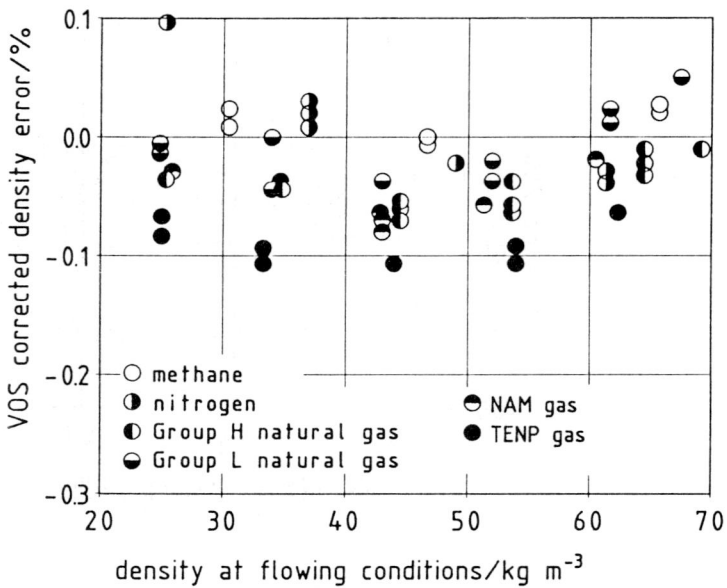

Fig. 8   Velocity of Sound (VOS)-Corrected Density Measurement Error

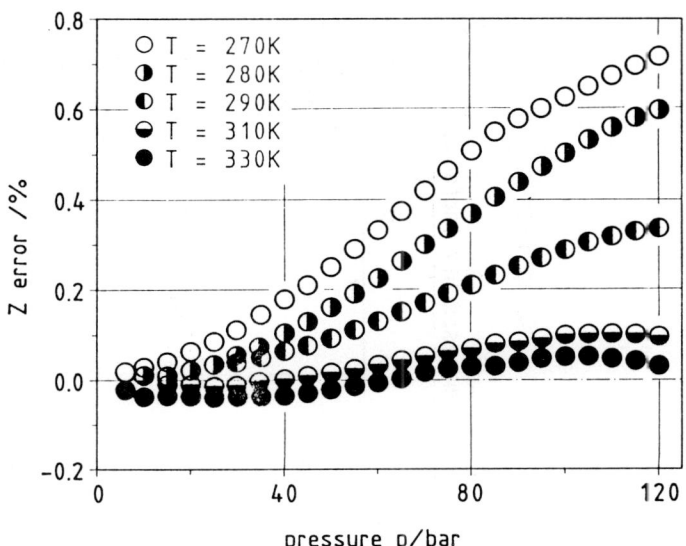

Fig. 9   Z-Error, Difference between Calculated Z-Values (AGA NX-19-mod) and Measured Z-Values for Group L Natural Gas (NAM Gas, $HHV_n = 36.6$ MJm^{-3})

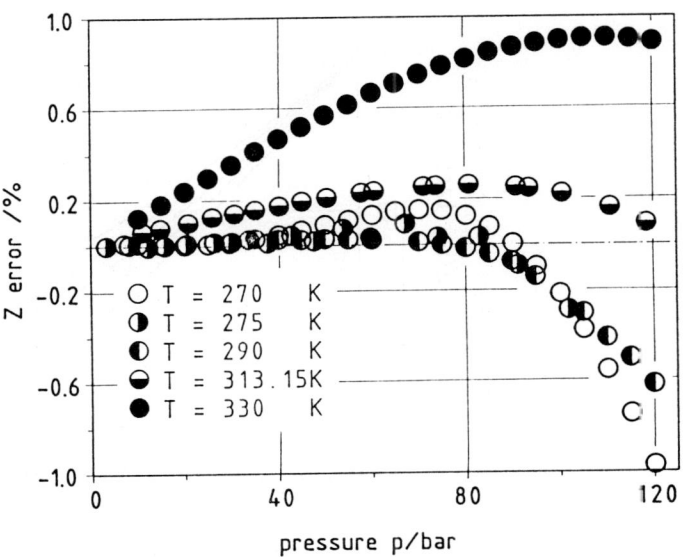

Fig. 10   Z Error, Difference Between Calculated Z-Values (AGA NX-19-mod/3H) and Measured Z-Values for Group H Natural Gas (Ekofisk Gas, $HHV_n = 44.3$ MJm^{-3})

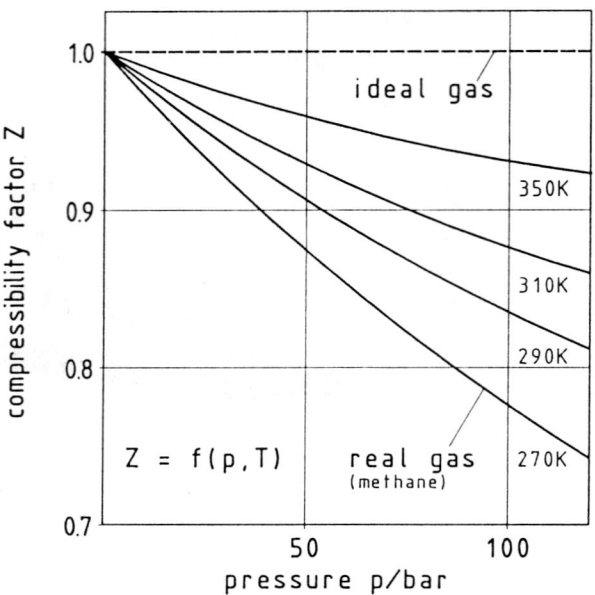

Fig. 11   Real Gas Behaviour of Natural Gas. Effect of Temperature on the Compressibility Factor of Methane

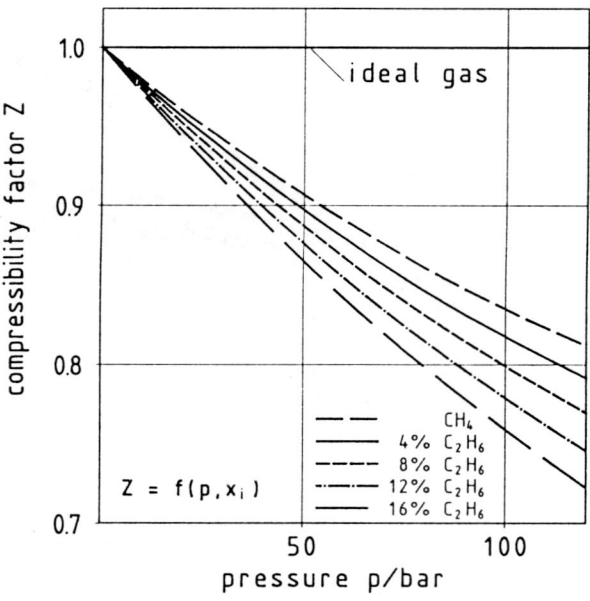

Fig. 12   Real Gas Behaviour of Natural Gas. Effect of Ethane Concentration on Compressibilty Factor at 290 K

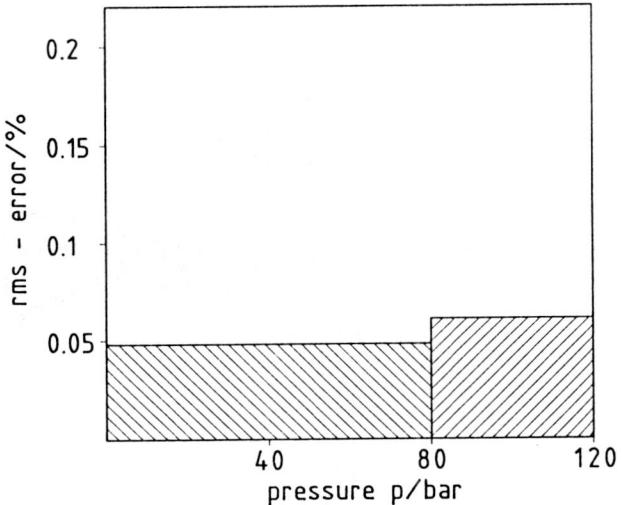

Fig. 13 Root-Mean-Square Errors of the GERG Virial Equation for all Natural Gases

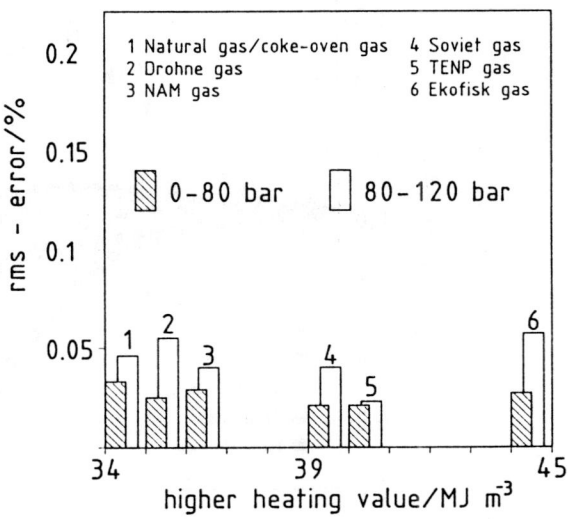

Fig. 14 Root-Mean-Square Errors of the GERG Virial Equation for Specific Natural Gases

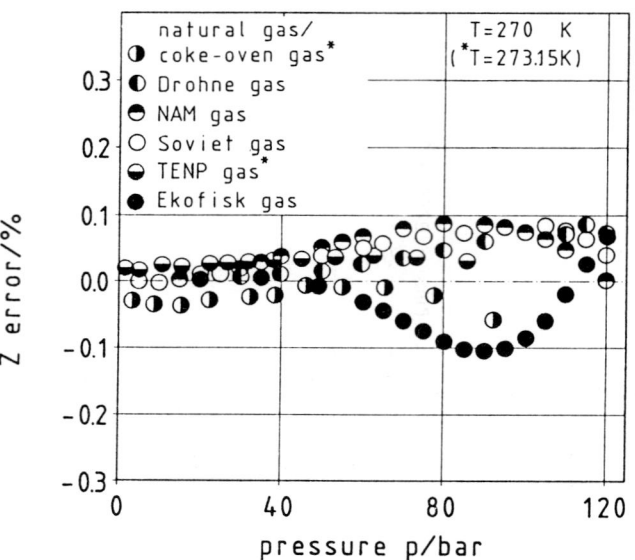

Fig. 15 Influence of Pressure on Z Error, the Difference between Calculated Z-Values (GERG Virial Equation) and Measured Z-Values for Specific Natural Gases at 270 K or 273.15 K.

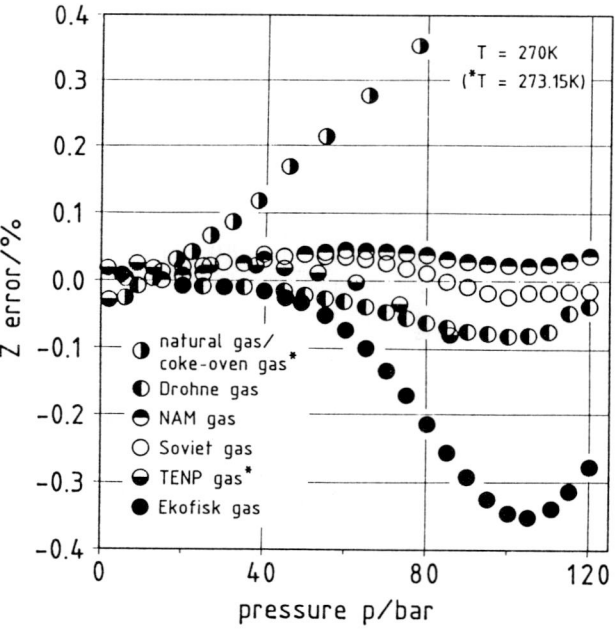

Fig. 16 Influence of Pressure on Z Error, the Difference between Calculated Z-Values (GRI Super Z Equation) and Measured Z-Values for Specific Natural Gases at 270 K or 273.15 K.

POSTER SESSIONS
SÉANCES D'AFFICHAGE

MICROWAVE GROUND THAWING DEVICE

G.E. COBURN
INHITEK SYSTEMS LTD., ONTARIO CANADA

W. RAHMAN
THE CONSUMERS' GAS CO., LTD., ONTARIO

November 1987

FROZEN GROUND PROBLEM

Each winter in Canada, Northern United States and certain Northern European Countries significant additional costs are incurred when handling frozen soil. The following is a description of a number of areas where frozen ground poses operational problems.

Frost makes repair work to utilities time consuming and expensive. The utilities can be damaged by excavation when jack hammers or backhoes are used. In Calgary coal and straw as well as propane heaters have been tried to thaw the soil. These techniques generally take five to seven days to thaw the soil. The exposed flames from the coal or propane can be hazardous. Very shallow utilities can also be damaged by excessive surface heating.

The Public Works Departments also experience difficulties regarding digging up and installing sewage systems and waterpipes in the winter.

Installation or replacement of hydro poles in the winter can be a serious problem. Augering frozen soil can be ineffective in the winter particularly in rocky soil conditions. In certain permafrost areas of Canada hydro poles must be installed in the winter in order to protect the environment.

Companies mining the permafrost gravels containing gold are attempting to melt the gravel through the use of steam which is slow and expensive. Explosives are ineffective in frozen soil and if they are used underground may cause caving of the underground workings.

Cemetery operators generally wait until spring to bury the dead because of frozen ground problems. Storage of the bodies must be arranged, which is expensive.

Nursery operators currently do not plant trees or shrubs in the winter because of frozen ground conditions. The trees are dormant in the winter and therefore could be transplanted without damage done to them.

The military also have problems in the winter digging trenches, fox holes, etc. in the frozen soil.

MICROWAVE HEATING

Microwaves are electromagnetic waves produced from commercially available magnetrons. They are absorbed by moisture which results in its temperature increase. Microwave heating is established technology and is most commonly used in small household microwave ovens.

Microwaves do not penetrate or heat up metals but they do easily penetrate plastic, dry wood and ice. Plastic is transparent to microwaves and as a result microwaves do not heat plastic or affect the properties of plastic. Soils, particularly clay rich soils and water do absorb microwaves.

When wet soil freezes, the main process is the physical change of soil water from liquid to solid that turns the soil into a hard mass resembling concrete. Its relatively high strength can be attributed in part to the binding together of soil particles with ice. In a porous body like soil, water exists in a network of interconnecting pores; when it freezes, this network becomes rigid and encloses the soil particles in a solid block. If the soil is dry it cannot "freeze" in the accepted sense although its temperature may well be below 32°F.

It has been found that all the water in soil does not freeze at the same temperature due to the presence of minerals and soil pressure gradient. The strength of frozen soil increases as the temperature is lowered and more water freezes.

Microwaves will be strongly absorbed by the water that remains unfrozen in the soil causing the temperature of the water and the soil to rise. Clay soil also absorbs microwaves. A certain amount of heating by conduction also takes place as the soil temperature rises.

MICROWAVE GROUND THAWING UNIT

Inhitek Systems Ltd. under the sponsorship of Consumers Gas Co. has developed microwave ground thawing units. In these units microwaves are transmitted directly from the bottom of a housing, containing a magnetron into a vertical antenna (probe). These waves propagate into the soil through horizontal slots in the antenna. Vertical holes have to be drilled in frozen soil to accommodate the units.

The unit is designed to be rugged, durable and easily portable by hand. The 1,400W output unit utilizes 'off the shelf' magnetron, transformer and capacitor found in commercial microwave ovens. It works on a 115 volt supply. The following is a description of the design of several components.

HOUSING DESIGN

The material used for the 1400W Output Power Unit is aluminum alloy 1/4 inch thick. The power unit consists of two separate castings, the Housing (which forms the base of the unit) and the Cover. The two castings, which are of equal size are held together by 12 screws.

The magnetron is located in the Housing and the rest of the components including the transformer, capacitor, blower, switches and other electronic components are bolted on to a metal plate located in the cover of the unit. (Please refer to Appendix A-1 for a photograph of the housing)

All of the intake and exhaust louvres are located in the cover of the unit rather than the Housing in order to minimize accidental water entry into the power unit. Watertight switch, running light, and fuseholder are used in the construction of the unit.

"Cast-In" handles were used in the construction of the unit. These handles are very sturdy and the design allows plenty of room for grasping the handles even with heavy work gloves. The handles do not protrude from the side of the Housing and therefore the units can be placed very close together if desired.

ANTENNA DESIGN

The radiating antenna is constructed from an inner and outer brass tube conductor. When the antenna is connected to the housing the inner conductor or brass tube fits directly over the radiating tip of the magnetron, inside the housing. The outer tubing has an outside diameter of 1-1/2 inches, and the inner brass tube has an outside diameter of 5/8 of an inch. The inner conductor is kept centred by teflon spacers. The inner and outer brass tubes are capped and soldered at the bottom of the antenna. (Please refer to Appendix A-1 for a photograph of the antenna). The length of the antenna is 3.33 feet and is covered with heat resistant teflon sleeve to prevent entry of dirt and water. These antennas can be produced in different lengths to suit a specific application.

Slots are cut at intervals down the length of the outer brass conductor. Uniform energy distribution, was achieved from the antenna by rotating alternate slot pairs 90° around the circumference of the brass conductor. This uniform transmission of microwave energy radially creates even thawing of the frozen soil.

The depth of the slots in the brass conductor determines how much microwave energy is transmitted at any location.

Extensive testing was conducted in cold rooms and in actual field conditions in order to match the energy output of the antenna to the soil temperature profile.

POWER REQUIREMENTS

Inhitek has chosen an "off-the-shelf" 2300W input magnetron with a frequency of 2450mHz generally used in commercial microwave ovens. These magnetrons are durable, available and relatively inexpensive and use 115 volt power source.

Ten Microwave Thawing Units have a power requirement of 23kW. These power requirements can be easily met with a trailer mounted generator.

SAFETY DEVICES

The design of the all metal lower housing and the radiating antenna, which fits over the tip of the magnetron, eliminates any back scatter of microwave energy into the interior of the housing of the unit. The antenna is locked in place after it has been tightly screwed onto the power unit.

A water-tight red light located on the cover of the power unit warns the operator that the microwave unit has been connected to the power source and has been turned on. The on and off switch is also water-tight.

A sealed pressure activated "cut-off" switch is located on the bottom of the power unit. This switch completes the circuit from the power source to the transformer and magnetron. If the microwave unit is accidentally lifted while in operation, the "cut-off" switch will automatically break the circuit to the magnetron after the unit has been lifted approximately one inch.

An externally sealed fuse protects the power unit from power surges. A switch located on the magnetron protects the magnetron from overheating.

CO-AXIAL CABLE SYSTEM

In order to improve the flexibility and ease of operation, a variation of this concept, a Co-axial Cable System was designed and developed.

This System allows the power units and antenna to be connected with a 7/8 inch diameter cable fifteen to twenty feet in length. The advantage of this concept are as follows:

1. The power units could be mounted on a generator, trolly or truck, which would minimize the amount of handling of these units by workers.

2. The power units could be locked in place which would minimize theft.

3. The housing of the power unit is made out of sheet metal which is robust and less expensive than the cast aluminum housing.

The housing of the power unit is constructed out of welded 1/4 inch sheet metal and is designed to bolt onto an angle iron rack. This rack could be mounted on a truck, compressor or generator. The on-off switch, running light, power connection and cutoff switch, connected to the mounting plate by a cord, are all located on the front panel for easy access.

The Co-axial Cable screws onto the threaded connection on the front panel. The other end of the co-axial cable is connected to a $90°$ elbow which in turn is connected to a transition connection which is attached to a mounting plate. The antenna screws onto the threaded connection at the bottom of the mounting plate. The cutoff switch will automatically shut the unit off if the mounting plate is accidentally lifted when the unit is in operation.

The metal sheathed co-axial cable is relatively stiff and is not designed for multiple flexing. It can be coiled into three foot diameter loops, however. Please refer to Appendix A-2 for photographs of the unit.

MICROWAVE HEAT TREATMENT OF GROUND

Six 1,400W output microwave thawing units were built for the field testing carried out in March and April of 1986 and the winter of 1986-87. A 1400W output Co-Axial Cable System was also built and tested in the field. Field testing in 1986 was conducted in North Bay, Sturgeon Falls and Timmins, due to the lack of frost in the Toronto area. Thawing tests were conducted in sandy as well as clay rich areas. The objective of the testing was to test the microwave units in the worst field conditions possible. (eg. in dense, greasy super-saturated clay). We succeeded in finding such a test site in Timmins that had a frost depth of six feet in early April of 1986.

Inhitek and Consumers Gas Co. also carried out ground thawing tests using the units on road sites in Peterborough and Ottawa during the winter of 1987.

THAWING RATE OF MICROWAVE UNITS

The thawing rate of the microwave units varies according to:

1. **Ground Temperature.** The colder the temperature, the longer it takes to thaw the soil.

2. **Volume of soil being thawed.** The greater the volume of soil being thawed the longer it takes to thaw the soil. Conversely a decrease in thawing time can be achieved by reducing the volume of soil being thawed.

3. **Soil Type.** The silty clay soil takes longer to thaw than permeable sand or gravel.

4. **Soil Moisture.** Extremely wet soils take longer to thaw than dry soils. (Microwaves can travel further in dry soils than wet soils before being absorbed.)

5. **Distribution of microwave energy down the length of the antenna.** For maximum thawing efficiency most of the transmitted microwave energy should be directed at the coldest section of the soil profile.

6. **Power output of the magnetron.** Decreases in thawing time were obtained by increasing the magnetron size from 850 W output to 1400 W output.

FIELD TESTS

During late winter of 1986, Inhitek conducted tests in the clay belt near Timmins, Ontario. The frost depth was approximately 6 feet and the ground was dense, greasy water saturated clay.

The microwave units even under these adverse conditions each thawed a volume of frozen soil 14 inches in diameter by 40 inches deep in a period of 2-1/4 hours.

Further thawing rate tests were conducted in Peterborough and Ottawa during the winter of 1987. Tests in Peterborough were conducted in soil conditions ranging from rocky-sandy soil containing 30% to 60% clay and the remainder silty sand and rock boulders. The ambient air temperature was -5°C and the frost depth ranged from 32 to 36 inches.

The modular and co-axial microwave units each thawed a volume of frozen soil 16 to 18 inches in diameter by 40 inches deep in 2-1/2 hours.

In the tests in Ottawa, again, both the co-axial and the modular units were used. Tests were conducted on roadways with soil conditions varying from sandy to hard plastic clay. The frost depth was 40 inches.

In one of the tests which was in very plastic clay, the units were placed on top of the pavement to determine the effect of pavement on the thawing pattern. The units were run for 2 hours and 10 minutes and the hole was dug the following morning. Each unit thawed a 15 inch diameter hole 40 inches deep. The pavement had no effect on the thawing pattern and waiting overnight actually increased the thawing diameter of the units.

The testing proved that even under the worst possible soil conditions a single 1400W output microwave unit will thaw at least a 12 inch diameter by 40 inch deep cylinder of frozen soil in 2-1/4 hours.

POTENTIAL BENEFITS

Straw-coal burning techniques are still used by utilities in Alberta. This method takes three or four days to thaw down to three or four feet and presents environmental problems such as sparks, open flames and obnoxious fumes.

The propane technique consists of a five hundred gallon propane tank mounted on a trailer. Five burners can be run off the trailer. The burners are placed in 4 inches steel pipes that are buried in a sand pit. This method is slower than the straw-coal technique and has the drawback of open flames and therefore cannot be used around leaking gas lines.

Electrical resistance heating rods have also been tried in Alberta but are less effective than the straw-coal or propane techniques.

The results of thawing tests conducted by the City of Calgary using the above techniques are outlined in the following tables.

TABLE 1

Time Required to Thaw Gravel to Three Foot Depth

Thawing Type

Coal & Straw	39.5 Hrs.
Propane	32.5 Hrs.
Electrical Resistance Rods	76.5 Hrs.
Microwave	1.5 Hrs.

TABLE 2

Time Required to Thaw Clay to Three Foot Depth

Thawing Type

Coal & Straw	73.5 Hrs.
Propane	61.5 Hrs.
Microwave	2.25 Hrs.

Due to the lack of adequate and consistant frost depths during the 1986 and 1987 winters, no direct comparison could be made with conventional excavation methods. However, the thawing rate tests so far have demonstrated that the microwave thawing unit can thaw soil effectively which should result in savings in winter excavation costs. This unit also provides additional benefit by avoiding accidental damage to underground utilities which can be caused by conventional methods such as jack hammers. Furthermore, excavating in thawed soil will reduce maintenace costs on conventional equipment. By avoiding the use of jackhammers for a long duration, in frost, the physical strain on workers is significantly reduced. Further field testing is planned during the upcoming winter to quantify the benefits derived from this unit.

CONCLUSIONS

The tests conducted so far show that the Microwave Thawing Unit can thaw soil much faster than other conventional methods such as: straw-coal; propane; and electrical resistance heating rods.

As the excavation time for thawed soil is significantly lower than in frozen soil conditions this development offers the potential for cost savings in winter operation.

An earlier limited market study and Inhiteks' communication with a number of companies indicate that there is a very good market for the Microwave Thawing Unit. The retail price of the unit will be based on a detailed market study.

APPENDIX

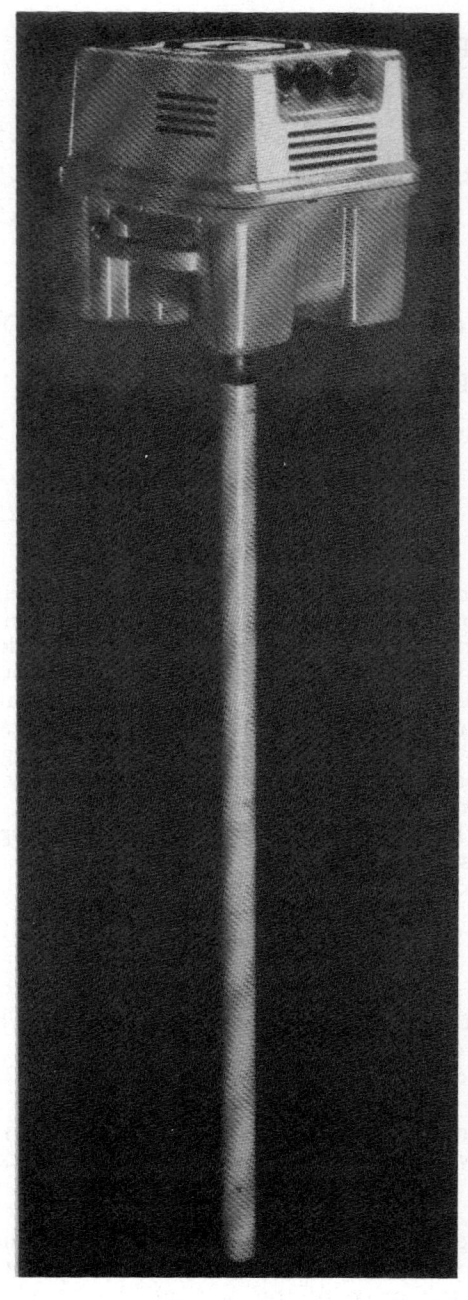

1400W OUTPUT MICROWAVE UNIT WITH ANTENNA

APPENDIX

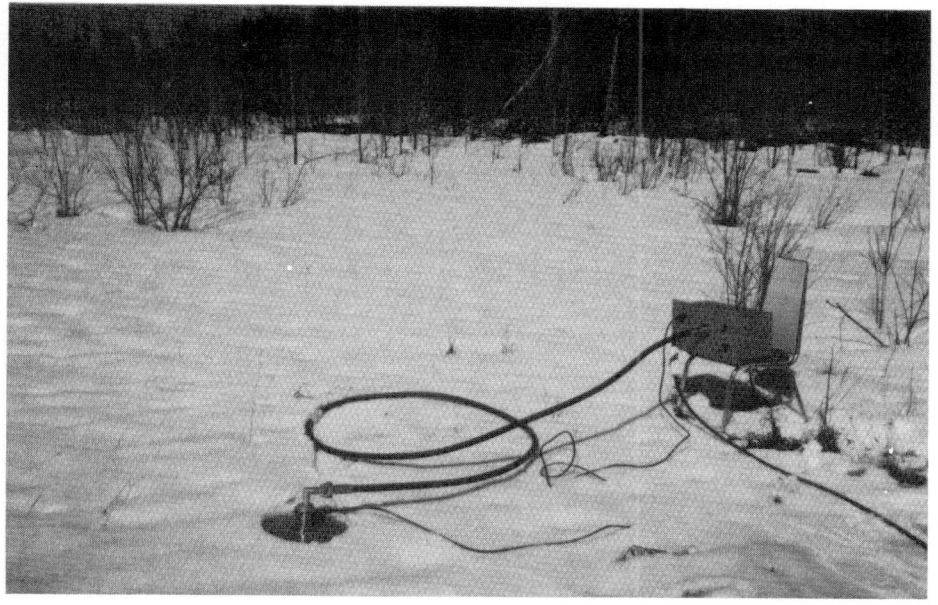

CO-AXIAL CABLE UNIT

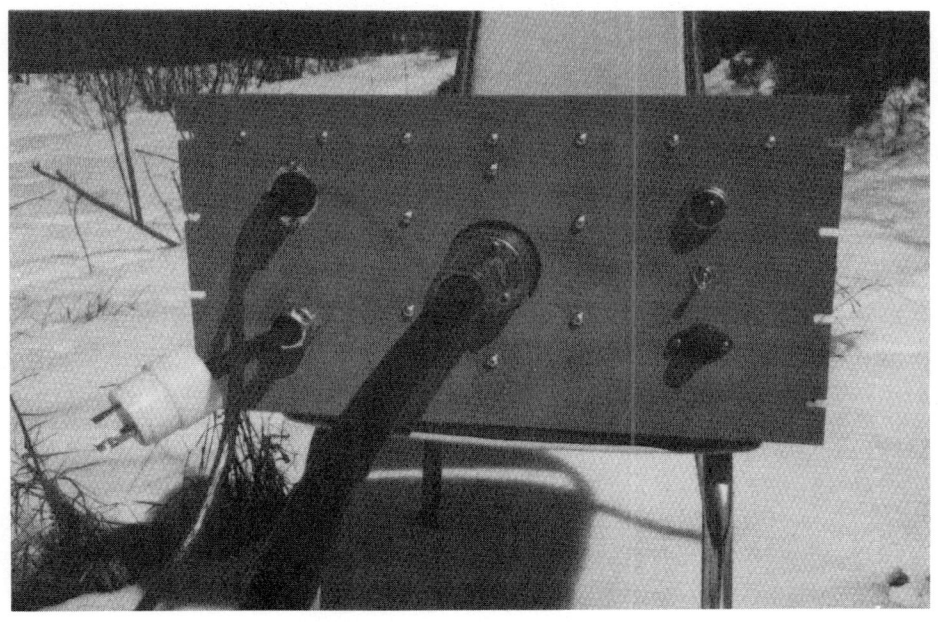

FRONT VIEW OF CO-AXIAL POWER UNIT

Simulation des Installations de Combustion Submergée
Martin Fournier, Christophe Guy,
Pierre J. Carreau et Jean R. Paris
Département de génie chimique, Ecole Polytechnique
Montréal, Québec, H3C 3A7

Le design d'installations de combustion submergée est réalisée de façon très empirique. Pour cette raison, un logiciel ayant pour objectifs de permettre la conception assistée par ordinateur de ces installations et de déterminer les conditions opératoires optimales a été mis au point.

Les calculs, les hypothèses, la structure interne, le fonctionnement et les développements futurs du logiciel sont présentés. De plus, deux exemples d'utilisation sont donnés.

INTRODUCTION:

La combustion submergée est un procédé de transfert de chaleur et de matière dans lequel les gaz de combustion provenant d'un brûleur sont mis en contact direct avec un liquide à chauffer, à évaporer ou à traiter chimiquement.

En dépit de ses performances énergétiques et économiques élevées et de ses multiples applications industrielles envisageables, ce n'est que depuis une quinzaine d'années que ce procédé a été appliqué industriellement. La combustion submergée, particulièrement adaptée au chauffage et à l'évaporation de bains industriels à basse température ($100^{\circ}C$ et moins) a été essentiellement utilisée jusqu'à ce jour pour des opérations de chauffage.

Deux articles ont traité en profondeur des caractéristiques massiques et thermiques, des avantages, des inconvénients et des applications de la combustion submergée [1,2]. Ainsi, seuls les éléments principaux de chacun de ces points sont rapportés ci-après.

CARACTERISTIQUES MASSIQUES ET THERMIQUES:

Le diagramme thermique théorique de la combustion submergée appliquée à l'eau a été présenté par Thouault [1] (Fig. 1). Le diagramme concerne la combustion stoechiométrique d'un gaz naturel (pouvoir calorifique supérieur = 40.5 MJ/NM^3) avec de l'air sec. Thouault fait l'hypothèse que les fumées s'échappant du bain ont atteint l'équilibre massique et thermique avec ce dernier. Il convient de s'assurer que la profondeur à laquelle est placé le distributeur soit suffisante pour que cette hypothèse soit valable.

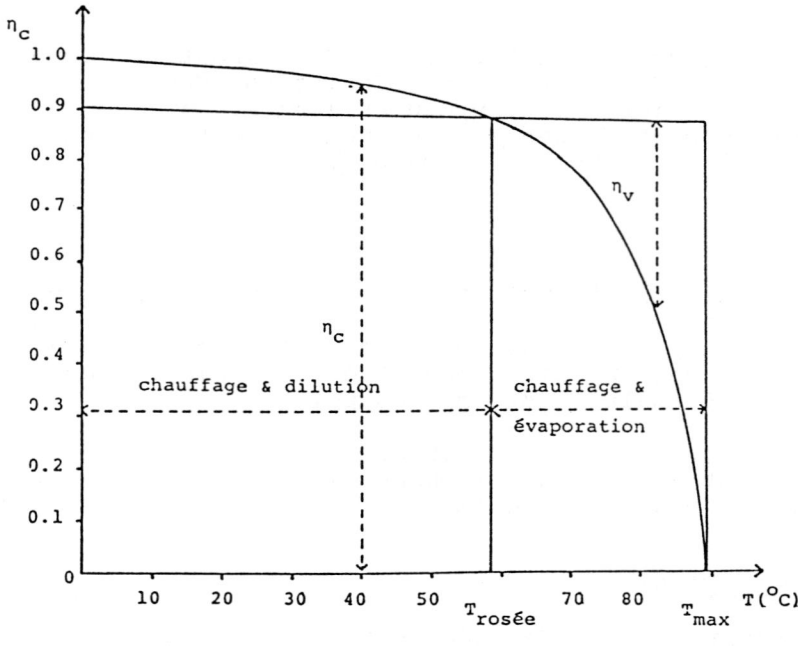

FIGURE 1

Pour une température inférieure à la température de rosée des produits de combustion, un rendement de chauffage élevé est atteint et une partie de l'eau de combustion se condense dans le bain. Pour une température du bain supérieure à la température de rosée, le rendement de chauffage chute et il y a évaporation du bain. La température maximale de chauffage est atteinte lorsque toute l'énergie de combustion est évacuée avec les fumées. A cette température, le rendement thermique est nul et le rendement d'évaporation est maximal.

Thouault a aussi étudié l'influence des divers paramètres de fonctionnement. Il a ainsi déterminé que:

- le rendement thermique, le rendement limite d'évaporation, la température de rosée et la température maximale de chauffage diminuent lorsque la taux d'aération augmente;

- le rendement thermique et la température de rosée augmentent lorsque l'hygrométrie du comburant augmente.

AVANTAGES :

Les principaux advantages de la combustion submergée sont:

- efficacités thermique et d'évaporation très élévées dû à une surface d'échange très grande entre les produits de combustion et le liquide et à l'absence de parois métallique se traduisant par un transfert de chaleur optimal;

- bonne homogénisation du liquide résultant du mouvement des bulles;

- installation relativement simple se traduisant par des coûts d'investissement et d'opération faibles.

INCONVENIENTS :

Les inconvénients majeurs de la combustion submergée sont:

- température optimale de chauffage du bain relativement basse (65-70°C), puisque pour une température supérieure à la température de rosée des produits de combustion, une quantité de plus en plus grande de l'énergie fournie sert à évaporer le liquide;

- acidification du liquide dû à la dissolution du dioxyde de carbone particulièrement notable pour des systèmes fonctionnant en circuit fermé.

APPLICATIONS :

Les applications de la combustion submergée se classifient parmi trois domaines:

- chauffage de bains pour des températures modérées (70-80°C et moins):
    - production d'eau chaude,
    - chauffage de liquides chargés, corrosifs et incrustants,
    - chauffage de boues ou lisiers,...

- évaporation et concentration de solutions:
    - concentration d'acides,
    - concentration de saumures,
    - concentration de rejets industriels, ...

- traitement d'effluents:
    - carbonatation de l'eau,
    - neutralisation de solution bassiques,
    - oxydation de rejets industriels, ...

Au Québec, la combustion submergée est utilisée notamment pour concentrer des solutions d'électrolyses dans le but de récupérer des sels, chauffer des solutions d'acides pour le traitement de surface des métaux et chauffer des bains de traitement aérobique d'effluents industriels.

CONCEPTION DES INSTALLATIONS:

A l'exception du brûleur, la conception d'une installations de combustion submergée et, plus particulièrement, du distributeur des produits de combustion et de la cuve est très empirique. Pour cette raison, la conception d'un logiciel a été entreprise. Il a pour objectifs, d'une part, de permettre la conception assistée par ordinateur d'installations de combustion submergée et, d'autre part, de déterminer les conditions optimales d'opération. De plus, le logiciel est de type intéractif amical et exécutable sur ordinateur personnel.

CALCULS ET HYPOTHESES:

Les rendements thermique et d'évaporation et les températures caractéristiques sont calculés en fonction des conditions opératoires. A partir des propriétés thermodynamiques du gaz et des liquides traités, les bilans massique et enthalpique sont effectués sur l'installation toute entière. Le rendement thermique est défini comme le rapport entre la charge thermique du bain et le pouvoir calorifique supérieur du carburant. Dans le cas du chauffage de solutions aqueuses, le rendement d'évaporation est défini comme le rapport de l'enthalpie de l'eau effectivement évaporée du bain et le pouvoir calorifique supérieur du carburant. Les températures caractéristiques sont la température de rosée des produits de combustion et la température maximale de chauffage du bain.

Quelques hypothèses et limitations interviennent dans les modules de calculs du logiciel. Parmi les plus importantes, notons que:

- les fumées s'échappant du bain sont considérées en équilibre massique et thermique avec le liquide;

- les pertes énergétiques de l'installation de combustion submergée ne sont pas calculées.

MODULES:

Le logiciel, conçu de façon modulaire, est constitué de quatre composantes: un aide, un démonstrateur, un module de calcul en régime permanent et un module de calcul en régime transitoire. Sa structure interne est présentée à la figure 2.

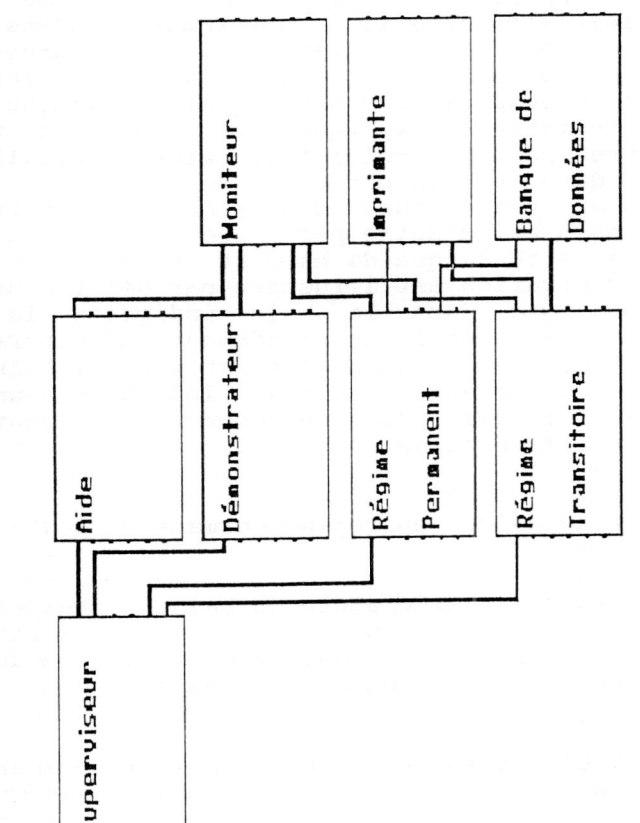

FIGURE 2

Le module d'aide, accessible en tout temps durant l'exécution, fournit à l'usager, de façon concise, les informations pertinentes concernant le logiciel en général et ses modules.

Le module de démonstration met en évidence les interactions qui existent entre les rendements thermique et d'évaporation et la température du bain pour une installation fonctionnant en régime permanent. Plus particulièrement, l'installation considérée dans ce module utilise une combustion stoechiométrique du gaz naturel avec de l'air sec à 15°C pour maintenir un bain d'eau à la température spécifiée par l'usager. Des pièces métalliques initialement à 15°C sont immergées dans le bain et chauffées jusqu'à la température de ce dernier. Pour une température de bain choisie par l'usager, les rendements thermique et d'évaporation sont qualitativement illustrés à l'aide d'une animation graphique. Le rendement thermique est ainsi illustré par un volume de pièces métalliques traité thermiquement dans le bain par unité de temps, car, d'une part, l'élévation en température des pièces constitue la charge thermique du bain et, d'autre part, une relation directe existe entre la charge thermique du bain et le rendement thermique. Le rendement d'évaporation est illustrée par des flèches en surface des bulles de gaz dans le bain indiquant la direction du transfert net d'eau. Ainsi, un rendement d'évaporation négatif est illustré par des flèches pointant vers le bain. Des flèches pointant en direction opposée indiquent un rendement d'évaporation positif. Un rendement d'évaporation nul est représenté par l'absence de flèche.

Le module de calcul en régime permanent peut traiter deux types de situations:

- connaissant la température du bain, la température de l'air comburant, son hygrométrie, le taux d'aération et la puissance du brûleur, le module calcule les rendements thermique et d'évaporation, les températures caractéristiques et la charge thermique du bain;

- connaissant la température du bain, la température de l'air comburant, son hygrométrie, le taux d'aération et la charge thermique du bain, le module calcule les rendements thermique et d'évaporation, les températures caractéristiques et la puissance du brûleur.

Les calculs relatifs a une installation de chauffage ou d'évaporation, dont la charge thermique du bain est nulle, dont la température du bain évolue d'une valeur initiale vers une valeur finale et dont les conditions d'opération du brûleur sont constantes dans le temps, sont effectués dans le module de calcul en régime transitoire. Le module peut traiter deux types de situations:

- connaissant la masse initiale du bain, la température

de l'air comburant, son hygrométrie, le taux d'aération et
le temps de chauffe, le module calcule, d'une part, les
rendements thermique et d'évaporation ainsi que la masse du
bain aux différentes températures de ce dernier et,
d'autres part, les températures caractéristiques et la
puissance du brûleur;

- connaissant la masse initiale du bain, la température
de l'air comburant, son hygrométrie, le taux d'aération et
la puissance du brûleur, le module calcule, d'une part, les
rendements thermique et d'évaporation ainsi que la masse du
bain aux différentes températures de ce dernier et,
d'autres part, les températures caractéristiques et le
temps de chauffe.

Pour les modules de calcul en régime permanent et en régime
transitoire, les données et les résultats sont affichés et
présentés sous forme graphique à l'écran. Un menu rappelle les
commandes disponibles, dont une commande d'impression d'écran qui
s'avère très utile pour la préparation de dossiers. Enfin,
l'exécution rapide des calculs permet à l'usager d'envisager
plusieurs conditions opératoires en très peu de temps.

EXEMPLES DE CALCULS:

1) Bain d'échaudage de porc [3]:

L'opération de l'épilage de porc nécessite préalablement
l'échaudage de l'animal dans une cuve de forme allongée remplie
d'eau maintenue à une température de 62°C. Un taux d'aération de
1.2 est utilisée, car, d'une part, l'opération d'épilage est
facilité par l'agitation de l'eau et, d'autre part, le rendement
thermique n'est pas significativement affecté. La température de
l'air comburant et l'humidité relative de ce dernier sont
supposées constantes et égales, respectivement, à 15°C et 50%.

Quelle puissance de brûleur est nécessaire pour traiter 80
porcs à l'heure équivalent à une charge thermique de 300 kW?

Le problème a été soumis au logiciel et la sortie est
présenté à la figure 3. D'après les calculs, un brûleur de 360 kW
est nécessaire pour permettre l'opération d'échaudage de porcs
sous les conditions opératoires spécifiées. L'installation de
combustion submergée permet d'obtenir un rendement thermique de
83.6% sur PCS.

Outre les rendements, les températures caractéristiques et
la puissance du brûleur, le logiciel calcule les concentrations
en dioxide de carbone, en oxygène et en azote des produits de
combustion, les débits volumiques des fumées sèches quittant le
bain et de gaz naturel nécessaire et le débit massique d'eau
entrainé par les fumées.

Enfin, un graphique résume les comportements des rendements

thermique et d'évaporation pour des températures de bain comprises entre 0°C et la température maximale de chauffage du bain. Les valeurs négatives sont représentées graphiquement par une courbe en pointillé. Ainsi, pour une température de bain inférieure à la température de rosée des produits de combustion, soit 56°C, un rendement thermique supérieur à 90% sur PCS et un rendement d'évaporation négatif sont obtenus. La valeur négative du rendement d'évaporation signifie qu'une partie de l'eau contenue dans les produits de combustion est condensée dans le bain. Pour une température supérieure à la température de rosée, le rendement thermique chute et une quantité d'eau du bain est évaporée par les fumées.

2) Pré-chauffage du bain d'échaudage:

Les opérations du procédé d'échaudage de porcs sont interrompues les fins de semaines.

Quel est le temps de chauffe nécessaire pour reprendre les opérations d'échaudage des porcs le lundi matin et donc pour amener le bain d'eau (13m^3) de 15°C à 62°C?

Le problème a été soumis au logiciel et la sortie est présenté à la figure 4. D'après les calculs, un temps de chauffe de 2 heures et 8 minutes est nécessaire pour chauffer le bain.

Outre les rendements, les températures caractéristiques et le temps de chauffe, le logiciel calcule les concentrations en dioxide de carbone, en oxygène et en azote des produits de combustion, le débit volumique des fumées sèches quittant le bain, le débit volumique de gaz naturel nécessaire et la masse du bain après l'opération de chauffage. De plus, le temps nécessaire pour chauffer le bain jusqu'à sa température maximale depuis la température initiale et la masse du bain sont calculés.

Enfin, un graphique résume les évolutions des rendements thermique et d'évaporation et de la température du bain dans le temps.

3) Conclusion

Pour la capacité de traitement et les conditions opératoires décrites ci-dessus, l'abattoir municipal de Douai en France, a installé un équipement de combustion submergée de puissance 370kW sur leur installation d'échaudage de porcs.

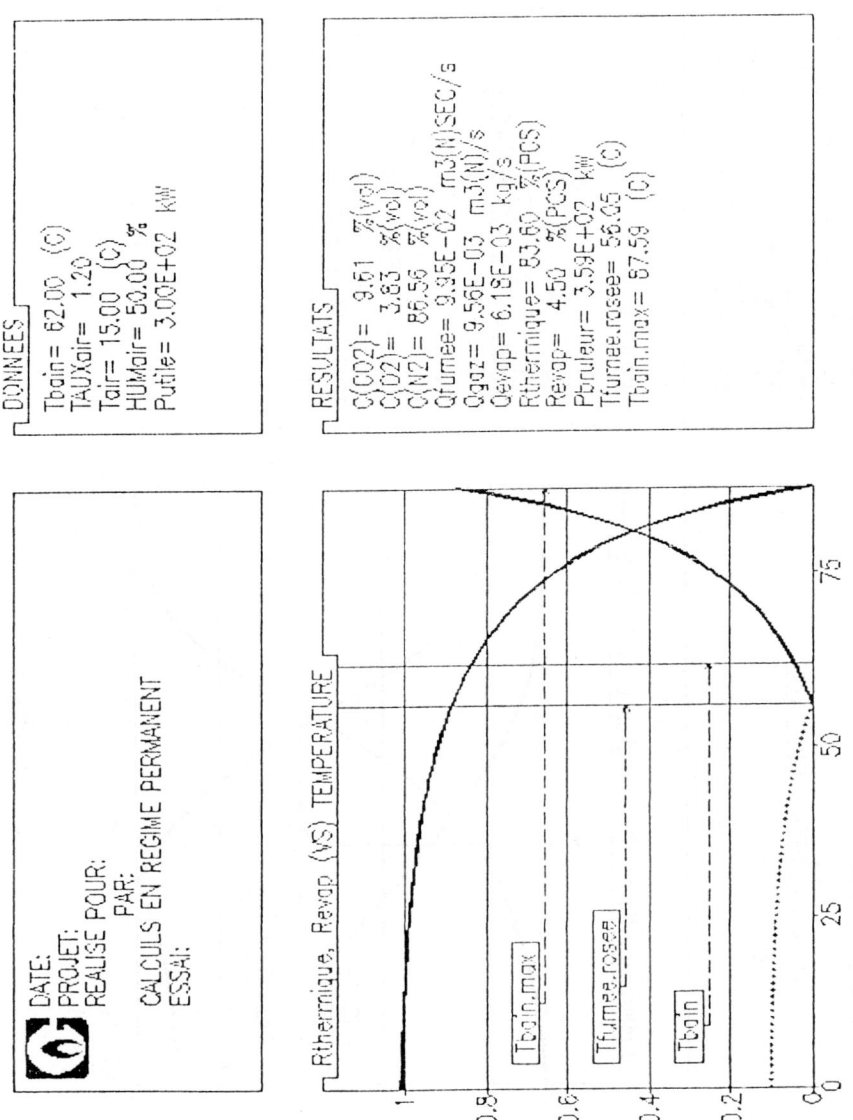

FIGURE 3

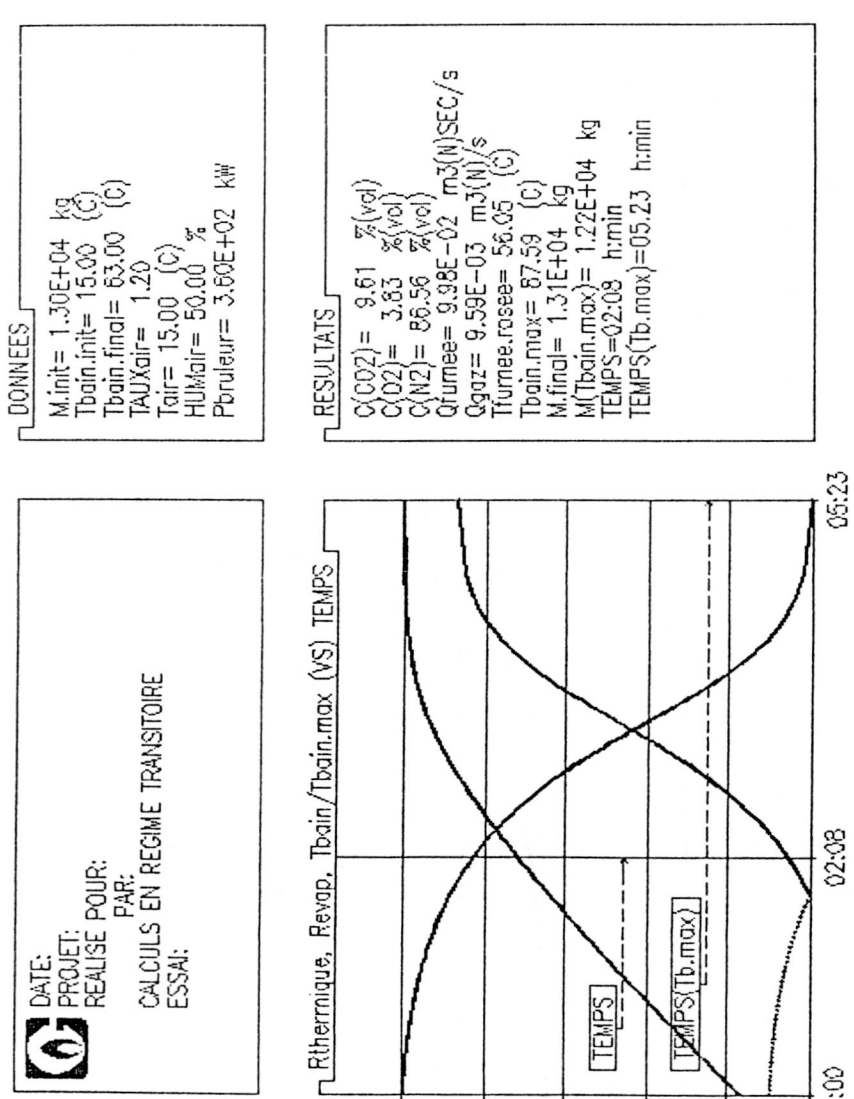

FIGURE 4

DEVELOPPEMENTS FUTURS:

Les développements futurs du logiciel concernent notamment la conception:

- d'une banque de données de propriétés de liquides d'intérêts industriels,

- d'un module de design de la cuve et du distributeur et de calcul des pertes thermiques,

- d'un module de calcul de l'évolution physico-chimique du liquide chauffé, évaporé ou traité,

- d'un module de calcul pour des conditions de non-équilibre: des études effectuées sur un montage expérimental à l'Ecole Polytechnique montrent que des efficacités thermiques améliorées peuvent être ainsi obtenues [4,5].

BIBLIOGRAPHIE:

1) Thouault, A., Proc. 96e Congr. Ind. Gas, 809 (1979)
2) Guy, C. et Carreau, P.J., Act. Chim. Can., 38, 19-23 (1986)
3) Fardeau, M.D., Gaz de France, D.E.T.N., Rapport M463 (1983)
4) Guy, C., Carreau, P.J. et Paris, J., Int. Gas Research Conf., Toronto, 3, 181-190 (Sept. 21-25, 1986)
5) Guy, C., Carreau, P.J. et Paris, J., 37th Can. Chem. Eng. Conf., Montréal, 116-118 (mai 18-21, 1987)

REMERCIEMENTS:

Nous tenons à remercier la compagnie Gaz Métropolitain Inc. qui grâce à sa subvention de recherche, nous a permis d'aborder ce sujet et de poursuivre les travaux en cours.

GNV: SYSTEME D'INJECTION A COMMANDE ELECTRONIQUE

Mathieu Perrault, Ing., M.Sc.A.
Michel Gou, Ing., M.Sc.A.
Gilles Allard, Ing.
Claude Guernier, Ing. M.Sc.

Ecole Polytechnique de Montréal
Département de Génie Mécanique
C.P. 6079, Succ. "A"
Montréal, Qué.   H3C 3A7

L'utilisation du gaz naturel comme carburant dans les véhicules permet de de réduire les coûts de transports et la dépendance vis-à-vis des pays producteurs de pétrole.

Au Canada, près de 10 000 véhicules ont été convertis au gaz naturel depuis 7 ans. En Italie, pays où le gaz naturel est utilisé depuis fort longtemps dans les transports, on compte 300 000 véhicules utilisant le gaz naturel et, en Nouvelle-Zélande, pays où des efforts importants ont été consentis par divers paliers de gouvernement, 80 000 véhicules ont été convertis en moins de 8 ans.

La technologie requise pour le développement du GNV (Gaz Naturel pour Véhicules) en est encore dans son adolescence et même si des efforts de recherche sont réalisés de plus en plus rapidement, le fonctionnement parfois inadéquat des dispositifs de conversion actuels diminue souvent l'attrait de ce nouveau carburant.

Cet article décrit les résultats d'une recherche effectuée à l'Ecole Polytechnique de Montréal dans le but d'améliorer les techniques d'utilisation du gaz naturel comme carburant. Les principaux objectifs de cette recherche étaient de concevoir un dispositif de conversion qui:
- a) permettrait l'utilisation du gaz naturel comme carburant,
- b) offrirait une performance égale au fonctionnement à l'essence,
- c) pourrait être adapté facilement à un grand nombre de moteurs divers.

Il fallait, en général, pallier aux déficiences des systèmes actuels et comparer la performance obtenue, au gaz naturel, avec celle obtenue à l'essence; la puissance du moteur, sa consommation, son niveau de pollution et sa souplesse étaient donc les facteurs les plus importants à considérer.

Certaines caractéristiques physiques du gaz naturel le rendent théoriquement attrayant en tant que carburant; en particulier, il faut citer:

- un indice d'octane d'environ 130 permettant l'utilisation d'un taux de compression plus élevé;
- un état gazeux favorisant une combustion plus complète, un mélange plus facile avec l'air même à basse température et une diminution de la formation des polluants;
- une densité plus faible que l'air contribuant à la sécurité, en cas de fuite.

Par contre, l'état actuel de la technologie de conversion et le faible développement du réseau de distribution ne permettent pas toujours de profiter de ces avantages. Au contraire, l'utilisateur doit faire face à plusieurs inconvénients qui ne sont pas tous inhérents au carburant. Citons par ordre d'importance:

- une diminution du rendement volumétrique et de la puissance (18 à 20%) causée en grande partie (10 à 12%) par l'état gazeux et (8%) par la présence d'un mélangeur introduit en amont du carburateur et jouant pour le gaz le même rôle que le carburateur pour l'essence;
- une diminution du rendement thermique causée par une vitesse de combustion plus lente; afin de réduire cette perte, il faut avancer l'allumage de façon significative;
- une consommation spécifique élevée, des difficultés de démarrage par grand froid du fait des limites étroites d'inflammabilité et même des ratés à chaud, tous ces problèmes étant causés par un contrôle inadéquat du débit du carburant, dans l'état actuel de la technologie.

Même si les dispositifs présentement utilisés ont été développés au début des années 50, ils fonctionnent relativement bien à température constante. Pourtant, ce n'est pas toujours le cas dans les conditions climatiques canadiennes. En général pour assurer le meilleur fonctionnement du moteur, le dispositif doit:

- fournir le débit de gaz requis à une pression constante, et ce, quelles que soient les conditions ambiantes et celles du stockage; or il faut rappeler que la détente provoque une forte variation de la température d'alimentation du GN. Les conditions d'opération peuvent varier dans les limites indiquées ci-dessous [1]:
    - pression de stockage: de 1,35 à 20,5 MPa
    - températures: air ambiant: de -40° C à 120° C
                    GNC: de -140° C à 120° C.
- admettre au moteur un mélange adéquat or à cause des régimes transitoires de fonctionnement d'un moteur d'automobile, le rapport stoechiométrique est normalement appelé à varier dans le temps suivant le régime et la charge;
- mélanger l'air et le gaz naturel de façon homogène;
- occasionner une perte de charge minimale afin de ne pas trop pénaliser le fonctionnement à l'essence;
- commander l'avance d'allumage pour obtenir la puissance maximale.

Afin de rencontrer les critères énoncés précédemment, nous avons envisagé la conception d'un dispositif d'injection à commande électronique basé sur un système en boucle fermée, audo-adaptatif [2]. Cette stratégie permettrait éventuellement, et à partir d'un nombre restreint d'essais en laboratoire pour caractériser le moteur, d'adapter continuellement et de façon autonome la demande en carburant tout au cours de la vie du moteur.

Dans un premier temps, afin de simplifier le problème et faute d'une sonde à oxygène adéquate, il fut décidé d'opérer au mélange stoechiométrique. Ainsi, le processus de commande en boucle ouverte décrit à la figure 1, basé sur une caractérisation préalable du moteur, fut utilisé.

Il s'agit donc de mesurer, sur banc d'essais, des intrants qui permettront, à l'aide de programmes d'interpolation, de dresser une cartographie tri-dimensionnelle du moteur, les coordonnées considérées étant le débit d'air, la pression du collecteur d'admission et la vitesse de rotation. Afin de limiter le temps d'essais et le temps de calcul en temps réel, les valeurs obtenues furent soumises au système SAS

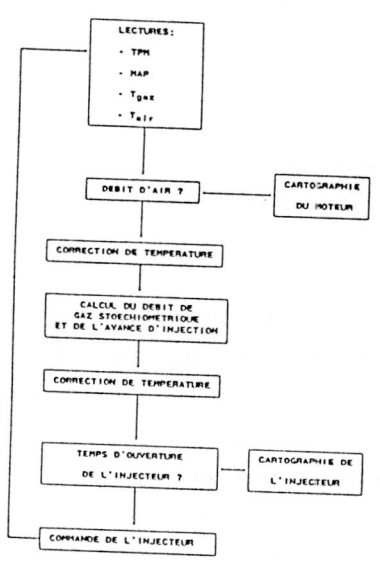

Figure 1 -Séquence de la commande (tiré de [3])

(Statistical Analysis System) à l'Ecole Polytechnique de façon à générer, par interpolation splinaire bi-dimensionnelle, les points intermédiaires et la cartographie fine montrée à la figure 2.

Cette cartographie est ensuite emmagasinée dans l'espace

d'étalonnage de l'injecteur Solex choisi ayant montré un comportement non linéaire, sa cartographie fut établie tel que montré à la figure 3 et emmagasinée en mémoire vive.

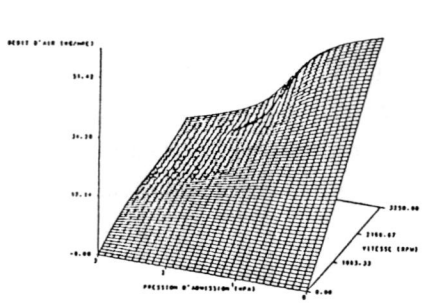

Figure 2
Cartographie du moteur
Ricardo (tiré de [3]).

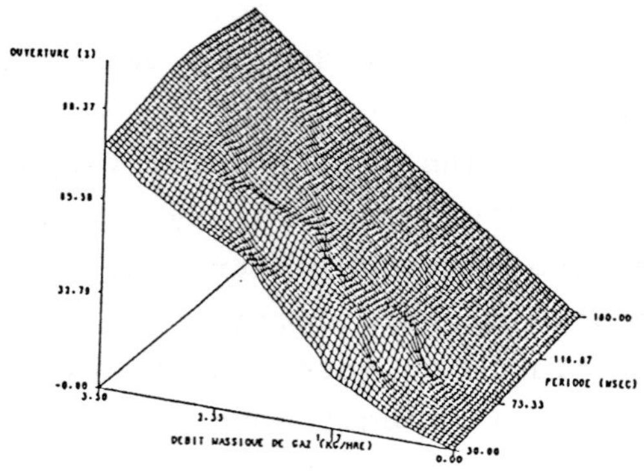

Figure 3
Cartographie de
l'injecteur (tiré de [3])

En opération, comme il existe un couple distinct TPM-MAP (régime moteur-pression d'air à l'admission) pour chaque état de charge du moteur, la vitesse de rotation du moteur, la pression du collecteur d'admission ainsi que les températures de l'air d'admission et du gaz détendu sont mesurées au moins une fois par cycle du moteur. A partir de ces données et des cartographies, il est alors possible de déterminer le débit massique d'air admis au moteur et de le corriger suivant la température ambiante. Le débit théorique de gaz naturel requis est ensuite calculé avec le rapport stoechiométrique choisi puis corrigé pour la température du gaz détendu. Le logiciel de commande calcule finalement la période et le pourcentage d'ouverture requis à l'injecteur pour admettre le débit adéquat et envoie le signal, par l'intermédiaire d'un circuit de commande, à l'injecteur. Le processus se répète ainsi à chaque cycle moteur et assure donc un contrôle adéquat du débit de gaz.

Les résultats en laboratoire permettent de constater que la stratégie employée, même si elle est encore imparfaite, offre les avantages suivants:

- elle permet de réduire les essais de caractérisation à leur plus simple expression,
- elle élimine toute restriction à l'admission,
- elle permet la maîtrise du mélange,
- elle offre la possibilité d'utiliser une sonde Lambda pour:
    a) varier le mélange en fonction des conditions d'opération et
    b) affiner la cartographie sur une base continuelle par une boucle fermée auto-adaptative,
- elle offre la possibilité d'ajouter la commande de l'allumage.

De plus, les résultats ont permis de confirmer qu'il est possible de caractériser le fonctionnement du moteur par la pression du collecteur et le régime.

En conclusion, et même si le développement en est encore au stage du prototype de laboratoire ne pouvant être embarqué dans un véhicule, il est permis de croire que les objectifs de conception ont été atteints.

REMERCIEMENTS

Les auteurs tiennent à remercier les compagnies Gaz Métropolitain Inc. et Gaz de France qui ont subventionné ces travaux de recherche et ont ainsi contribué au développement de l'équipe de recherche sur le GNV de l'Ecole Polytechnique.

[1] Carter, Stephen, "New under the hood CNG Fuel System or GEN II, Non Petroleum Vehicular Fuels V: CNG Fuels," Arlington Virginie, 1985.

[2] Allard, Gilles, "Projet d'un système d'injection électronique pour un moteur monocylindre à allumage commandé fonctionnant au gaz naturel", Mémoire de maîtrise ès Sciences Appliquées, présenté à l'Ecole Polytechnique 1986.

[3] Gou, Michel, Perrault, Mathieu et Guernier, Claude, "Simulation et analyse du comportement d'un système de carburation pneumatique pour véhicules à gaz naturel sous différentes conditions de température et de pression", Rapport technique EPM/RT-86-2, Ecole Polytechnique 1986.

PERFORMANCE OF ORIFICE METERS IN FIELD CONDITIONS

W. Studzinski, J. Szabo, J. Eastwood
Nova Husky Research Corporation
R. Rans, D. Bell
NOVA Corporation of Alberta
Calgary, Alberta, Canada

Abstract

Experimental studies into the performance of orifice meters performance in natural gas flows indicate that a small nicks at the orifice edge, gas contamination with small amounts of liquids and gasket protrusion/recess do not cause any significant measurement errors. Existing stringent orifice plate rejection criteria can now be quantified to avoid unnecessary plate rejections. Investigations into the effects of the centering of the orifice plate show quite substantial measurement errors caused by eccentric plate position and confirm previous results obtained at lower Reynolds number.

1. Introduction

The orifice plate is probably the most widespread type of flowmeter used by the natural gas industry. Its simplicity, reliability and relatively low cost ensures that this measurement method will still be used in the near future. The basic studies of the orifice flow coefficient should be complemented by investigation of operational factors which could alter metering accuracy. Subsequent review of industry standards and regulations related to meter station design, maintenance and operation is necessary to ensure construction and operating costs are minimized while maintaining overall accuracy.

In the case of a large gas transmission company such as NOVA Corporation of Alberta, which handles over 75 percent of Canadian natural gas, measurement problems always require cautious and thorough investigation. At the moment among the 681 receipt meter stations and 93 major delivery points over six hundred are based on the orifice plate meters. With volumes of 6.0 $10^{10} m^3$ (2.13Tcf) per year small differences between receipt and delivery metering can represent significant dollar values.

The main purpose of this study was to characterize the most common deviations from ideal conditions which can be encountered in the field, and to establish relationships between given metering errors and various characteristic parameters.

Although the installation requirements for the orifice meter are specified by standard, not all are quantified. For example, the upstream edge conditions are loosely defined. The common method of checking edge conditions is to run a fingernail around the leading edge of the plate to check for small nicks and burrs. This technique is very subjective and often results in plates being rejected with very minor defects.

The first attempts to quantify the influence of small nicks on the accuracy of the orifice meter were done by Hoch (1) and Burgin (2). Unfortunately, the data obtained was not extensive enough to develop any relationship between the size of the nick and the error. In some cases, two different effects like a nick and scratch were investigated in the same test. The experiments were run on natural gas with two 0.1 m ID (four inch) meters in series which normally compared within 0.25%.

Much more detailed studies were carried out on the effects of orifice plate centering (eccentricity) on measurement error. The results of laboratory measurements done by Miller and Kneisel (3), Norman et al (4) and Husain and Teyssandier (5) indicated that the eccentricity limits allowable by the ISO-5167 standard are too restrictive. The effects of eccentricity are related to the orifice diameter ratio β, the magnitude and the direction of the plate center shift. The largest change in flow coefficient is caused by the eccentricity toward the pressure tap. This rule is valid only for relatively small eccentricities.

The most comprehensive studies related to the gasket protrusion and recess were done by Zedan and Teyssandier (6) on a 0.05 m ID pipe using water and a dynamic weigh tank. The effects of the protrusion were more pronounced for orifice plates with larger β-ratio. Surprisingly, even quite a large recess did not cause any significant measurement error.

In some cases natural gas can be contaminated with condensate, glycol, compressor oil and water. Orifice plate standards exclude any extraneous materials on the plate surface and in the flow but in the field it is important to know what liquid concentration levels can be tolerated without a deterioration of measurement accuracy. Lin's (7) review of various correlations for orifice metering in two-phase flows stresses limitation of all formulas to the range of experimental conditions.

Unlike the papers discussed our study was carried out on natural gas at conditions very similar to field measurements. The basic goal was to quantify relative changes in the orifice meter readings due to various damages and nonstandard operational conditions. The orifice fittings and meter runs utilized were exactly the same as in typical meter stations. The maximum Reynolds number was close to 10 million and therefore, the data obtained can be readily applied to many real life situations.

2. Experimental Set Up

All experimental data presented here was obtained at NOVA's Gas Dynamic Test Facility in Didsbury, Alberta. The general layout of the facility is shown in Fig. 1 and the schematic of orifice plate arrangement in Fig. 2. Two orifice meters of nominal size 0.25 m ID (10 inch) were installed in series, 53 pipe diameter apart. Some of the tests were performed on 0.2 m ID (8 inch) piping and 0.1 m ID (4 inch) meter runs. The nondimensional distance between the orifice meters was the same as for 0.25 m ID piping. The upstream orifice fitting was always preceded by a straight length of pipe at least 60 pipe diameters long. Penetration of external acoustic disturbances and generation of a standing wave in the test section was prevented by anechoic terminations located at the inlet and outlet of the test section. The straightening vanes were located 11 pipe diameters upstream of each orifice plate.

Since relative differences in flow rate readings were of main interest, it was important to ensure good measurement repeatability. The static and differential pressure transducers had accuracies of $\pm$ 0.1% of span and the temperature transducers $\pm$ 0.2% of the calibrated range. The uncertainty of calibration for the static and differential pressure transducers was $\pm$ 0.025% and for the temperature transducers $\pm$ 0.1%. In order to minimize errors only static pressure was measured, the second was evaluated by subtracting the differential pressure between the plates from this static pressure. The calibration procedure used included the entire data acquisition system. In order to eliminate the small systematic errors due to daily changes of ambient conditions the transducers were frequently set up to check zero values. Additionally each measurement was preceded by an on-line calibration of the differential pressure transducers by connecting them all to the differential pressure across the upstream orifice plate. The transmitters were insulated and the piping was kept wet to minimize any temperature gradients between the test and reference meter.

Each data point results from averaging of 9 or 10 data blocks, each containing up to 1024 measurements. Utilized sampling rate did not exceed 100 Hz.

3. Test of Two Standard Orifice Meters

The first task in this study was to find a bias and random error of the system consisting of two orifice meters in series. Theoretically, they should measure equal flows but the orifice fittings and meter runs as well as the orifice plates themselves are never perfectly identical. This is one of the reasons why the orifice flow coefficient has uncertainty at least $\pm 0.5\%$.

The flow rate calculations for the upstream orifice meter Q_0 (used as a reference) and the downstream meter Q_1 were based on AGA-3 standard (8). The results of all tests are presented in the form of a nondimensional difference in flow reading

$$\Delta Q = (Q_1 - Q_0)/Q_0 = Q_1/Q_0 - 1$$

as a function of the Reynolds number based on pipe diameter. The cross-sectional area of the orifice bore used in flow rate calculations was always based on the nominal orifice diameter without any correction for V-notches. Because gas composition was the same for both meters and static pressure and temperature differences were very small, the main factors defining ΔQ were changes of differential pressure across the orifice plate.

Extensive measurements of flow rates through different but standard orifice plates established a so called baseline measurement for each β-ratio. One example of such a baseline consisting of 16 points (nine hundreds measurements each) is presented in Fig. 3. This type of measurement was taken during each test with damaged orifice plates and it ensured the accuracy and confidence in the data obtained. The observed bias of the baseline is within 0.1%. The repeatability R of a single orifice plate at 95% confidence level was defined as follows:

$$R = 2\,\sigma/\sqrt{2}$$

where σ is a standard deviation of measured difference ΔQ. As it can be seen from Fig. 3, these particular orifice meters have repeatability in the range $\pm 0.15\%$.

The sign and magnitude of the bias varied with β-ratio (Fig. 4) but did not exceed $\pm 0.25\%$. The repeatability of a single orifice plate was always better than $\pm 0.16\%$.

4. Effects of V-notch nicks on orifice meter accuracy

Preliminary field tests of rejected orifice plates with small nicks and burrs at the edge did not indicate any significant measurement errors caused by these real damages. It was also obvious that any effects which are smaller than the magnitude of the orifice plate repeatability ($\pm 0.15\%$ from the baseline measurement) cannot be detected in the system with two orifice in series. Therefore, it was decided to inspect typical damages and to identify basic geometrical parameters which could be scaled up to obtain meaningful results.

Microscopic investigation of rejected orifice plates revealed three basic geometrical features of orifice edge damage:
- change of the cross-sectional area of orifice bore
- displacement of material forming a protruding bump or burr
- oblique groove

To model the first effect, equilateral triangle V-notches of various sizes were machined at the orifice edge. Evaluation of the influence of such damage on orifice readings was done at various Reynolds numbers. The circumfrential position of the notch in relation to the tap holes did not have any significant effect on the measurement error (Fig. 3). Rotation of the orifice plate with a very large V-notch did not indicate any distinct error maximum and all error changes were almost within the repeatability band.

Comparison of the tests with the orifice diameter ratio $\beta = 0.6$ (Fig. 6) and $\beta = 0.2$ (Fig. 7) shows that the same size of a nick (e.g. 6.4 mm) can cause a much larger difference in flow reading for smaller orifice bore. It is also quite surprising that relatively large damage (3.2 mm triangle, Fig. 6), which will probably never occur in the field, does not cause any meaningful change of the orifice reading. The influence of Reynolds number (up to 10 million) on nick effects is negligible.

The data obtained required some kind of a generalization to extrapolate and utilize it for very small damage of the orifice edge. As is shown in Fig. 8, the observed errors are much higher for small β- ratio. Therefore, it was convenient to plot all collected measurement data as a function of a ratio of two cross-sectional areas: V-notch area to nominal orifice bore area (Fig. 9). Linear regression of the data (thin straight line) does not differ significantly from a line relating the error directly to the change of the orifice bore cross-sectional area. At least two thirds of the total error can be explained by this simple effect and the rest by changes in the orifice flow coefficient.

This finding was supported by an additional test (0.25 m ID, $\beta = 0.6$) using a 12 mm V-notch and an equivalent size triangle mounted on the opposite side in the orifice bore. The effective change of the cross-sectional area was zero and the notch error decreased from -0.6% to -0.05% (i.e. within the repeatability band).

5. Orifice Eccentricity Effects

As it was already mentioned in the literature review, for small eccentricities the greatest error was caused by the movement of the orifice bore center towards the tap. Introducing the nondimensional scale of $(0.1 + 2.3 \beta^4)/D$ Hussain and Teyssandier (5) obtained essentially a single line such that for all β-ratios the bias error was identical. The validity of this generalization is limited to smaller eccentricities, the case of primary interest. Our test with an eccentricity of e/D = 2.95% (7.5 mm) indicated a similar trend.

Quite opposite results were obtained for orifice plates with large eccentricity e/D = 5.9% (15 mm) which were tested at β =0.2 and 0.6. The influence of the orifice bore position relative to pressure tap location was investigated by plate rotation. The greatest deviation occurred with the orifice bore center away from the tap (Fig. 10). Similar to the results reported in ref. (3) and (4), at larger eccentricity we noticed quite strong differential pressure fluctuations. Measurement errors proved to be more significant for β =0.2 than for β =0.6. It seems that for β =0.6 there is an increase of eccentricity effect at higher Reynolds number. This observation should be taken with caution because of the unstable flow behaviour. It has been well proven for smaller eccentricities that Reynolds number does not effect measurement error (4), (5).

A practical evaluation of the eccentricity effects indicate that a slight carrier movement within the play in the orifice fitting can cause changes in the readings by as much as 1.2%.

6. Liquid Injection Test

The main purpose at this test was to find out how much liquid contamination is needed to cause significant measurement errors.

A simple arrangement of the test facility with liquid injection nozzle located between the two orifice meters (upstream of the straightening vane) did not allow any measurement of liquid distribution in gas flow and on the pipe wall. Some insight into this problem was obtained from orifice plate inspection.

The first tests were carried out on 0.25 m ID piping with gas condensate injection (density 695 kg/m^3). Even at the maximum mass concentration of injected liquid (0.37%) there was no detectable change of the orifice reading. This concentration is equivalent to seven barrels a day. The tests were conducted at orifice diameter ratio $\beta = 0.2$. The orifice plate when inspected after the injection tests, was wet but without any distinct streaks or liquid collection spots. Therefore, it can be assumed that gas condensate was in the form of a mist and Lin's (6) formula can be applied for estimation of possible measurement error. A simple calculation shows that the expected error for 0.37% of liquid should be in the range of 0.07%. Such a deviation in flow reading could not be detected by the measurement system.

A different type of liquid injection test was carried out on 0.10 m ID piping and $\beta = 0.6$. The compressor oil (density 885 kg/m^3) used for these tests was probably separating onto the pipe wall and flowing along the wall toward the downstream orifice plate. Visual inspection of the plate revealed traces of liquid collection at the bottom of the pipe on the upstream side of the orifice plate as well as radial liquid streaks towards the orifice bore. The orifice reading was changing over time and approached a steady value after some delay. This was probably related to the observed collection of liquid in the front of the orifice. The difference in flow readings (steady value) increased with higher injection rates (i.e. oil concentration in the natural gas). As it is shown in Fig. 11, slightly less than 0.07% (by mass) of oil in a gas-oil mixture can cause an error of almost -1.1% in the flow measurement. This value is well over the prediction based on any correlation and should be investigated further.

The main conclusion from this test is that the liquid contamination effect depends strongly on two-phase flow pattern and homogeneous liquid dispersion gives negligible measurement errors for small liquid concentrations.

7. Improper Size of the Orifice Gasket and Backward Installation of the Bevelled Orifice Plate

Two simple tests ($\beta = 0.2$) were carried out to evaluate the influence of the oversized or undersized orifice gasket. This type of operating error can cause gasket protrusion or recess, however, in our test it was impossible to measure the size of it. In both cases there was no meaningful change in the orifice reading.

Extrapolation of Zedan and Teyssandier (6) results shows that the step or cavity at the orifice plate required to cause a 0.2% error (detectable by our method) is so large that in practice it is not possible to install such gaskets.

The bevelled orifice plate installed backwards indicates 12.5% lower reading at $\beta = 0.2$ than a properly installed plate. This result is consistent with Hoch's (1) measurement indicating a 13.8% lower reading at $\beta = 0.5$.

8. Conclusions

Quantitative determination of measurement errors due to various operational problems indicates that to ensure the accuracy of the orifice meters special care should be taken regarding the center position of the orifice bore, liquid separation and collection at the bottom of the pipe and proper orientation of bevelled orifice plates.

Only in very extreme situations do orifice nicks cause significant measurement errors. Orifice plate rejection criteria can now be quantified and the number of rejected plates can be limited without sacrificing orifice meter accuracy.

Contamination of natural gas with small amounts of liquids in the form of a fine mist cannot cause significant measurement errors unless it forms distinct streaks on the orifice plate front surface. It is also highly improbable that any operational mistake in the orifice gasket size can cause significant measurement errors.

9. Acknowledgement

Presented results are based on a research project sponsored by NOVA Corporation of Alberta, permission to publish these results is gratefully acknowledged.

10. References

1. Hoch, K.A.: "Effects of rounded orifice edges, dirt and other foreign materials on orifice meter measurement accuracy". In: Proc. of the 57th Int. Okla. Univ. Hydrocarbon Measurement Sch. 1982, pp. 298-306.

2. Burgin, E.J.: "Factors affecting accuracy of orifice measurement (primary element)". In: Proc. of the 32nd Ann. Gas Measurement Short Course, 1971, pp. 198-205.

3. Miller, R.W., Kneisel, O.: "Experimental study of the effects of orifice plate eccentricity on flow coefficients". In: Trans ASME J. Basic Engineering, March 1969, pp. 121-131.

4. Norman, R., Rawat, M.S., Jepson, P.: "Buckling and eccentricity effects on orifice metering accuracy". In: Proc. of Int. Gas Res. Conf. (London, U.K., 1983) pp. 128-138.

5. Husain, Z.D., Teyssandier, R.G.: "Orifice eccentricity

effects for flange, pipe and radius (D-D/2) taps". ASME paper 86WA/FM-1, presented at Winter Annual Meeting, Anaheim, California, Dec. 7-12, 1986.

6. Zedan, M.F., Teyssandier, R.G.: "The effects of recess and protrusions on the discharge coefficient of a flange tapped orifice plate". In: "Mass Flow Measurements - 1984" ed. T.R. Hedrick, R.H. Reimer, Winter Ann. Mtg. of ASME,(New Orleans, 1984), pp. 17-23.

7. Lin, Z.H.: "Two-phase flow measurements with orifices". In: "Encyclopedia of Fluid Mechanics", ed. N.P. Cheremisinoff, Gulf Publ. Co. 1986, pp. 841-862.

8. "Orifice Metering of Natural Gas and Other Related Hydrocarbon Fluids". A.G.A. Report No. 3 - ANSI/API 2530, Sept. 1985.

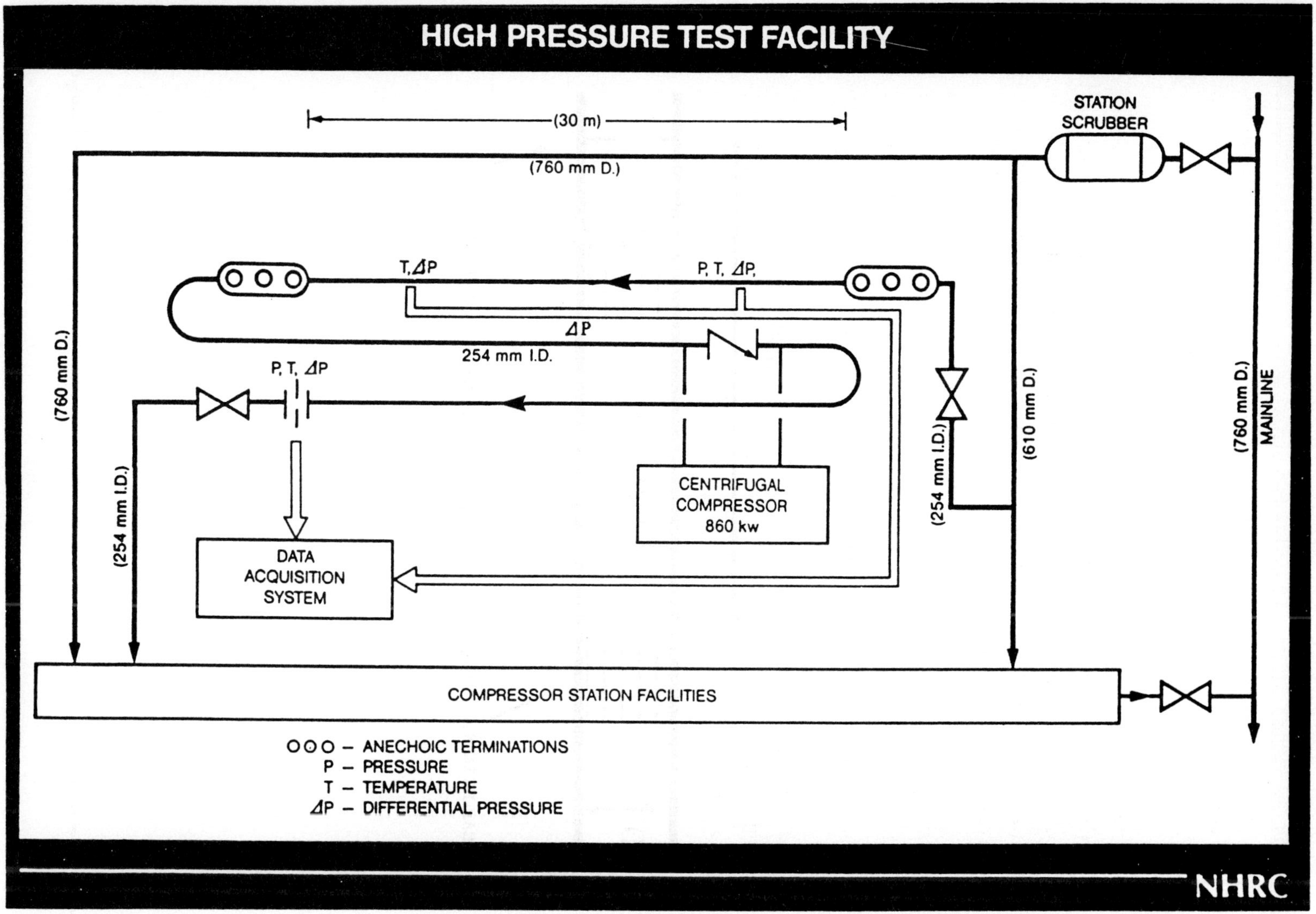
HIGH PRESSURE TEST FACILITY
(30 m)
STATION
SCRUBBER
(760 mm D.)
MAINLINE
(760 mm D.)
(610 mm D.)
(254 mm I.D.)
T, ΔP
P, T, ΔP,
ΔP
254 mm I.D.
P, T, ΔP
(760 mm D.)
(254 mm I.D.)
CENTRIFUGAL
COMPRESSOR
860 kw
DATA
ACQUISITION
SYSTEM
COMPRESSOR STATION FACILITIES
OOO – ANECHOIC TERMINATIONS
P – PRESSURE
T – TEMPERATURE
ΔP – DIFFERENTIAL PRESSURE
NHRC

FIGURE 1

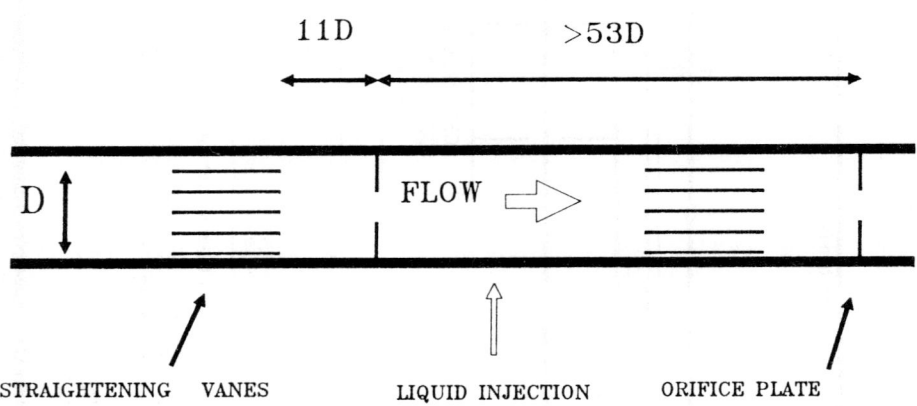

FIGURE 2

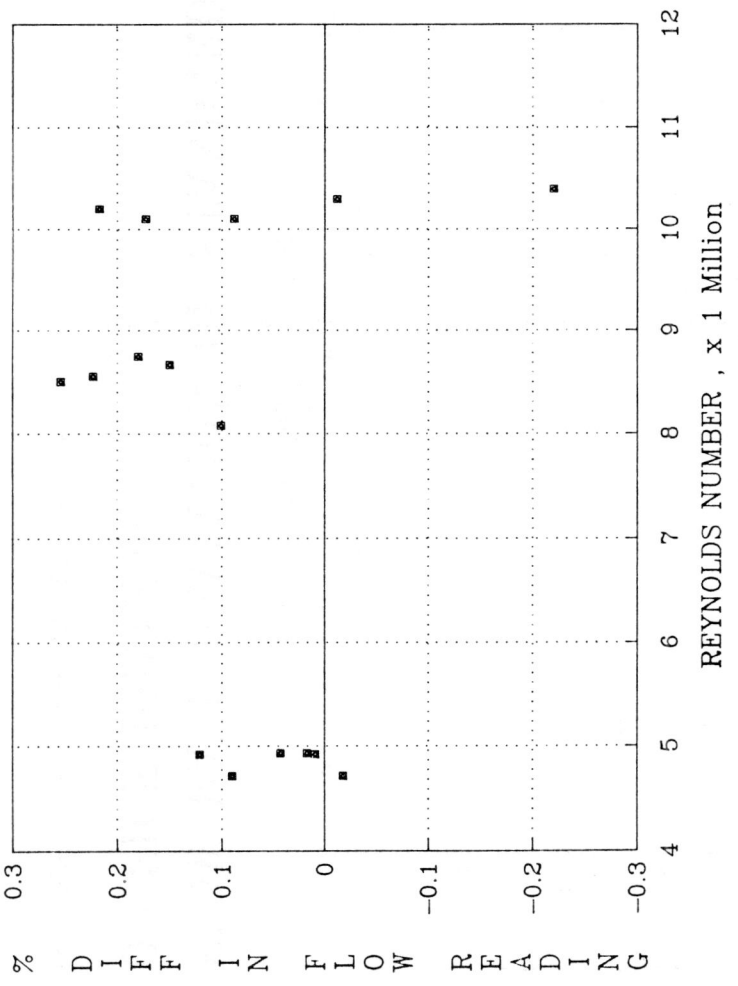

FLOW RATE DEVIATION OF STANDARD ORIFICE PLATES
FOR PIPE ID = 0.25 m AND BETA = 0.6

FIGURE 3

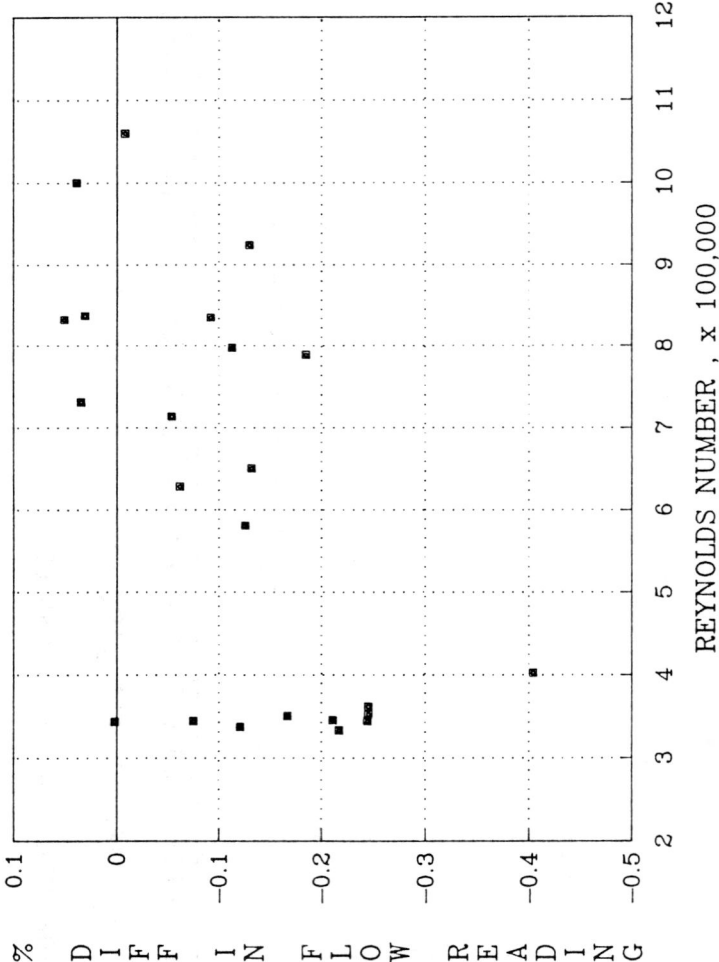

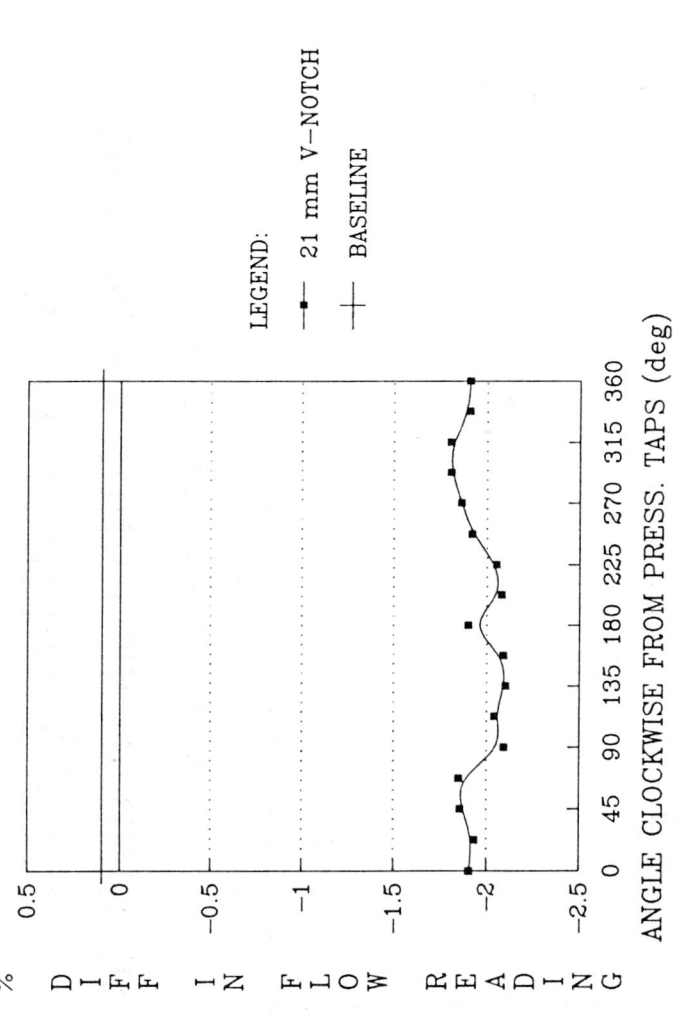

FIGURE 5

EFFECT OF A RELATIVE V-NOTCH POSITION ON MEASUREMENT ERROR

FOR PIPE ID = 0.2 m AND BETA = 0.6

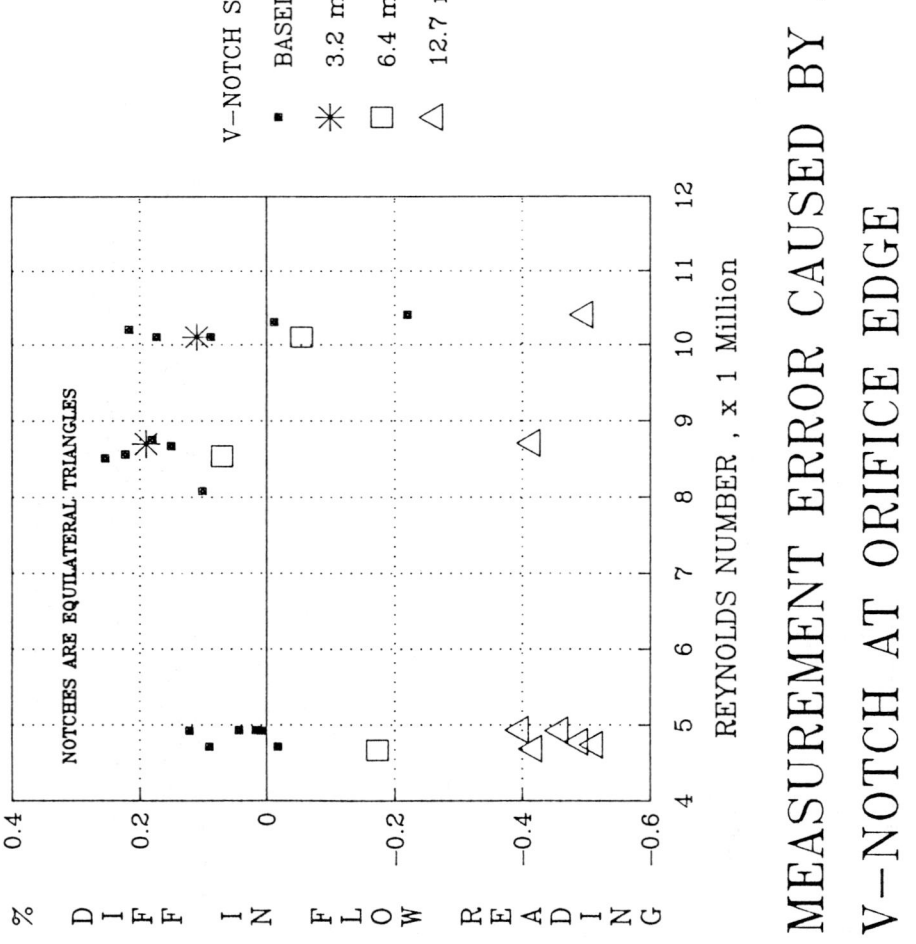

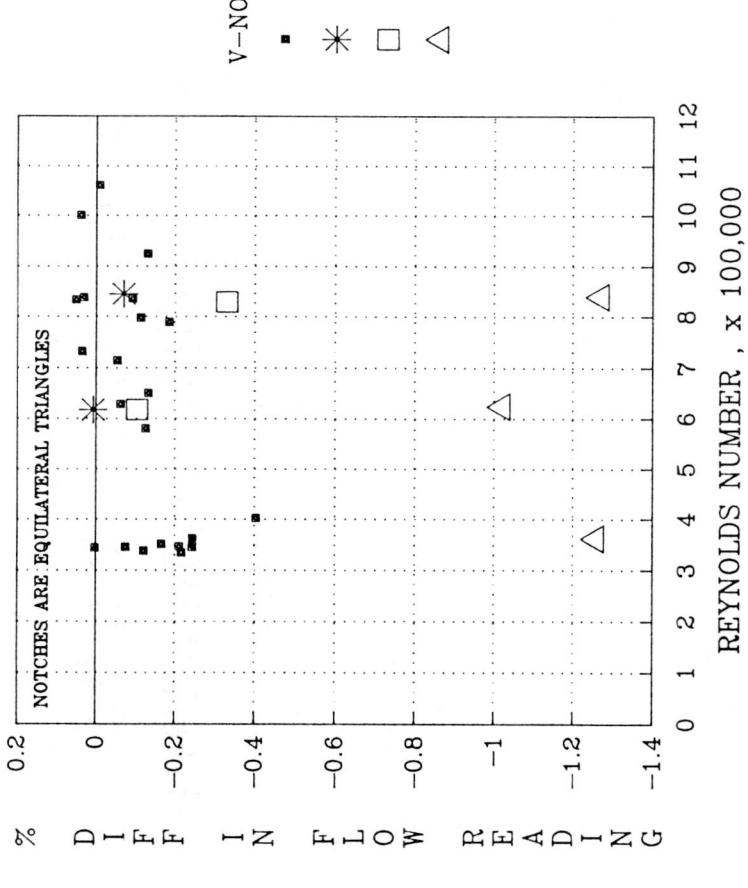

FIGURE 7

MEASUREMENT ERROR CAUSED BY A
V-NOTCH AT ORIFICE EDGE
FOR PIPE ID = 0.25 m AND BETA = 0.2

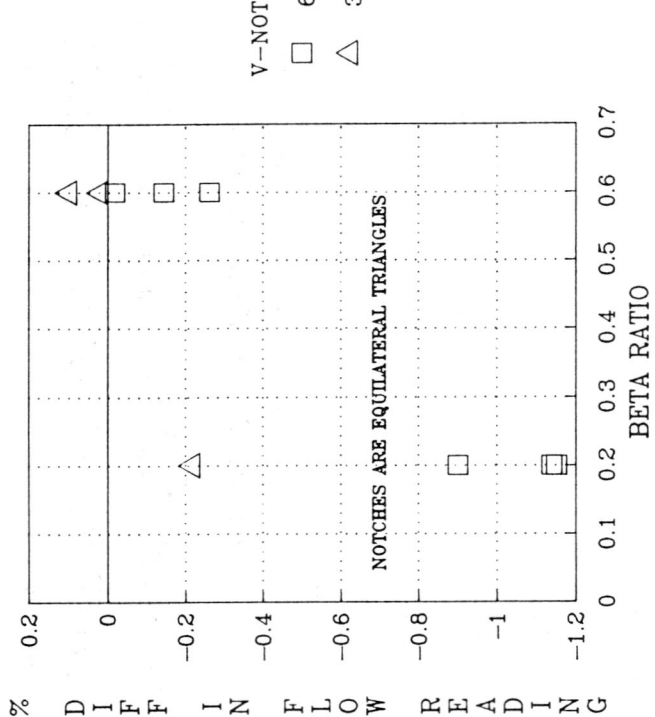

INFLUENCE OF BETA RATIO ON V-NOTCH MEASUREMENT ERROR

FOR PIPE ID = 0.25 m

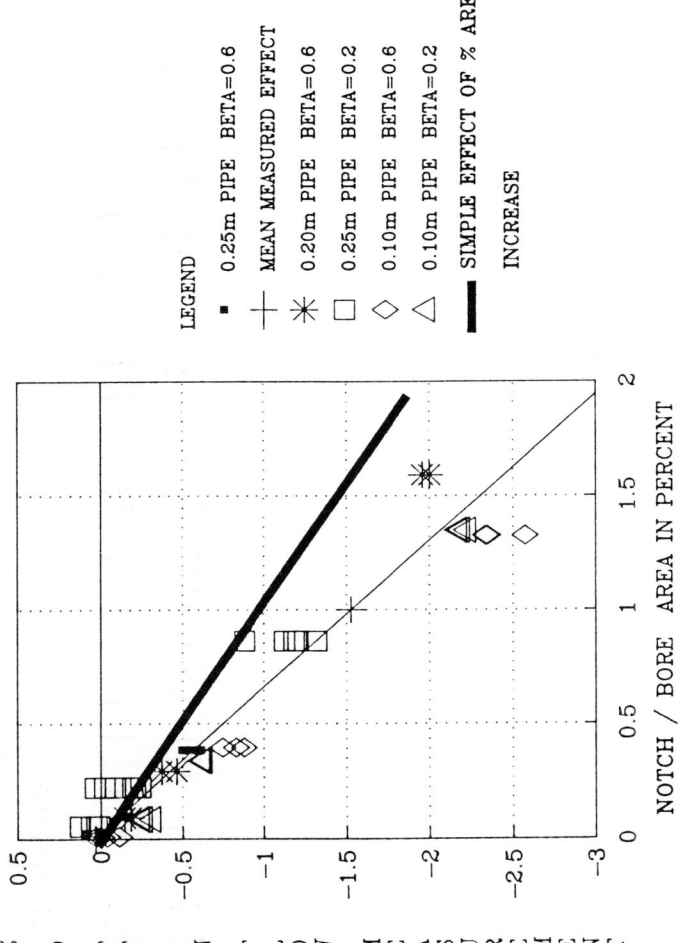

FIGURE 9

MEASUREMENT ERRORS FROM RELATIVE CHANGE OF THE ORIFICE BORE AREA

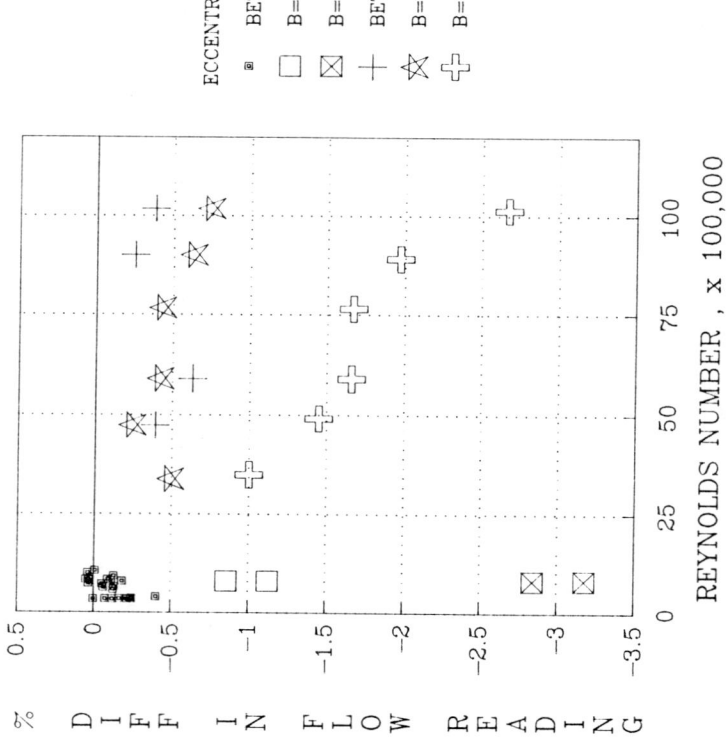

FIGURE 10

FLOW MEASUREMENT ERROR FROM ECCENTRIC ORIFICE PLATE BORES

FOR PIPE ID = 0.25 m AND ECCENTRICITY OF 15 mm

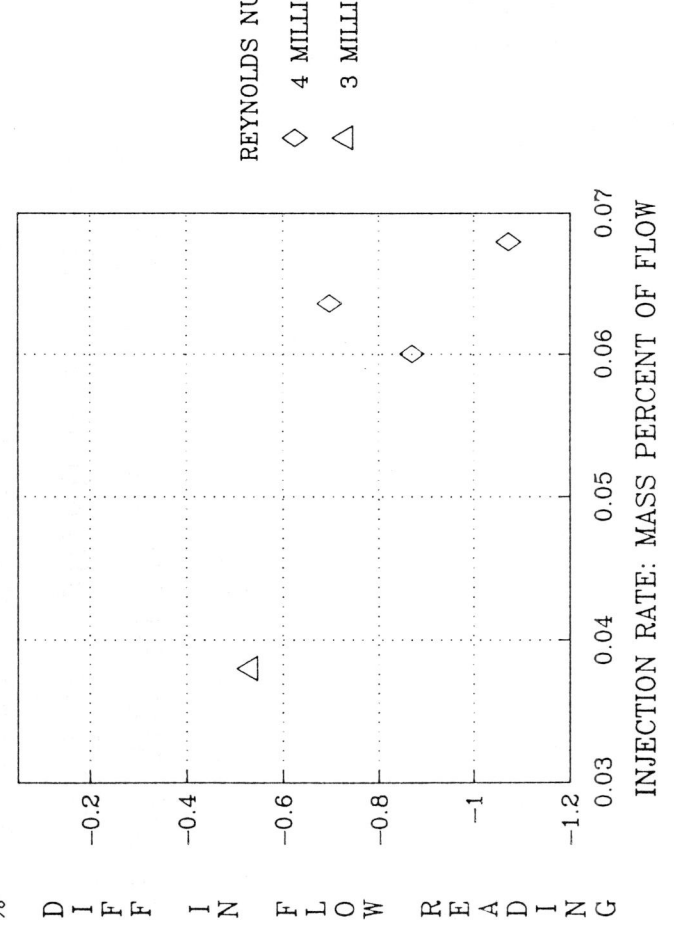

FIGURE 11

L'UTILISATION DU GAZ NATUREL DANS LES PROCEDES D'INCINERATION

Illustration par la présentation de l'équipement fourni par PILLARD chez GENERAL MOTORS (OSHAWA) Canada

Xavier d'Hubert
PILLARD INC
10401 Linn Station Road
Louisville, KY 40223
U.S.A.

La diversité des techniques d'incinération interdit d'en faire la liste exhaustive. Cependant, que ce soit pour la destruction d'effluents gazeux, de liquides résiduaires ou de déchets solides et ce, par le moyen d'un incinérateur statique, à grille, tournant, d'une chaudière ou même d'un four de cimenterie, il est presque toujours fait appel à un combustible "noble".

Celui-ci, qu'il s'agisse de charbon, de fuel-oil ou de gaz naturel, est utilisé pour plusieurs fonctions et á differentes situations dans une installation.

A) - En premier lieu pour le préchauffage du foyer, (dans le cas d'un incinérateur briqueté), afin de porter les réfractaires à température en suivant une courbe préétablie.
B) - Ensuite pour préchauffer l'ensemble de l'installation, principalement l'unité de traittement des fumées à l'aval de l'incinérateur.(Mise en température des filtres ...)
C) - Pour maintenir une température suffisante dans l'incinérateur dans le cas de produits à trop faible pouvoir calorifique ou brûlant avec difficulté.
D) - Pour produire une flamme dans laquelle le produit à détruire est injecté; que ce soit à partir du même brûleur ou d'un dispositif séparé.
E) - Enfin en post-combustion, que ce soit pour brûler les gaz produits dans le but de réduire leur taux en produits polluants, ou pour augmenter la température de ces gaz afin d'obtenir un rendement satisfaisant dans la chaudière de récupération.

Ces différentes fonctions sont donc réalisées par des brûleurs mais avec une efficacité et une souplesse accrue lorsque le gaz naturel est employé comme combustible. C'est ce qui est présenté au paragraphe suivant.

D'une manière générale, les avantages apportés par le gaz naturel sont bien connus, ce sont ceux obtenus dans sur les chaudières, à savoir:

- Il permet de réaliser des économies de combustible,
    - grâce à la réduction de l'excès d'air de combustion,
    - du fait du non encrassement des surfaces d'échange.

- Par rapport au fuel-oil ou au charbon pulvérisé il entraine la suppression,
    - des équipements de préparation tels que réchauffeurs, pompes, broyeurs, filtres...
    - du fluide de transport ou de pulvérisation.

- S'ajoute également,
    - un entretien réduit,
    - une possibilité d'automatisation poussée,
    - des rejets dans l'atmosphère de particules et de SO2 nuls, ce qui autorise la récupération de calories sur la chaleur sensible des fumées.

Cependant, il est d'autres avantages qui sont plus particulièrement liés aux procédés d'incinération, et qu'il convient de détailler en les mettant en regard de chacune des applications que les brûleurs réalisent en incinération.

A&B) - Le préchauffage du foyer et de l'installation en générale peut se faire trés progressivement grâce aux grandes variations de charge qui peuvent être obtenues (de 1 à 50 par utilisation de plusieurs circuits d'injection par exemple). Il est également possible d'obtenir des fumées à température basse grâce à des brûleurs ayant des flammes stables sous 800% d'excès d'air. Brûleur à prémélange partiel par exemple. (Induction d'une partie de l'air de combustion dans le brûleur, en amont de la zône de combustion.)

C) - En soutien, pour maintenir une température d'incinération suffisante la souplesse et la facilité d'arrêt et de redémarrage sont des points essentiels que permet d'obtenir le gaz naturel.
Ces brûleurs peuvent également être conçus pour être placés dans des endroit sensibles (faible encombrement, exposition auxs hautes températures) sans diminution de leur performances.

D) - Parce qu'il peut être injecté soit par une canne centrale, soit par une couronne ou des buses ou autre moyen, le gaz naturel permet de concevoir des brûleurs à deux, trois, voir même quatre combustibles, ainsi les produits à incinérer peuvent ils être injecter dans un brûleur unique.
Le gaz naturel peut parfois être mélangé à un gaz pauvre pour en augmenter le pouvoir calorifique.
Enfin, il peut servir de fluide de pulvérisation dans des injecteurs de résidus liquides.

E) - En post-combustion la location d'un brûleur à gaz est facilitée par le fait que l'on dispose de brûleurs soit à flamme longue et étroite ou au contraire courte et large. On peut également utilise un système appelé " brûleur en veine " avec lequel le brûleur est directement placé dans la gaine des gaz à réchauffer.

Cette énumération peut apparaitre un peu superficielle, mais entrer dans le détail de chacun des cas avec calculs, schémas, résultats et photos conduirait à un développement excessif pour ce type d'ouvrage qui se veut la synthèse des échanges réalisés au cours du Salon International TRANSTECH 87.

Les données d'une des dernières réalisation du groupe PILLARD en matière d'incinération illustrent en partie la présentation ci-dessus.

<u>Location</u>: Usine General Motors d'Oshawa, Canada.

<u>Date</u>: Réalisation et mise en route en 1987.

<u>Objet</u>: Incinération des résidus générés par l'usine. Ils sont composés de bois, plastique, papiers, boues de peinture et pneus. 90 T/J sont à incinérer.

<u>Installation</u>, elle comprend:

- Une unité de récupération, broyage, manutention et chargement des déchets.
- Un incinérateur tournant d'une capacité de 12×10^6 kcal/hr.
Diamètre extérieur 3.4m.
Longueur 10.5m.
Cet incinérateur est équipé d'un brûleur à gaz naturel, à haute turbulence, de 4×10^6 kca l/hr qui assure le préchauffage de l'installation, en particulier l'unité de dépollution située en aval.

En opération, il apporte le complément calorifique nécessaire au maintien d'une température d'incinération (environ 850°C) imposée à la fois par le process et la législation.
- Une chaudière de récupération qui produit 30 t/hr de vapeur à 12 bar.
Cette chaudière est équipée de deux brûleurs gaz naturel, à haute turbulence, de chacun 6×10^6 kcal/hr.
Ils servent également au préchauffage de l'installation et à élever la temoérature des gaz dans le foyer (environ 1,100°C) afin que les échanges calorifiques soient satisfaisants.
- Une unité de traitement des fumées par réacteur venturi, filtres à manches, ventilateur de tirage et cheminée.

Cette installation a atteint sa marche nominale au début de l'année 1988.

USING NATURAL GAS IN THE INCINERATION PROCESS

ILLUSTRATED BY THE EQUIPMENT PROVIDED BY PILLARD
TO GENERAL MOTORS (OSHAWA) CANADA

Xavier d'Hubert
PILLARD, INC.
10401 Linn Station Road
Louisville, KY 40223
U.S.A.

It is almost impossible to enumerate all the incineration systems. However, there is a need for a burner with fossil fuel such as natural gas, fuel oil, or coal in almost each system. The need is there, whatever the system (static or rotary incinerator, boiler, or cement kiln) and whatever the waste (liquid, gaseous, or solid).

The high LHV fuels are burnt by means of burners at different stages of the incineration process.

   A) First, preheat the furnace (when it has a refractory lining) to heat the refractory according to a defined curve.

   B) Second, preheat the entire installation, particularly the depollution unit downstream of the incinerator. (heating of the baghouse filters, etc...).

   C) Third, maintain a sufficient temperature inside the incinerator in case of a waste with a low LHV or burning with difficulties.

   D) Fourth, produce a flame in which the matter to be incinerated is directly injected from the same burner or a separate burner.

   E) Last, in post-combustion either burn the exhaust gas to reduce the polluting contents, or increase the temperature of these flue gas to obtain a better efficiency in the recovery boiler.

These applications are enhanced by the use of natural gas versus other fuels such as fuel oil or pulverized coal (more versatility and efficiency). The following explains why.

The major advantages of natural gas have been known for several years by the users of boilers. These are mainly:

- Saving fuel by increased efficieny due to:
  - an excess air reduction
  - cleaner heat exchange surfaces

- Compared with other fuels it avoids:
  - a preparation unit such as a heater, pumps, mills, and filters
  - the air transport (with the use of coal) and pulverized fluid (with the use of fuel oil)

- Furthermore you get:
  - a decrease in maintenance cost
  - an easier computerized control
  - clean exhaust gas which allows the setting of a heat exchanger on the flue gas

Other advantages may be noted considering the incineration process. They are described hereafter in regard to each particular application.

A&B) Thanks to the large turn down ratio (from 1-50 with multi channel special burners for example) the preheating of the installation can be achieved very smoothly.

It is possible to get low temperature flue gas by means of burners able to withstand 800% excess air. This is very useful during the very first step of the preheating of a new installation. (This can be realized by introducing a part of the combustion air into the gas burner upstream the combustion zone).

C) As a complementary burner to maintain a necessary temperature of incineration, the versatility and easy shut-off/start-up of gas burners are a great advantage.

The design of these burners can be made in order to suit critical surroundings (lack of available space, high temperature, thermal shock) without affecting their performance.

D) The natural gas can be injected through different devices: rings, spuds, central gun, etc... Therefore, one can design multi-fuel burners suitable to burn waste in a natural gas burner providing a sustaining flame.

Natural gas can also be blended with a low BTU gas to increase its low calorific value.

E) In post-combustion the ability of a gas burner to have its flame shape changed easily (changing of the outlet section, increasing or decreasing the upstream pressure, adding more or less combusiton air, etc...) permits it to be set in almost any location.

There is also the possiblity of setting an "in-duct burner". This is a device where the burner is fitted inside the flue gas pipe.

This enumeration may look a bit superficial, but to provide more explanation with calculations, drawings, pictures, and the results on each case would require a complete textbook which is not the objective of this synthesis on the exchange of the points of view that occured during TRANSTECH 87.

The abstract of the engineering data from one of the latest PILLARD realizations in the field of incineration illustrates the above paragraph.

Location: General Motors, Oshawa plant, CANADA

Date: Erection and start-up in 1987

Objective: Incinerate the waste and refuse generated by the plant, ie. wood, plastics, papers, painting sludges, tires. 90 t/day to be destroyed

Installation: Including,

- A collecting unit with grinding, handling, and feeding up device
- A rotary kiln incinerator, 48 x 10^6 BTU/hr capacity, External diameter: 11'4"
Length: 35'
A natural gas, high velocity type, 16 x 10^6 BTU/hr burner is fitted on the incinerator. It achieves the preheating of the installation. During nominal charge running, it provides the complementary BTU to maintain the necessary temperature of 1,560°F according to the process and the regulation
- A recovery boiler producing 67,000 lbs/hr of steam at 180 PSI. Two natural gas, high velocity, 24 x 10^6 BTU/hr each, burners are fitted on the boiler. These burners are firing during the preheating, as well as during normal operation to raise the flue gas temperature to 2,010°F to enable the heat exchange in the boiler furnace to be efficient enough.
- A depollution unit including reactor venturi, baghouse filters, exhaust fans, and stack.

This installation reached its nominal load at the beginning of 1988.

THERMAL PERFORMANCE STUDIES OF GAS HEATING SYSTEMS

M. Zaheer-Uddin, P. Fazio and P. Roozmon
Centre for Building Studies, Concordia University
1455 de Maisonneuve Boulevard West
Montreal, Quebec H3G 1M8

ABSTRACT

A study is made of the thermal performance of three different types of gas heating strategies. The heating systems range a conventional warm air system to the most modern concepts in gas heating as self contained modular system and the Combined Boiler. These gas heating systems also employ condensing technology and therefore are classified as high efficiency systems. In order to evaluate their performance and compare their relative merits, they are installed and fully instrumented, one on each floor of a three story apartment building in Montreal. The building is unoccupied and therefore offers great flexibility in performing controlled tests. From the data gathered, calculations will be made of cycle, daily and seasonal efficiencies.

Also, tests will be performed to study the effects of supply and return temperatures, rate of condensation at various thermostat settings. Combustion product analysis will be carried out to determine what effects the excess air supply has on the cycle efficiency.

THE INFLUENCE OF TYPE OF HEATING SYSTEMS ON THERMAL COMFORT

P. Fazio, F. Haghighat, and M. Auger
Centre for Building Studies
Concordia Univesity
Montreal, Quebec   H3G 1M8

The growing industrialization of society has forced man to spend the greater part of his life in an artificial environment, at the office, at home, at the movies or during transportation. Thermal comfort in artificial environments is provided by heating and cooling systems and up to one third of the world's energy consumption is used for this purpose. ASHRAE defines thermal comfort as that "state of mind that expresses satisfaction with the thermal environment". Therefore, thermal comfort is an important factor to the overall success of a building for human occupancy.

The main objective of this study is to investigate experimentally the relationship between type of heating systems and thermal environment, and its effect on human comfort. Various type of heating systems provide different thermal conditions in a space. For example, in a room heated by a warm air system, the room air temperature is usually higher than walls surface temperatures. This causes heat loss from the body to the walls by radiation. In order to compensate for this effect on thermal comfort, the room air temperature should be increased. In the case of hydronic heating systems, heat is provided to the space by radiator. The mechanism of heat transfer in this case is mostly by radiation, which causes the temperature of the inside wall surfaces be higher than the space air temperature. But in this case, the air velocity is low, therefore, the evaporation heat loss from the body is low, and occupants can achieve thermal comfort in lower space air temperature.

The thermal comfort depends on the following environmental factors such as; mean air temperature around the human body, and mean air velocity around the human body (convection film coefficient). The heating method affect the air velocity around the human body. In an experiment with a radiator a mean air velocity of 0.27 m/s was observed, which could produce a subjective sensation of draught (thermal discomfort).

These experimental studies are underway in a three story house. The first set of heating systems to be studied are: the forced air heating system, which has been installed on the first floor, the modular air heating system, installed on the second floor, and the hydronic heating system, installed on the third floor.

To determine air temperature distribution in the room, shielded thermocouples are used to measure the room air temperature at five levels above the floor and at nine locations. The mean radiant temperature is measured using a two-sphere radio-meter. The velocity of the air at these locations is measured by the automated flow analysis system. The average temperature of the inside and outside surfaces of the exterior wall is used to measure the combined effect of the thermal parameters. The relative humidity is measured using common types of hygrometers.

INDOOR EMISSIONS FROM COMBUSTION APPLIANCES:
DEVELOPMENT OF A PREDICTIVE MODEL

F. Haghighat, P. Fazio and J. Payer
Centre for Building Studies
Concordia University
Montreal, Quebec   H3G 1M8

Canadians are spending up to 90% of their time in the built environment due to the severity of the climate. Therefore, the indoor climate has a significant role on their performance and health. The current trends in conservation measures, particularly related to reduced ventilation, have caused health problems for occupants due to increased levels of pollutants. It is now apparent that concentrations of combustion pollutants found within built environments are much higher than those outdoors. Although these issues are applicable to all types of appliances, they are particularly relevant to gas appliances. There are a wide variety of indoor combustion pollutant sources. Combustion sources can be grouped as smoking sources (i.e. cigarettes, cigars and pipes) or combustion appliances (space heaters, stoves, water heaters, fire places and gas dryers). Indoor combustion has been found to contribute to indoor concentrations of carbon monoxide, nitric oxide and nitrogen dioxide. Nitrogen oxide and carbon monoxide are of significant hazard to health. The impact on health of indoor combustion products is well documented.

There have been several studies aimed at investigating indoor pollutant levels from combustion sources. There are yet many gaps in the knowledge of indoor combustion pollutant concentrations and factors that affect them (air change, volume, source strength, reactivity), and these studies have not been able to fill these gaps. As an example, there is not yet enough information for modelling source strength. This model could be used to extend the results of indoor environment studies to a variety of houses and types of appliances. This study is aimed at filling some of these gaps by carrying out specifically designed studies.

The major objectives of this research are: 1) to determine the emission rates of combustion products from gas appliances under various operation conditions, 2) to determine how the level of contaminants vary with ventilation strategies, 3) to develop a mathematical model, 4) to carry-out on-site measurements and evaluation of several gas appliances, and 5) to validate the computer model.

To investigate the problem, a comprehensive study on the gas appliances is required. These appliances must be evaluated and ways and means to minimize the combustion products must be found. Mathematical modelling and computer simulation techniques will be excellent tools in predicting the combustion products in built environment. Detailed models can provide data to not only identify the problem areas but to seek optimum solutions to see how the ventilation technique can be designed more efficiently. To answer these questions, actual field installation and continuous monitoring is required. Computer model predictions can, then, be verified with the field measurement to develop a validated model.

This experimental study is underway in a three story house with a full basement. Combustion appliances being considered are: space heaters, stoves, fire-places and gas dryers. In this study, two basic combustion products - carbon monoxide and nitrogen dioxide will be monitored in the kitchen, living room and bedrooms under various operating conditions. Multi-tracer gas techniques will be used to simultaneously determine the air exchange rates for various rooms in a building. Simultaneous measurements are important for this study in order to come up with a possible solution to control the level of contaminants.

MESURE PRECISE DU FACTEUR DE SUPERCOMPRESSIBILITE DU GAZ NATUREL PAR UNE METHODE OPTIQUE.

J.M. St-Arnaud[1], T.K. Bose[1] et H.J. Achtermann[2]

(1) Groupe de recherche sur les diélectriques
 Département de physique
 Université du Québec à Trois-Rivières
 Trois-Rivières, Québec, Canada, G9A 5H7

(2) Institut für Thermodynamik
 Universität Hannover
 Federal Republic of Germany

Résumé

A l'aide d'une méthode optique, nous avons mesuré le facteur de supercompressibilité d'un gaz naturel fourni par Gaz Métropolitain Inc. sur trois isothermes (35°F, 55°F et 70°F) pour des pressions jusqu'à 3000 PSIG. Nos valeurs expérimentales sont en accord avec la formule NX-19.

Abstract

Using an optical method, we have measured the supercompressibility factor of a natural gas supplied by Gaz Metropolitain Inc. along three isotherms (35°F, 55°F and 70°F) for pressures up to 3000 PSIG. Our experimental values agree well with NX-19 formula.

Introduction

La loi idéale des gaz est donnée par

$$PV = nRT \qquad (1)$$

où P est la pression, V le volume, n le nombre de moles, R la constante universelle du gaz et T la température absolue.

Dans le cas d'un gaz réel soumis à de hautes pressions, l'équation (1) n'est plus valide. Dans un tel cas, l'équation d'état la plus représentative prend la forme

$$PV = ZnRT \qquad (2)$$

où Z est le facteur de compressibilité qui mesure la déviation entre le gaz réel et le gaz idéal. Ce facteur de compressibilité est une fonction de la température, de la pression et de la composition du gaz. En raison de ces divers facteurs et de la précision requise, la détermination exacte de Z requiert une expérience élaborée et soigneuse.

Dans l'industrie gazière, la quantité de gaz vendue ou achetée se calcule selon la masse totale ou selon le volume standard de ce gaz. Or, la masse totale m du gaz se déduit du facteur de compressibilité, selon la relation

$$m = MPV/ZRT \qquad (3)$$

où M est le poids moléculaire. Si on opte pour le volume standard (V_S), on le calcule en mètre cube à une température standard (T_S) et une pression standard (P_S). Dans ce cas, on procède à partir de

$$V_S = PVZ_S T_S / ZTP_S \qquad (4)$$

où Z_S est le facteur de compressibilité aux températures (T_S) et pressions (P_S) standards. Dans l'industrie gazière, la coutume est d'utiliser plutôt le facteur de supercompressibilité (F_{PV}) défini par

$$F_{PV} = (Z_S/Z)^{1/2} \qquad (5)$$

Plusieurs méthodes existent pour obtenir Z. Nous présentons ici une méthode nouvelle[1] basée sur la mesure précise de l'indice de réfraction du gaz. Après avoir présenté le développement mathématique pour illustrer comment nous pouvons déduire Z à partir de la détermination par interféromètre de l'indice de réfraction, nous discuterons de notre méthode expérimentale, présenterons nos résultats pour le gaz naturel étudié et montrerons l'accord entre nos résultats et les valeurs obtenues de l'équation[11] NX-19.

Développement mathématique

Partant du fait que la densité molaire d égale n/V, l'équation (2) peut s'écrire

$$Z = P/dRT. \qquad (6)$$

Dans le domaine optique, le lien entre l'indice de réfraction n et d est donné par l'équation de Lorentz-Lorenz:

$$[(n^2-1)/(n^2+2)d] = A_n + B_n d + C_n d^2 + \ldots \qquad (7)$$

où A_n, B_n et C_n sont respectivement le premier, le deuxième et le troisième coefficient du viriel de l'indice de réfraction du gaz étudié.

L'équation précédente peut cependant être réécrite sous la forme de

$$L = (n^2-1)/(n^2+2) = A_n d + B_n d^2 + C_n d^3 + \ldots \qquad (8)$$

qui conduit à une première approximation de la densité

$$d_1 \sim (L/A_n) \qquad (9)$$

laquelle permet d'obtenir, en première approximation

$$Z_1 = (P/RT)(A_n/L) \qquad (10)$$

En procédant de la même manière pour une seconde et une troisième approximation de la densité, on obtient une seconde et une troisième approximation de Z, cette dernière prenant la forme de

$$Z_3 = (P/RT)[\, A_n/L + B_n/A_n + C_n L/A_n^2 - B_n^2 L/A_n^3 \,] \qquad (11)$$

Nous avons déjà utilisé[1] l'équation (11) en mesurant le facteur de compressibilité du méthane selon notre méthode optique. Nos valeurs de Z concordent,, jusqu'à la pression maximum de nos mesures (286 bar) avec les meilleures mesures de Z réalisées par Douslin et al.[2] et Trappeniers et al.[3].

Nous avons obtenu le Z du gaz naturel selon l'équation (11) par la méthode optique qui consiste essentiellement à mesurer par interférométrie l'indice de réfraction du gaz en fonction de la pression et ce, sur diverses isothermes.

Méthode expérimentale

La détermination exacte du facteur de compressibilité implique, selon l'équation (11), les mesures précises de L, P, T, A_n, B_n et C_n. Dans notre approche expérimentale, nous voulons être aussi précis que la méthode de Burnett mais plus rapide. Pour ce faire, nous préconisons la mesure simultanée de l'indice de réfraction du gaz étudié et de la pression suivant la même méthode interférométrique décrite en détail dans une publication antérieure[1]. De fait, nous employons deux interféromètres à réseaux de diffraction. Le premier nous permet de déduire L par la mesure de n du gaz naturel. Le second, relié au premier et préalablement calibré, nous permet d'obtenir la pression P à partir des mesures de n de l'azote. Notons que l'interféromètre de pression a été calibré avec une jauge à l'huile construite par Ruska U.S.A.. La précision de la mesure de P est estimée à .04% entre 1 et 10 bar et à .01% pour P > 10 bar. D'autre part, la température a été mesurée avec un thermistor calibré par rapport à un thermomètre à cristal de quartz (Hewlett Packard 2801 A). La précision sur T est de l'ordre de 1×10^{-5} °C.

Dans le cas de nos interféromètres à réseaux, l'indice de réfraction est calculé à partir de la mesure du nombre de franges (K) défilant en diminuant la pression jusqu'au vide obtenu par une pompe mécanique. La relation

$$n = (K\lambda/l) + 1 \qquad (12)$$

permet de déduire n en mesurant K, en multiples de $\lambda/256$, pour $\lambda = 632,899$ nm (laser $He-Ne$) lorsque le gaz est contenu dans une cellule de longueur (l). Les précisions sur K, λ et l sont respectivement de ± λ/256, ± 1 X 10^{-11} m et ± 1 X 10^{-6} m.

Les valeurs de A_n sont obtenues par des mesures à basse pression (P < 15 bar) alors que celles de B_n et C_n sont acquises directement par la technique de l'expansion. Décrivons ces deux méthodes expérimentales.

La valeur du premier coefficient viriel A_n est déterminée par une mesure absolue de l'indice de réfraction du gaz naturel en fonction de la pression. Sachant que la densité d est reliée au deuxième coefficient du viriel de pression (B_P) par la relation

$$P/RT = d + B_P d^2 \qquad (13)$$

on peut remplacer d en termes de P dans l'équation (7) et nous obtenons

$$[(n^2-1)/(n^2+2)] (RT/P) = A_n + (B_n - A_n B_P)(P/RT) \qquad (14)$$

Une mise en graphique du côté gauche de l'équation (14) en fonction de P/RT permet, par les moindres carrés, d'obtenir A_n à partir de l'intercepte. Notons que si B_n apparaît dans le terme de la pente, cette méthode absolue ne s'avère pas valable pour une détermination précise de B_n. En effet, B_n est normalement une très faible fraction du deuxième terme dans l'équation (14). Conséquemment, une erreur aussi minime que 2% dans ($B_n - A_n B_P$) peut produire une erreur aussi grande que 100% dans la détermination[4] de B_n. Nous avons donc choisi d'obtenir directement B_n en utilisant la méthode de l'expansion qui a fait ses preuves antérieurement[1].

La technique de l'expansion, appliquée à la mesure optique, consiste[1,5-10] à mesurer la somme des chemins optiques de deux cellules similaires (Fig.1) dont une est remplie de gaz à la densité d et l'autre est sous vide. Lorsque la valve entre les deux cellules est ouverte (Fig. 1), la densité diminue de moitié et on mesure à nouveau le chemin optique total. Comme le terme de densité reste le même avant et après l'expansion (d/2 + d/2 = d) et que seulement les termes quadratiques et d'ordres plus élevés changent, on peut déterminer B_n et C_n directement à partir du changement de chemin optique.

Examinons en détail la procédure mise de l'avant pour déduire directement B_n et C_n par la technique de l'expansion appliquée au domaine optique. En fait, la procédure repose sur la mesure de n par une méthode interférométrique.

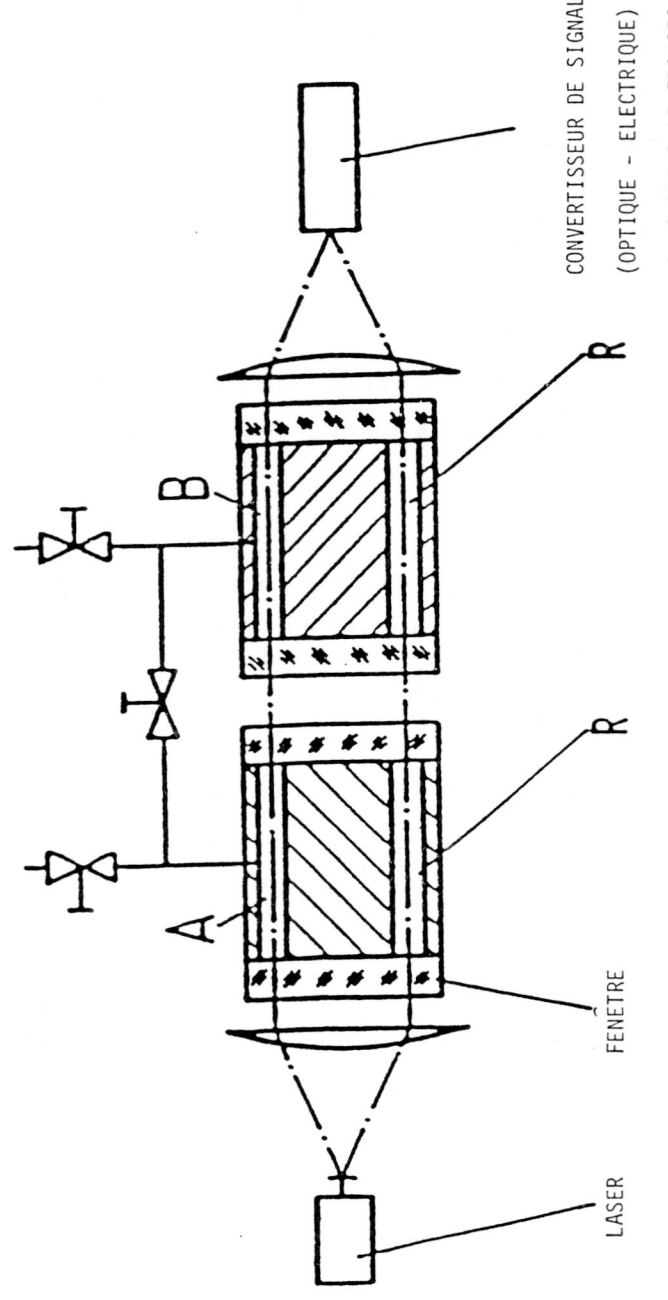

Figure 1 Disposition des cellules pour la méthode de l'expansion et la mesure de l'indice de réfraction du gaz.

Technique de l'expansion appliquée à l'optique

Le développement de $(n-1)d^{-1}$ en fonction de la densité est donné par

$$(n-1)d^{-1} = A_m + B_m d + C_m d^2 + \dots \qquad (15)$$

Les coefficients A_m, B_m et C_m sont liés aux A_n, B_n et C_n de l'équation (7) par des relations

$$A_n = (2/3)A_m \qquad (16)$$

$$B_n = (2/3)B_m - (1/9)A_m^2 \qquad (17)$$

$$C_n = (2/3)C_m - (2/9)A_m B_m - (4/27)A_m^3 \qquad (18)$$

Considérons que les volumes A et B (Fig.1) sont donnés par $V_A = V(1+\delta)$ et $V_B = V(1-\delta)$ où δ est petit. Les chemins optiques des volumes A et B sont donnés par $l_A = l(1+\Delta)$ et $l_B = l(1-\Delta)$ où Δ est petit. Si la cellule A est initialement remplie avec un gaz d'indice de réfraction n_A et de densité d_A et si la cellule B est sous vide, on observe un changement dans l'indice de réfraction (D_A) lorsqu'on ouvre la valve entre A et B. D_A est donné par la relation

$$D_A = (n_A-1)(1+\Delta) - 2(n_{AB}-1) \qquad (19)$$

où n_{AB} est l'indice de réfraction dans les deux cellules après l'expansion et à l'équilibre thermodynamique. L'équation (19) peut être exprimée en termes des coefficients A_m, B_m et C_m comme suit

$$D_A = A_m(\Delta-\delta)d_A + \frac{B_m}{2}\left[1 + 2(\Delta-\delta)\right]d_A^2 + \frac{C_m}{4}\left[3 + (4\Delta-3\delta)\right]d_B^3 + \dots \qquad (20)$$

De façon similaire, si B contient du gaz d'indice n_B et de densité d_B et si A est vide, l'expansion du gaz de B à A produira un changement D_B dans l'indice de réfraction. Défini de la même façon que D_A, D_B est donné par

$$D_B = -A_m(\Delta-\delta)d_B + \frac{B_m}{2}\left[1 - 2(\Delta-\delta)\right]d_B^2 + \frac{C_m}{4}\left[3 - (4\Delta-3\delta)\right]d_B^3 + \ldots \tag{21}$$

De l'équation (18) on peut exprimer d_A et d_B en termes de $n_A - 1$ et $n_B - 1$ par les relations

$$d_A = (n_A-1)/A_m - (n_A-1)^2 (B_m/A_m^3) + (n_A-1)^3 (2B_m^2 - A_m C_m)/A_m^5 + \ldots \tag{22}$$

$$d_B = (n_B-1)/A_m - (n_B-1)^2 (B_m/A_m^3) + (n_B-1)^3 (2B_m^2 - A_m C_m)/A_m^5 + \ldots \tag{23}$$

Si on remplace d_A et d_B dans les équations (20) et (21) par les équations (22) et (23), nous obtenons par la combinaison des équations (20) et (21)

$$D_A/(n_A-1) + D_B/(n_B-1) = (B_m/2A_m^2)\left[(n_A-1) + (n_B-1)\right]$$

$$+ \left[(3A_m C_m - 4B_m^2)/4A_m^4\right]\left[(n_A-1)^2 + (n_B-1)^2\right] + \ldots \tag{24}$$

On peut transformer l'équation (24) en une forme plus pratique à l'aide de l'équation (12). On obtient alors

$$F = (\Delta K_{AB})/K_A + (\Delta K_{BA})/K_B$$

$$= (B_m/2A_m^2)(\lambda/l)(K_A + K_B)$$

$$+ \left|(3A_m C_m - 4B_m^2)/4A_m^4\right|(\lambda/l)^2(K_A^2 + K_B^2) + \ldots \qquad (25)$$

où K_A et K_B correspondent aux nombres absolus de franges dans les cellules A et B avant l'expansion; ΔK_{AB} et ΔK_{BA} sont respectivement les nombres de franges observés durant l'expansion de A à B et de B à A. Les mesures sont entreprises de telle sorte que K_A est presqu'égal à K_B. La variable dans le deuxième terme, $K_A^2 + K_B^2$, peut ainsi être écrite comme $[(K_A + K_B)^2/2]$.

Si on trace F contre $(K_A + K_B)$, on obtient B_n et C_n selon la méthode des moindres carrés à partir d'un polynôme de la forme

$$Y = ax + bx^2 + cx^3 + \ldots \qquad (26)$$

Les erreurs sur F diminuent avec la pression parce que les mesures à haute pression ont plus de poids statistique.

Les valeurs de B_n et C_n sont déduites en tenant compte des transformations (16), (17) et (18).

Résultats

Nous avons obtenu des valeurs de A_n, B_n et C_n qui sont indépendantes de la température dans les limites mesurées (35°F à 70°F). Ces valeurs de $A_n = 6.639 \pm .004$ L/KMol, $B_n = 5.1 \pm 0.4$ L^2/KMol^2 et $C_n = -272 \pm 26$ L^3/KMol^3 ont été utilisées pour déduire le Z suivant l'équation (11) et obtenir le facteur F_{pv} selon l'équation

(5) où $Z_S = 1.0$. Les tableaux 1, 2 et 3 donnent respectivement à 35°F, 55°F et 70°F nos valeurs expérimentales (M) de P et F_{PV}, les valeurs de F_{PV} calculées selon la formule NX-19 et pourcentage d'écart $|(M - NX.19)/M| \cdot 100$

On constate qu'aux basses pressions nos valeurs expérimentales de F_{PV} concordent bien avec les valeurs calculées selon NX-19 pour les trois isothermes. On note cependant que l'écart est plus important aux grandes pressions, particulièrement à la température de 35°F.

La composition molaire du gaz naturel a été déterminée par chromatographie avec spectromètre de masse. Les résultats sont présentés au tableau 4.

Remerciements

Nous tenons à remercier particulièrement Gaz Métropolitain Inc. pour sa participation financière, l'analyse et la fourniture du gaz naturel.

BIBLIOGRAPHIE

1- T.K. Bose, J.M. St-Arnaud, H.R. Achtermann et R. Scharf, Rev. Sc. Instr., 57, 26 (1986).

2- D.R. Douslin, R.H. Harrison, R.T. Moore et J.P. McCullough, J. Chem. Eng. Data, 9, 358 (1964).

3- N.J. Trappeniers, T. Wassenaar et J.C., Abels, Physica, 98A, 289 (1979).

4- T.K. Bose, "A Comparative Study of the Dielectric, Refractive and Kerr Virial Coefficients" NATO Advanced Research Workshop on "Collision induced absorption", Ed. G. Birnbaum, Plenum. (1985), page 49.

5- J.M. St-Arnaud and T.K. Bose, Bull. Am. Phys. Soc., 17, 68 (1972)

6- A.D. Buckingham and C. Graham, Proc. R. Soc. London, A 336, 275 (1974).

7- J.M. St-Arnaud and T.K. Bose, J. Chem. Phys., 65, 4854 (1976).

8- J.M. St-Arnaud and T.K. Bose, J. Chem. Phys., 68, 2129 (1978).

9- J.M. St-Arnaud and T.K. Bose, J. Chem. Phys., 71, 4951 (1979).

10- H.J. Achtermann, R. Scharf and G. Magnus, VDI-Forsch.-Heft, 619, 11 (1983).

11- American Gas Association, Catalog No L00340, (1976).

TABLEAU 1

- Facteur de supercompressibilité du gaz naturel à 35°F
- Comparaison entre les mesures optiques (M) et les valeurs calculées selon NX-19.

Pression PSIG	Mesures optiques [M]	Valeurs calculées [N X 19]	$\left[\dfrac{M - NX19}{M}\right] 100$
50	1.00458	1.00414	.0439
100	1.00887	1.00830	.0562
200	1.01739	1.01680	.0583
300	1.02614	1.02550	.0624
400	1.03501	1.03437	.0618
500	1.04416	1.04340	.0723
700	1.06281	1.06183	.0922
800	1.07236	1.07114	.1137
900	1.08173	1.08045	.1183
1000	1.09051	1.08963	.0807
1100	1.10044	1.09874	.1548
1200	1.10947	1.10755	.1732
1300	1.11818	1.11755	.0563
1400	1.12637	1.12531	.0941

TABLEAU 2

- Facteur de supercompressibilité du gaz naturel à 55°F
- Comparaison entre les mesures optiques (M) et les valeurs calculées selon NX-19.

Pression PSIG	Mesures optiques [M]	Valeurs calculées [NX19]	$\left[\dfrac{M - NX19}{M} \right] 100$
50	1.00357	1.00361	-.0040
100	1.00712	1.00724	-.0115
200	1.01451	1.01459	-.0079
300	1.02195	1.02205	-.0096
400	1.02945	1.02960	-.0146
500	1.03709	1.03721	-.0111
600	1.04486	1.04485	+.0008
700	1.05256	1.05251	+.0047
800	1.06026	1.06012	+.0140
900	1.06786	1.06766	+.0187
1000	1.07534	1.07507	+.0251
1100	1.08268	1.08229	+.0360
1200	1.08977	1.08927	+.0459

TABLEAU 3

. Facteur de supercompressibilité du gaz naturel à 70°F
. Comparaison entre les mesures optiques (M) et les valeurs calculées selon NX-19.

Pression PSIG	Mesures optiques [M]	Valeurs calculées [NX19]	$\left[\dfrac{M - NX19}{M}\right] 100$
50	1.00353	1.00327	+.0259
100	1.00660	1.00654	+.0596
200	1.01311	1.01315	-.0039
300	1.01976	1.01981	-.0049
400	1.02644	1.02652	-.0078
500	1.03313	1.03323	-.0097
600	1.03986	1.03994	-.0077
700	1.04652	1.04662	-.0090
800	1.05315	1.05323	-.0076
900	1.05971	1.05974	-.0028
1000	1.06612	1.06611	+.0009
1100	1.07239	1.07229	+.0093
1200	1.07842	1.07824	+.0167
1300	1.08419	1.08391	+.0258
1400	1.08945	1.08925	+.0183
1500	1.09470	1.09421	+.0448
1600	1.09941	1.09875	+.0600
1700	1.10352	1.10284	+.0616
1800	1.10718	1.10643	+.0667
1900	1.11034	1.10951	+.0748
2000	1.11291	1.11209	+.0737
2100	1.11479	1.11420	+.0529
2200	1.11615	1.11563	+.0466
2300	1.11689	1.11640	+.0439
2400	1.11711	1.11654	+.0510
2500	1.11676	1.11609	+.0600
2600	1.11579	1.11509	+.0627
2700	1.11431	1.11358	+.0655
2800	1.11242	1.11161	+.0728
2900	1.11013	1.10922	+.0820
3000	1.10742	1.10645	+.0876

TABLEAU 4

Composition du gaz naturel fourni par Gaz Métropolitain Inc.

GAZ	% PAR MOLE
CH_4	95.9770
C_2H_6	1.9050
C_3H_8	0.0770
$i-C_4H_{10}$	0.0210
$n-C_4H_{10}$	0.0140
N_2	1.6200
CO_2	0.3760
$i-C_5H_{12}$	.0060
$n-C_5H_{12}$	.0040
TOTAL	100.0000

MODELISATION DE L'ODORISATION D'UNE CONDUITE

J. Goyette et J. Sochanski

Université du Québec à Trois-Rivières
Groupe de recherche sur les diélectriques
Département de physique
C.P. 500, Trois-Rivières, Québec, Canada, G9A 5H7

RESUME

Nous avons développé un modèle pour étudier le comportement dynamique de la concentration de l'odorant rajouté au gaz naturel. Notre modèle, basé sur le principe de la conservation de la masse appliqué à l'odorant circulant dans une conduite, suppose que les molécules d'odorant réagissent sur des sites actifs sur la paroi de la conduite. Ce modèle nous permet de calculer la concentration d'odorant en tout temps et en tout point de la conduite pour un patron d'injection d'odorant donné. Il nous permet aussi de voir comment la concentration de l'odorant contenu dans du gaz naturel au repos dans une conduite va décroître avec le temps.

ABSTRACT

We have developed a model in order to study the dynamical evolution of the concentration of the odorant added to natural gas. Our model is based on the mass conservation principle applied to the odorant flowing inside a gas line and assumes that the odorant molecules react on active sites on the interior surface of the gas line. This model allows us to compute the odorant concentration at any time and any point along the line for a given injection pattern of odorant and the decay of the odorant concentration in a line where there is no gas flow.

INTRODUCTION

Le gaz naturel est intrinsèquement inodore. Dans le but de protéger le public dans l'éventualité d'une fuite, des composés sulfureux (thiols et sulfides) sont ajoutés au gaz naturel afin de lui donner une odeur désagréable bien caractéristique. Ce processus d'odorisation du gaz naturel a fait ses preuves et est en général efficace. Cependant, il existe des situations particulières où il est difficile d'ajuster le taux d'injection des composés sulfureux afin d'obtenir une odorisation adéquate du gaz naturel. On peut penser à deux cas particuliers: - la mise en service d'une nouvelle conduite où il faut un certain temps avant d'obtenir une concentration suffisante de composés sulfureux dans la conduite et - les lignes antennes où la consommation et, par conséquent, le débit de gaz est limité; dans ce cas, du gaz bien odorisé tend, après quelques temps, à perdre son odorisation.

Les composés sulfureux utilisés comme odorant sont stables aux températures et pressions rencontrées dans une conduite. Bien qu'ils puissent réagir avec les thiols légers[1] contenus dans certains gaz, ils sont chimiquement inertes par rapport aux molécules de méthane et autres composants du gaz naturel. Dans le cas d'un gaz qui, comme le gaz canadien, ne contient pratiquement pas de thiols légers, la perte d'odorisation doit nécessairement provenir d'interactions sur la paroi de la conduite sous la forme de réactions chimiques ou d'adsorption. Par exemple, le 2-methyl-2-propanethiol (tertiary butyl mercaptan ou TBM, un des odorants les plus largement utilisés dans l'industrie du gaz) peut s'oxyder sur les molécules d'oxyde de fer qui recouvrent l'intérieur d'une conduite en acier[2].

Afin d'assurer une odorisation adéquate du gaz naturel, il faut donc tenir compte de ces interactions possibles entre l'odorant et la paroi. Nous avons développé un modèle qui simule le comportement dynamique de la concentration d'un odorant dont les molécules subissent des interactions avec la paroi telles qu'elles sont définitivement perdues. Ces molécules peuvent être perdues à la suite de réactions chimiques sur la paroi dont les produits ont une odeur moins forte que l'odorant originel ou, encore, à la suite d'un phénomène d'adsorption où les liens entre les molécules d'odorant adsorbées et la paroi sont tellement forts qu'il n'y a pratiquement pas de probabilité que ces molécules ne se désorbent et retournent dans le gaz de la conduite.

LES EQUATIONS DU MODELE

Considérons une conduite de gaz de rayon R et de longueur L. Prenons une section de la conduite de longueur dx située à une distance x de l'origine de la conduite.

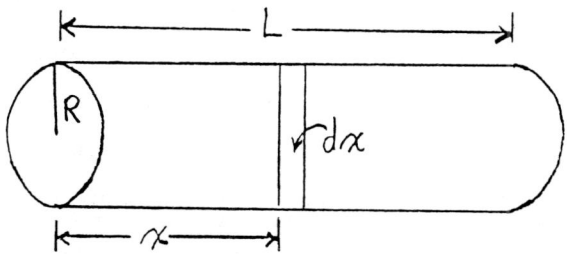

Soit C(x,t) la concentration de l'odorant au point x le long de la conduite et au temps t. Le nombre total de molécules d'odorant contenu dans la longueur dx de conduite est

$$dN = \pi R^2 C(x, t) \, dx.$$

A cause de phénomènes tels que le débit du gaz et les interactions avec la paroi, le nombre de molécules d'odorant à l'intérieur de la section dx variera et

$$\frac{dN}{dt} = \pi R^2 \frac{\partial C}{\partial t} \, dx. \tag{1}$$

Le flux de molécules au point x est $\pi R^2 C(x,t) v_d$ où v_d est la composante de la vitesse des molécules parallèles à l'axe de la conduite. Si on suppose v_d constant, le flux à x + dx sera $\pi R^2 C(x+dx,t) v_d$. Le changement dans le nombre de molécules à l'intérieur de la section dx dû au débit de gaz naturel sera

$$\left. \frac{dN}{dt} \right|_{\text{débit}} = \pi R^2 v_d (C(x,t) - C(x+dx,t)) = -\pi R^2 v_d \frac{\partial C}{\partial x} \, dx. \tag{2}$$

S(x,t) est la fonction qui décrit le nombre de molécules d'odorant qui interagissent avec la paroi de la conduite par unité de temps et par unité de longueur de la conduite. On pourra donc écrire

$$\left. \frac{dN}{dt} \right|_{\text{interaction}} = -S(x,t) \, dx. \tag{3}$$

Donc, d'après le principe de conservation de la masse, on a

$$\frac{\partial C}{\partial t} = -\frac{S(x,t)}{\pi R^2} - v_d \frac{\partial C}{\partial x}. \tag{4}$$

A) Calcul de S(x,t)

Des études sur les réactions chimiques à l'interface gaz-solide montrent qu'en général les réactions n'ont pas lieu n'importe où sur l'interface mais plutôt à des endroits bien précis de la surface où les conditions énergétiques sont favorables aux réactions. Une surface est donc caractérisée par des sites actifs sur lesquels les molécules d'un gaz peuvent réagir. Une fois que la réaction chimique a eu lieu, la configuration moléculaire de la surface va changer de telle façon qu'il ne pourra plus s'y produire de réactions chimiques. Considérons donc un modèle où les molécules d'odorant ont des collisions avec une paroi de la conduite sur laquelle elles peuvent réagir. Le nombre de molécules d'odorant qui vont réagir par unité de temps dans l'élément de la conduite sera

$$S(x,t)\,dx = N_c\,K_c\,(2\pi R dx) \qquad (5)$$

où N_c: nombre de molécules qui frappent une unité de surface de la conduite par unité de temps,

K_c: probabilité qu'une collision amène une réaction chimique,

$2\pi R dx$: surface de la conduite sur laquelle les collisions ont lieu.

Si on utilise la fonction de distribution de Boltzmann pour les vitesses radiales (les vitesses perpendiculaires à l'axe de la conduite)

$$F(v_r) = \frac{mv_r}{kT}\,\exp-\left(\frac{mv_r^2}{2kT}\right)$$

où m est la masse d'une molécule d'odorant, T la température absolue et K la constante de Boltzmann, on peut trouver que

$$N_c = C\bar{v}_r = \frac{C}{2}\left(\frac{2\pi KT}{m}\right)^{1/2} \qquad (6)$$

où $\bar{v}_r$ est la vitesse radiale moyenne.

Pour qu'il y ait une réaction chimique sur la paroi de la conduite, il faut que deux évènements indépendants se produisent: il y a d'abord une collision sur un site actif, ensuite la molécule doit réagir. On peut donc écrire

$$K_c = K_a K_e \qquad (7)$$

où K_a: probabilité que la collision sur la paroi ait lieu sur un site actif

K_e: probabilité que la collision soit efficace.

On peut aussi poser

$$K_a = D_a a \qquad (8)$$

où D_a: nombre de sites actifs par unité de surface (densité de sites actifs)

a: surface moyenne d'un site actif

Considérant le produit aK_e comme une surface effective, c'est-à-dire posant

$$S_e = aK_e, \qquad (9)$$

on peut finalement écrire

$$K_c = D_a S_e \tag{10}$$

Les équations (6), (8) et (12) nous donnent donc

$$S(x, t) = \pi R \left(\frac{2\pi KT}{m} \right)^{1/2} D_a S_e C \tag{11}$$

et l'équation (5) devient:

$$\frac{\partial C}{\partial t} = - \left(\frac{2\pi KT}{m} \right)^{1/2} \frac{S_e D_a C}{R} - v_d \frac{\partial C}{\partial x} \tag{12}$$

Cette équation reproduit bien les résultats expérimentaux exposés dans la littérature[3] où il est trouvé que le taux d'oxydation du TBM dépend de la concentration de TBM, de la pression totale (elle est proportionnelle à la température), du débit, de la surface intérieure de la conduite et du temps. Une augmentation de la concentration d'odorant, de la pression ou du débit augmente le taux d'oxydation. D'un autre côté, une augmentation de la surface (i.e. R) ou du temps amène une diminution du taux de conversion.

B) **Comportement dynamique de D_a.**

L'équation (12) contient un terme, D_a, qui est une fonction du temps. Il faut donc compléter l'équation (12) avec une équation qui décrit la façon dont D_a varie dans le temps. Puisque le nombre de sites actifs sur la paroi d'une section de conduite de longueur dx est

$$dN_a = 2\pi R\, D_a\, dx,$$

on peut écrire

$$\frac{dN_a}{dt} = 2\pi R \frac{\partial D_a}{\partial t} dx . \tag{13}$$

On peut supposer que pour chaque molécule qui réagit sur la paroi, il y a un site actif qui disparait, on a donc

$$\frac{dN_a}{dt} = - S(x,t) dx \tag{14}$$

et l'équation qui décrit le comportement dynamique de Da est

$$\frac{\partial D_a}{\partial t} = -\left(\frac{2\pi KT}{m}\right)^{1/2} \frac{S_e D_a C}{2} . \tag{15}$$

C) Solutions

Les équations (12) et (15) forment un système qui décrit le comportement dynamique de la concentration d'odorant dans une conduite. On peut solutionner ce système relativement facilement[4]. En effet, posons

$$u = t - \frac{x}{v_d} \qquad w = -\frac{x}{v_d} ,$$

$$F = \left(\frac{2\pi KT}{m}\right)^{1/2} S_e , \tag{16}$$

on obtient alors

$$\frac{\partial C}{\partial w} = -\frac{2}{R} \frac{\partial D_a}{\partial w} .$$

Les solutions de ce système auront la forme

$$C = \frac{f'(u)}{g(w) + Ff(u)} , \qquad D_a = -\frac{R}{2F}\left(\frac{g'(w)}{g(w) + Ff(u)}\right) \tag{17}$$

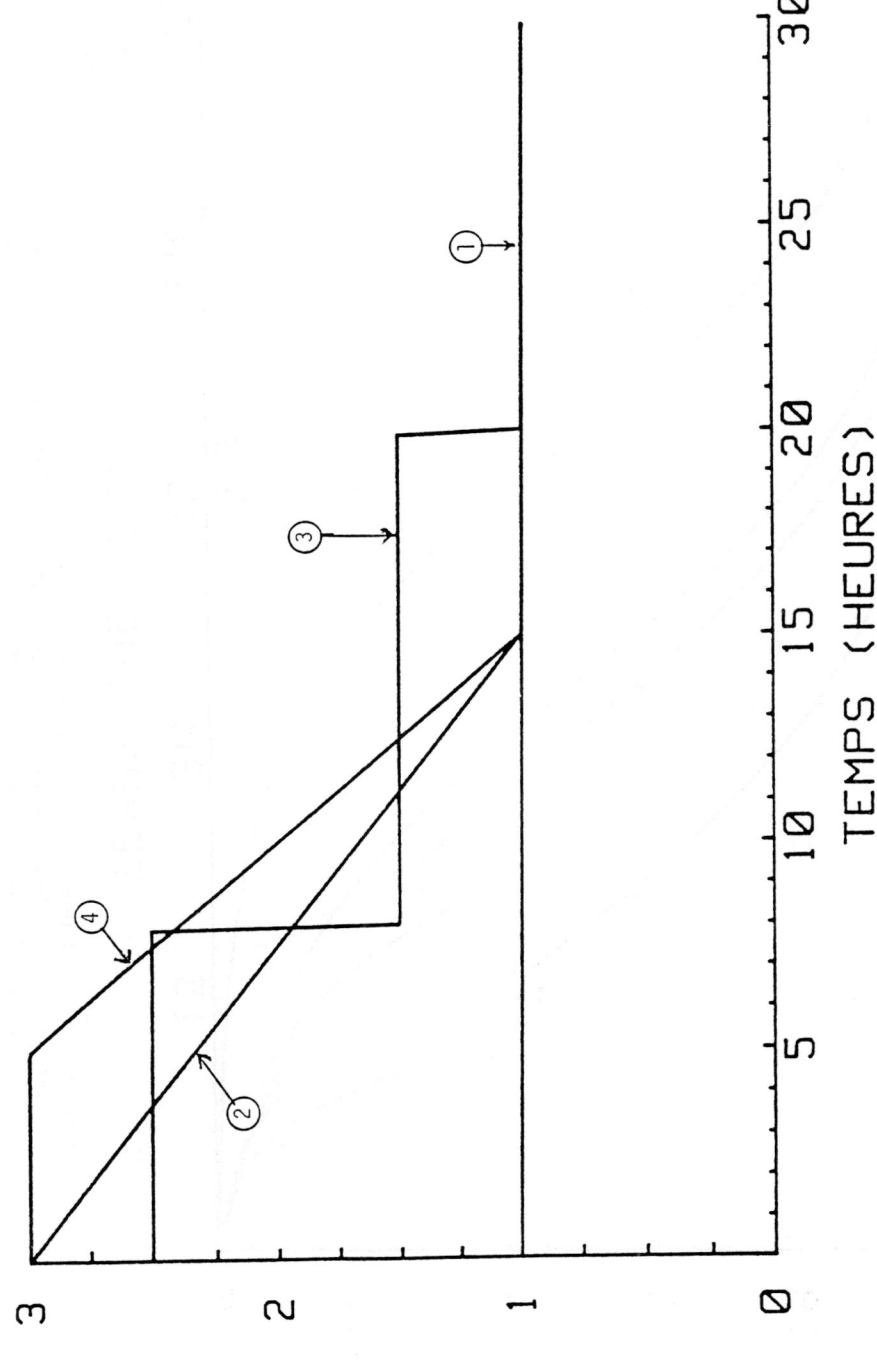

Figure 1a. Concentration d'odorant injectée à l'entrée de la ligne en fonction du temps. Chaque unité de concentration d'odorant correspond a 1. x 10²⁰ molécules par mètre cube de gaz.

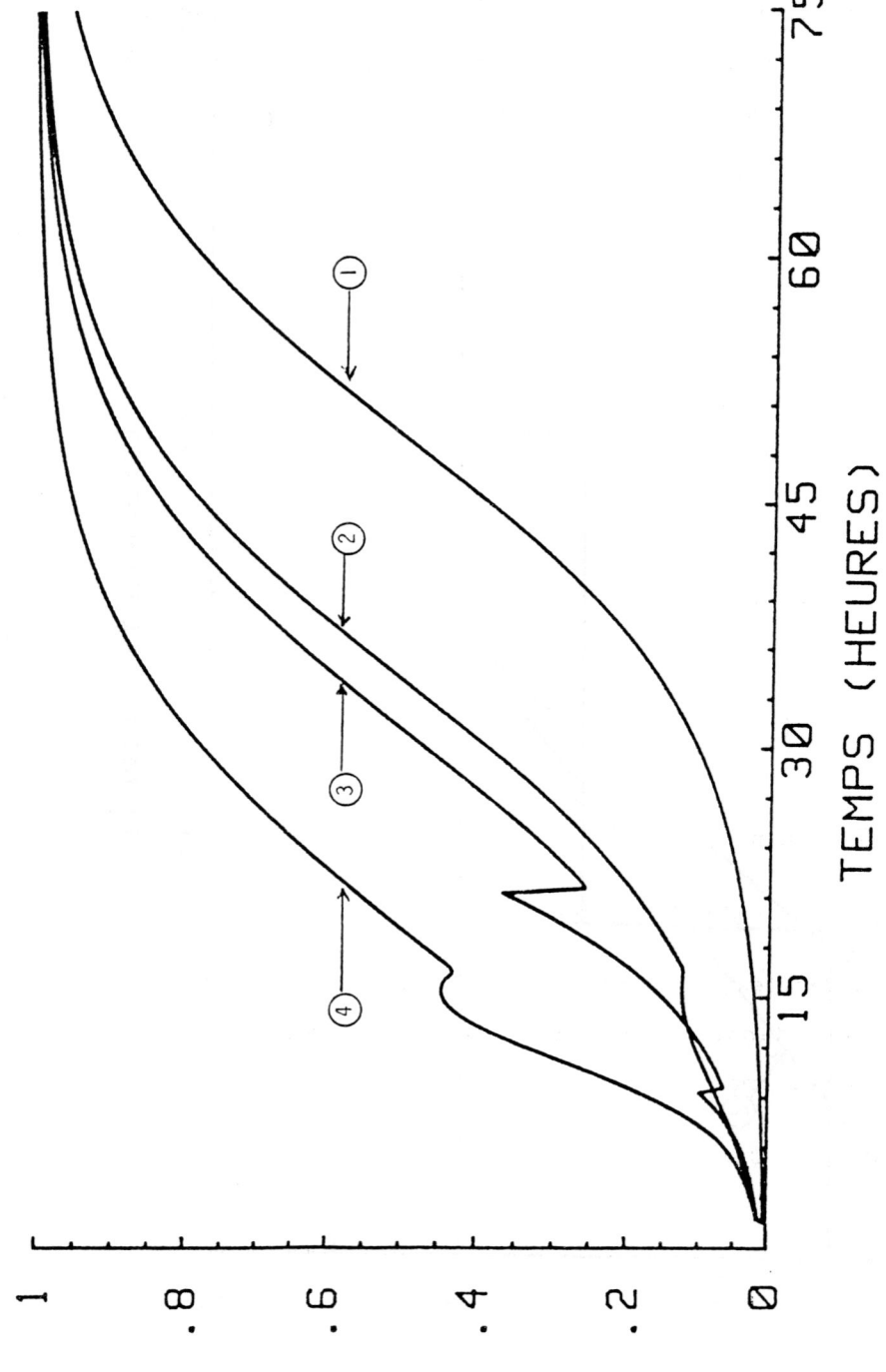

Figure 1b. Concentration d'odorant en bout de ligne en fonction du temps pour les patrons d'injection décrits sur la figure 1a. Longueur de la ligne: 35 km, rayon: 4 cm, débit: 100 m^3/hr, pression: 100 KPa, Dao: 3. x 10^{19}/m^2, Se: 1.5 x 10^{-27} m^2. Chaque unité de concentration d'odorant correspond à 1. x 10^{20} molécules par mètre cube de gaz.

où f et g sont des fonctions que l'on peut déterminer à partir des conditions de frontière. Considérons le cas d'une nouvelle conduite ayant une densité initiale de sites actifs D_{ao}. Pendant qu'on la remplit de gaz, la concentration d'odorant à l'entrée est donnée par $C_0(t)$, et les conditions de frontière deviennent:

a) a $x = 0$ ou $w = 0$

$$C(0,u) = C_0(u) \qquad (18)$$

La concentration d'odorant vu par les sites actifs à l'entrée de la ligne est $C_0(u)$, ils obéissent donc à l'équation suivante:

$$\frac{\partial D_a(0,u)}{\partial u} = -\frac{F}{2} D_a(0,u) C(0,u).$$

On a donc

$$D_a(0,u) = D_{ao} \exp -\left(\frac{FH(u)}{2}\right) \qquad (19)$$

où $$H(u) = \int_0^u C_0(u') \, du'. \qquad (20)$$

b) a $t = \dfrac{x}{v_d}$ ou $u = 0$

$$D_a(w,0) = D_{ao}. \qquad (21)$$

Pour les molécules d'odorant circulant à l'avant de la vague d'odorant, la densité de sites actifs demeure constante. La concentration d'odorant subit donc une décroissance exponentielle et

$$C(w,0) = C_0(0) \exp\left(\frac{FD_{ao}w}{R}\right) \qquad (22)$$

avec les équations (17) à (22) on peut finalement obtenir

$$C = 0 \qquad t < \frac{x}{v_d}$$

$$C = \frac{C_0 \left(t - \frac{x}{v_d} \right)}{1 - \left[\exp - \frac{FH}{2} \left(t - \frac{x}{v_d} \right) \right] \left(1 - \exp \left(- \frac{FD_{ao}x}{Rv_d} \right) \right)} \qquad t \geq \frac{x}{v_d} \qquad (23)$$

Il y a plusieurs modes d'injection qui semblent à prime abord, intéressants. Mentionnons, par exemple, l'injection à une concentration élevée suivie d'une injection à une concentration plus basse; diminution graduelle de l'injection à partir d'une valeur maximum jusqu'à la concentration C_0; une forte injection au début suivie d'une diminution; etc... . L'équation (23) nous permet de calculer quel est l'effet sur l'odorisation d'une conduite de différents patrons d'injection. Les figures Ia et Ib illustrent comment la concentration en bout de ligne est affectée par le taux d'injection d'odorant à l'entrée de la ligne et laissent entrevoir qu'il est probablement possible de choisir un patron d'injection d'odorant pour obtenir une odorisation efficace d'une conduite.

D) Ligne antenne

Dans le réseau d'exploitation d'une compagnie de gaz, on a souvent à faire face à des conditions de sous-odorisation dans des conduites antennes c'est-à-dire dans des conduites qui ne desservent que quelques clients et dans lesquelles, à certaines périodes de l'année (en été par exemple), il y a un débit pratiquement nul. Notre modèle

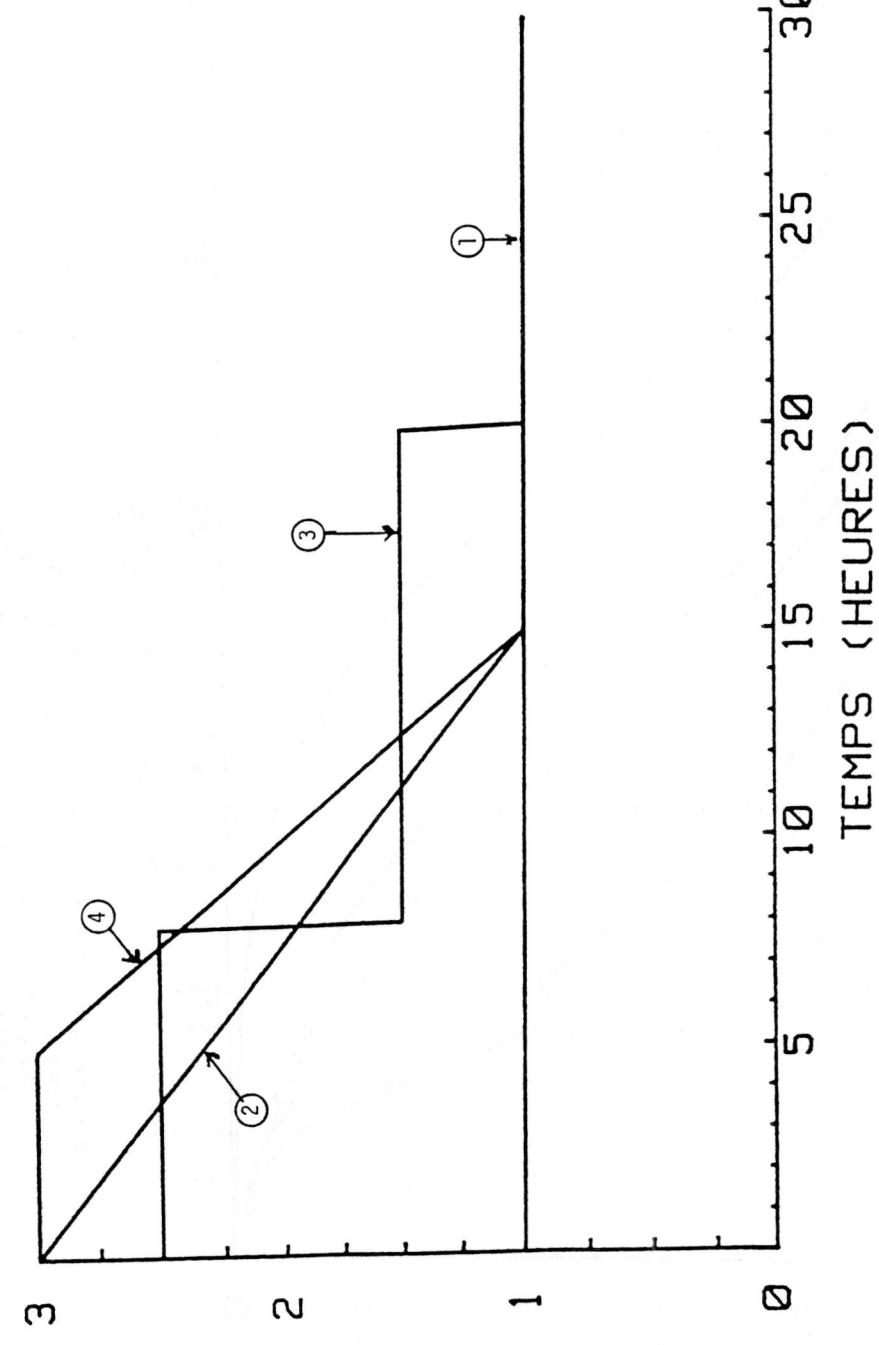

Figure Ia. Concentration d'odorant injectée à l'entrée de la ligne en fonction du temps. Chaque unité de concentration d'odorant correspond à 1. x 10^{20} molécules par mètre cube de gaz.

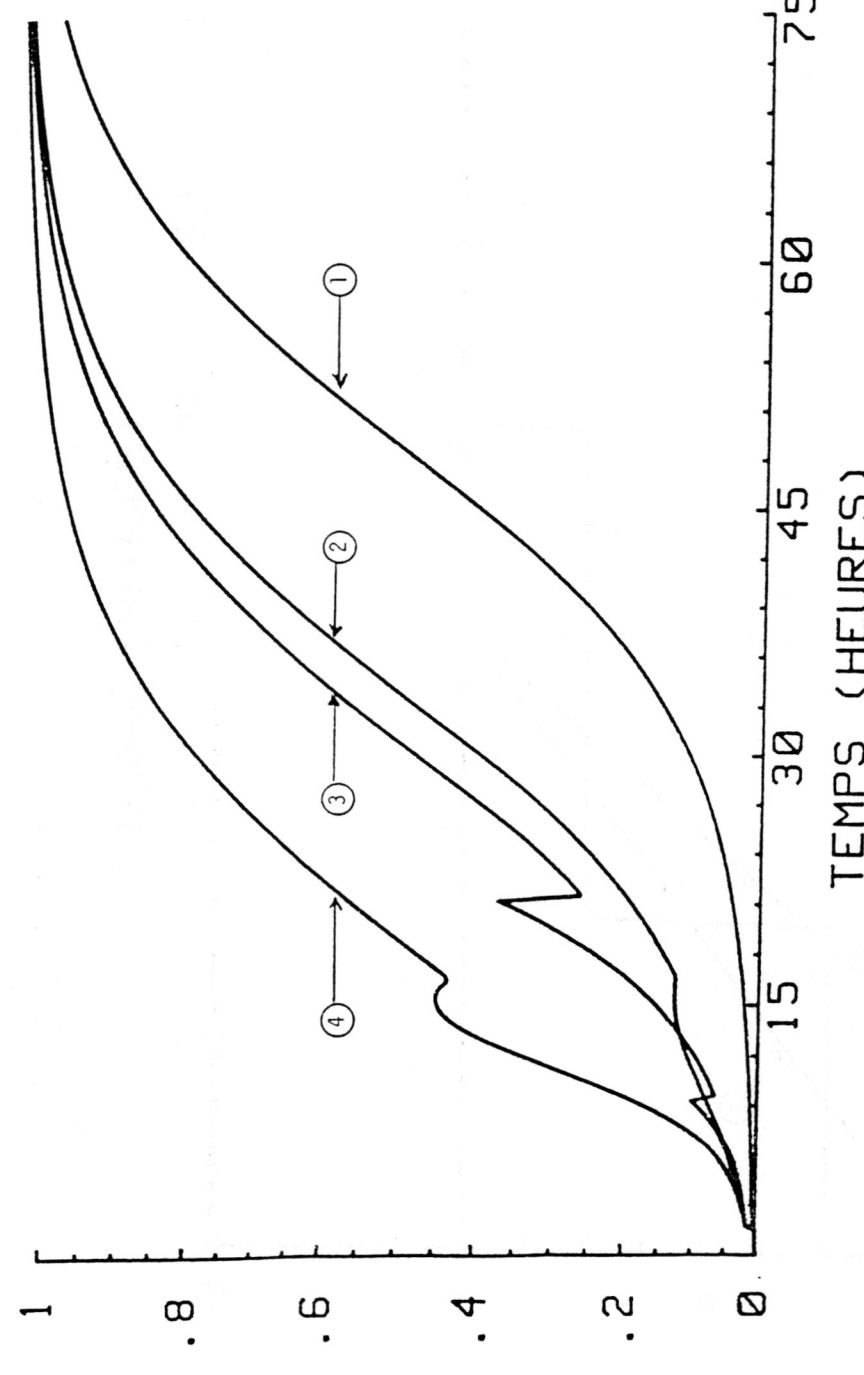

Figure 1b. Concentration d'odorant en bout de ligne en fonction du temps pour les patrons d'injection décrits sur la figure 1a. Longueur de la ligne: 35 km, rayon: 4 cm, débit: 100 m^3/hr, pression: 100 kPa, Dao: 3. x 10^{19}/m^2, Se: 1.5 x 10^{-27} m^2. Chaque unité de concentration d'odorant correspond à 1. x 10^{20} molécules par mètre cube de gaz.

peut expliquer comment, en de telles circonstances, le gaz peut perdre son odorisation. Posant $v_d = 0$ dans l'équation (14) et utilisant aussi l'équation (12) et les conditins initiales

$$C(0) = C_o \qquad D_a(0) = D_{ao}$$

on peut trouver

$$C(t) = \frac{C_o \left(C_o - \frac{2D_{ao}}{R} \right)}{C_o - \frac{2D_{ao}}{R} \left(\exp \frac{Ft}{2} \left(\frac{2D_{ao}}{R} - C_o \right) \right)} \qquad (24)$$

On voit donc que du gaz bien odorisé laissé au repos dans une conduite sur laquelle il y a des sites actifs va, à la longue, perdre son odorisation. Les lignes antennes dans lesquelles il n'y a pas eu une circulation de gaz odorisé suffisante pour neutraliser les sites actifs qui se trouvaient originellement sur la paroi et celles qui ont subi des réparations amenant le remplacement de certaines sections de conduite seront donc susceptibles aux problèmes de sous-odorisation.

CONCLUSION

Nous avons developpé un modèle qui permet de calculer la concentration d'odorant en tout temps et en tout point d'une conduite pour un patron d'injection d'odorant donné. Ce modèle explique de façon relativement simple comment des conditions de sous-odorisation peuvent se produire dans des conduites nouvellement installées et des conduites antennes et suggère des patrons d'injection qui peuvent corriger ces situations. Notre modèle est basé sur le concept de sites actifs localisés sur la paroi intérieure de la conduite sur lesquels les molécules d'odorant peuvent réagir. Il se sert de deux paramètres pour décrire l'état microscopique de la paroi. D_{ao}, la densité initiale de sites actifs, est une mesure de la quantité d'odorant qui sera ultimement perdue sur les parois de la conduite tandis que S_e, la surface effective d'un site actif, est une mesure de la vitesse à laquelle l'odorant sera perdu sur la paroi.

Notre modèle a aussi l'avantage d'expliquer pourquoi les problèmes de sous-odorisation semblent souvent si imprévisibles et aléatoires. Ainsi, il arrive souvent que deux conduites semblent opérer pratiquement sous les mêmes conditions; mais, tandis que dans l'une le gaz est bien odorisé, dans l'autre il y a des problèmes. Une explication possible est que l'état microscopique de leur surface est différent. En effet, prenons le cas du TBM dans une conduite en acier. Puisque le TBM réagit sur le molécules d'oxyde de fer, on peut considérer que D_{ao} dépend de la quantité de rouille qui s'est formée sur la surface intérieure de la conduite. Mais cette quantité de rouille va varier dépendant si on vient de recevoir les sections de conduite de l'aciérie, si on les a entreposées dans un endroit sec, si on les a laissées dans un champ pendant un certain temps, etc... . Il faut donc s'attendre à une variation importante de D_{ao} d'une conduite à l'autre et donc d'un comportement différent de l'odorant dans les différents conduites.

Le modèle exposé dans cette communication ne s'applique qu'au cas où l'odorant est définitivement perdu à la suite des interactions avec la paroi. Cependant, il est relativement facile de modifier notre modèle[5] pour tenir compte d'un phénomène d'adsorption où, après avoir été adsorbées pendant quelque temps sur la paroi de la conduite, les molécules d'odorant peuvent se désorber et retourner dans le gaz. Il suffit d'ajouter à la fonction $S(x,t)$ qui décrit les interactions entre la paroi et les molécules d'odorant le terme $(D_a(x,t) - D_{ao})\nu_d$ qui est le produit de la densité de molécules adsorbées sur la paroi $(D_a(x,t) - D_{ao})$ et de la probabilité qu'une molécules adsorbée se désorbe (ν_d). Les équations ainsi obtenues sont plus complexes que les équations (12) et (15) traitées ici et ne peuvent être solutionnées analytiquement. Cependant, l'équation (17) pourrait servir de première approximation à un calcul de perturbation. Ceci devrait donner de bons résultats dans le cas où ν_d est petit. Pratiquement c'est la seule situation d'intérêt puisque, lorsque ν_d est grand, les molécules d'odorant demeurent peu de temps sur la paroi de la conduite ce qui ne devrait pas amener une situation de sous-odorisation.

REMERCIEMENTS

Nous remercions Gaz Métropolitain Inc. pour son support financier.

REFERENCES

1. Roberson, S.T., 1987. "Factors to Consider when Choosing a Gas Odorant" in Odorization Symposium, Chicago.

2. Kniebes, D.V., 1980, "Odorant Stability in Natural Gas Systems" in Odorization Symposium, Chicago, p. 197.

3. Scott, P.M. et Lipinski, E.S., 1987, "Reducing Odorant Fade due to Absorption / Adsorption of Mercaptan Odorants by the Iron Oxide Mill Scale Found Inside New Steel Pipes" Batelle, Colombus, 11 pages.

4. Danby, C.J. et al., 1946, "The Kinetics of Absorption of Gases from an Air Stream by Granular Reagents", J. Chem. Soc., p. 918.

5. Goyette, J. et Bose, T.K., Janvier 1988, "Dosage de l'odorant", Rapport présenté à Gaz Métropolitain Inc.

ADSORPTION DU METHANE A HAUTE PRESSION SUR LES CHARBONS ACTIFS

R. Chahine et T.K. Bose

Université du Québec à Trois-Rivières
Groupe de recherche sur les diélectriques
Département de physique
C.P. 500, Trois-Rivières, Québec, Canada, G9A 5H7

ABSTRACT

Physical adsorption of methane on activated carbons is studied as a function of pressure (0 to 12 MPa) and temperature (-30 to +60 C). Measurements were done using an automated volumetric method and a new dielectric method for the determination of gas adsorption at high pressure. The latter is based on dielectric virial coefficients and it takes advantage of the dielectric technique for the precise measurement of the density of real gases. Comparative results of the two methods are given and the primary factors affecting the amount of natural gas that can be stored by an adsorbent are discussed.

RESUME

L'adsorption physique du méthane sur les charbons actifs est caractérisée en fonction de la pression (0 à 12 MPa) et de la température (-30 à + 60 C). Les mesures ont été effectuées à l'aide d'une méthode volumétrique automatisée et d'une nouvelle méthode diélectrique pour déterminer l'adsorption des gaz à haute pression. Cette dernière est basée sur les coefficients du viriel de la constante diélectrique (CVCD) et elle prend avantage de la technique diélectrique pour mesurer avec précision la densité d'un gaz réel. Des résultats obtenus par les deux méthodes sont comparés et les principaux facteurs affectant la quantité de gaz naturel qu'un adsorbant peut emmagasiner sont discutés.

INTRODUCTION

L'emploi du gaz naturel comme carburant de véhicules automobiles (GNV) offre plusieurs avantages. Des inconvénients majeurs ont toutefois, jusqu'à présent, sérieusement freiné son utilisation massive. Ces inconvénients sont causés, en grande partie, par le faible contenu énergétique du GN sous sa forme gazeuse. En effet, pour assurer aux véhicules une autonomie routière raisonnable, il est nécessaire de comprimer le gaz naturel dans des cylindres de haute pression. Les pressions utilisées sont nettement élevées et elles varient généralement entre 16.5 MPa (2400 psi) et 20.7 MPa (3000 psi). Or, l'équipement nécessaire pour comprimer et manipuler le GN à de telles pressions est très cher. Le coût du compresseur et du système de mesure s'élève à environ 50% du coût total requis pour convertir et desservir une flotte automobile typique au gaz naturel comprimé (GNC).

La disponibilité d'un mode de stockage du GNV à plus faible pression assurerait une percée accrue du GN sur le marché de l'énergie et faciliterait son rôle de substitut au pétrole importé. En effet, un tel mode de stockage offrirait des avantages économiques et techniques. Parmi les premiers, notons en particulier la baisse du coût élevé des stations de service et la réduction du coût de compression et de maintien des compresseurs. Du point de vue technique, on note que l'équipement requis pour comprimer et manipuler le GN à une pression d'environ 3.6 MPa plutôt que 21 MPa, est beaucoup moins sophistiqué et donc plus fiable.

A l'heure actuelle, le stockage par adsorption semble être la technologie la plus prometteuse pour emmagasiner le gaz naturel à faible pression[1]. En effet, des adsorbants capables de stocker à 3.5 MPa une quantité de gaz trois à quatre fois supérieure à celle stockée dans un cylindre vide à la même pression sont déjà disponibles[2]. Les efforts pour améliorer ces performances se multiplient un peu partout dans le monde.

Les travaux de recherche sur le stockage du GN par adsorption démontrent bien que les charbons actifs sont les meilleurs adsorbants existant à l'heure actuelle. Ces travaux démontrent aussi que la performance d'un adsorbant, en terme de capacité de stockage, dépend principalement de sa surface spécifique et de sa densité en vrac. Les résultats expérimentaux révèlent[3] que cette capacité est généralement proportionnelle à la surface spécifique par unité de masse de l'adsorbant. Par ailleurs, une grande valeur de la densité en vrac de l'adsorbant permet de minimiser le volume d'un système de stockage du GNV.

A température constante, la quantité de gaz adsorbé dans un solide poreux augmente avec la pression et cette augmentation est relativement beaucoup plus rapide à basse pression qu'à haute pression. D'autre part, à pression fixe, la quantité de gaz adsorbé diminue à mesure que la température augmente et vice versa. La plupart des expériences reliées aux systèmes de stockage du gaz naturel par adsorption, ont été, jusqu'à présent, menées au voisinage de 25 C. Il y a donc très peu d'information reliée aux températures opérationnelles de stockage dictées par les variations climatiques et les effets thermiques de l'adsorption.

Le but principal du présent travail est d'étudier l'effet de la température sur les isothermes d'adsorption du méthane, constituant principal du GN, sur les charbons actifs. Dans ce qui suit, nous décrivons notre méthodologie expérimantale et nous comparons les résultats obtenus par la méthode volumétrique et la méthode diélectrique. Dans un deuxième temps, nous donnons un exemple des paramètres intrinsèques affectant la capacité d'un système de stockage du GN par adsorption. Finalement nous discutons de la variation de cette capacité en fonction de la température.

Méthodologie expérimentale

Pour un gaz et un adsorbant donnés, la quantité de gaz adsorbé N_a est fonction de la pression et de la température[4]. De façon générale, on fixe la température et on mesure la quantité de gaz adsorbé en fonction de la pression. Les résultats ainsi obtenus peuvent être représentés graphiquement à l'aide de courbes appelées isothermes d'adsorption.

Avant d'aller plus loin, il est nécessaire de bien spécifier ce qu'on entend par "quantité de gaz adsorbé". Supposons que le solide et le gaz occupent un contenant fermé de volume V et que le gaz lui-même occupe un volume V_g de sorte que le volume du solide est $(V-V_g)$. La quantité de gaz adsorbé (en moles) est égale au nombre total de moles de gaz dans le contenant en présence du solide, moins le nombre de moles de gaz qui occuperaient le volume V_g aux mêmes température et pression. Cela dit, il est clair que, pour déterminer expérimentalement N_a (en moles), nous devons connaître deux quantités: d'abord, le nombre total N_t de moles de gaz dans le contenant (i.e. celles en phase gazeuse et celles adsorbées), puis le volume V_g occupé par la phase gazeuse.

Méthode volumétrique

Pour mesurer les isothermes d'adsorption des charbons étudiés, nous avons conçu et construit un montage expérimental géré par ordinateur et basé sur la méthode volumétrique traditionnelle (voir Fig. 1). La méthode de mesure est complètement automatique, elle peut fonctionner continuellement et d'une façon autonome. Par le biais d'un système d'acquisition de données, l'ordinateur contrôle les opérations de remplissage et d'expansion du gaz dans les cellules grâce à des valves pneumatiques. De plus, il réalise la prise de mesures à l'équilibre et il effectue les calculs relatifs à l'adsorption. Afin de bien visualiser le principe de cette méthode, considérons tout d'abord le cas d'un gaz idéal. Nous avons deux cellules vides A et B reliées par une valve permettant le libre passage du gaz d'une cellule vers l'autre. Après avoir fermé cette valve, on remplit la cellule A avec du gaz comprimé à la pression P_1 et à la température absolue T. Préalablement, on a inséré, dans la cellule B, l'adsorbant qu'on veut caractériser pour ce gaz en particulier. Le nombre initial N_1 de moles dans la cellule A ayant un volume V est donné, d'après la loi idéale des gaz, par

$$N_1 = (P_1) V/R T, \qquad (1)$$

où R est la constante universelle du gaz.

On ouvre ensuite la valve entre les deux cellules. Alors, les moles du gaz se répartissent entre les deux cellules et à l'équilibre thermodynamique (à T constante) une nouvelle pression P_2 inférieure à P_1 s'établit également dans les deux cellules. Le nombre de moles N_2 restant dans la cellule A devient

$$N_2 = (P_2) V/R T \qquad (2)$$

et le nombre de moles (N_t) passées vers la cellule B où il y a l'adsorbant, est alors donné par la différence (N_1-N_2). Comme nous l'avons expliqué plus haut, N_t est la somme (N_a+N_g), N_a étant le nombre de moles adsorbées et N_g étant donné par

$$N_g = (P_2) V_g/R T. \qquad (3)$$

Pour mesurer V_g, il suffit de répéter la même procédure, mais pour un gaz comme l'hélium qui ne serait pas adsorbé à ces température et pression. Dans ce cas, N_t devient égal à N_g et V_g est simplement donné par

$$V_g = N_g R T/ P_2. \qquad (4)$$

Ayant mesuré ainsi le nombre total de moles de gaz N_t dans la cellule contenant l'adsorbant solide et le nombre de moles en phase gazeuse N_g, on déduit alors la quantité (en moles) de gaz adsorbé N_a à la pression P_2, soit

$$N_a = N_t - N_g. \qquad (5)$$

La loi idéale des gaz, exprimée par l'équation (1), n'est pas valable pour exprimer le comportement d'un gaz réel à haute pression.

On peut cependant modifier l'équation (1) par l'inclusion du facteur de compressibilité Z pour décrire le comportement d'un gaz réel à haute pression. Dans un tel cas, l'équation d'état est donnée par

$$PV = ZNRT. \qquad (6)$$

Le facteur de compressibilité est une fonction de la température, de la pression et de la spécifité du gaz considéré (sa composition entre autres). Etant donné que le facteur Z du méthane est bien caractérisé, la précision expérimentale est alors dictée par la précision sur P, V, et T uniquement.

Méthode diélectrique

En l'absence de valeurs précises de Z couvrant le champ des températures et pressions désirées, la méthode volumétrique est sujette à des erreurs. Nous avons alors conçu une nouvelle méthode (voir Fig. 2) basée sur la technique d'expansion diélectrique[5] que nous avons développée dans nos laboratoires. Cette méthode nous permet de mesurer la densité réelle du gaz aux mêmes conditions de pression et de température que l'expérience. Notre approche expérimentale devient ainsi autosuffisante. Dans ce qui suit, nous présentons brièvement la base scientifique de la méthode. La description détaillée de la méthode expérimentale est présentée ailleurs[6].

Dans un premier temps, nous établissons le lien entre la densité d'un gaz, sa constante diélectrique statique et les coefficients du viriel de la constante diélectrique (CVCD). Par la suite, nous montrons brièvement comment nous déduisons les CVCD d'un gaz à haute pression.

Les CVCD sont définis par le développement de la fonction Clausius-Mossotti en série de puissances de la densité. On obtient

$$(\varepsilon - 1)/(\varepsilon + 2)d = A_\varepsilon + B_\varepsilon d + ... \qquad (7)$$

ou ε est la constante diélectrique statique, $d = N/V$ est la densité molaire et A_ε, B_ε sont respectivement le premier et le deuxième CVCD. Bien que notre méthode expérimentale puisse déterminer ces deux coefficients, seulement la mesure de A_ε est suffisante dans le cas du méthane. En effet, ce gaz étant non polaire, il en résulte que le terme B_ε devient négligeable devant A_ε et l'équation (7) se réduit à

$$L_\varepsilon = (\varepsilon - 1)/(\varepsilon + 2) = A_\varepsilon d \qquad (8)$$

et la densité est alors simplement donnée par

$$d = L_\varepsilon / A_\varepsilon. \qquad (9)$$

L'examen de cette relation nous permet de conclure que, pour obtenir la densité d'un gaz tel que le méthane, il suffit de mesurer la constante diélectrique ε aux mêmes conditions de pression et température. Il faut cependant obtenir expérimentalement la valeur de A_ε qui, pour les gaz non polaires, est indépendente de la température.

La constante diélectrique est donnée par l'équation

$$\varepsilon = C/C_0, \qquad (10)$$

ou C_0 représente la capacité d'un condensateur dans le vide et C

représente la capacité du même condensateur rempli de gaz. Pour mesurer C et Co, on utilise un pont de capacitances à transformateur très précis. Ceci nous permet d'évaluer la valeur de ϵ avec une précision d'une partie par million.

Le premier CVCD est obtenu en faisant une mesure absolue de la constante diélectrique en fonction de la pression jusqu'à environ 1.38 MPa (200 psi).

Remplaçant d en fonction de P, l'équation (7) est modifiée par

$$[(\epsilon-1)/(\epsilon+2)] [RT/P] = A\epsilon + (B\epsilon - A\epsilon B_p) (P/RT), \qquad (11)$$

où B_p est le second coefficient du viriel de la pression et provient de

$$P/RT = d + B_p d^2 + \ldots \qquad (12)$$

Une mise en graphique du terme de gauche dans l'expression (11) en fonction de P/RT permet de déterminer $A\epsilon$ à partir de l'intercepte (voir Fig. 3).

Le protocole expérimental de la méthode diélectrique est semblable à celui de la méthode volumétrique sauf le fait qu'on mesure directement la densité du gaz (plutôt que la pression) dans la cellule A qui forme maintenant le condensateur. Alors que la méthode volumétrique appliquée sur les gaz réels se base sur l'équation (6)

$$N = P V / Z R T, \qquad (6')$$

la méthode diélectrique se base sur l'équation suivante:

$$n = (L_E/A_E) \, V. \qquad (13)$$

On remarque immédiatement que la quantité de gaz recherchée ne comprend que de facteurs que l'on mesure directement alors que dans la méthode volumétrique nous sommes dépendents des valeurs tabulées du facteur Z en fonction de la pression et de la température.

Résultats et discussions

La Figure 4 montre l'isotherme d'adsorption du charbon actif BPL mesurée avec la méthode diélectrique et celles obtenues avec la méthode volumétrique avec corrections ($Z \neq 1$) et sans corrections ($Z=1$) pour la non idéalité du gaz. On remarque qu'à basse pression où la phase gazeuse se comporte presque comme un gaz idéal, les résultats sont sensiblement les mêmes. Cependant, à plus haute pression où la phase gazeuse dévie de l'idéalité, les résultats de la méthode volumétrique deviennent de plus en plus erronés si on ne tient pas compte du facteur de compressibilité.

Avant d'aller plus loin, nous tenons à commenter l'allure de l'isotherme d'adsoption qui comme le montre la Figure 4 présente un maximum à environ 7 MPa. Ce comportement tout à fait normal à haute pression résulte de la définition de l'adsorption, selon laquelle la quantité adsorbée sur la surface et dans les pores de l'adsorbant est l'excès relatif à la quantité de gaz qui remplirait normalement et simultanément ces pores aux mêmes conditions de pression et de température et sans adsorption. L'adsorption absolue croît toujours avec l'augmentation de la pression, mais la quantité en excès ou l'adsorption différentielle atteint un maximum. En augmentant davantage la pression, la densité de la phase gazeuse approche graduellement celle de la phase adsorbée. Cette approche est reflétée par la décroissance de l'isotherme d'adsorption. En principe, cette décroissance peut continuer jusqu'au moment où les deux densités deviennent égales. En ce point l'adsorption mesurée expérimentalement devient nulle.

On pourrait, en principe, calculer l'adsorption absolue à partir des mesures expérimentales si nous pouvions attribuer un volume quelconque à la phase adsorbée plutôt que de le considérer comme étant nul. Par exemple, si l'on tient compte du volume de la phase adsorbée en supposant que sa densité est la même que celle du gaz liquéfié, on obtient une isotherme sans cesse croissante jusqu'à une valeur maximale de saturation. Mais étant donné la complexité du problème, ces calculs sont plus approximatifs que rigoureux et les résultats sont souvent controversés.

La Figure 5 montre les isothermes d'adsorption de deux charbons actifs disponibles commercialement et hautement microporeux. Le produit Super-A, en poudre (AX-21) ou en grains (AX-31), est la version commerciale du produit de développement Amoco GX-32 qui possède la plus grande capacité d'adsorption spécifique (par unité de masse) de tout les charbons connus à ce jour. Ce charbon est produit par la reaction du coke avec l'hydroxide de potassium. Le produit CNS-201 fourni par A.C. Carbone Canada Inc., est un charbon à base de coquilles de noix de coco activé à la vapeur d'eau. Bien que ces deux charbons possèdent sensiblement la même surface spécifique (environ 3000 m²/g), la nature chimique de cette surface et les dimensions des pores formant cette surface font, en principe, du Super-A un meilleur candidat pour le stockage du gaz naturel. Cependant quand on tient compte de leur densité en vrac, celle du CNS étant deux fois supérieure, nous remarquons que leurs capacités de stockage volumique à l'alentour des pressions d'intérêt (< 3.5 MPa) deviennent sensiblement égales (voir Fig. 6).

Les Figures 5 et 6 montrent clairement que la capacité d'adsorption par unité de masse n'est qu'un seul des importants paramètres contribuant à la performance du système de stockage. En effet, même si une grande capacité massique est désirable afin de minimiser le poids du système, il est aussi important que l'adsorbant ait une densité apparente élevée afin de minimiser le volume du système de stockage.

Les Figures 7 et 8 montrent les effets de la température sur les isothermes d'adsorption du méthane sur le CNS-201. On constate que la capacité de stockage par adsorption augmente à mesure que la température diminue et que cette augmentation est plus forte dans le cas de l'adsorption que dans le cas de stockage par pure compression. Ainsi, pour une pression de stockage de 3.5 MPa et dans la plage des températures saisonnières allant de -30 C à +30 C, cette augmentation est de l'ordre de 50% comparée à 35% pour la pure compression. D'un autre côté, on constate que la montée initiale des isothermes se fait plus rapidement à basse température. Ceci pourrait constituer un désavantage pour l'adsorption dans les temps froids, car la quantité de carburant non livrable devient importante par rapport à la quantité totale emmagasinée.

Les résultats présentés ci-haut, sont des résultats d'équilibre thermodynamique et, par conséquent, ne tiennent pas compte des effets transitoires des réactions exothermiques et endothermiques engendrées par le cycle adsorption/désorption. En effet, la chaleur d'adsorption du méthane sur les charbons actifs est d'environ 4 K cal/mole. Alors quand on charge l'adsorbant avec du GN, une quantité substantielle d'énergie est normalement générée. Si cette énergie n'est pas dissipée vers l'extérieur, la température de l'adsorbant augmente et favorise ainsi la désorption accompagnée d'un effet de refroidissement. Le phénomène inverse se produit lors de la désorption.

Les variations de température, produites lors d'un cycle adsorption/désorption plus ou moin rapide, ajoutées aux températures ambiantes peuvent amener l'adsorbant à opérer dans une plage de température beaucoup plus étendue que celle des températures saisonnières. La courbe de la Figure 9 donne un exemple de la variation de la capacité de stockage d'un adsorbant opérant à 3.5 MPa et dans une grande plage de température.

REMERCIEMENTS

Ce travail à été supporté par le conseil de recherches en sciences naturelles et en génie (CRSNG) et par la société québécoise d'initiatives pétrolières (SOQUIP). Nous remercions Monsieur Réal Julien pour sa participation aux mesures expérimentales.

REFERENCES

1- R.J. Remick et A.J. Tiller, dans <u>Symposium papers on Nonpetroleum Vehicular Fuels V: CNG Fuel</u>, IGT, (1985).

2- S.S. Barton, J.A. Holland et D.F. Quinn, <u>Rapport No AF-85-01</u>, Publié par Ontario Ministry of Transportation and Communication, Mai (1984).

3- R.J. Remick, R.H. Elkins, E.H. Camara et T. Bulicz, U.S. Department of Energy and NASA Report 0327-1, Juin (1984).

4- S.J. Gregg et K.S.W. Sing, <u>Adsorption, Surface Area and Porosity</u>, 2ième édition, (Academic Press, New York 1982).

5- T.K. Bose, J.M. St-Arnaud, H.J. Achterman et R. Scharf, Rev. Sci. Instrum., <u>57</u>, 26 (1986).

6- T.K. Bose, R. Chahine, L. Marchildon et J.M. St-Arnaud, Rev. Sci. Instrum., <u>58</u>, 2217 (1987).

LISTE DES FIGURES

Figure 1   Méthode volumétrique automatique.

Figure 2   Méthode diélectrique.

Figure 3   La courbe des moindres carrés donne l'intercepte $A\epsilon$ et la pente ($B\epsilon - A\epsilon B_p$).

Figure 4   Isothermes d'adsorption obtenues par la méthode diélectrique et la méthode volumétrique.

Figure 5   Capacité d'adsorption massique de divers charbons actifs.

Figure 6   Capacité d'adsorption volumique de divers charbons actifs.

Figure 7   Adsorption du méthane sur le charbon actif CNS-201 en fonction de la pression et de la température.

Figure 8   Adsorption du méthane sur le charbon actif CNS-201 en fonction de la pression et de la température.

Figure 9   Variation de la capacité d'adsorption du CNS-201 en fonction de la température et à 3.5 MPa.

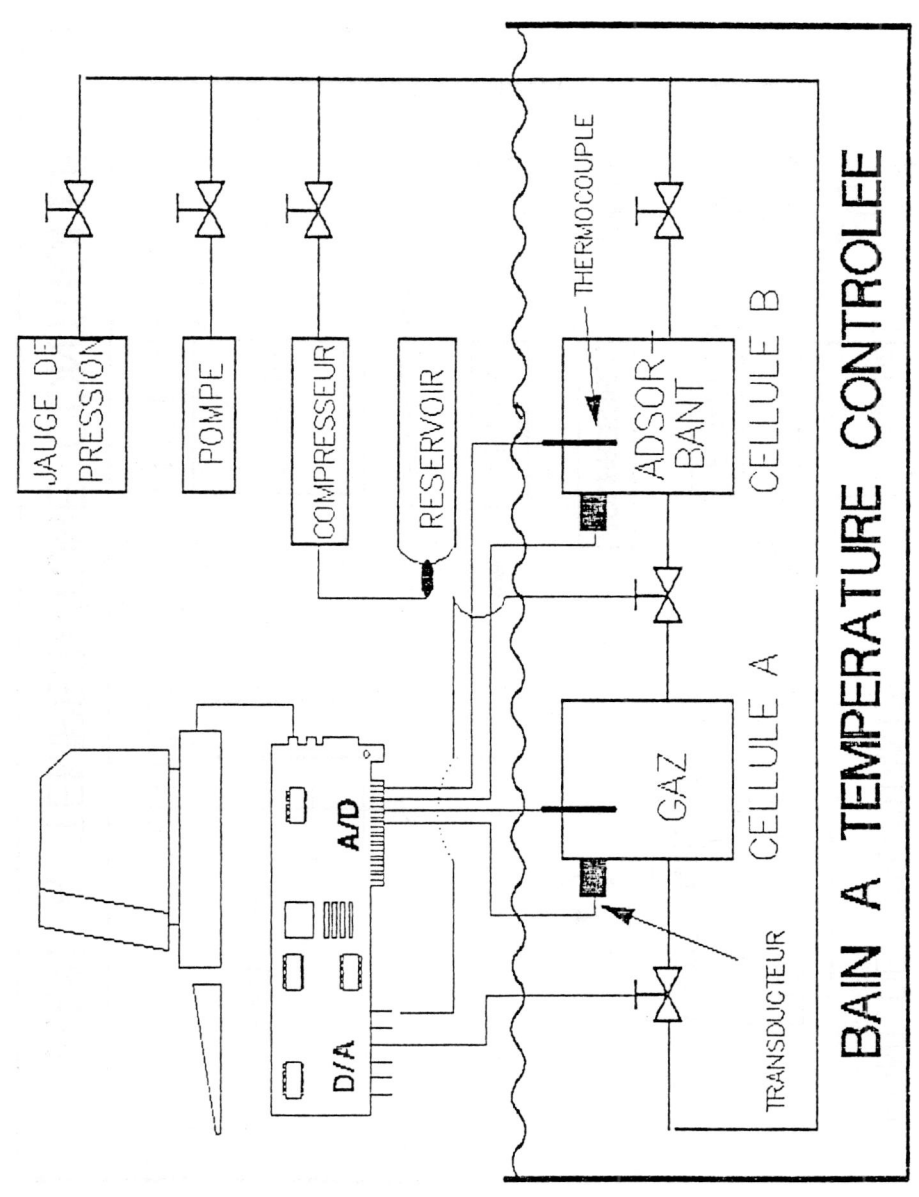

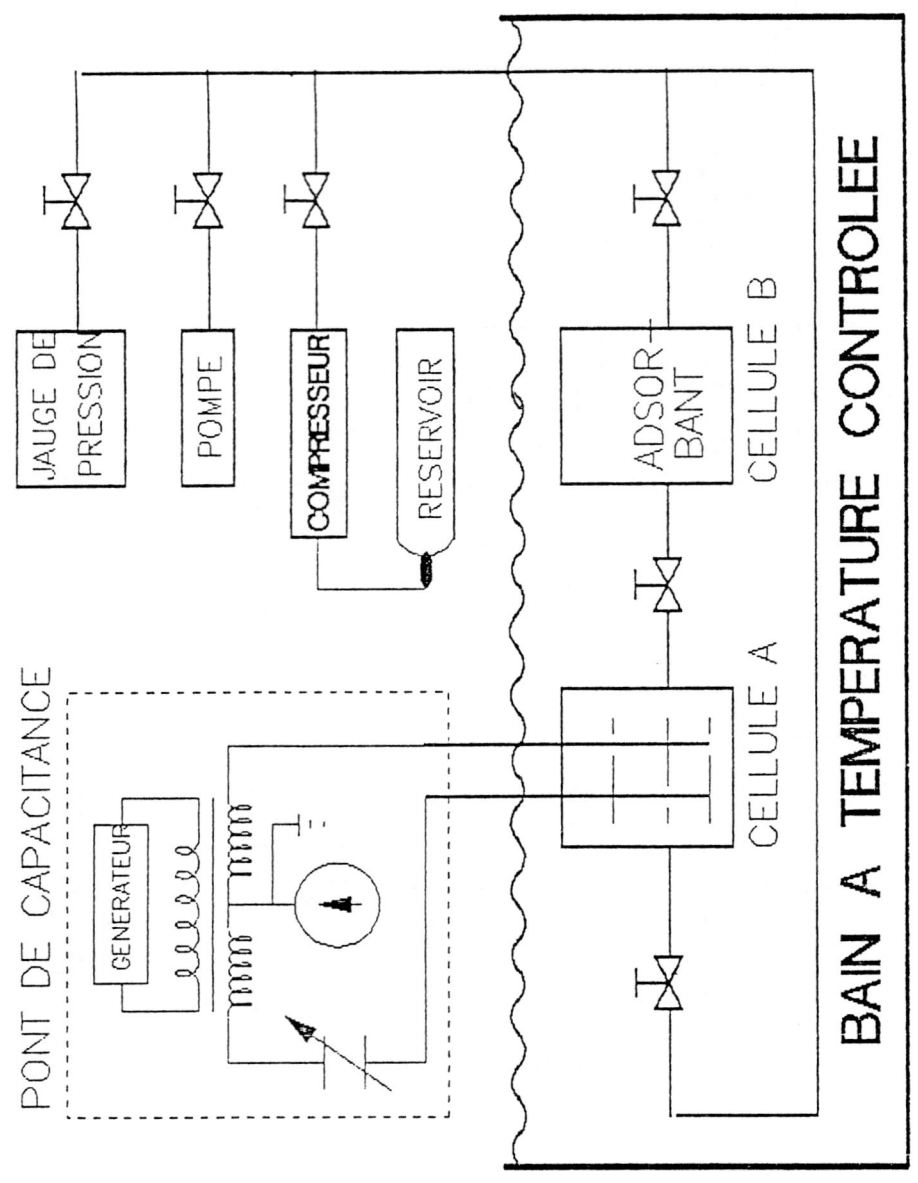

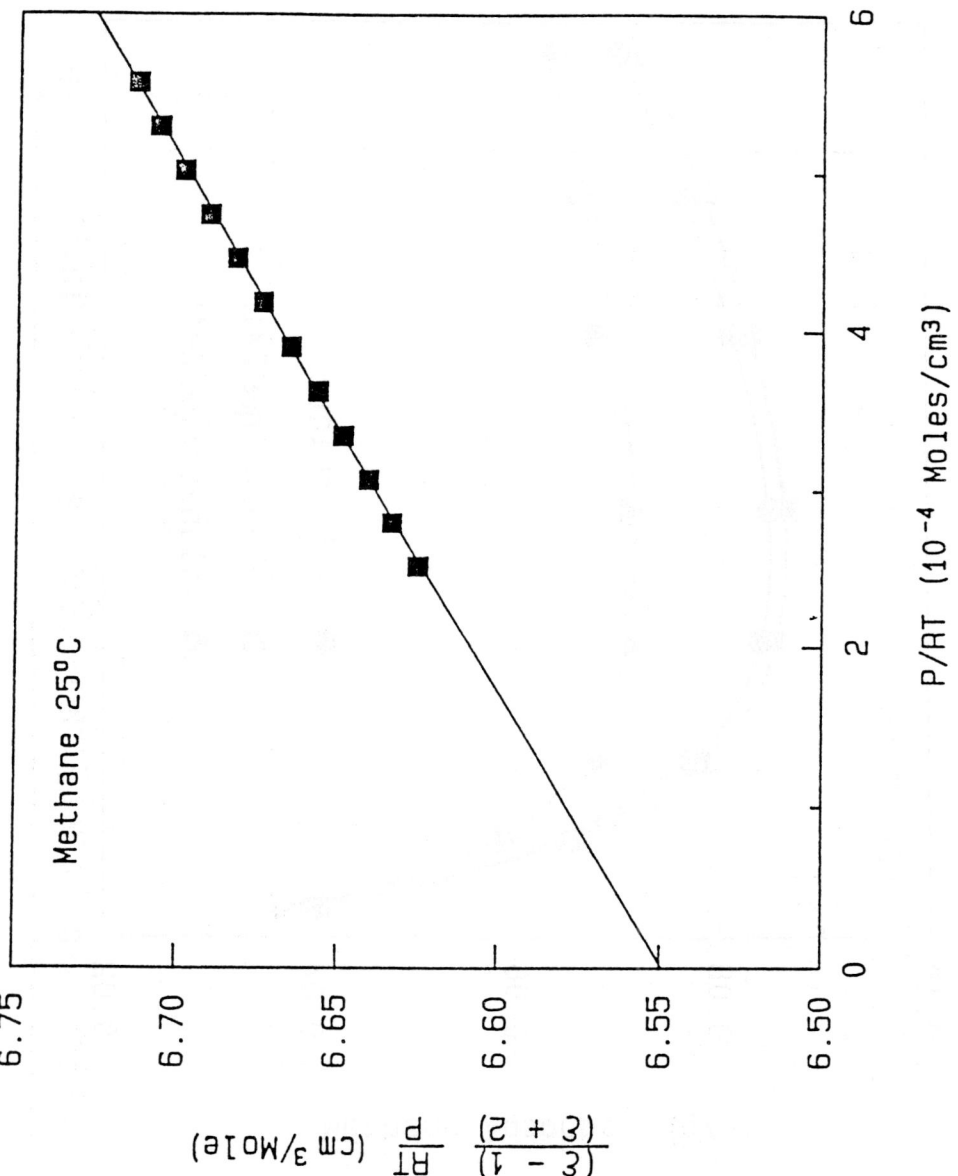

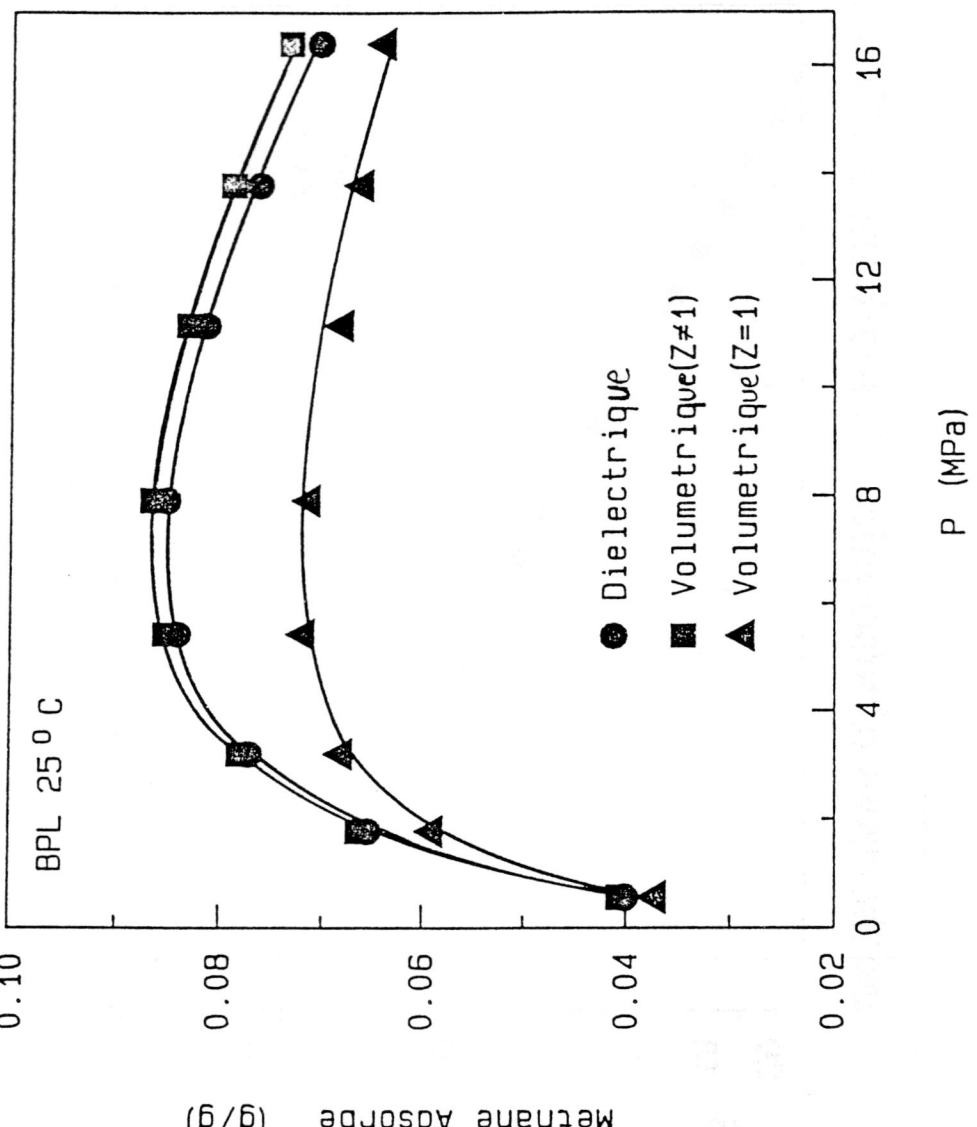

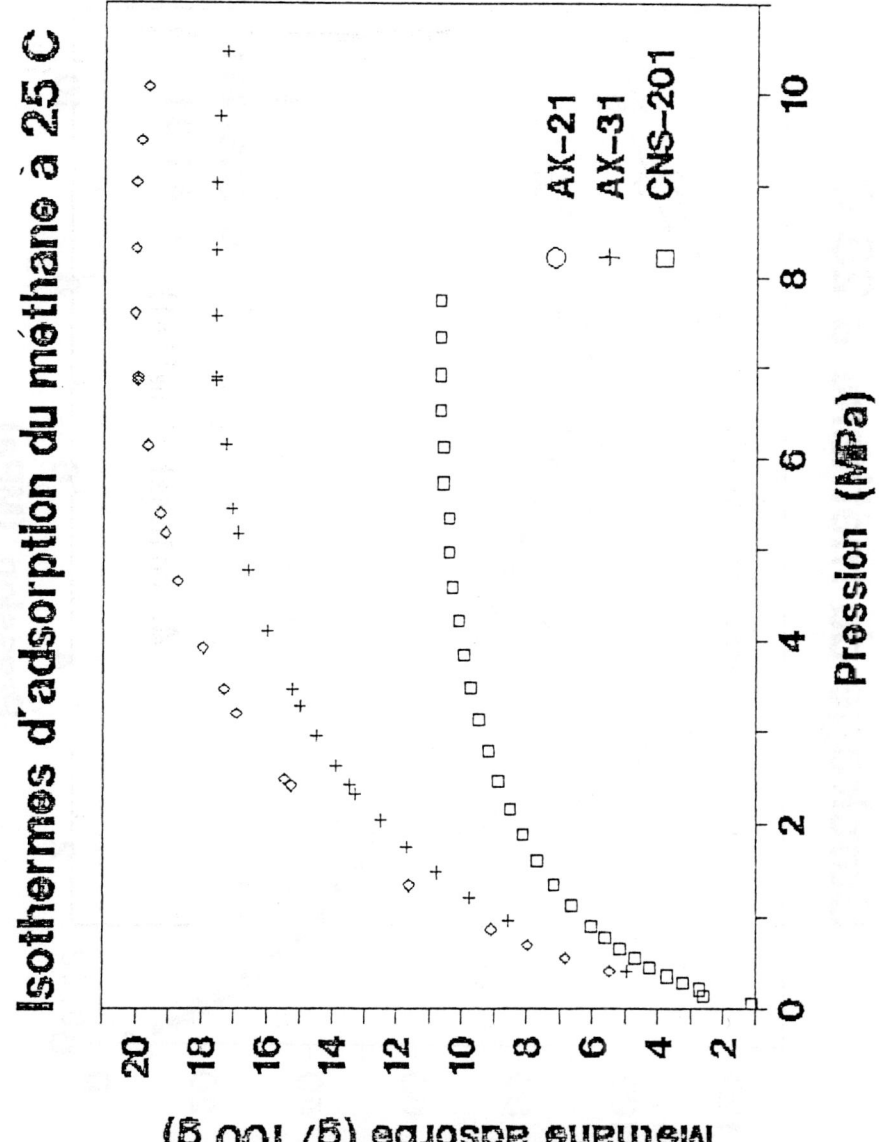

Stockage du méthane à 25 C

- ○ AX-21
- ■ CNS-201
- + AX-31

Méthane stocké (g/l) vs Pression (MPa)

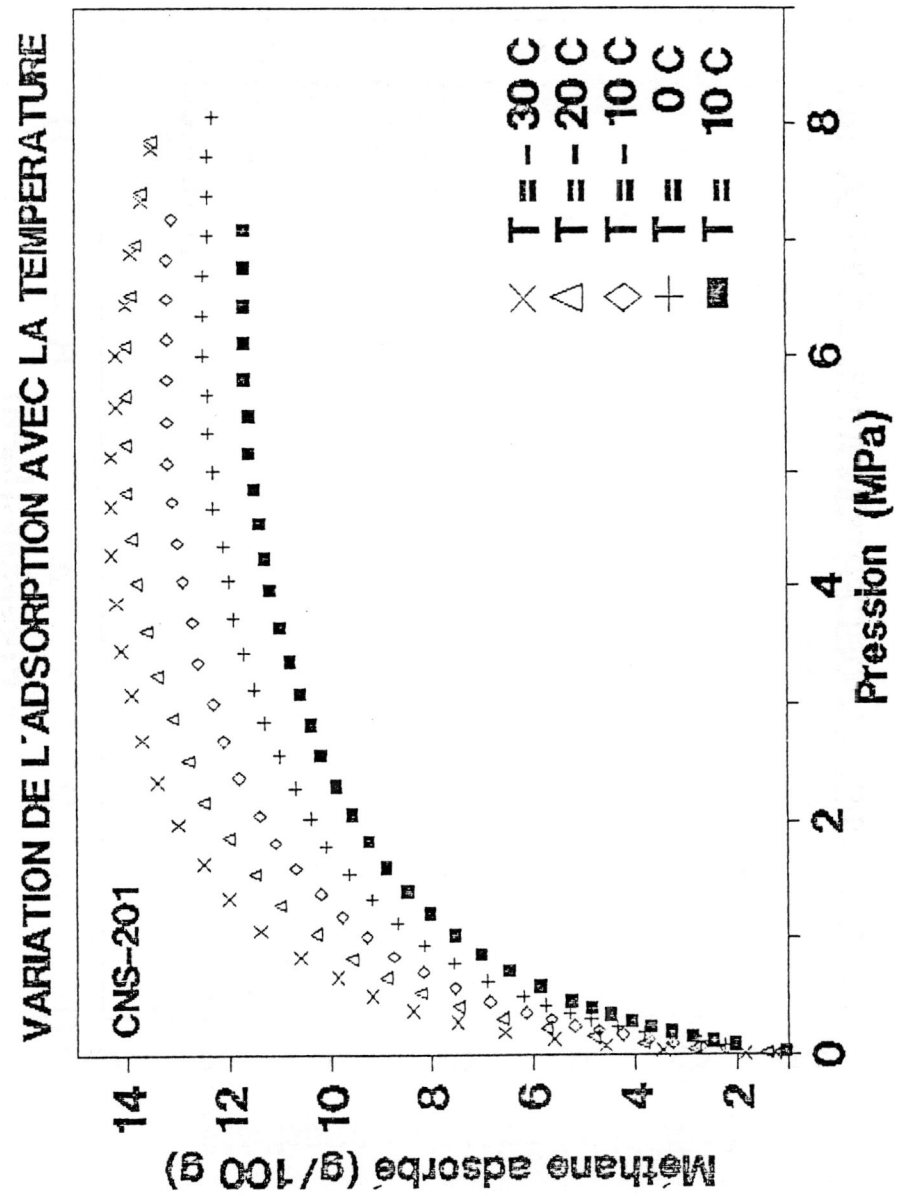

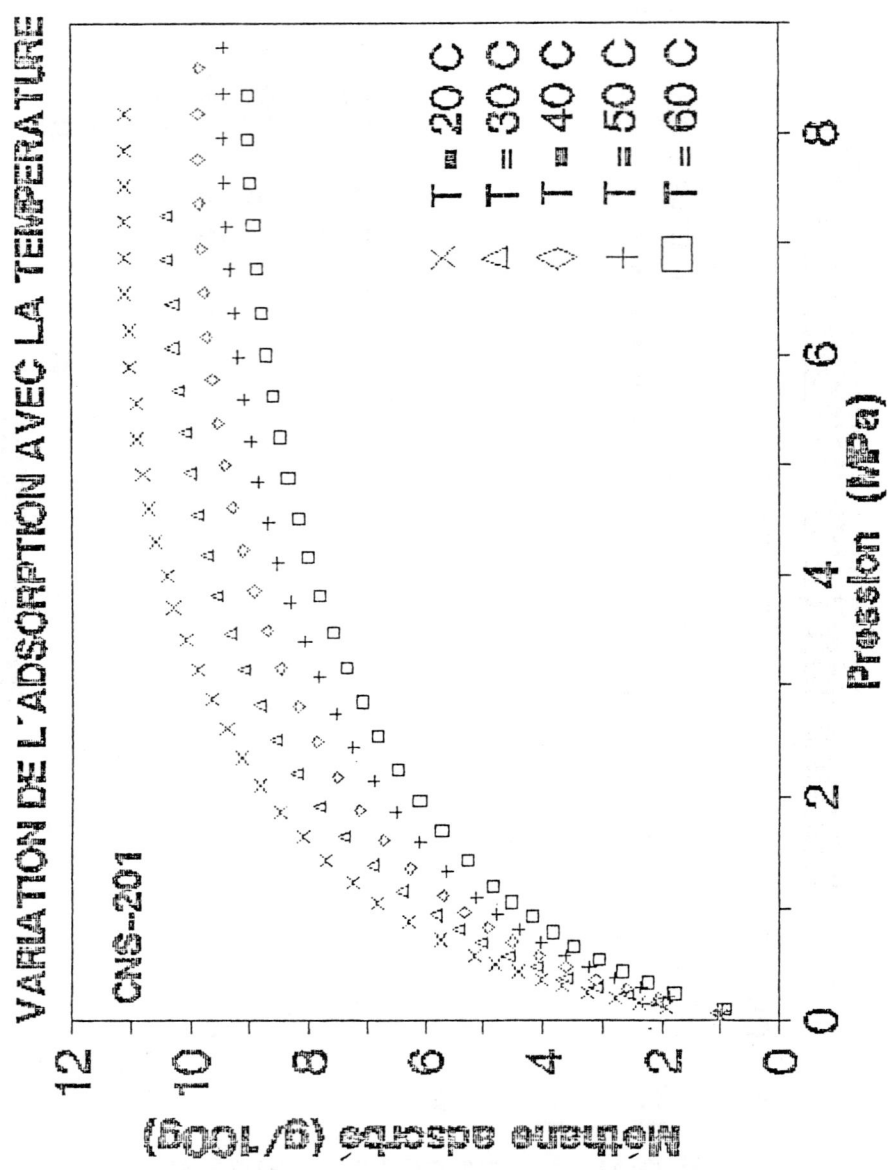

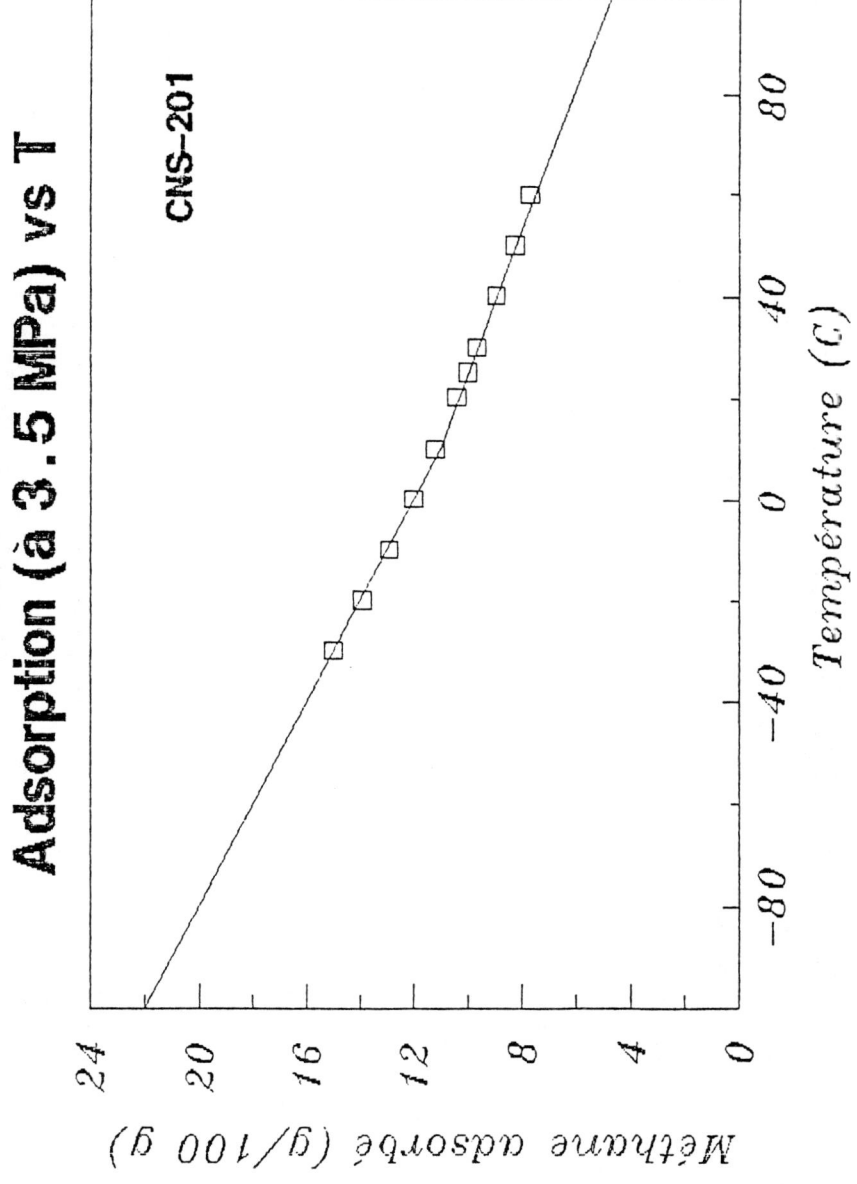

A SIMPLIFIED VIRIAL EQUATION APPLIED TO NATURAL GAS MIXTURES

D.R. McGregor, J.C. Holste, and K.R. Hall

Department of Chemical Engineering
Texas A&M University, College Station, Texas 77843 USA

INTRODUCTION

In a recent publication, McGregor *et al.* (1986) propose a relation between the cross third virial coefficients of a binary mixture and use the result to derive a simplified form of the virial equation of state applicable to multi-component mixtures. This equation (MHEMHS equation) is applicable for mixtures that require at most the third virial coefficient to predict accurately the compressibility factor (real gas factor). The ability of the MHEMHS equation to predict compressibility factors was shown to rival that of the virial equation, at least at moderate densities. However, a rigorous evaluation of the error associated with using the MHEMHS equation has not been performed, partially because accurate experimental measurements of the virial coefficients of either a pure compound or a mixture have been limited to the second virial coefficient (either pure or cross virials). Recently, extremely precise compressibility data for several mixtures of light components of natural gas have yielded reasonably accurate values of the cross third virial coefficients. With these data, a more rigorous evaluation of the MHEMHS equation can be performed.

DEVELOPMENT

The virial equation of state accurately predicts the compressibility factor of a pure compound or a mixture provided that all relevant virial coefficients are known. For this development, we work with the density virial equation and consider the virial equation only through densities where the third virial coefficient is of importance. The virial equation for this case is

$$Z = 1 + B_m \rho + C_m \rho^2 \tag{1}$$

where

$$B_m = \sum_{i=1}^{n} \sum_{j=1}^{n} x_i x_j B_{ij} \tag{2}$$

$$C_m = \sum_{i=1}^{n} \sum_{j=1}^{n} \sum_{k=1}^{n} x_i x_j x_k C_{ijk} \ . \tag{3}$$

For a binary mixture, Eqs. 2 and 3 become

$$B_m = x_1^2 B_{11} + 2 x_1 x_2 B_{12} + x_2^2 B_{22} \tag{4}$$

$$C_m = x_1^3 C_{111} + 3 x_1^2 x_2 C_{112} + 3 x_1 x_2^2 C_{122} + x_2^3 C_{222}. \tag{5}$$

According to McGregor *et al.* (1986), the excess cross second and third virial coefficients are

$$B_{12}^e = B_{12} - \left(\frac{B_{11} + B_{22}}{2} \right) \tag{6}$$

$$C_{112}^e = C_{112} - \left(\frac{2 C_{111} + C_{222}}{3} \right) \tag{7}$$

$$C_{122}^e = C_{122} - \left(\frac{C_{111} + 2 C_{222}}{3} \right) \tag{8}$$

and

$$Z^e = Z(T, \rho, x_i) - \sum_{i=1}^{n} x_i Z_i(T, \rho) \ . \tag{9}$$

If a mixture is a model solution, then $Z^e = 0$ and

$$B_{12}^e = C_{112}^e = C_{122}^e = 0 \tag{10}$$

If a real mixture obeys Eq. 10 then model solution behavior applies, and Eqs. 6-8 yield the cross virial coefficients.

Model solution behavior for a real mixture is atypical; McGregor *et al.* (1987) have produced a new simplified form of the mixture third virial coefficient by assuming that non-model behavior of the cross third virial coefficients is related by

$$C_{112}^e = C_{122}^e. \tag{11}$$

Substituting Eq. 11 into Eq. 5 yields

$$C_m = x_1 C_{111} + x_2 C_{222} + x_1 x_2 \delta C_{12} \tag{12}$$

where $\delta C_{12} = 3C_{112}^e = 3C_{122}^e$. For multi-component mixtures, applying Eq. 12 to Eq. 1-3 yields a general expression for the compressibility factor

$$Z = 1 + \rho \left[\sum_{i=1}^{n} x_i B_{ii} + \sum_{i=1}^{n} \sum_{j=i+1}^{n} x_i x_j \delta B_{ij} \right] + \rho^2 \left[\sum_{i=1}^{n} x_i C_{iii} + \sum_{i=1}^{n} \sum_{j=i+1}^{n} x_i x_j \delta C_{ij} \right] \tag{13}$$

where $\delta C_{ij} = 3C_{iij}^e = 3C_{ijj}^e$ and $\delta B_{ij} = 2B_{ij}^e$. Equation 13 is the general form of the MHEMIIS equation. In this analysis, either Eq. 12 or Eq. 13 are referred to as the MHEMHS equation.

The goal of this work is to examine the prediction error associated with using the MHEMHS equation in place of the virial equation. Although the virial equation is rigorous, it requires two cross third virial coefficients to predict the compressibility factor of a binary mixture. Experimental determination of the cross third virial coefficients requires extensive, precise P-ρ-T measurements on at least three mixtures at a given temperature. By using the MHEMHS equation, the number of cross parameters required to describe a multi-component mixture is significantly reduced (Table 1). This effect becomes more pronounced as the number of components increases. For a binary mixture, the interaction parameter can be obtained from a single isotherm, greatly reducing time and expense of measurement. In addition, if the mixture obeys closely Eq. 11, then accurate values of the cross third virial coefficients can be derived from the MHEMHS third virial interaction parameter.

The relationship between δC_{12} and the excess cross third virial coefficients is

$$\delta C_{12} = 3x_1 C^e_{112} + 3x_2 C^e_{122}. \tag{14}$$

Note that for a single experimental isotherm, the MHEMHS equation can fit data with error similar to the virial equation because through Eq. 14, the two cross third virials combine into a single independent statistical variable. Because the mole fraction is bounded between 0 and 1, it is apparent from Eq. 14 that δC_{12} is bounded between $3C^e_{112}$ and $3C^e_{122}$. If $x_1 = 0.5$, then δC_{12} is simply the average of the two excess cross third virial coefficients. In applying the MHEMHS equation, x_1 should be chosen to minimize the difference between the MHEMHS and virial equations over the entire range of mole fractions

$$\Delta C_m = C_m^{Virial} - C_m^{MHEMHS}. \tag{15}$$

Substituting Eqs. 5 and 12 into Eq. 15 yields

$$\Delta C_m = x_1 x_2 \left[x_1(3C_{112} - 2C_{111} - C_{222}) + x_2(3C_{122} - C_{111} - 2C_{222}) - \delta C_{12} \right]$$

or

$$\Delta C_m = x_1 x_2 [3x_1 C^e_{112} + 3(1-x_1) C^e_{122} - \delta C_{12}]. \tag{16}$$

Eq. 16 provides the basis for evaluating deviations of the MHEMHS equation from the virial equation.

ANALYSIS

The deviation (ΔC_m) of the MHEMHS equation from the virial equation is examined for three cases (three choices of the mole fraction, x_1).

CASE I $x_1 \Rightarrow 1$

If the mole fraction of component 1 approaches 1, then Eq. 14 shows that $\delta C_{12} \Rightarrow 3C^e_{112}$. Assuming $\delta C_{12} = 3C^e_{112}$ and substituting into Eq. 16 yields

$$\Delta C_m = -3x_1(1-x_1)^2 [C^e_{112} - C^e_{122}] \tag{17}$$

or in dimensionless form

$$\frac{\Delta C_m}{[C^e_{112} - C^e_{122}]} = -3x_1(1-x_1)^2. \tag{18}$$

Equation 17 shows that if the difference between the excess cross third virial coefficients is small, then the deviation between the MHEMHS and virial equations is negligible. The maximum dimensionless deviation occurs when $x_1 = \frac{1}{3}$, and this deviation is $-\frac{4}{9}$.

CASE II $x_1 \Rightarrow 0$

If the mole fraction of component 1 approaches 0, then Eq. 14 shows that $\delta C_{12} \Rightarrow 3C^e_{122}$. Assuming $\delta C_{12} = 3C^e_{122}$ and substituting into Eq. 16 yields

$$\Delta C_m = -3x_1^2(1-x_1)[C^e_{112} - C^e_{122}] \tag{19}$$

or in dimensionless form

$$\frac{\Delta C_m}{[C^e_{112} - C^e_{122}]} = 3x_1^2(1 - x_1). \tag{20}$$

The maximum dimensionless deviation occurs when $x_1 = \frac{2}{3}$, and this deviation is $\frac{4}{9}$. Case II is simply the reciprocal of Case I.

CASE III $x_1 = 0.5$

If the mixture is equimolar, then Eq. 14 becomes

$$\delta C_{12} = \frac{1}{2}(3C^e_{112} + 3C^e_{122}) \tag{21}$$

Substituting Eq. 21 into Eq. 16 yields

$$\Delta C_m = -3x_1(1 - x_1)(0.5 - x_1)[C^e_{112} - C^e_{122}] \tag{22}$$

or

$$\frac{\Delta C_m}{[C^e_{112} - C^e_{122}]} = 3x_1(1 - x_1)(0.5 - x_1). \tag{23}$$

The maximum deviation occurs when $x_1 = \frac{1}{2} \pm \frac{\sqrt{3}}{6}$, and this deviation is ± 0.14434.

Plotting the dimensionless deviation of the MHEMHS from the virial equation for each of the three cases shows that over the entire range of mole fractions, the least deviations occur if the interaction parameter for the MHEMHS equation is determined at an equimolar composition (Figure 1), and at the equimolar composition the deviation is identically zero. As the mixture becomes less equimolar, the average deviation increases to a maximum. Also, if the MHEMHS equation is applied to an isothermal set of compressibility factor data at a given mixture composition, then the deviation will be zero at that composition, and greater than zero away from that composition. Finally, note that the dimensionless deviation depends only upon mole fraction and choice of δC_{12}, while the absolute deviation depends upon the validity of Eq. 11.

Next, we consider the application of the MHEMHS equation to prediction of the mixture third virial coefficient and of the compressibility factor using experimentally determined second and third virial coefficients for three binary mixtures of four light components of natural gas (T=300 K). For these mixtures, extremely precise compressibility factor data were measured by the Thermodynamics Group at Texas A&M University. The mixtures are: $CO_2 - N_2$, $CO_2 - CH_4$, and $CO_2 - C_2H_6$. From the mixture data, cross second and third virial coefficients were statistically determined.

The deviation of the mixture third virial coefficient calculated from the MHEMHS equation as opposed to the virial equation depends upon the accuracy of Eq. 11. Throughout these calculations, we use the δC_{12} that is the average of the two cross third virial coefficients (Eq. 21) because this gives the minimum average deviation from the virial equation (as seen in Figure 1). The deviation depends upon the difference between $3C^c_{112}$ and $3C^c_{122}$, not upon the non-model behavior of the mixture, as shown by Eqs. 18, 20, and 23. Figure 2 shows that for the mixtures considered, the CO_2-CH_4 system deviates the least from the virial equation. This system most closely obeys the MHEMHS assumption.

The propagation of the deviation in the mixture third virial coefficient to the prediction of the compressibility factor depends upon the relative influence of the mixture third virial coefficient. This influence depends only upon the reduced density of the mixture. Figure 3 shows this effect, and shows the relative deviations from using the MHEMHS equation versus the virial equation. For Figure 3, a mole fraction of 0.788 is used because it gives the maximum deviation in the third virial coefficient when the average δC_{12} is used in the MHEMHS equation. At any other mole fraction, the deviation in the compressibility factor must be less.

CONCLUSIONS

The deviation of the MHEMHS equation from the virial equation depends upon the composition at which δC_{12} is determined, the composition of the mixture under consideration, and the difference between the excess cross third virial coefficients. If the difference in the excess cross third virials is zero, then the MHEMHS and virial equations predict the same fluid behavior.

For the mixtures of light gases considered, the $CO_2 - CH_4$ mixture best obeys the underlying assumption of the MHEMHS equation, and thus best predicts the mixture third virial coefficient. The propagation of deviation in the mixture third virial coefficient to the compressibility factor depends upon the density of the mixture. For the systems considered, the compressibility factor is predicted using the MHEMHS equation with a maximum deviation of $\sim 0.5\%$ up to 1/2 of the critical density. At compositions away from the one that provides the maximum deviation, the deviations in the compressibility factor are less.

The MHEMHS equation predicts well the fluid behavior of binary mixtures of light components of natural gas. For multi-component mixtures such as natural gas, the MHEMHS equation predicts fluid behavior nearly as well as the virial equation, but with many fewer interaction parameters.

REFERENCES

McGregor, D.R., J.C. Holste, P.T. Eubank, K.N. Marsh, and K.R. Hall, "Simple Solution Models Applied to Virial Coefficients," AIChE J., 32, 1221 (1986).

McGregor, D.R., J.C. Holste, P.T. Eubank, K.N. Marsh, K.R. Hall, and J.Schouten, "An Interaction Model for Third Virial Coefficients which Provides Simplified Equations for Mixtures," Fluid Phase Equilibria, 35, 153 (1987).

Table 1. Number of Interaction Terms in Mixture Third Virial

Number of Components	Virial Equation	MHEMHS Equation	Interaction Terms Eliminated
1	0	0	0
2	2	1	1
3	7	3	4
4	16	6	10
5	30	10	20
⋮	⋮	⋮	⋮
10	210	45	165
⋮	⋮	⋮	⋮
n	$\frac{n(n-1)(n+4)}{6}$	$\frac{n(n-1)}{2}$	$\frac{n(n^2-1)}{6}$

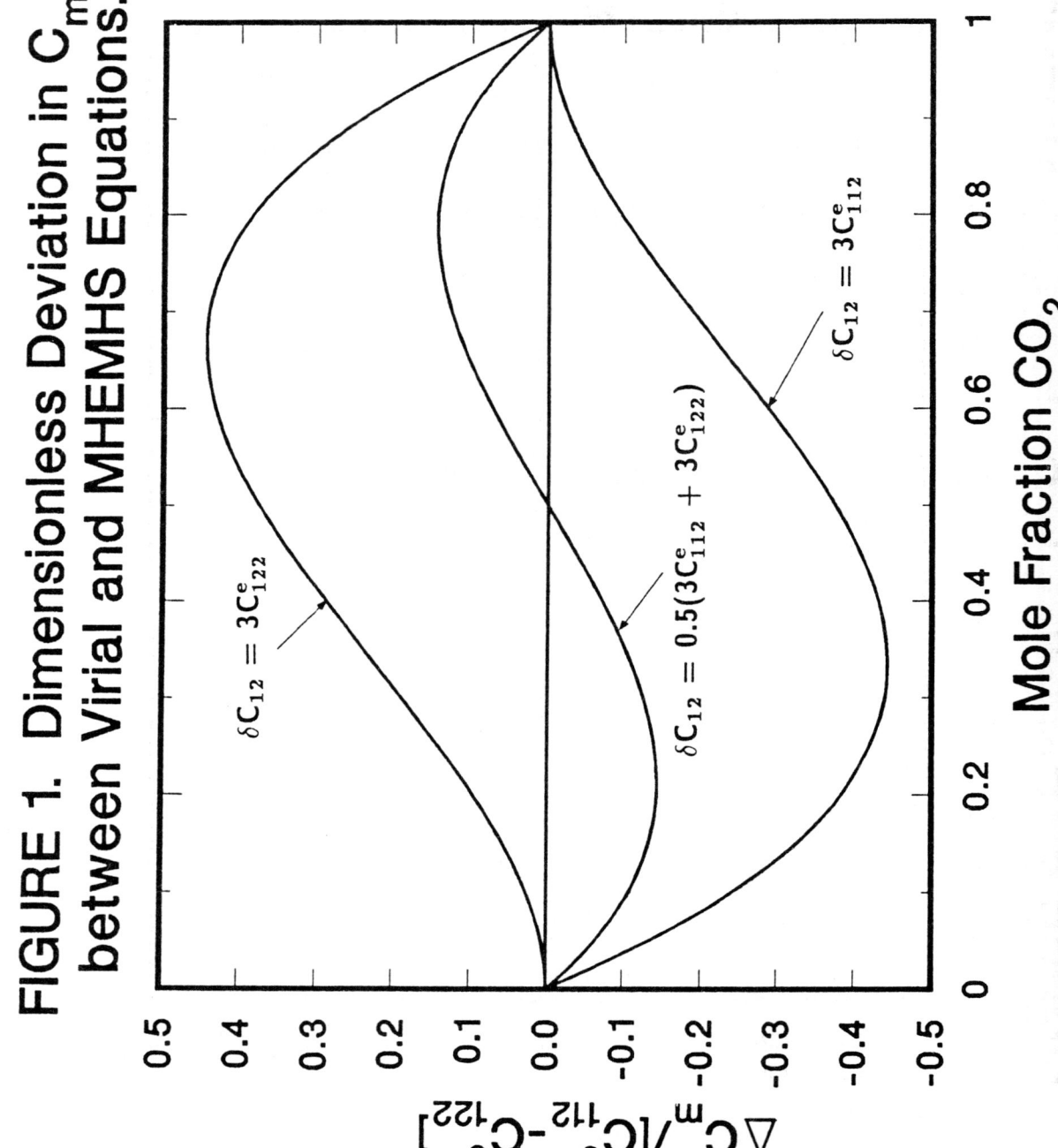

FIGURE 1. Dimensionless Deviation in C_m between Virial and MHEMHS Equations.

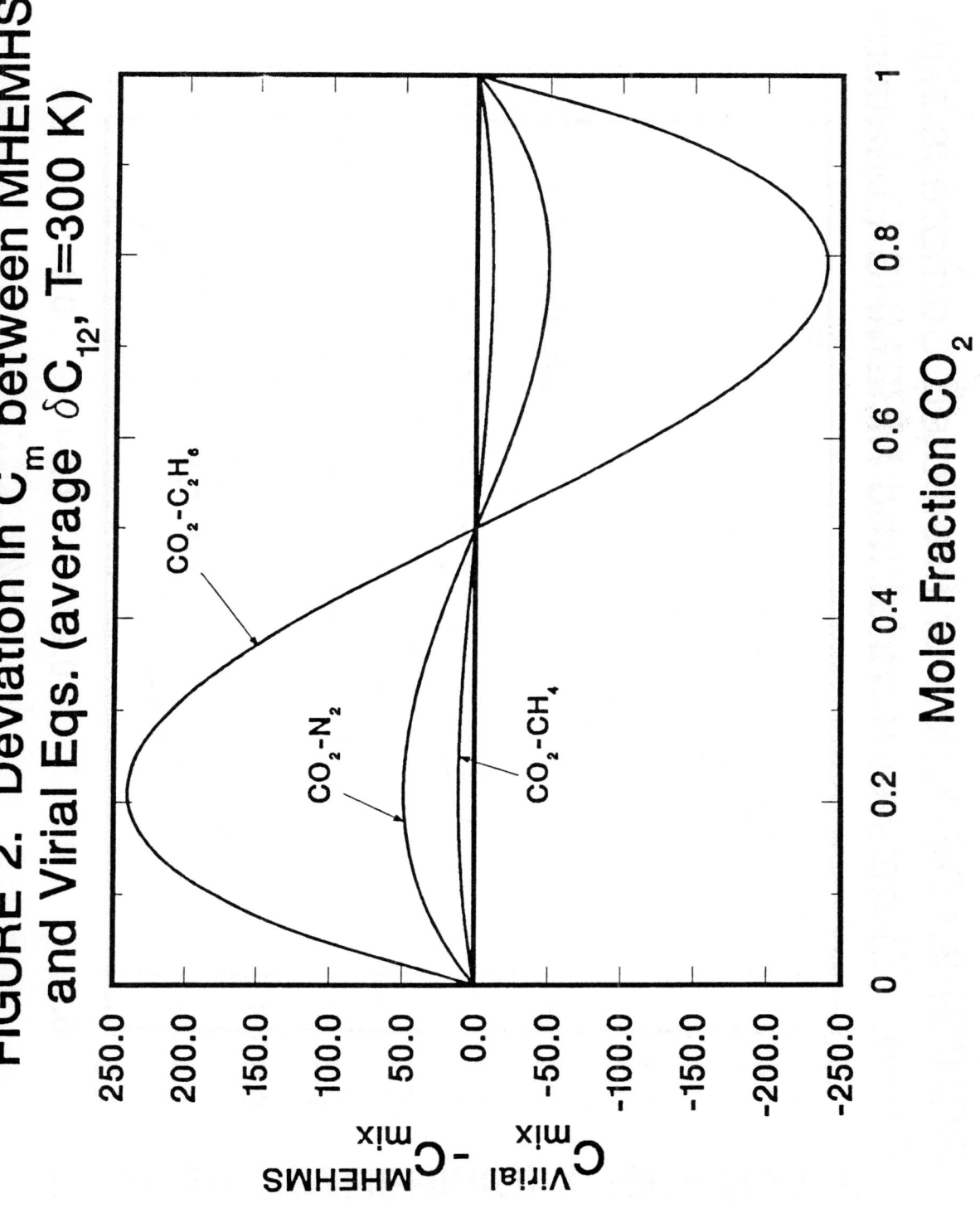

FIGURE 2. Deviation in C_m between MHEMHS and Virial Eqs. (average δC_{12}, T=300 K)

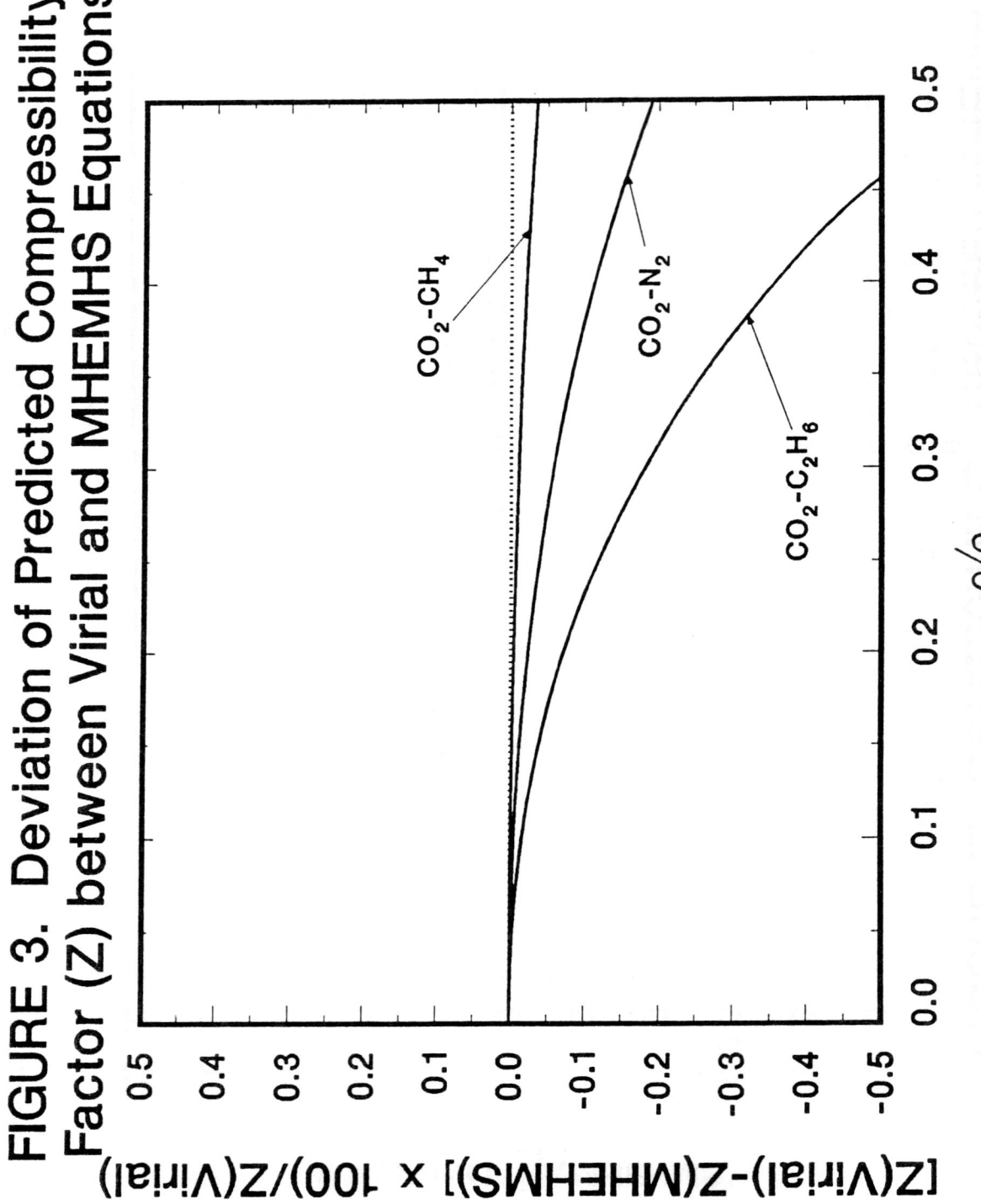

FIGURE 3. Deviation of Predicted Compressibility Factor (Z) between Virial and MHEMHS Equations.

PVT MEASUREMENTS OF CARBON DIOXIDE – METHANE MIXTURES

by

Chih-An Hwang, James C. Holste
Kenneth R. Hall, Kenneth N. Marsh

Chemical Engineering Department
and Thermodynamics Research Center
Texas A&M University
College Station, Texas 77843, USA

ABSTRACT

Accurate data on the thermophysical properties of fluid mixtures are required by the gas industry. Mixtures containing significant quantities of carbon dioxide are encountered in natural gas and petroleum reservoirs. The separation of various concentrations of carbon dioxide from light hydrocarbons becomes important because the presence of carbon dioxide will lead to lower energy content and to inefficiencies in combustion. Also, carbon dioxide has been widely used as an injecting fluid in the tertiary oil recovery for the petroleum industry. Data on carbon dioxide and hydrocarbon systems are applicable to prediction of well fluid behavior. Four different compositions of carbon dioxide – methane (CO_2–CH_4) mixtures were prepared. The continuously weighed pycnometer was used to measure the densities of CO_2–CH_4 mixtures between 225 and 350 K up to 35 MPa. Densities and cross second and third virial coefficients of CO_2–CH_4 mixtures at 300 and 320 K up to 10 MPa were obtained by using the Burnett apparatus.

INTRODUCTION

Accurate data on the thermophysical properties of fluid mixtures are important to the gas industry for efficient operation of existing plants, design of new plants, custody transfer of gaseous fuels, and efficient and profitable exploitation of natural gas and petroleum reservoirs. The gas industry faces severe problems in the near future because of the lack of data on the properties of fluid mixtures. From the standpoint of gas processing and separation operations, the most important properties are vapor-liquid equilibrium (VLE), enthalpy and density (PVT) data.

The increasing demand for natural gas has led to utilizing sources previously considered to be uneconomical because of carbon dioxide contamination. Because methane is the major component in natural gas, the separation of carbon dioxide from methane becomes an important problem to be solved. In addition, the cost of extracting crude oil from the earth has steadily increased over the past decade. This is largely because of the depletion of shallow well reserves. Instead of drilling high cost, new, deep wells, the petroleum industry tries to inject fluids such as carbon dioxide into existing wells for enhanced oil recovery to reduce the cost. Data on carbon dioxide and methane acts as a simple model for more complex well fluid behavior in the tertiary oil recovery.

Many different experimental techniques for determining the PVT behavior of fluid mixtures have been developed and improved in the past decade as reviewed by Holste *et al.* (1986). Among them, Burnett expansions provide the best measurements of densities less than half the critical density. This method also provides by far the best determinations of the virial coefficients. At higher densities, the continuously weighed pycnometer provides measurements more rapidly and with equivalent accuracy to the Burnett apparatus. These two experimental techniques are used to measure the PVT data.

APPARATUS

The pycnometer apparatus used for the density measurements is described fully by Lau (1986). The overall schematic of this apparatus and the cross section of the isothermal bath and of the balance chamber appear in Figures 1 and 2, respectively. The sample cell is filled and evacuated through a straight stainless-steel capillary that remains attached to the sample cell along an axis at a right angle to the axis of the wire leading to the balance. The entire balance and the sample cell are totally immersed in helium at a controlled pressure to eliminate changes in buoyancy. Helium is chosen for its high thermal conductivity and low density. The sample densities are determined from the measured masses and the known volume of the sample cell.

The 500 g capacity, electronic balance provides masses with a precision of 0.1 mg. Pressures are measured with a Rosemount (model 1333G10) strain gauge pressure transducer operated at room temperature or a Paroscientific (model 700) digiquartz pressure transducer located inside the isothermal bath. Both transducers have been calibrated against a DH Instruments (type 26000) automatic pressure standard (dead-weight gauge, DWG). Temperatures are measured with a four-lead platinum resistance thermometer (PRT, MINCO model S1059PA5X10) which is adjacent to the sample cell on the inside surface of the copper compartment used for controlling the sample cell temperature.

Figure 3 shows the schematic of the Burnett apparatus. This apparatus consists of essentially two thermostated cells, V_A and V_B, with unspecified volumes. Cell V_A is filled with sample fluid to a predetermined pressure — the highest pressure for the experiment. The pressure is measured after equilibrium is reached. The fluid then expands into a previously evacuated cell V_B. The pressure is again measured after equilibrium is reached. The sequence of evacuation of V_B, expansion into

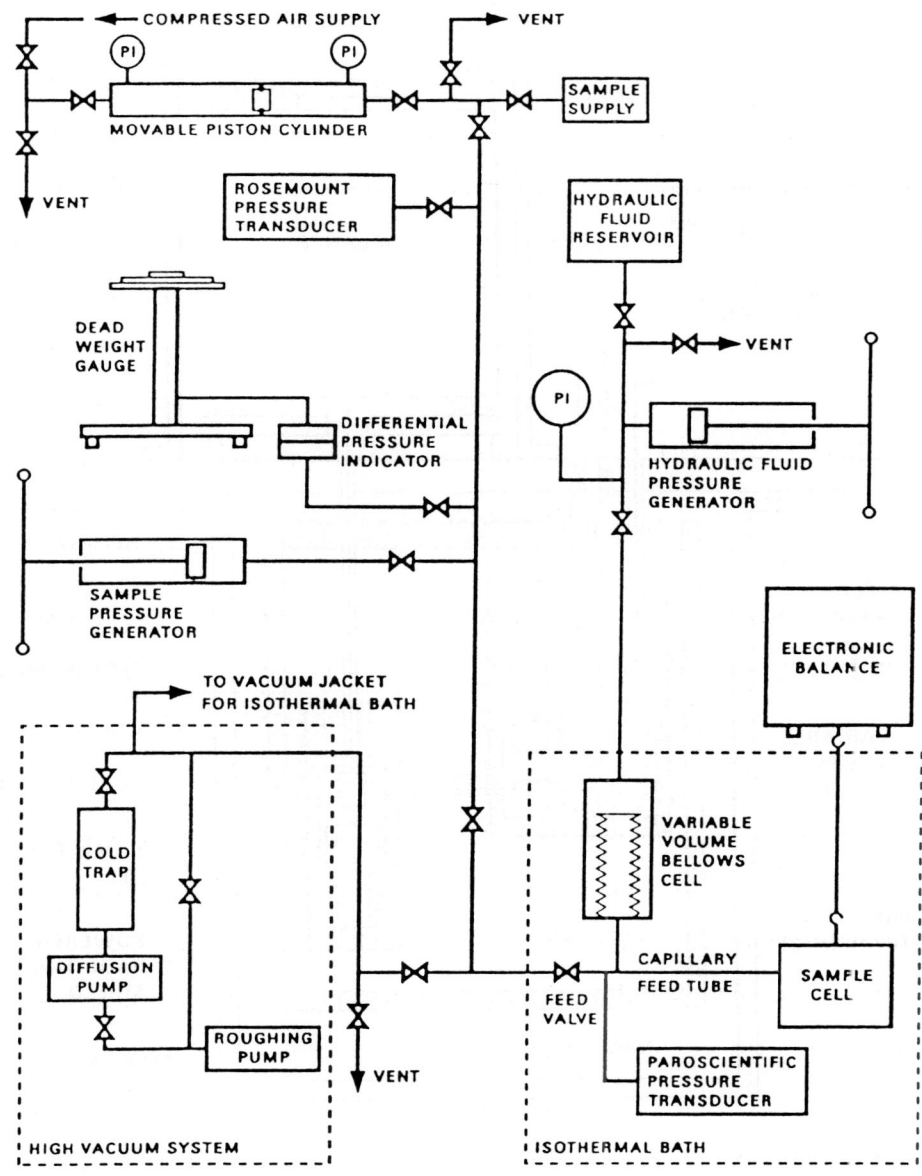

Figure 1. Overall schematic of pycnometer apparatus.

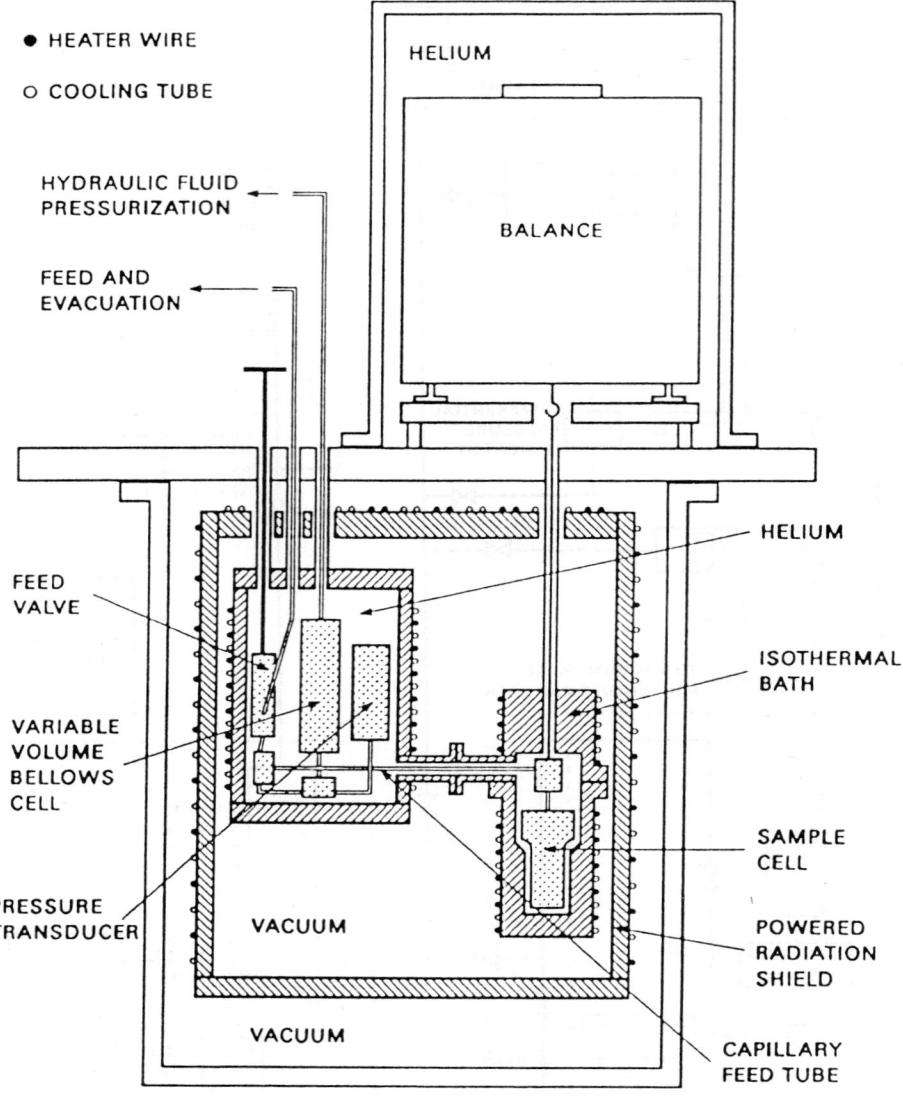

Figure 2. Cross section of isothermal bath and balance chamber.

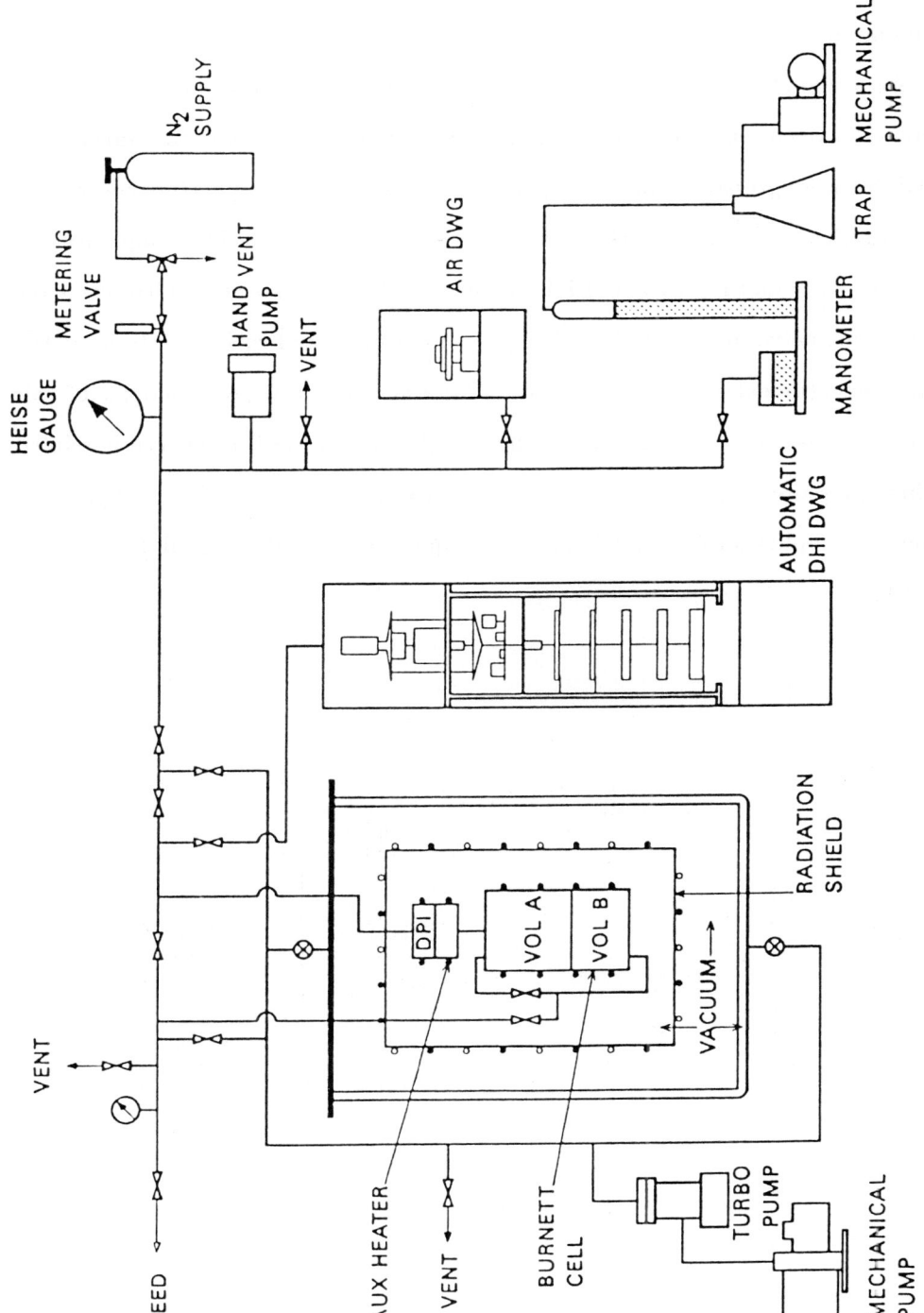

Figure 3. Overall schematic of Burnett apparatus.

V_B, and pressure measurement after equilibrium is continued till a predetermined minimum pressure has been reached.

An automatic digital temperature control system is used to control the temperatures of both the radiation shield and the auxiliary heaters around the Burnett cell and differential pressure transducer (DPT). This automatic temperature control can maintain the temperature within 3mK of the set temperature. The temperature is measured with another MINCO PRT (model S1059-2) which is embedded inside the Burnett cell between V_A and V_B. The pressure is measured with an automatic DH Instruments (model 50200) DWG above 4 MPa and with a Ruska (model 2465) air DWG below 4 MPa. The pressure of the sample fluid in the Burnett cell is related to these pressure gauges and compared to an external pressure medium supply (N_2) through a diaphragm-type DPT. This technique is described in detail by Holste *et al.* (1977).

RESULTS

Four different compositions of carbon dioxide + methane (CO_2–CH_4) mixtures were prepared using a gravimetric method. The continuously weighed pycnometer was used to measure the densities of CO_2–CH_4 mixtures between 225 and 350 K up to 35 MPa. Data analysis for the pycnometer apparatus is straightforward. Carbon dioxide and ethane were used previously to determine the sample cell volume as a function of temperature and pressure. The sample density is determined by dividing the measured mass of sample in the cell by the known cell volume. The absolute accuracy of the density measurements using the pycnometer apparatus is estimated to be 0.1 kg·m^{-3} or 0.1 %, whichever is the greater. Densities and cross second and third virial coefficients of CO_2–CH_4 mixtures at 300 and 320 K up to 10 MPa were obtained by using the Burnett apparatus. A Burnett-Isochoric data reduction procedure applying the Britt and Luecke maximum likelihood algorithm was developed by Embry (1980). The percentage deviation of the experimental pressures from the values calculated from the maximum likelihood estimates for the 0.30 CO_2 + 0.70 CH_4 mixture at 300 K is shown in Figure 4. We note that the maximum likehood estimates for the pressures differ from the experimental values by less than 0.005 % for all the mixtures. The second virial coefficients have an uncertainty of 0.07 cm^3·mole^{-1} for pure CH_4 and all the mixtures.

Figure 4. Relative deviation of experimental pressures from the maximum likelihood estimates for 0.30 CO_2 + 0.70 CH_4 mixture at 300 K.

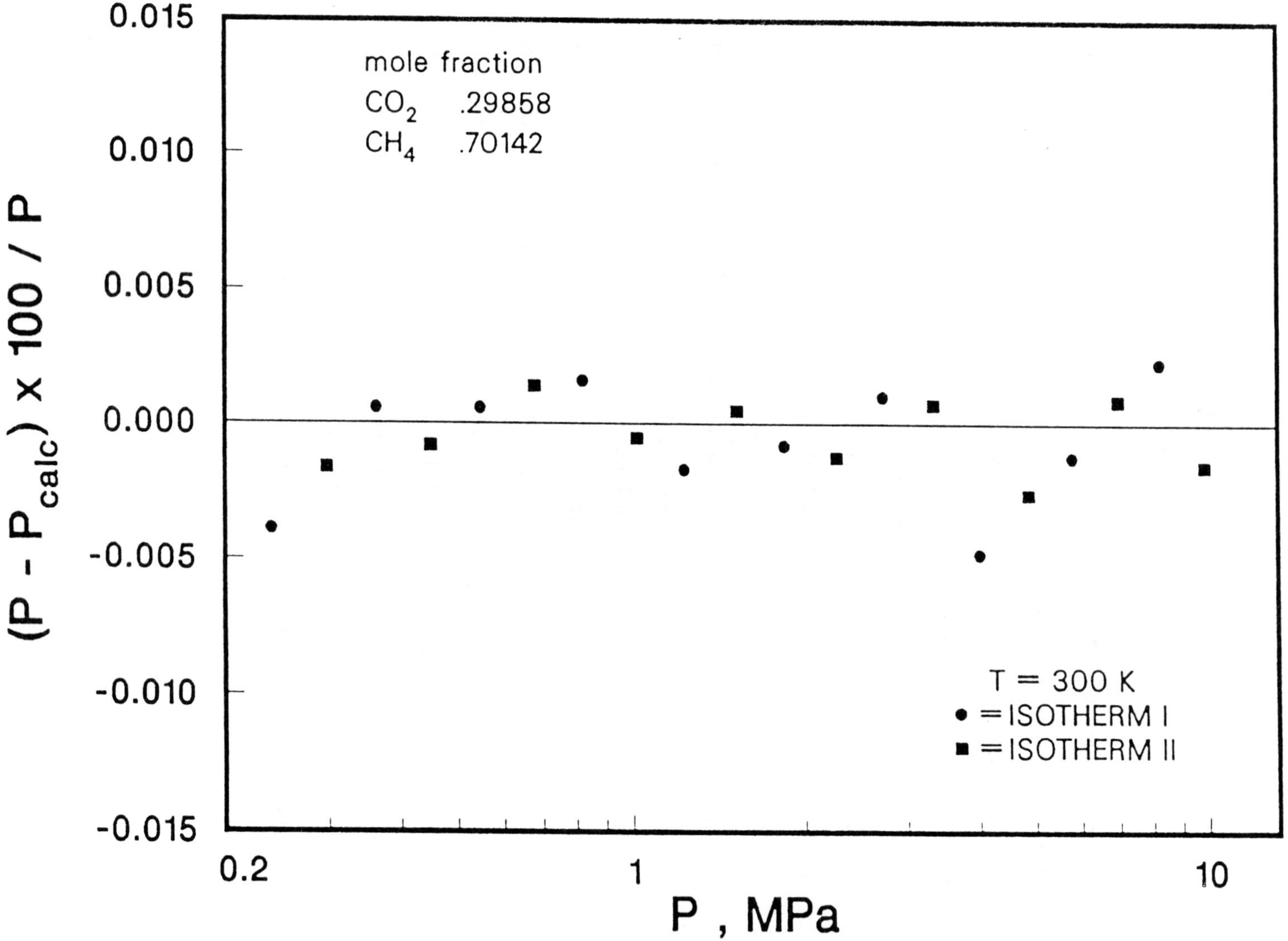

REFERENCES

Embry, D. L., "Analysis of Burnett-Isochoric Data," M.S. Thesis, Texas A&M Univ., College Station, TX (1980).

Holste, J. C., P. T. Eubank, and K. R. Hall, "Optimum Use of a Differential Pressure Transducer for High-Precision Measurements," *Ind. Eng. Chem., Fund.*, **16**, 378 (1977).

Holste, J. C., K. R. Hall, P. T. Eubank, and K. N. Marsh, "High Pressure PVT Measurements," *Fluid Phase Equil.*, **29**, 161 (1986).

Lau, W. R., "A Continuously Weighed Pycnometer Providing Densities for Carbon Dioxide + Ethane Mixtures between 240 and 350 K at Pressures up to 35 MPa," Ph.D. Dissertation, Texas A&M Univ., College Station, TX (1986).

GERG SAMPLE MEASUREMENTS

by

Hunter Brugge, Chih-An Hwang
James C. Holste, Kenneth R. Hall, Kenneth N. Marsh

Chemical Engineering Department
Texas A&M University
College Station, Texas 77843, USA

ABSTRACT

An accurate knowledge of densities is requested for nitrogen + methane and methane + ethane + propane mixtures to test the new GERG custody transfer equation. These two gas samples were prepared by Ruhrgas, Inc., and the gas composition has been marked. Also, these two mixtures are of considerable interest to those involved in the natural gas industry. We have measured two isotherms for each mixture up to 33 MPa.

INTRODUCTION

Experimental densities for two mixtures were measured using a Burnett apparatus (1) for pressures up to 10.7 MPa and a continuously weighed pycnometer for pressures up to 33.1 MPa. Coefficients of the density series virial equation were determined for the first mixture, 49.94 mol% nitrogen and 50.06% methane, at 280 and 300K. Virial coefficients were determined for the second mixture, 81.18% methane, 16.56% ethane, and 2.26% propane at 290 and 320K.

These particular mixtures were studied as part of a round-robin test conducted by Ruhrgas Aktiengesellschaft. The measured densities will provide an independent set of data to further prove the new GERG equation. Most of the data used in the development of the GERG equation were obtained from a commercial z-meter which is basically a single expansion Burnett device. Some of the complex mixtures analyzed with the z-meter may have passed through the two phase region during the expansion and there is some question about the accuracy of these data. The compositions of the two mixtures measured here were chosen so that the nitrogen + methane mixture would remain single phase in the z-meter while the methane + ethane + propane mixture would undergo a phase change if the z-meter technique were used.

EXPERIMENTAL SECTION

Burnett Apparatus

The Burnett apparatus used in this work was discussed in detail elsewhere (2, 3) and was modified recently (4). All temperature measurements were made with a MINCO capsule-type platinum resistance thermometer which had an accuracy better than 5 mK with respect to IPTS-68 based on a calibration traceable to the National Bureau of Standards. Temperature gradients across the two volumes were less than 10 mK. Pressure measurements were made with Ruska Instruments air dead-weight gauges, certified NBS-traceable with an accuracy of 0.015%, using helium as the pressure medium. A Ruska low temperature differential pressure indicator was used within the cell according to the method described by Holste, *et al.* (5).

Pycnometer Apparatus

Lau (6) has discussed the continuously weighed pycnometer used in this work. A known volume sample (pycnometer) cell is suspended from an electronic balance (7, 8). The sample cell is filled and evacuated through a straight, stainless-steel capillary, which is attached to the sample cell without affecting the precision of the balance. The entire balance and the sample cell are totally immersed in helium at a controlled pressure to eliminate changes in buoyancy. The sample densities are determined from the measured masses and the known volume of the sample cell.

The isothermal bath consists of two copper compartments (A and B) connected by a short copper tube. Compartment A is used for controlling the temperature of the sample cell which is fabricated from berylium copper to obtain high thermal conductivity and good mechnical strength. A feed valve is placed inside compartment B which is controlled at the same temperature as the sample cell, allowing the entire confined sample to be subjected to the same uniform temperature. This is especially important when the sample exists as one phase at room temperature and as a different phase at the isothermal bath temperature. A variable volume bellows cell is installed inside compartment B for the adjustment of sample density, even when the feed valve is closed. The isothermal bath is placed inside a powered aluminum radiation shield and a vacuum chamber to minimize heat transfer.

The balance, Arbor Laboratories model 507, measures the force required to maintain a null position of the weighing pan with the sample cell attached. This balance has a completely electronic mechanism, a capacity of 500 g, a precision of 0.1 mg, and allows vertical displacement less than 1 μm during the weighing operation. Pressures were measured using either a Rosemount pressure transducer operated at room temperature or a Paroscientific pressure transducer also located in the isothermal compartment B. Both transducers were calibrated against a DH Instruments (type 26000) automatic pressure standard (dead-weight gauge). The Rosemount and Paroscientific transducers also were compared at every operating temperature. The accuracy of the pressure measurements is within 0.006 MPa. Temperatures were measured with a MINCO four-lead platinum resistance thermometer identical to the one used in the Burnett apparatus, which was placed adjacent to the sample cell on the inside surface of compartment A. The absolute accuracy of the reported density measurements using the pycnometer apparatus is estimated to be 0.1 kg·m^{-3} or 0.1 %, whichever is greater.

The mixtures were furnished by Ruhrgas Aktiengesellschaft. Both samples were prepared gravimetrically and the compositions were comfirmed by chromatographic analysis at Ruhrgas.

RESULTS

A Burnett-Isochoric data reduction procedure applying the Britt and Luecke maximum likelihood algorithm was developed by Embry (9). The percentage deviation of the experimental pressures from the values calculated from the maximum likelihood estimates for the nitrogen + methane mixture at 280 K is shown in Figure 1. We note that the maximum likelihood estimates for the pressures differ from the experimental values by less than 0.005 % for both the nitrogen + methane mixture and methane + ethane + propane mixture.

Data analysis for the pycnometer is straightforward. The sample cell volume is calibrated with well known fluid as a function of temperature and pressure. The sample density is determined by dividing the measured mass of sample in the cell by the known cell volume.

Because the measurements were made along isotherms, an effort was made to correlate the pressure-density relationship at each isotherm. The virial equation in density

$$P = RT\sum_{i=1}^{n} B_i \rho^i \tag{1}$$

was used to correlate the combined data taken from both apparatus. The internal precision of the data using the pycnometer apparatus is illustrated by the small differences (less than 0.09 kg·m^{-3}) between the experimental and calculated values using equation (1).

Isotherms of compressibility factors (Z) for methane + ethane + propane mixture is shown in Figure 2. The percentage deviation of the experimental compressibility factors from the calculated values for the above mixture at 290 K is in Figure 3. The differences between the two various experimental apparatus

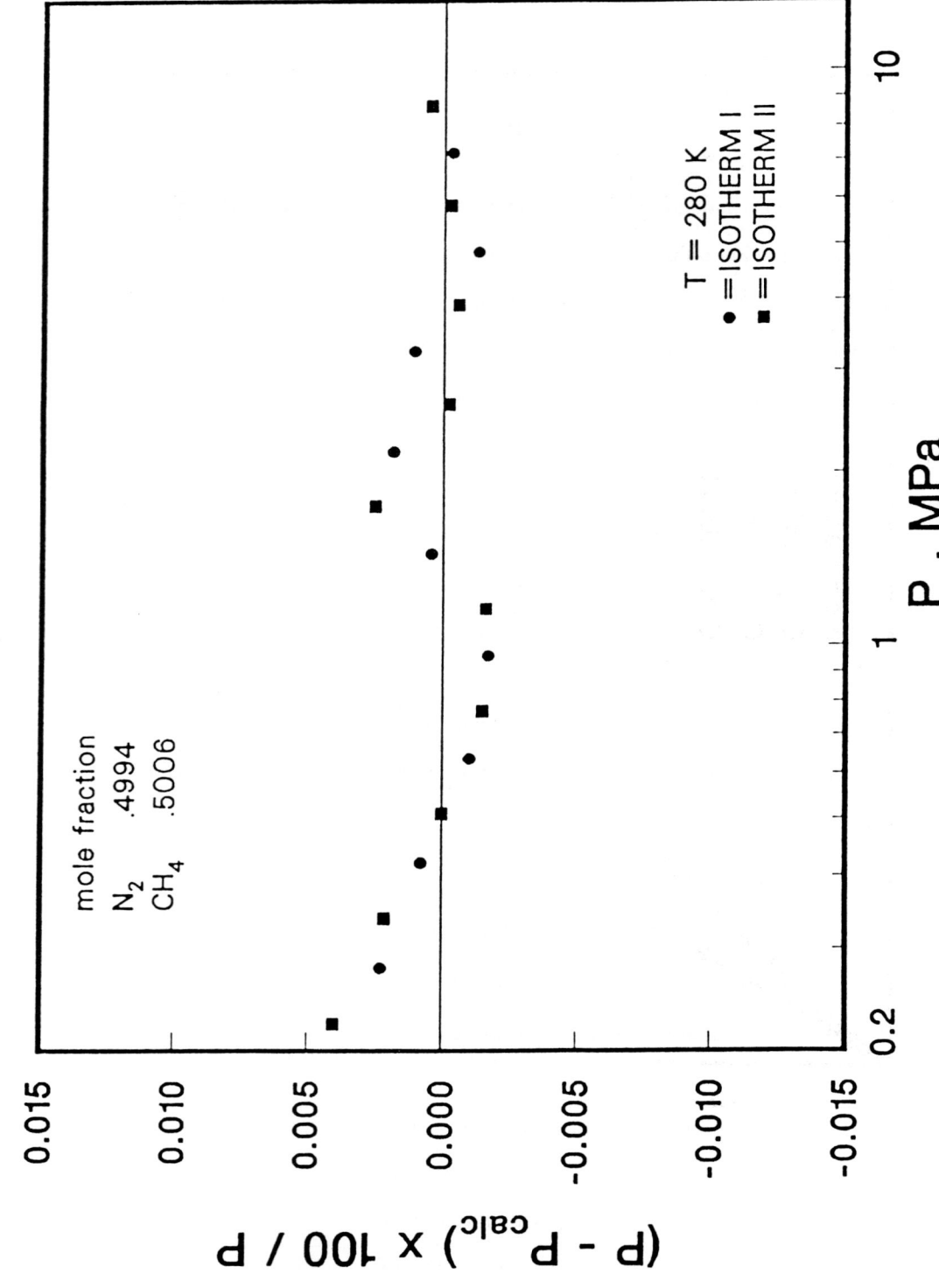

Figure 1. Relative deviation of experimental pressures from the maximum likelihood estimates for $N_2 + CH_4$ mixture at 280 K.

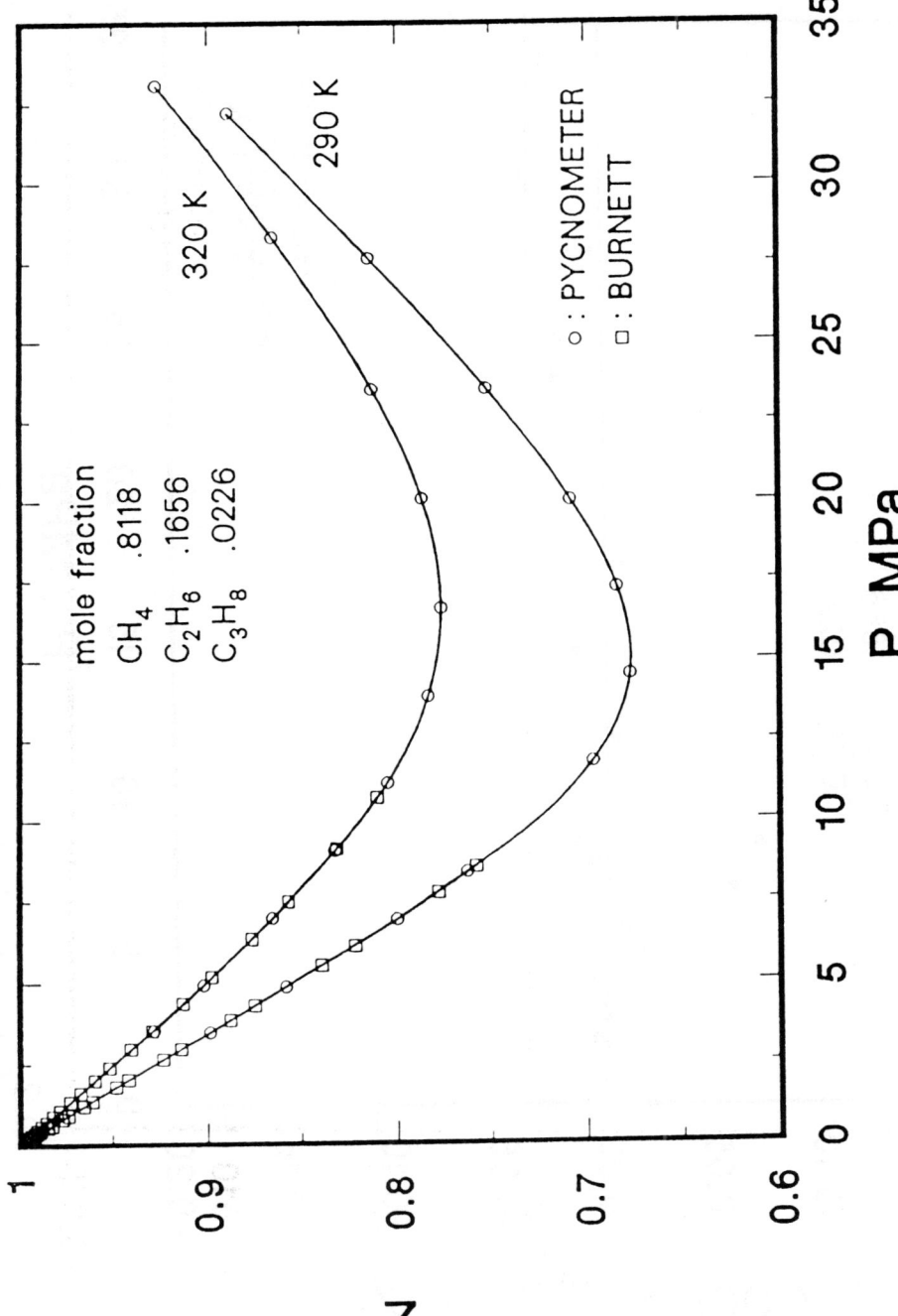

Figure 2. Isotherms of compressibility factors for $CH_4 + C_2H_6 + C_3H_8$ mixture.

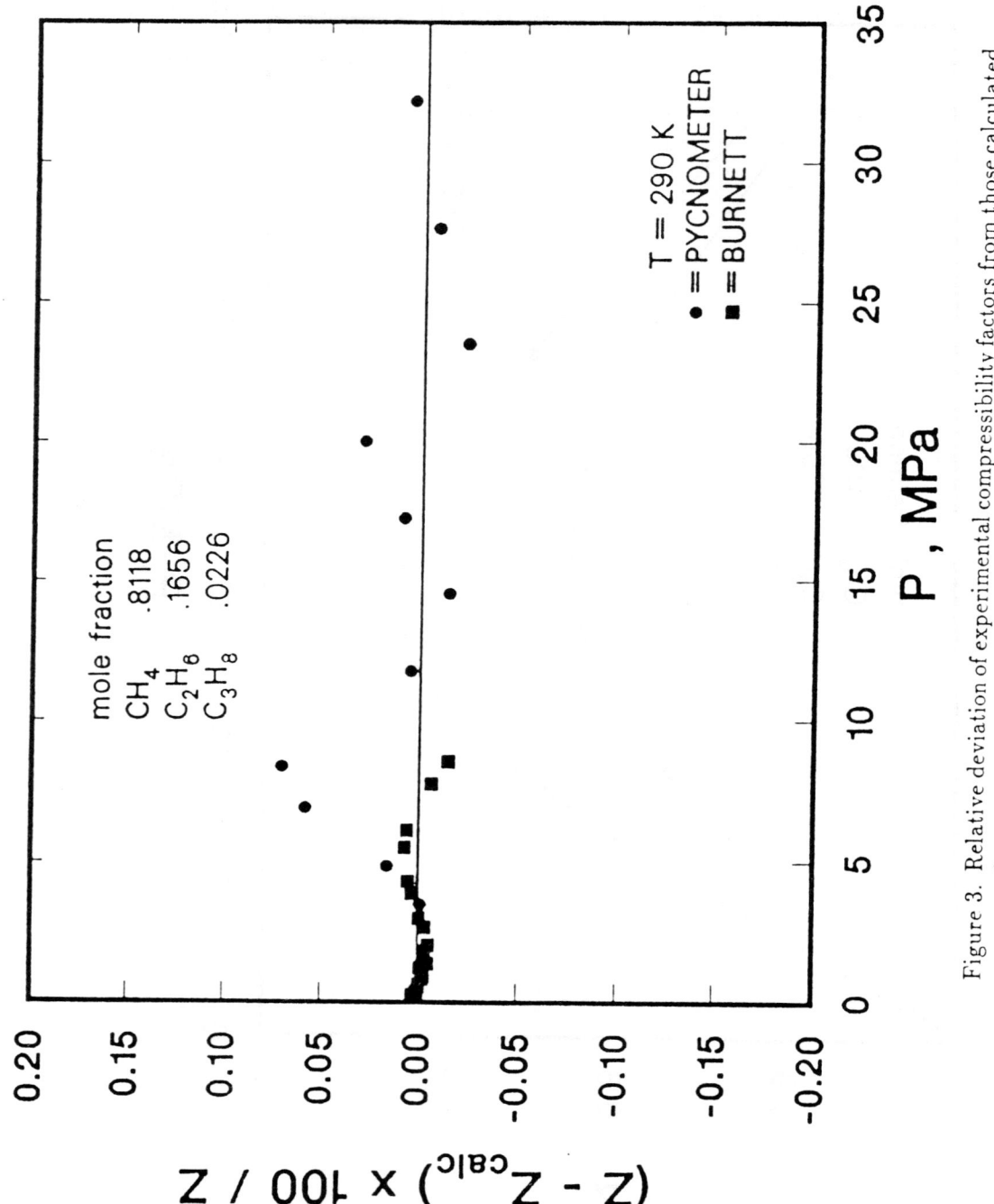

Figure 3. Relative deviation of experimental compressibility factors from those calculated from equation (1) for $CH_4 + C_2H_6 + C_3H_8$ mixture at 290 K.

do not exceed 0.1 % for both the nitrogen + methane mixture and methane + ethane + propane mixture. We also compare our compressibility factors with those obtained by Jaeschke at Ruhrgas Aktiengesellschaft. In all cases, the deviations among various apparatus in different laboratories are less than 0.1 %.

REFERENCES

[1] Burnett, B.S., "Compresibility Determinations Without Volume Measurements," *J. Appl. Mech.*, vol. 58, p. A136, 1936.

[2] Holste, J.C.; Watson, M.Q.; Bellomy, M.T.; Eubank, P.T.; Hall, K.R., *AIChE J.*, vol. 26, p. 954, 1980.

[3] Holste, J.C.; Young, J.G.; Eubank, P.T.; Hall, K.R., *AIChE J.*, vol. 28, p. 807, 1982.

[4] Holste, J.C. et al., "Experimental PVT Values for Pure Carbon Dioxide Between 220 and 448K," Chemical Engineering Department, Texas A&M University, submitted to Journal of Chemical Thermodynamics, April, 1985.

[5] Holste, J.C.; Hall, K.R.; Eubank, P.T., *Ind. Eng. Chem. Fundam.*, vol. 16, p. 378, 1977.

[6] Lau, W. R., "A Continuously Weighed Pycnometer Providing Densities for Carbon Dioxide + Ethane Mixtures Between 240 and 350 K at Pressures Up to 35 MPa," Dissertation, Department of Chemical Engineering, Texas A&M University, 1986.

[7] Van Witzenburg, W, and J.C. Stryland, "Density Measurements of Compressed Solid and Liquid Argon," *Can. J. of Physics*, vol. 46, p. 811, 1968.

[8] Machado, J.R.S. and W.B. Street, "Equation of State and Thermodynamic Properties of Liquid Methanol from 298 to 489 K and Pressures to 1040 bar," *J. Chem. Eng. Data*, vol. 28, p. 218, 1983.

[9] Embry, D.L., "Analysis of Burnett-Isochoric Data," Thesis, Department of Chemical Engineering, Texas A&M University, 1980.

Liquid Enthalpies of the C_8-Hydrocarbons Ethylbenzene and Isoctane

D. Möller, J.C. Holste, K.R. Hall, B.E. Gammon, K.N. Marsh

Department of Chemical Engineering and Thermodynamics Research Center
Texas A&M University, College Station, Texas 77843 USA

Introduction

The data presented in this paper are part of a larger effort at Texas A&M University to provide calorimetric data for improved heat exchanger design for process streams. There is also an interest in the thermodynamic properties of these substances in the context of the characterization of C_6+ components in natural gases.

The enthalpies are for 350, 400 and 450 K at two different pressures (20 and 50 bar). The apparatus is a thermoelectric flow calorimeter.

Calorimetric Technique

Castro-Gomez [1] described the thermoelectric flow calorimeter used for this work. Therefore, a brief description of its measuring principles and its features appear in this article. Figure 1 presents a schematic outline of this apparatus. It consists in its primary parts of a positive displacment pump, a fluid heater section, the calorimetric cell, a pressure control system and a discharge container placed on an electronic balance.

The fluid is introduced to the system by the high pressure pump at a volumetric flow rate which can be varied from 0.02 to 200 cm^3/hr, a typical value being 48 cm^3/hr. It passes first through the temperature controlled heater section. From there the fluid flows through an insulated tube into the calorimetric cell, which is cooled at a constant rate by a thermoelectric device while a controlled matching heater provides the heat needed to maintain a constant temperature in the cell. In this case the temperature is 25 °C.

The temperatures at the inlet and the outlet of the cell are measured by thermistor probes. After passing the outlet thermistor the fluid flows through a backpressure regulator and discharges into an appropriate container, which is on an electronic balance. This balance provides a measurement of the mass flow rate. The apparatus is fully automated and computer controlled for fast measurements.

The theory of this experiment can be explained briefly by looking at the energy balance of the calorimetric cell. When the sample fluid is not flowing the balance is:

$$MC\frac{dT_r}{dt} = \dot{Q}_{H_0} - \dot{Q}_{P_0} - \dot{Q}_{L_0} \qquad (1)$$

whereas with flowing sample fluid the heat introduced by it must be added:

$$MC\frac{dT_r}{dt} = \dot{Q}_f + \dot{Q}_{H_1} - \dot{Q}_{P_1} - \dot{Q}_{L_1} \qquad (2)$$

The subscripts 0 and 1 refer to the flow and non flow condition respectively.

At a steady state the reference temperature is constant. Hence

$$\frac{dT_r}{dt} = 0 \qquad (3)$$

Rearranging and combining of these three equations gives

$$\dot{Q}_f = (\dot{Q}_{H_0} - \dot{Q}_{H_1}) - (\dot{Q}_{P_0} - \dot{Q}_{P_1}) - (\dot{Q}_{L_0} - \dot{Q}_{L_1}) \qquad (4)$$

The heat losses $\dot{Q}_L$ are equal for both cases when the temperature of the calorimetric cell T_r is constant. The same applies to the heat withdrawn by the Peltier elements if they are run at a constant current. Therefore the last two expressions in Eqn.(4) become zero and the heat flux from the sample fluid simply equals the difference in the heater power between the flow and non-flow conditions.

Because the change in density of the sample between the inlet and the outlet is rather small for a liquid, the change in kinetic energy of the fluid is negligible. This leads to the following equation for the enthalpy

$$H(T_{in}, P_{in}) - H(T_{out}, P_{out}) = \frac{\dot{Q}_{H_0} - \dot{Q}_{H_1}}{\dot{m}} \qquad (5)$$

The pressure drop of the sample fluid flowing through the calorimeter is on-the-order-of 10^{-4} bar and has also been neglected. Therfore the working equation for this experiment is:

$$H(T_{in}, P) - H(T_{out}, P) = \frac{\dot{Q}_{H_0} - \dot{Q}_{H_1}}{\dot{m}} \qquad (6)$$

Thus the heat withdrawn from the fluid when it is cooled from the inlet to the outlet temperature is provided by the difference in power at the "flow" steady state to a non-flow one.

For a more detailed discussion of the measuring principle and the apparatus refer to Castro-Gomez [2]. In addition to the data evaluation procedure outlined above, minor corrections for the performance of the Peltier elements at the different stages of the experiment are necessary.

Samples

The ethylbenzene was provided by Eastman Kodak with a purity of 99.9%. The isooctane came from MCB Reagents with a purity of 99.9%. Both samples were degassed before use.

Results

The results appear in Tables I to IV. Tables I and III show the experimental values for the enthalpy difference, the pressures, the inlet and outlet temperatures. It was not possible to match the desired inlet temperature and the reference temperature at the outlet, so the data were used to estimate an overall heat capacity $\bar{c}_p$ to correct for those temperature differences. A correction for pressure deviations from an isobar was not done because there are not enough density data available and the pressure dependency of the enthalpy is small in the liquid region away from the critical region. An error propagation analysis by Castro-Gomez [2] gives an overall standard deviation for the experimental measurements of $\pm 0.64 \text{Jg}^{-1}$ in the region of these measurements; this was verified with water measurements.

The corrected or nominal values and literature data for comparision appear in Tables II and IV. In both tables, values for the enthalpies at saturation were taken from the ESDU-tables. The authors estimate uncertainties of $\pm 10\%$ for the ethylbenzene and $\pm 5\%$ for the isooctane. For ethylbenzene Sultanov and Akhundov [4] reported experimental enthalpies between 25 and 420° C and 0 to 250 bar. The values in Table IV are interpolated from tabulated ones [4] at pressures of 25 and 50 bar respectively.

Although the literature values are in all cases given for pressures different from ours they are comparable because the pressure dependency of the enthalpy lies within the estimated error of the measurement. For both substances the enthalpies compare well within the the given limits of error. The isooctane was measured twice at 450 K and about 50 bar. The resulting enthalpies agreed within 0.4%.

Cited Literature

[1] K. N. Marsh, R. C. Castro-Gomez, B. E. Gammon, J. C. Holste
"A thermoelectric total enthalpy flow calorimeter"
Presented at the Forth International Conference on Fluid Properties and Phase Equilibria for Chemical Process Design, Helsingor , Denmark, May 1986.

[2] R. C. Castro Gomez
Dissertation, Department of Chemical Engineering, Texas A&M University, 1987

[3] ESDU Tables, ESDU International Ltd.

[4] Ch. I. Sultanov, T. S. Akhundov
"Thermal Properties of Ethylbenzene"
Izv. Vyssh. Uchebn. Zaved., Neft Gaz 1985 28(12), 50-3

Symbols

H	Enthalpy
P	Pressure
T	Temperature
$\dot{Q}$	Heat flux
$\dot{m}$	Mass flow

Subscripts:

0	Non flow condition
1	flow condition
σ	saturation
L	Heat losses
P	Peltier element
f	Fluid
H	Heater

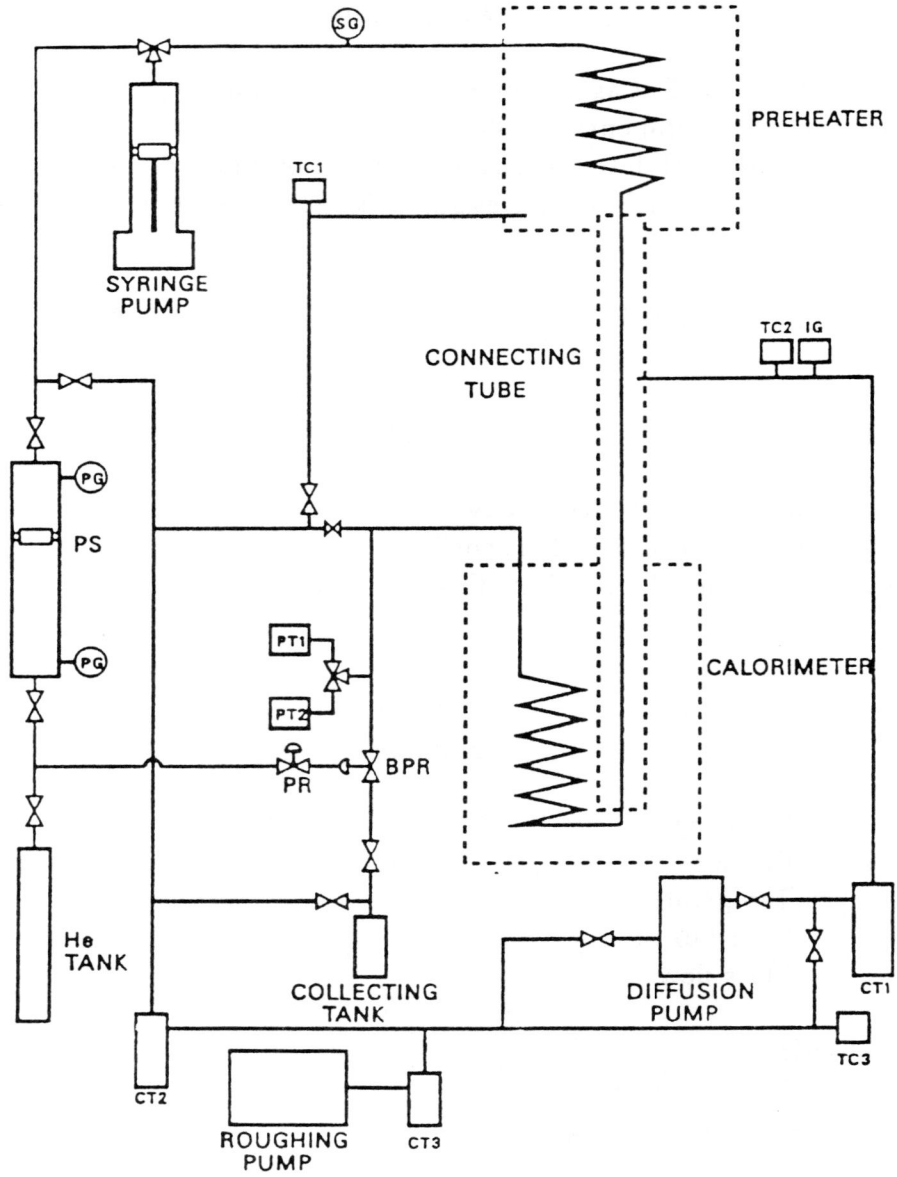

Figure 1. Flow Diagram of Calorimeter. BPR = Back Pressure Regulator; CT = Cold Traps; IG = Ionization Gauge; PG = Pressure Gauges; PR = Pressure Regulator: PS = Piston Sampler; PT = Pressure Transducers; SG = Switch Gauge; TC = Thermocouple Gauges.

Figure 2, Cross Section of the Flow Calorimeter

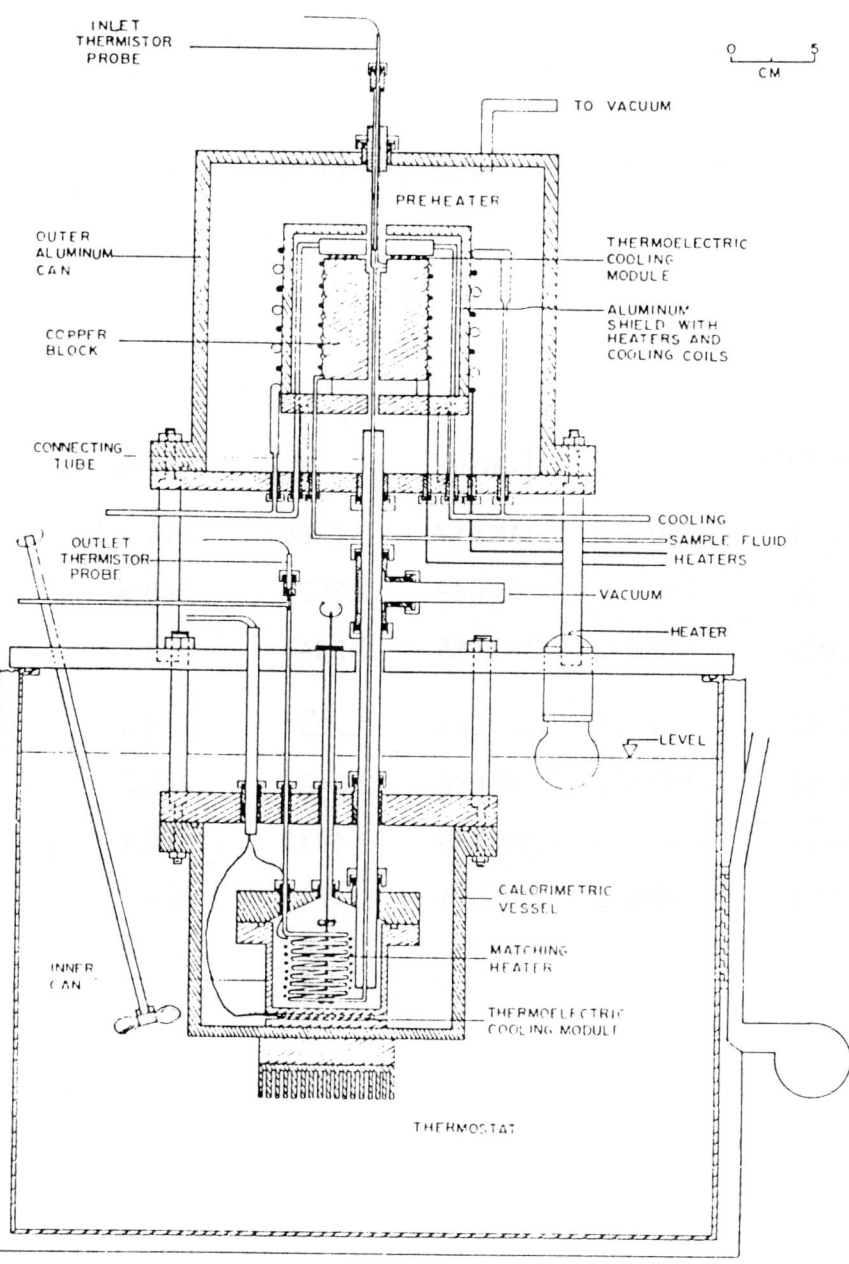

Table I

Experimental enthalpy differences for isooctane

p [kPa]	T_{in} [K]	T_{out} [K]	$\overline{c_p}$ [$\frac{kJ}{kgK}$]	Δh_{exp} [$\frac{kJ}{kg}$]
2021	350.708	298.617	2.2286	116.1
1980	400.277	298.649	2.3677	240.6
2009	449.873	298.585	2.5340	383.4
5212	349.688	298.655	2.2234	113.5
5162	400.938	298.670	2.3485	240.2
5199	450.140	298.588	2.4834	376.4
5053	450.635	298.594	2.4744	376.2

Table II

Nominal enthalpy differences * for isooctane

p [kPa]	T [K]	$\Delta h \left[\frac{kJ}{kg}\right]$	$\Delta h_\sigma^{**} \left[\frac{kJ}{kg}\right]$
2021	350	115.6	114
1980	400	241.2	237
2009	450	384.8	374
5212	350	115.3	114
5162	400	239.2	237
5199	450	377.1	374
5053	450	375.7	374

---

* $h_{ref} = h(298.15 K, p)$
** $Ref.: ESDU - Tables, Nr. 86007$

Table III

Experimental enthalpy differences for ethylbenzene

p [kPa]	T_{in} [K]	T_{out} [K]	$\overline{c_p}$ [$\frac{kJ}{kgK}$]	Δh_{exp} [$\frac{kJ}{kg}$]
2003	350.704	298.314	1.8333	96.1
2001	400.614	298.361	1.9197	196.3
1994	450.266	298.329	2.0080	305.1
5394	348.992	298.323	1.8425	93.4
5367	400.453	298.333	1.9327	197.4

Table IV

Nominal enthalpy differences * for ethylbenzene

p [kPa]	T [K]	$\Delta h \left[\frac{kJ}{kg}\right]$	$\Delta h_\sigma^{**} \left[\frac{kJ}{kg}\right]$	$\Delta h^{***} \left[\frac{kJ}{kg}\right]$
2003	350	95.1	94	95.8
2001	400	195.5	195	196.1
1994	450	304.9		305.4
5394	350	95.5	94	95.4
5367	400	196.9	195	195.7

* $h_{ref} = h(298.15 K, p)$
** Ref.: $ESDU - Tables, Nr.75015$
*** Ref.: Sultanov et al., Values for 25 and 50 bar respectively

IMPRIMERIE LOUIS-JEAN
Publications scientifiques et littéraires
05002   GAP   —   Tél. :   92.51.35.23
Dépôt légal : 488 — Septembre 1988